Knov

Pancreatic Cancer

John P. Neoptolemos, Raul Urrutia, James L. Abbruzzese,
Markus W. Büchler (Eds.)

Pancreatic Cancer

Volume 1
Chapters 1–25

With 253 Figures and 95 Tables

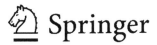 Springer

John P. Neoptolemos
University of Liverpool
Liverpool
UK

Raul Urrutia
Mayo Clinic
Rochester, MN
USA

James L. Abbruzzese
The University of Texas M. D. Anderson Cancer Center
Houston, TX
USA

Markus W. Büchler
University of Heidelberg
Heidelberg
Germany

Library of Congress Control Number: 2009937021

ISBN: 978-0-387-77497-8

This publication is available also as:
Electronic publication under ISBN: 978-0-387-77498-5 and
Print and electronic bundle under ISBN: 978-0-387-77499-2

springer.com

Printed on acid free paper   SPIN: 12037278 2109SPi– 5 4 3 2 1 0

This work is dedicated to our wives Linda, Gwen, Marie, and Hedi and to our patients and their relatives.

Foreword

For those of us immersed in cancer research, the last decade has been a fruitful one, with many significant achievements and real clinical advances. One needs to look only at the declining mortality rates in many malignancies such as breast and prostate cancer to appreciate that new discoveries have a positive impact on our patients. In some arenas, the advances have been transforming. For example, imatinib mesylate and successor drugs that target an enzyme called BCR/ABL in chronic myelogenous leukemia have turned this previously uniformly fatal disease into an easily manageable condition. Similarly, the work of the legendary Judah Folkman on the importance of the angiogenesis in malignancy spawned a number of agents that can interfere with the angiogenic pathway either by neutralizing ligands or inhibiting receptors. As a result, patients with breast, colon, kidney, lung, and other cancers are living longer and feeling better. Agents that target EGFR and HER2, among others, have also strengthened our therapeutic arsenal.

However, in reflecting on pancreatic cancers, especially pancreatic ductal adenocarcinoma, one is immediately struck by how little progress we have made. Incidence rates continue to rise because of an aging population, and patients still present primarily with locally advanced or metastatic disease because cost-effective early detection tools are not available. Our treatments, while clearly improved, have not yet had a major impact on the overall mortality rate.

Have we done anything to turn this warhead around? Most certainly! It has been almost ten years since we published *Pancreatic Cancer: An Agenda for Action, a Report of the Pancreatic Cancer Progress Review Group* sponsored by the US National Cancer Institute (NCI). In that document, we identified the gaps in our knowledge, laid out a scientific toolkit, and encouraged the NCI to support more research in this area, and to help train young investigators. Since then, new transgenic animal models that faithfully recapitulate human diseases have been developed, and we have a better understanding of the aberrant signaling networks in malignant pancreatic epithelium moving us closer to finding the critical nodes that comprise the Achilles heel for this tumor. An increased emphasis on understanding stromal biology is beginning to yield clues about potential new therapeutic targets, such as activated hedgehog signaling, and is allowing us to unravel the role of stroma on invasion and progression in this disease, which is characterized by its profound desmoplastic component. In the clinical arena, we now have more insight into inherited patterns of disease and have identified more genetic syndromes. Thanks to work within the NCI Cancer Cohort Consortium, genomic material from patients enrolled in large epidemiologic studies is now being shared and probed for further clues about genetic susceptibility. Screening, although not yet practical on a population-wide basis, is proving to be extremely useful for patients at high risk because of their family histories. Therapy is improving. Surgery is safe and the benefit of adjuvant therapy is now clearly apparent, supported by the highest level of medical evidence. Research activity aimed at identifying new drugs and new drug combinations has been robust, but unfortunately has yielded very few approved drugs. As a result, the NCI convened a state-of-the-science meeting last year which resulted in consensus on standardization in trial design and harmonization of eligibility criteria in an effort to minimize unintended bias in clinical trial conduct. Most assuredly, we have learned that large global adjuvant trials are feasible and that many patients are also willing to participate in large randomized trials in locally advanced and metastatic disease. Thus, the infrastructure is in place to do much more.

So how do we get to the next level? As we probe further into the biology of this disease, it is becoming increasingly clear that there is more diversity than we appreciated. Thus, there will be more need for an individualized management in this cancer as is now clearly appreciated in many other malignancies. Understanding the host genotype, gene–gene and gene–environment interactions, and the biological consequences of the many mutations that occur in pancreatic ductal adenocarcinoma will allow us to risk-adapt our management from surveillance and screening to the identification and selection of effective therapy. Developing large biorepositories of pancreatic cancer tissue and related specimens with exquisite clinical and molecular annotation will be one of the highest priorities. And investigators will need access to an appropriate context in order to advance knowledge.

This textbook, *Pancreatic Cancer*, is a carefully composed compendium of the state-of-the-science in all aspects of research in both pancreatic ductal adenocarcinoma and pancreatic neuroendocrine tumors. The experts who were selected to provide contributions are the best in their fields. The content is contemporary and comprehensive. This text will be a necessary reference for anyone already doing research in pancreatic cancer.

Although research funding for pancreatic cancer research has improved, the level of funding lags far behind other cancers, including much less lethal ones. In addition, the army of capable investigators is still too small. This text will also serve as a vehicle for change since its content will whet the appetite of highly competent investigators entrenched in other fields and encourage them to change direction. The book will also serve as a tremendous guide for young investigators to help them understand the landscape and plan their research strategy.

I am truly grateful to my colleagues around the world who have worked so hard and so tirelessly to create this reference. Disseminating what we know now will accelerate our progress, and there is no doubt in my mind that the scientific breakthroughs that will transform the lives of our patients are just round the corner.

Margaret A. Tempero, M.D.
University of California, San Francisco

Preface

Trying to advance the agenda for pancreatic cancer has always been a huge challenge but we are living in exciting times for cancer research as a whole. Although the numerous hurdles hindering the understanding, diagnosis and treatment of pancreatic cancer seem as daunting as ever, one by one these are now being dismantled. This has only been possible by bringing together large multi-disciplinary teams of world class scientists and clinicians in comprehensive cancer centres and specific centres of pancreas cancer excellence.

DNA sequencing has shown that pancreatic cancer has just over 1,000 somatic mutations involving 12 critical pathways: apoptosis, DNA damage control, regulation of the G_1/S transition, Hedgehog signalling, homophilic cell adhesion, integrin signalling, c-Jun N-terminal kinase signalling, KRAS signalling, other small GTPase-dependent signalling, regulation of invasion, TGFβ signalling and Wnt/Notch signalling. What is interesting is that there are a similar number of genetic mutations in breast cancer involving the identical number of pathways. Or at least that is how the vast amount of accumulated molecular data is perceived. How can two human cancers appear so similar at the genetic level yet behave so differently in the clinic? A few percent of patients with pancreatic cancer make it to five years and most are dead well within the year. What shocks so much in pancreatic cancer is the unerring predictability of the time of death.

Yet there is now some real hope emerging. Even a few years ago it seemed unthinkable that we could detect early pre-invasive pancreatic cancer. Yet now, pancreas units all over the world are resecting an increasing proportion of intraductal papillary mucinous neoplasms, often with the welcome 'no invasion seen' in the histopathology report. Pancreas cancer resection was once infrequently performed partly because of the technical difficulty and partly because there was a fearsome post-operative mortality rate (30–40%). Today, pancreas resection can be performed in 20% or so of pancreas cancer patients with localized disease with a very low mortality rate and producing a five year survival rate that readily exceeds 20% with adjuvant therapy. There is some evidence that we can also improve survival even in advanced pancreatic cancer. Moreover there is increasing optimism for successful novel therapies with over 200 therapeutic clinical trials underway, many using agents based on the concepts of the new biology.

Emulating the successes made in breast cancer over the past 30 years may still seem a long way off except it is important to recall that mortality then for breast cancer exceeded 50% at five years compared to an 80% ten year survival today. The clues as to why there is the gap between pancreas cancer and other tumour types are contained within these pages.

The contributors have been put together as much for their style of thinking as well as representing the best there is in their own areas of expertise. The outcome of this collective endeavour is that it has met and exceeded expectations and - much more importantly - with added value throughout.

This kind of labour becomes dated as soon as the keyboards are hit but by its very nature and quality is invaluable for all those involved in any aspect of pancreatic cancer.

John P. Neoptolemos
Raul Urrutia
James L. Abbruzzese
Markus W. Büchler

Acknowledgements

The Editors would like to dedicate their work to all the pancreatic cancer patients and their families.

The Editors wish to acknowledge Sarah Cottle in the office of Professor Neoptolemos (Liverpool, UK). Ms. Cottle provided incalculable time and effort overseeing the accuracy and timeliness of this publication.

We also acknowledge the significant support offered by our individual editorial assistants, who provided the day-to-day contacts, oversights, and management of manuscripts that were submitted in each international office. We specifically wish to thank the assistance of Professor Jens Werner and Irmgard Alffermann in the office of Professor Büchler (Heidelberg, Germany), Anne LeBourgeois in the office of Professor James Abbruzzese (MD Anderson Cancer Center, USA), and to Dr. Martin Fernandez-Zapico and Dr. Gwen Lomberk in the office of Professor Raul Urrutia (Mayo Clinic, USA).

All of these people provided an invaluable service that is appreciated highly by the Editors and allowed Springer to publish in a timely and organized fashion.

The Editors would also like to thank Rachel Warren at Springer.

Finally, the Editors acknowledge the assistance and organizational skills, and the extraordinary attention and diligence of Springer's Jennifer Carlson. Ms. Carlson's oversight allowed the assimilation of this book from its inception and ensured its completion.

Table of Contents

Editors . . . . **xix**
List of Contributors . . . . **xxiii**

Volume 1

Section 1 The Nature of Pancreatic Cancer 1

1   **Epidemiology and Prospects for Prevention of Pancreatic Cancer** 3
Li Jiao · Donghui Li

2   **Development and Structure of the Pancreas** 27
Roberto A. Rovasio

3   **Pathologic Classification and Biological Behavior of
Pancreatic Neoplasia** 39
Olca Basturk · Ipek Coban · N. Volkan Adsay

4   **Developmental Molecular Biology of the Pancreas** 71
Ondine Cleaver · Raymond J. MacDonald

5   **Molecular Pathology of Precursor Lesions of Pancreatic Cancer** 119
Georg Feldmann · Anirban Maitra

6   **Epigenetics and its Applications to a Revised Progression Model
of Pancreatic Cancer** 143
Gwen Lomberk · Raul Urrutia

7   **Molecular Pathology of Pancreatic Endocrine Tumors** 171
Gabriele Capurso · Stefano Festa · Matteo Piciucchi · Roberto Valente ·
Gianfranco Delle Fave

8   **Sporadic Pancreatic Endocrine Tumors** 199
Volker Fendrich · Peter Langer · Detlef K. Bartsch

9   **Molecular Pathology of Ampullary, Intra-Pancreatic Bile Duct and
Duodenal Cancers** 233
Patrick Michl · Albrecht Neesse · Thomas M. Gress

10   Miscellaneous Non-Pancreatic Non-Endocrine Tumors 255
John D. Abad · Keith D. Lillemoe

11   Molecular Relationships Between Chronic Pancreatitis and Cancer 285
Craig D. Logsdon · Baoan Ji · Rosa F. Hwang

12   Pancreatic Cancer Stem Cells 317
Chenwei Li · Diane M. Simeone

13   Cell Cycle Control in Pancreatic Cancer Pathogenesis 333
Brian Lewis

14   Apoptosis Signaling Pathways in Pancreatic Cancer Pathogenesis 369
David J. McConkey

15   EGFR Signaling Pathways in Pancreatic Cancer Pathogenesis 387
Caroline R. Sussman · Gwen Lomberk · Raul Urrutia

16   Hedgehog Signaling Pathways in Pancreatic Cancer Pathogenesis 403
Marina Pasca di Magliano · Matthias Hebrok

17   Smad4/TGF-β Signaling Pathways in Pancreatic Cancer Pathogenesis 419
Alixanna Norris · Murray Korc

**18   Notch Signaling in Pancreatic Morphogenesis and Pancreatic Cancer
Pathogenesis** 441
Gwen Lomberk · Raul Urrutia

19   Molecular Characterization of Pancreatic Cancer Cell Lines 457
*David J. McConkey · Woonyoung Choi · Keith Fournier ·
Lauren Marquis · Vijaya Ramachandran · Thiruvengadam Arumugam*

20   Mouse Models of Pancreatic Exocrine Cancer 471
Michelle Lockley · David Tuveson

**21   Principles and Applications of Microarray Gene Expression in
Pancreatic Cancer** 497
Malte Buchholz · Thomas M. Gress

22   Principles and Applications of Proteomics in Pancreatic Cancer 509
Sarah Tonack · John Neoptolemos · Eithne Costello

23   Tumor-Stromal Interactions in Invasion and Metastases 535
Mert Erkan · Irene Esposito · Helmut Friess · Jörg Kleeff

24   Genetic Susceptibility and High Risk Groups for Pancreatic Cancer 565
William Greenhalf · John Neoptolemos

25   **Inherited Pancreatic Endocrine Tumors** 601
      Jens Waldmann · Peter Langer · Detlef K. Bartsch

Volume 2

Section 2 Clinical Management of Pancreatic Cancer 623

26   **Clinical Decision Making in Pancreatic Cancer** 625
      Robert A. Wolff

27   **Paraneoplastic Syndromes in Pancreatic Cancer** 651
      Jens Werner · Stephan Herzig

28   **Diagnostic and Therapeutic Response Markers** 675
      Anne Marie Lennon · Michael Goggins

29   **CT and Fusion PET-CT for Diagnosis, Staging and Follow-Up** 703
      Aparna Balachandran · Priya Bhosale · Chuslip Charnsangavej

30   **MRI and MRCP for Diagnosis and Staging of Pancreatic Cancer** 731
      Eric P. Tamm · Aparna Balachandran · Priya R. Bhosale · Leonardo P. Marcal

31   **EUS for Diagnosis and Staging of Pancreatic Cancer** 763
      Ioannis S. Papanikolaou · Thomas Rösch

32   **Laparoscopy and Laparoscopic Ultrasound for Diagnosis and**
      Staging 801
      Nicholas Alexakis · Robert Sutton

33   **Palliative Management of Pancreatic Cancer** 813
      Milind Javle · Michael Fisch

34   **Diagnostic and Therapeutic Endoscopy in Pancreatic Cancer** 839
      Folasade P. May · Field F. Willingham · David L. Carr-Locke

35   **Interventional Radiology for Pancreatic Cancer** 859
      Ferga C. Gleeson · Michael J. Levy

36   **Palliative Surgery in Advanced Pancreatic Cancer** 895
      Dirk J. Gouma · O. R. C. Busch · T. M. Gulik

37   **Chemotherapy for Advanced Pancreatic Cancer** 913
      Alicia Okines · Gihan Ratnayake · Ian Chau · David Cunningham

38   **Developments in Chemoradiation for Advanced Pancreatic Cancer** 951
      Stephen H. Settle · Jeffrey J. Meyer · Christopher H. Crane

39   Surgical Resection for Pancreatic Cancer 971
*Nuh N. Rahbari · Nathan Mollberg · Moritz Koch · John P. Neoptolemos · Jürgen Weitz ·
Markus W. Büchler*

40   Venous Resection in Pancreatic Cancer Surgery 997
Yuji Nimura

**41   Pathological Reporting and Staging Following Pancreatic Cancer
Resection** 1015
Irene Esposito · Diana Born

42   Japanese Pancreas Society Staging Systems for Pancreatic Cancer 1035
Satoshi Kondo

43   Adjuvant Chemotherapy in Pancreatic Cancer 1051
Paula Ghaneh · John P. Neoptolemos · David Cunningham

44   Adjuvant Chemoradiation Therapy for Pancreatic Cancer 1079
Naimish Pandya · Michael C. Garofalo · William F. Regine

45   Neoadjuvant Treatment in Pancreatic Cancer 1093
Alysandra Lal · Douglas B. Evans

46   Borderline Resectable Pancreatic Cancer 1109
Gauri R. Varadhachary

47   Management of Cystic Neoplasms of the Pancreas 1125
Cristina R. Ferrone · Carlos Fernandez-del Castillo · Andrew L. Warshaw

48   Laparoscopic Surgery for Pancreatic Neoplasms 1141
Laureano Fernández-Cruz

49   Modern Japanese Approach to Pancreas Cancer 1153
Masao Tanaka

Section 3 New Directions 1173

50   Development of Novel Pancreatic Tumor Biomarkers 1175
Michael Goggins

51   Inherited Genetics of Pancreatic Cancer and Secondary Screening 1203
William Greenhalf · John Neoptolemos

52   Gene Therapy for Pancreatic Cancer 1237
Han Hsi Wong · Nicholas R. Lemoine

53   Vaccine Therapy and Immunotherapy for Pancreatic Cancer 1269
Lei Zheng · Elizabeth M. Jaffee

54   Emerging Therapeutic Targets for Pancreatic Cancer 1319
Rachna T. Shroff · James L. Abbruzzese

Color Insert 1337
Subject Index 1385

About the Editors

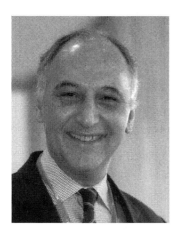

John P. Neoptolemos

Professor John P. Neoptolemos is Professor of Surgery, Head of the Division of Surgery and Oncology, and Head of School of Cancer Studies (The Owen and Ellen Evans Chair of Cancer Studies) at the University of Liverpool, and Honorary Consultant Surgeon at the Royal Liverpool University Hospital.

He studied Natural Sciences and then Philosophy at Cambridge before completing his clinical undergraduate training at Guys Hospital. He completed his academic and clinical training in Leicester under Professor Sir Peter Bell and was awarded a Doctorate in Medicine for his research thesis. In 1981, he became a Fellow of the Royal College of Surgeons in England. He also trained in San Diego, Paris, and Ulm before being appointed senior lecturer at the University of Birmingham in 1987. He became a Full Professor of Surgery in 1994 and then moved to the University of Liverpool and Royal Liverpool University Hospital in 1996 as the Head of the Department of Surgery, followed by the Head of the Division of Surgery and Oncology in 2004.

In 2005, Professor Neoptolemos was appointed as the Head of the School of Cancer Studies and in 2009 became the Chairman of the Cancer Research UK Cancer Centre. He is also Director of the Cancer Research UK Liverpool Cancer Trials Unit, Co-Director of the Liverpool Experimental Cancer Medicine Centre, and Scientific Director of the National Institute for Health Research Liverpool Pancreas Biomedical Research Unit.

He has been the President of the Pancreatic Society of Great Britain and Ireland; Secretary and then President of the European Pancreatic Club; and President of the International Association of Pancreatology.

Professor Neoptolemos is the Chairman of the Pancreatic Cancer Sub-Group, National Cancer Research Institute (UK) Committee on Upper GI Cancer; Chairman of the European Study Group for Pancreatic Cancer (ESPAC); and member of the Cancer Research UK Science Strategy Advisory Group. In 2007, he was elected as a Fellow of the Academy of Medical Sciences (UK).

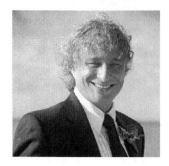

Raul Urrutia

Raul Urrutia, M.D., is the Professor and Chair of the GI Unit and Director of the Epigenetics and Chromatin Dynamics Laboratory at the Mayo Clinic. Over the years at Mayo, he has served as the Director of the Ph.D. Program in Tumor Biology, Associate Director for Genomics at the Mayo Clinic General Clinical Research Center (GCRC), and Director of the GI Cancer Research Program at the Mayo Cancer Center.

Born in Mendoza, Argentina, Dr. Urrutia graduated Magna Cum Laude in 1987 from the University of Cordoba Medical School in Cordoba, Argentina, as a surgeon. During medical school, he did research at the Cell Biology Institute of the University where he studied pancreatic cancer. Immediately following graduation, he traveled to the United States where he was a visiting fellow at the Laboratory of Molecular Otology at the NIDCD-National Institutes of Health in Bethesda, MD. He worked at the National Institutes of Health for three years in various titles including guest researcher, visiting fellow, and visiting associate. In 1993, Dr. Urrutia joined the faculty at the Mayo Clinic for Basic Research in Digestive Diseases. He is married and has two children, twins.

Dr. Urrutia has published over 300 publications among peer-reviewed articles, chapters, and reviews. He has prided himself on a commitment to scientific mentorship, with over 30 researchers ranging from graduate students to postdoctoral students, as well as junior faculty members. Currently, he is the Director of the Mayo Clinic GI Unit, which accommodates the research of 10 independent faculty members, all of whom have space adjacent to the Epigenetics and Chromatin Dynamics Laboratory on the tenth floor of the Guggenheim research building. In addition, he is the PI for an Institutional Research Grant for the Mayo Clinic Cancer Center awarded by the American Cancer Society, which administers funds for career development of young investigators. Dr. Urrutia has participated in multiple teaching activities since 1993 at the Mayo Graduate School. His current teaching capacity includes the course on Transcription, Chromatin, and Epigenetics.

He is currently the Editor-in-Chief of three journals, including *Pancreatology, Case Reports in Gastroenterology,* and *Journal of Gastrointestinal Cancer,* and member of several other editorial boards including past service for the *Journal of Biological Chemistry* and *Pancreas* Dr. Urrutia is a manuscript reviewer for *Gastroenterology, Pancreas, Pancreatology, Oncogene, Journal of Clinical Investigation, Journal of Biological Chemistry, EMBO, Nature Cell Biology, Nature Medicine, PNAS, Cancer Research and Cancer Cell.*

Dr. Urrutia has served on various national and international society governments. He is the past chair for Pancreatic Diseases Section of the American Gastroenterological Association, the past president of the American Pancreatic Association (2007), and member of the International Association of Pancreatology board.

Dr. Urrutia's research program focuses on the epigenetics and chromatin dynamics in normal pancreas development and pancreatic cancer.

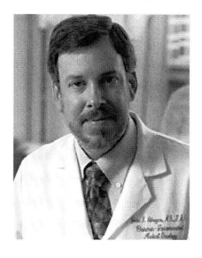

James L. Abbruzzese

James L. Abbruzzese, M.D., F.A.C.P. is the M.G. and Lillie A. Johnson Chair for Cancer Treatment and Research and Chairman of the Department of Gastrointestinal Medical Oncology at the University of Texas M. D. Anderson Cancer Center in Houston, Texas. He is a member of a number scientific advisory boards including the external scientific advisory board for the University of Massachusetts, The Arizona Cancer Center, The University of Colorado, and The Lustgarten Foundation for Pancreatic Cancer Research.

Born in Hartford, Connecticut, he graduated from medical school with honors from the University of Chicago, Pritzker School of Medicine, Chicago, IL. He completed his residency in internal medicine at The Johns Hopkins Hospital in Baltimore, MD, and fellowship in medical oncology at the Dana-Farber Cancer Center, Harvard Medical School in Boston, MA. He is married and has one child.

Dr. Abbruzzese has published over 350 peer-reviewed articles, numerous chapters and reviews. In 2004 he co-edited a book entitled *Gastrointestinal Oncology* published by Oxford University Press. His research group has been awarded a SPORE in pancreatic cancer and U54 grant on angiogenesis. In 2001 he served as a Co-chair for the American Association for Cancer Research Program Committee and was the Program Chairman for the ASCO Annual Meeting in 2007. He has recently served as a member of the AACR Board of Directors. He is a past member of the AACR Research Fellowships Committee, the ASCO Grant Awards, and Nominating Committees and currently serves on the newly constituted NCI Clinical Trials Advisory Committee.

He is a Deputy Editor of *Clinical Cancer Research*, and a member of several other editorial boards including the past service for the *Journal of Clinical Oncology*. His scholarly interests center on clinical and translational research for pancreatic cancer.

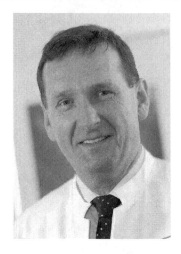

Markus W. Büchler

Professor Markus W. Büchler is Professor of Surgery and Chairman of the Department of Surgery at the University Hospital, University of Heidelberg, Germany.

He studied medicine at the Universities of Heidelberg and Berlin and was trained in surgery at the Department of Surgery, University of Ulm, where he was appointed as Consultant Surgeon in 1987 and Vice-Chairman in 1991. In 1993, Büchler became the Chairman and Professor of Surgery of the Department of Visceral and Transplantation Surgery at the Inselspital, University of Bern, Switzerland. From Switzerland, he moved back to Germany in 2001 where he became the Chairman of the Department of General, Visceral, and Transplantation Surgery at the University Hospital, Heidelberg.

Professor Büchler is a specialist in hepato–pancreato–biliary surgery (HPB) and, in particular, pancreatic surgery. He has a substantial curriculum of scientific publications in the field of HPB diseases, especially in the translational research of pancreatic cancer.

He is member of the Editorial Boards of many journals in general and gastrointestinal surgery, translational and molecular research in pancreatology, and other gastrointestinal diseases.

He has been the President of the European Pancreatic Club (EPC) in 2002 and President of the International Hepato–Pancreato–Biliary Association (IHPBA) in 2006–2008 and is the elected President of the German Surgical Association.

List of Contributors

John D. Abad
Indiana University School of Medicine
Indianapolis, IN
USA

James L. Abbruzzese
University of Texas M.D. Anderson
Cancer Center
Houston, TX
USA

N. Volkan Adsay
Emory University School of Medicine and
Winship Cancer Institute
Atlanta, GA
USA

Nicholas Alexakis
University of Athens
Athens
Greece

Thiruvengadam Arumugam
University of Texas M.D. Anderson
Cancer Center
Houston, TX
USA

Aparna Balachandran
University of Texas M.D. Anderson
Cancer Center
Houston, TX
USA

Detlef K. Bartsch
University Hospital Marburg and Giessen
Marburg
Germany

Olca Basturk
New York University School of Medicine
New York, NY
USA

Priya R. Bhosale
University of Texas M.D. Anderson
Cancer Center
Houston, TX
USA

Diana Born
University of Bern
Bern
Switzerland

Malte Buchholz
University Hospital Marburg
Marburg
Germany

O. R. C. Busch
Academic Medical Center from the
University of Amsterdam
Amsterdam
The Netherlands

Markus W. Buchler
University of Heidelberg
Heidelberg
Germany

Gabriele Capurso
University of Rome
Rome
Italy

David L. Carr-Locke
Brigham and Women's Hospital
Boston, MA
USA

Chuslip Charnsangavej
University of Texas M.D. Anderson
Cancer Center
Houston, TX
USA

Ian Chau
The Royal Marsden Hospital
London and Surrey
UK

Woonyoung Choi
University of Texas M.D. Anderson
Cancer Center
Houston, TX
USA

Ondine Cleaver
The University of Texas Southwestern
Medical Center
Dallas, TX
USA

Ipek Coban
Emory University School of Medicine and
Winship Cancer Institute
Atlanta, GA
USA

Eithne Costello
Royal Liverpool University Hospital
Liverpool
UK

Christopher H. Crane
University of Texas M.D. Anderson
Cancer Center
Houston, TX
USA

David Cunningham
The Royal Marsden Hospital
London and Surrey
UK

Gianfranco Delle Fave
University of Rome
Rome
Italy

Mert Erkan
Technical University of Munich
Munich
Germany

Irene Esposito
Helmholtz Zentrum Munich
Munich
Germany
Technical University of Munich
Munich
Germany

Douglas B. Evans
The Medical College of Wisconsin
Milwaukee, WI
USA

Georg Feldmann
Johns Hopkins University School of Medicine
Baltimore, MD
USA

Volker Fendrich
University Hospital Marburg and Giessen
Marburg
Germany

Laureano Fernandez-Cruz
University of Barcelona
Barcelona
Spain

Carlos Fernandez-del Castillo
Massachusetts General Hospital
Boston, MA
USA

Cristina R. Ferrone
Massachusetts General Hospital
Boston, MA
USA

Stefano Festa
University of Rome
Rome
Italy

Michael Fisch
University of Texas M.D. Anderson
Cancer Center
Houston, TX
USA

Keith Fournier
University of Texas M.D. Anderson
Cancer Center
Houston, TX
USA

Helmut Friess
Technical University of Munich
Munich
Germany

Michael C. Garofalo
University of Maryland School of Medicine
Baltimore, MD
USA

Paula Ghaneh
University of Liverpool
Liverpool
UK

Ferga C. Gleeson
Mayo Clinic College of Medicine
Rochester, MN
USA

Michael Goggins
Johns Hopkins Medical Institutions
Baltimore, MD
USA

Dirk J. Gouma
Academic Medical Center from the University
of Amsterdam
Amsterdam
The Netherlands

William Greenhalf
Liverpool of University
Liverpool
UK

Thomas M. Gress
Philipps-University of Marburg
Marburg
Germany

T. M van Gulik
Academic Medical Center from the University
of Amsterdam
Amsterdam
The Netherlands

Matthias Hebrok
University of California
San Francisco, CA
USA

Stephan Herzig
German Cancer Research Center
Heidelberg
Germany

Rosa F. Hwang
University of Texas M.D. Anderson
Cancer Center
Houston, TX
USA

Elizabeth M. Jaffee
The Sidney Kimmel Cancer Center at
Johns Hopkins
Baltimore, MD
USA

Milind Javle
University of Texas M.D. Anderson
Cancer Center
Houston, TX
USA

Baoan Ji
University of Texas M.D. Anderson
Cancer Center
Houston, TX
USA

Li Jiao
National Cancer Institute
Rockville, MD
USA

Jorg Kleeff
Technical University of Munich
Munich
Germany

Moritz Koch
University of Heidelberg
Heidelberg
Germany

Satoshi Kondo
Hokkaido University Graduate School
of Medicine
Sapporo
Japan

Murray Korc
Dartmouth-Hitchcock Medical Center
Lebanon, NH
USA

Alysandra Lal
The Medical College of Wisconsin
Milwaukee, WI
USA

Peter Langer
University Hospital Marburg and Giessen
Marburg
Germany

Nicholas R. Lemoine
University of London
London
UK

Anne Marie Lennon
Johns Hopkins Medical Institutions
Baltimore, MD
USA

Michael J. Levy
Mayo Clinic College of Medicine
Rochester, MN
USA

Brian Lewis
University of Massachusetts Medical School
Worcester, MA
USA

Chenwei Li
University of Michigan
Ann Arbor, MI
USA

Donghui Li
University of Texas M.D. Anderson
Cancer Center
Houston, TX
USA

Keith D. Lillemoe
Indiana University School of Medicine
Indianapolis, IN
USA

Michelle Lockley
University of Cambridge
Cambridge
London

Craig D. Logsdon
University of Texas M.D. Anderson
Cancer Center
Houston, TX
USA

Gwen Lomberk
Mayo Clinic
Rochester, MN
USA

Raymond J. MacDonald
The University of Texas Southwestern
Medical Center
Dallas, TX
USA

Anirban Maitra
Johns Hopkins University School of Medicine
Baltimore, MD
USA

Leonardo P. Marcal
University of Texas M.D. Anderson
Cancer Center
Houston, TX
USA

Lauren Marquis
University of Texas M.D. Anderson
Cancer Center
Houston, TX
USA

Folasade P. May
Massachusetts General Hospital
Boston, MA
USA

David J. McConkey
University of Texas M.D. Anderson
Cancer Center
Houston, TX
USA

Jeffrey J. Meyer
University of Texas M.D. Anderson
Cancer Center
Houston, TX
USA

Patrick Michl
Philipps-University of Marburg
Marburg
Germany

Nathan Mollberg
University of Heidelberg
Heidelberg
Germany

Albrecht Neesse
Philipps-University of Marburg
Marburg
Germany

John P. Neoptolemos
University of Liverpool
Liverpool
UK

Yuji Nimura
Aichi Cancer Center
Nagoya
Japan

Alixanna Norris
Norris Cotton Cancer Center
Lebanon, NH
USA

Alicia Okines
The Royal Marsden Hospital
London and Surrey
UK

Naimish Pandya
University of Maryland School of Medicine
Baltimore, MD
USA

Ioannis S. Papanikolaou
Attikon University General Hospital
Athens
Greece

Marina Pasca di Magliano
University of Michigan
Ann Arbor, MI
USA

Matteo Piciucchi
University of Rome
Rome
Italy

Nuh N. Rahbari
University of Heidelberg
Heidelberg
Germany

Vijaya Ramachandran
University of Texas M.D. Anderson
Cancer Center
Houston, TX
USA

Gihan Ratnayake
The Royal Marsden Hospital
London and Surrey
UK

William F. Regine
University of Maryland School of Medicine
Baltimore, MD
USA

Thomas Rosch
Eppendorf University Hospital of Hamburg
Hamburg
Germany

Roberto A. Rovasio
National University of Cordoba
Córdoba
Argentina

Stephen H. Settle
University of Texas M.D. Anderson
Cancer Center
Houston, TX
USA

Rachna T. Shroff
University of Texas M.D. Anderson
Cancer Center
Houston, TX
USA

Diane M. Simeone
University of Michigan
Ann Arbor, MI
USA

Caroline R. Sussman
Mayo Clinic
Rochester, MN
USA

Robert Sutton
University of Liverpool
Liverpool
UK

Eric P. Tamm
University of Texas M.D. Anderson
Cancer Center
Houston, TX
USA

Masao Tanaka
Kyushu University
Fukuoka
Japan

Sarah Tonack
Royal Liverpool University Hospital
Liverpool
UK

David Tuveson
Cancer Research UK
Cambridge
UK

Raul Urrutia
Mayo Clinic
Rochester, MN
USA

Roberto Valente
University of Rome
Rome
Italy

Gauri R. Varadhachary
University of Texas M.D. Anderson
Cancer Center
Houston, TX
USA

Jens Waldmann
University Hospital Marburg and Giessen
Marburg
Germany

Andrew L. Warshaw
Massachusetts General Hospital
Boston, MA
USA

Jurgen Weitz
University of Heidelberg
Heidelberg
Germany

Jens Werner
University of Heidelberg
Heidelberg
Germany

Field F. Willingham
Massachusetts General Hospital
Boston, MA
USA
Brigham & Women's Hospital
Boston, MA
USA

Robert A. Wolff
University of Texas M.D. Anderson
Cancer Center
Houston, TX
USA

Han Hsi Wong
Queen Mary, University of London
London
UK

Lei Zheng
The Sidney Kimmel Cancer Center at
Johns Hopkins
Baltimore, MD
USA

The Nature of
Pancreatic Cancer

1 Epidemiology and Prospects for Prevention of Pancreatic Cancer

Li Jiao · Donghui Li

1	**Epidemiology**	**4**
2	**Established Risk Factors**	**5**
2.1	Age	5
2.2	Hereditary Risk Factors	5
2.3	Cigarette Smoking	7
2.4	Obesity	8
2.5	Diabetes Mellitus	9
3	**Suspected Risk Factors**	**10**
3.1	Alcohol	10
3.2	Pancreatitis	11
4	**Dietary Factors**	**12**
4.1	Meat	12
4.2	Fruits and Vegetables	13
4.3	Flavonoinds, Folate, Lycopene	13
4.4	Carbohydrate, Glycemic Index/Load	14
5	**Other Factors**	**14**
5.1	Infectious Agents	14
5.2	Occupation	15
5.3	Allergy	16
5.4	Non-Steroidal Anti-Inflammatory Drugs	16
5.5	Statins and Metformin	17
6	**Conclusion**	**17**

J. P. Neoptolemos, R. Urrutia, J. L. Abbruzzese, M. W. Büchler (eds.), *Pancreatic Cancer*,
DOI 10.1007/978-0-387-77498-5_1, © Springer Science+Business Media, LLC 2010

Abstract: The overall incidence of pancreatic cancer in the United States is approximately 8–10 cases per 100,000 person-years. African Americans have higher incidence rate than other ethnic groups. Men have a slightly higher incidence than women. Age is the most significant risk factor for pancreatic cancer. Genetic predispositions account for 5–10% of cases. Cigarette smoking is the only confirmed environmental risk factor and long-term smoking cessation reduces the risk. The causal relationship between high body mass index and risk has been established. Diabetes could be the manifestation of pancreatic cancer, but long-standing type II diabetes mellitus has been implicated as a risk factor. Other suspected risk factors for pancreatic cancer include alcohol and pancreatitis. Heavy alcohol use, especially heavy liquor use, may serve as a cofactor in pancreatic cancer development. However, the confounding effect by smoking cannot be excluded. Chronic pancreatitis may increase the risk for pancreatic cancer but the confounding effect of alcohol cannot be excluded. Dietary factors that have been suggested to associate with increased risk of pancreatic cancer include: high intake of total energy, total fat, red meat, animal protein and dietary mutagens. Dietary intake of folate and flavonoid may be protective against pancreatic cancer but the results are inconclusive. The association of pancreatic cancer with passive smoking, non-cigarette tobacco product use, carbohydrate intake, coffee consumption, physical activity, infectious factors, allergy, occupation and use of NSAIDs or statins are all inconclusive. Other than tobacco carcinogen, epidemiologic studies support that insulin resistance, energy imbalance and inflammation may be the underlying mechanisms in pancreatic cancer development. In view of the high mortality of pancreatic cancer, an appropriate strategy for reducing the burden of this cancer is to reduce exposure to known risk factors such as cigarette smoking, obesity and diabetes. Lifestyle changes hold the hope for primary prevention of pancreatic cancer. Well-designed epidemiologic studies will speed up our understanding on the etiology of pancreatic cancer.

1   Epidemiology

Worldwide, pancreatic cancer is the 13th most common type of cancer. Its poor prognosis makes it the eighth major form of cancer-related death causing more than 227,000 deaths annually [1]. Age-adjusted incidence rates range from 10–15 per 100,000 people in parts of Northern, Central, and Eastern Europe to less than 1 per 100,000 in areas of Africa and Asia [2]. The highest incidence rates were observed among African American in the United States and New Zealand Maoris; the lowest rates were reported for India and Thailand [3]. Pancreatic cancer incidence and mortality statistics are similar throughout the world. In the United States, based on cases diagnosed in 2001–2005 from 17 Surveillance Epidemiology and End Results (SEER) geographic areas, the age-adjusted incidence rate for all races was 13.0 per 100,000 men and 10.3 per 100,000 women [4]. Based on patients died in 2001–2005, the age-adjusted death rate per 100,000 for pancreatic cancer was 12.2 for men, 9.3 for women, 15.4 for black men, 12.4 for black women, 12.1 for white men, and 9.0 for white women. Worldwide, pancreatic cancer occurs slightly more frequently in men than in women and in urban areas more than in rural regions. In the United States, while the incidence in women has increased slightly over the past two decades, the incidence in men has dropped slightly. Now the incidence is about the same for both sexes, probably as a result of the increased use of tobacco by women [5]. The reasons for the regional and ethnic differences in the incidence of pancreatic cancer are unknown. The higher incidence in most developed countries probably reflects diagnostic capacity rather than etiology [6]. The fact that the rates in African

Americans are considerably higher than in native Africans suggests an environmental influence. Among men, the established risk factors (mainly cigarette smoking and diabetes mellitus) explain almost the entire black/white disparity in incidence. Among women, moderate/heavy alcohol consumption and elevated body mass index appear to contribute to the racial disparity [7].

2   Established Risk Factors

2.1   Age

Age is the most established predictor of pancreatic cancer incidence and death. The risk of pancreatic cancer is low in the first three to four decades of life but increases sharply after age 50 years, with most patients between the ages of 60 and 80 years and the median age at diagnosis of 72 years [5] (Table I–11 (http://seer.cancer.gov/csr/1975_2005/results_single/sect_01_table.11_2pgs.pdf)). Approximately 0.0% was diagnosed under age 20; 0.4% between 20 and 34; 2.4% between 35 and 44; 9.6% between 45 and 54; 18.9% between 55 and 64; 26.6% between 65 and 74; 29.5% between 75 and 84; and 12.5% 85+ years of age [4].

2.2   Hereditary Risk Factors

Inherited pancreatic cancers represent approximately 5–10% of all pancreatic cancers [8]. Pancreatic cancer may be inherited as part of a known cancer syndrome or in association with hereditary pancreatitis or cystic fibrosis [9].

Hereditary breast-ovarian cancer syndrome is associated with mutations in BRCA1 or BRCA2. BRCA2 is a tumor suppressor gene on chromosome 13q12 and its protein product is involved in the repair of DNA strand breaks. Deleterious germline mutations in the BRCA2 gene have been found in 17% of patients with familial pancreatic cancer [10] and in 7% of patients thought to have sporadic pancreatic cancer [11]. Such germline BRCA2 mutations represent the most common inherited predisposition to pancreatic cancer and are associated with an up to 10 times greater risk of pancreatic cancer than exists in the general population [12].

The *familial atypical multiple-mole melanoma* (FAMMM) syndrome is a rare autosomal dominant genetic disorder with incomplete penetrance caused by germline mutations in the CDKN2A (p16) tumor suppressor gene on chromosome 9p21 and is associated with the development of multiple nevi, including malignant melanoma [13]. Among 159 families collected in the Creighton University registry of familial pancreatic cancer, 19 (12%) showed FAMMM and 8 with ascertained mutations within CDKN2A [14]. Both early-onset and late-onset pancreatic cancer have been seen in the affected families.

Peutz-Jeghers syndrome is rare and inherited as an autosomal dominant genetic disorder characterized by the presence of multiple hamartomatous gastrointestinal polyps and mucocutaneous pigmentation and is associated with an increased risk of several gastrointestinal cancers [15]. It is often caused by mutations in the LKB1/STK11 tumor suppressor gene on chromosome 19p13. Although patients with Peutz-Jeghers syndrome are at significant higher risk of pancreatic cancer, the exact magnitude of the risk is unclear. One study showed relative risk (RR) is 132 (95% confidence interval (CI), 44–261) with a cumulative lifetime risk of 36% [16].

Interestingly, biallelic inactivation of the LKB1/STK11 gene was also found in 4% of patients with resected sporadic pancreatic cancers [17]. Lim et al. analyzed the incidence of cancer in 240 individuals with Peutz-Jeghers syndrome possessing germline mutations in STK11. All pancreatic cancers were diagnosed between age 34 and 49 years. The risk of developing pancreatic cancer was 5% at age 40, increasing to 8% at age 60 years [18].

Li-Fraumeni syndrome occurs among carriers of mutations within TP53 gene [19]. TP53 is an extensively studied tumor suppressor protein with a critical role in controlling cell-cycle arrest and apoptosis. Germline mutation of *p53* is known to be the underlying genetic defect in the Li-Fraumeni syndrome of childhood malignancies, bone and soft-tissue sarcomas, premenopausal breast carcinoma, brain tumors, adrenocortical carcinoma, and leukemias. Pancreatic adenocarcinoma is the only adult epithelial malignancy that has been proven to be associated with Li-Fraumeni syndrome, other than breast cancer [20].

Hereditary nonpolyposis colon cancer (HNPCC), also known as Lynch syndrome, is an autosomal dominant genetic disorder caused by germline mutations in mismatch repair genes resulting in an increased risk of colorectal cancer and other cancers, including cancer of the breast, endometrium, and ovary. Patients with HNPCC may also have an increased risk of pancreatic cancer. However, the magnitude of the increased risk is not clear because the numbers of cases often are not adequate for an appropriate assessment of the risk.

Familial adenomatous polyposis (FAP) is the most common adenomatous polyposis syndrome. It is an autosomal dominant inherited disorder characterized by the early onset of hundreds to thousands of adenomatous polyps throughout the colon. The genetic defect in FAP is a germline mutation in the adenomatous polyposis coli (APC) tumor suppressor gene, located on chromosome 5q21. *APC* encodes a multi-domain protein that plays a major role as a tumor suppressor by antagonizing the wingless-type (Wnt) signaling pathway. A study of 197 FAP pedigrees found a RR of 4.46 (95% CI, 1.2–11.4) [21].

Hereditary pancreatitis is a rare form of pancreatitis. It has an autosomal dominant pattern of transmission with 80% penetrate. It is characterized by the development of recurrent episodes of severe chronic pancreatitis starting at an early age. The symptoms usually arise by age 40 years, but can occur before age 5 years. In approximately one-third of all cases, no etiologic factor can be found, and these patients are classified as having idiopathic disease. Mutations in the cationic trypsinogen gene (PRSS1) on chromosome 7q35 have been identified in patients with hereditary or idiopathic chronic pancreatitis [22]. Lowenfels and colleagues [23] obtained data on 246 patients with hereditary pancreatitis from pancreatologists in 10 countries. They found that the estimated cumulative risk of pancreatic cancer developing by age 70 was approximately 40% in this patient population. The mean age at the diagnosis of pancreatic cancer was 57 years. Idiopathic pancreatitis has been found to be associated with mutations in the cystic fibrosis gene (CFTR) [24]. Compared with the background population, the risk of pancreatic cancer is approximately 50 to 60 times greater than expected [25].

Familial pancreatic cancer kindreds have also been identified that are not affected by an inherited cancer syndrome. At-risk patients for familial pancreatic cancer include those with a minimum of two first-degree relatives with pancreatic cancer [26]. A meta-analysis identified 7 case-control and 2 cohort studies involving 6,568 pancreatic cancer cases [27]. This analysis found a significant increase in risk associated with having an affected relative, with a summary RR of 1.80 (95% CI, 1.48–2.12). Individuals with a family history of pancreatic cancer have nearly a two-fold increased risk of pancreatic cancer compared with those without such a history. The study suggested that families with two or more pancreatic cancer cases might benefit from comprehensive risk assessment that involves collection of detailed information on family history and environmental exposure, especially smoking history. Previous studies of a well-known family of familial pancreatic cancer suggested that the susceptibility locus for autosomal dominant pancreatic cancer is on chromosome 4q32–34 [28] and Palladin might be the responsible gene [29]. However, two later studies failed to confirm these findings in other study populations [30,31].

More details on this topic can be found in the Chapter "Genetic susceptibility – High risk groups, chronic and hereditary pancreatitis, familial pancreatic cancer syndromes" of this book.

2.3   Cigarette Smoking

The risk factor most firmly associated with pancreatic cancer is cigarette smoking [5]. A meta-analysis of 82 independent studies published between 1950 and 2007 containing epidemiologic information on smoking and pancreatic cancer across four continents. This analysis found the overall risk of pancreatic cancer estimated from the combined results for current and former smokers was, respectively, 1.74 (95% CI, 1.61–1.87) and 1.20 (95% CI, 1.11–1.29), compared with never smokers. For former cigarette smokers, the risk remains elevated for a minimum of 10 years after cessation and long-term smoking cessation (>10 years) reduces the risk by approximately 30% relative to the risk in current smokers [32]. It is currently estimated that approximately 25% of cases of pancreatic cancer are due to cigarette smoking.

In animals, pancreatic malignancies can be induced through the long-term administration of tobacco-specific N-nitrosamines or the parenteral administration of other N-nitroso compounds. These carcinogens are metabolized to electrophiles that readily react with DNA, leading to the miscoding and activation of oncogenes. Indeed, the detections of carcinogen-DNA adducts in human pancreas tissues and tobacco-specific compounds in pancreatic juice further support the link between cigarette smoking and pancreatic cancer [33–35]. Recent molecular epidemiological studies have also shown that individual genetic variability in carcinogen metabolism and DNA repair may partially determine the susceptibility to smoking-related pancreatic cancer [36–40]. Previous studies have also shown an association of K-ras mutation in pancreatic tumors with cigarette smoking [41,42]. Information generated from such studies may facilitate the development of strategies in identifying high-risk individuals for the primary prevention of pancreatic cancer.

Noncigarette tobacco use has been increasing in the United States [43]. Several previous studies have reported significant associations between use of pipe [44], smokeless tobacco [45], or cigar [43,46–48] and risk for pancreatic cancer. Compared with never smokers, the risk of pancreatic cancer for current and former pipe and/or cigar smokers was respectively 1.47 (95% CI, 1.17–1.83) and 1.29 (95% CI, 0.68–2.45) in the recent meta-analysis report [32].

Few studies have investigated the relation of passive smoking or environmental tobacco smoke (ETS) with risk of pancreatic cancer. A Canadian population-based cases control study including 583 pancreatic cancer cases and 4,813 controls first reported a statistically nonsignificant moderate increased risk of developing pancreatic cancer (odds ratio [OR], 1.21; 95% CI, 0.60–2.44) when childhood and adult exposure to ETS compared to non-exposure among never smokers [49]. A hospital-based case-control study conducted at the University of Texas M. D. Anderson Cancer Center included 808 cases and 808 controls [48] found passive smoking was significantly associated with risk of pancreatic cancer among ever smokers (OR, 1.7; 95% CI, 1.0–2.6) but not among never smokers (OR, 1.1; 95% CI, 0.8–1.6).

Similarly, one study, including two prospective cohorts, did not observe an association between passive smoking and risk among never smokers [50]. Overall these data do not support a significant role of passive smoking in pancreatic cancer.

2.4   Obesity

The positive association between obesity, as measured by high body mass index (BMI), and risk for pancreatic cancer has been observed in at least 16 out of the 27 prospective studies and 3 meta-analyses [51–53]. The first meta-analysis [51] identified 6 case–control and 8 cohort studies involving 6,391 cases of pancreatic cancer from 1966 to 2003. The summary RR per unit increase in body mass index was 1.02 (95% CI, 1.01–1.03). The second meta-analysis of 21 independent prospective studies involving 3,495,981 individuals and 8,062 pancreatic cancer patients showed that the RR of pancreatic cancer per 5 kg/m^2 increase in BMI was 1.16 (95% CI, 1.06–1.17) in men, and 1.10 (95% CI, 1.02–1.19) in women [52]. The latest meta-analysis [53] includes 16 prospective studies involving 3,338,001 individuals and 4,443 cases. The RR of pancreatic cancer per 5 kg/m^2 increase in BMI was 1.07 (95% CI, 0.93–1.23) in men, and 1.12 (95% CI, 1.03–1.23) in women. It has been estimated that the population attributable fraction of obesity-associated pancreatic cancer is 26.9% for the U.S. population [54]. In 2007, the World Cancer Research Fund (WCRF) and American Institute for Cancer Research (AICR) concluded that the evidence that greater body fatness is a cause of pancreatic cancer is convincing [2].

Abdominal fatness is probably also a cause of pancreatic cancer. Central adiposity is associated with glucose intolerance and is a risk factor for diabetes; hence concomitantly increased insulin levels may be the mechanism through which central adiposity increases pancreatic cancer risk. A few studies have investigated central adiposity in association with risk of pancreatic cancer [55–59]. In the American Cancer Society Cancer Prevention Study II Nutrition Cohort, men and women who reported "central" weight gain had a RR of pancreatic cancer of 1.45 (95% CI, 1.02–2.07) compared with men and women who reported peripheral weight gain, independent of BMI [56]. Central weight gain was defined as reported weight gain in chest and shoulders or waist, and peripheral weight gain was defined as reported weight gain in hips and thighs or equally all over [56]. In the European Prospective Investigation into Cancer and Nutrition study (EPIC), 324 incident cases of pancreatic cancer were diagnosed in the cohort over an average of 6 years of follow-up. Larger waist-to-hip ratio and waist circumference were both associated with an increased risk of pancreatic cancer (RR per 0.1, 1.24; 95% CI, 1.04–1.48; and RR per 10 cm, 1.13; 95% CI, 1.01–1.26, respectively) [57]. In the NIH-AARP Diet and Health study, 654 pancreatic cancer cases were identified in 495,035 AARP cohort members during an average of 5 years of follow-up. Waist circumference was positively associated with pancreatic cancer (fourth vs. first quartile: RR, 2.53; 95% CI, 1.13- 5.65) in women but not men [58]. In the Women's Health Initiative study [59], women in the highest quintile of waist-to -hip ratio after adjusting for potential confounders had 70% (95% CI, 10–160%) excess risk compared with women in the lowest quintile. When waist-to-hip ratio was analyzed as a continuous variable, risk increased by 27% (95% CI, 7–50%) per 0.1 increase. This observation was made on the basis of 251 cases after following up 138,503 women for average of 7.7 years [59]. In a pooled analysis of 30 cohort studies involving 519,643 Asian-Pacific participants and 324 deaths from pancreatic cancer, the RR (95% CI) was 1.08 (1.02–1.14) for every 2-cm increase in waist circumference [60].

Physical activity has been associated with improved glucose metabolism, increased insulin sensitivity, and decreased insulin, independent of its effects on weight [61]. Increased physical activity may confer a reduced risk for pancreatic cancer [62]. However, a recent systematic review found total physical activity (occupational and leisure time) was not significantly associated with risk for pancreatic cancer (4 prospective studies; summary RR, 0.76; 95% CI, 0.53–1.09). A decreased risk for pancreatic cancer was observed for occupational physical activity (3 prospective studies; RR, 0.75; 95% CI, 0.58–0.96) but not for leisure-time physical activity (14 prospective studies; RR, 0.94; 95% CI, 0.83–1.05). Measurement of physical activity is subjected to error, and the non-differential misclassification would bias the risk estimate towards the null.

2.5   Diabetes Mellitus

In addition to cigarette smoking and obesity, type II diabetes is likely to be a third modifiable risk factor for pancreatic cancer. Diabetes mellitus has been implicated both as an early manifestation of pancreatic cancer and as a predisposing factor [63,64]. Related to this is the observation that pancreatic adenocarcinoma of duct cell origin can induce peripheral insulin resistance [65]. In addition, a putative cancer-associated diabetogenic factor has been isolated from the conditioned medium of pancreatic cancer cell lines and from patient serum [66]. From the standpoint of clinical observations, a cohort study showed that patients were at increased risk of pancreatic cancer after an initial hospitalization for diabetes, and this risk persisted for more than a decade [67]. Two meta-analyses have investigated the risk of pancreatic cancer in relation to diabetes. The first meta-analysis conducted in 1995 and identified 20 of a total of 30 case-control and cohort studies [68]. The second meta-analysis was conducted in 2005 that included 17 case-control and 19 cohorts or nested case-control studies published from 1996 to 2005 [69]. The summary OR (95% CI) of pancreatic cancer for diabetics relative to nondiabetics was 2.1 (1.6–2.8) and 1.82 (1.66–1.89) in the first and second meta-analysis, respectively. The first meta-analysis found requiring diabetes duration of at least 5 years resulted in an RR of 2.0 (95% CI, 1.2–3.2). The authors concluded that pancreatic cancer occurs with increased frequency among persons with long-standing diabetes. The second meta-analysis found that individuals in whom diabetes had only recently been diagnosed (<4 years) had a 50% greater risk of pancreatic cancer compared with individuals who had diabetes for ≥5 years (OR, 2.1 vs. 1.5; P = 0.005). These results support a modest causal association between type II diabetes and pancreatic cancer.

It has been estimated that approximately 1% of diabetics aged ≥50 years will be diagnosed with pancreatic cancer within 3 years of first meeting criteria for diabetes [70]. Pancreatic cancer-induced hyperglycemia occurs up to 24 months prior to the diagnosis of pancreatic cancer [71]. Therefore, it has been suggested that diabetes itself may act as a biomarker of early pancreatic cancer [72]. Identifying the patients with cancer-associated diabetes at their diabetes onset would offer an opportunity for early detection of pancreatic cancer.

The studies on type I diabetes and risk of pancreatic cancer are rare. A systematic review and meta-analysis conducted in 2007 identified 3 cohort studies and 6 case-control studies [73]. Based on 39 cases, the summary RR for pancreatic cancer in young-onset or type I diabetes versus no diabetes was 2.00 (95% CI, 1.37–3.01). Since this study indicates a similarly elevated risk in type I as in type II diabetes, this weighs against the involvement of β-cell activity in the etiology of pancreatic cancer in diabetes.

The causal relationship between diabetes and risk of pancreatic cancer is supported by findings from biomarker studies. Prediagnostic elevations in post-load plasma glucose [74,75], serum and plasma glucose [76], insulin [77,78], and plasma C-peptide levels [79] have been associated with greater risk of pancreatic cancer. These observations suggest that insulin plays an important role in pancreatic carcinogenesis. High insulin concentrations in the microenvironment of the pancreatic duct cell may contribute to malignant transformation. In addition, the insulin-like growth factors (IGFs) may also play a role in promoting pancreatic tumor development. The prediagnostic biomarkers of IGF axis have been investigated in association with pancreatic cancer in a few prospective cohort studies [80]. A study of 93 pancreatic cancer cases and 400 randomly selected cohort controls from the Alpha-Tocopherol, Beta-Carotene (ATBC) Cancer Prevention Study [81] found no association between IGF-I, or IGF binding protein-3 (IGFBP-3), or IGF-1:IGFBP-3 molar ratio and the risk of pancreatic cancer in male smokers. In a Japanese nested case-control study [82] including 69 cases and 207 controls, there was a positive, but statistically insignificant association between serum levels of IGF-I and risk of death from pancreatic cancer. In a pooled nested case-control study in the United States [80], plasma levels of IGF-1, IGF-2, or IGFBP-3 were not associated with risk of pancreatic cancer among 212 incident cases and 635 matched controls. In the same study setting [83] including 144 pancreatic cancer cases that occurred ≥ 4 years after plasma collection and in 429 controls, lower plasma IGFBP-1 level was significantly associated with an increased risk of pancreatic cancer in never smokers (RR, 2.07; 95% CI, 1.26–3.39). The strength of the association was not substantially attenuated by the inclusion of plasma IGF-I, C-peptide, and IGFBP-3 in the multivariate models, suggesting an independent effect for IGFBP-1 on pancreatic cancer risk.

3   Suspected Risk Factors

3.1   Alcohol

Alcohol consumption is an established risk factor for pancreatitis and type II diabetes mellitus, both of which are associated with increased risk of pancreatic cancer. However, only a few studies have shown significant increased risk in association with total alcohol intake more than 30 g per day among more than 60 analytic studies [84–87]. In 2007, a panel sponsored by the WCRF and AICR concluded that the current data on the relationship between alcohol intake and pancreatic cancer risk were too inconsistent to reach a judgment on the association between alcohol intake and risk of pancreatic cancer. A recent pooled analysis of the primary data from 14 prospective cohort studies [88] has shown a slight positive association of pancreatic cancer risk with alcohol intake (summary multivariate RR, 1.22; 95% CI, 1.03–1.45 comparing >30–0 grams/day). This association was statistically significant among women only. A recent EPIC study of 555 non-endocrine pancreatic cancer cases showed that high lifetime ethanol intake from spirits/liquor at recruitment tended to be associated with a higher risk (RR, 1.40; 95% CI, 0.93–2.10 comparing 10+ g/day vs. 0.1–4.9 g/day), but no associations were observed for wine and beer consumption [89]. In the NIH-AARP Diet and Health Study [90], the authors identified 1,149 eligible exocrine pancreatic cancer cases among 470,681 participants during average 7.3 years of follow-up, the RR of pancreatic cancer was 1.45 (95% CI, 1.17–1.80) for heavy total alcohol use (≥ 3 drinks/day, ~40 g alcohol/day) and 1.62 (95% CI, 1.24–2.10) for heavy liquor use, compared to the light alcohol use

(<1 drink per day among ever drinkers). The increased risk was not statistically significant in women due to the fact that women tended to drink less. However, the confounding effect of smoking cannot be excluded because heavy alcohol users were more likely to be smokers. Additional large studies or meta-analysis of pooled data from existing studies are required to demonstrate the association of alcohol consumption and risk independent of smoking. Overall, moderate alcohol consumption is not a risk factor of pancreatic cancer. Heavy alcohol use, in particular heavy drink of liquor, may play a role in pancreatic cancer development. Alcohol consumption may sensitize the pancreas to inflammatory, immune, and fibrosing responses induced by genetic and environmental predisposing factors and functions as a co-factor in the development of pancreatic disease.

3.2   Pancreatitis

Alcohol is the dominant identified cause for chronic pancreatitis, although a significant number of individuals may have chronic pancreatitis of idiopathic origin [91]. As pancreatic cancer may obstruct pancreatic enzyme flow, pancreatitis may be a consequence of pancreatic cancer. Even after exclusion of individuals diagnosed with pancreatitis in close proximity to pancreatic cancer, some have reported a continued association between a remote history of pancreatitis and/or chronic pancreatitis and pancreatic cancer, whereas others have not. For example, in a cohort study of 2,015 patients with chronic pancreatitis from six countries, Lowenfels et al. reported an increased risk of pancreatic cancer in patients with chronic pancreatitis, with the cumulative incidence of pancreatic cancer increasing with the longer duration of follow-up [92]. Talamini and colleagues [93] made similar observations in a study of 715 patients with chronic pancreatitis and found a 13- to 18-fold increase in the incidence of pancreatic cancer. They also observed that patients with a short duration between pancreatitis and pancreatic cancer diagnosis were older, had a lower percentage of men, infrequently used tobacco and alcohol, and were more likely to be noninsulin-dependent diabetics compared to patients without pancreatic cancer or patients in whom pancreatic cancer developed late after the diagnosis of chronic pancreatitis. The authors therefore hypothesized that the cancer causes pancreatitis in some cases (as may be the case with hyperglycemia) and emphasized that, for this reason, cancer should be strongly considered in a patient diagnosed with idiopathic chronic pancreatitis without a history of significant alcohol or tobacco use, especially in the context of hyperglycemia. Somewhat in contrast, however, were the findings of Karlson and colleagues [94], who identified 230 patients with pancreatic cancer among 29,530 patients in the Swedish national registry discharged 1 year or more after a hospital admission for pancreatitis. Although they found that the standardized incidence ratio (observed/expected) for pancreatic cancer increased in patients with pancreatitis (2.8; 95% CI, 2.5–3.2), after 10 years or more, the excess risk declined and was of borderline significance. The authors concluded that their data thus did not support a causal association between pancreatitis and pancreatic cancer; instead, alcohol consumption and smoking were thought to contribute significantly to the increased cancer risk associated with chronic pancreatitis. As inflammation has been implicated in the causal pathway of many other malignancies, a causal relationship between pancreatitis and pancreatic cancer is plausible, possibly through increased cell-proliferation due to chronic inflammation in the presence of growth factors. Additional studies are required to clarify the association between pancreatitis and pancreatic cancer.

4   Dietary Factors

Various dietary factors have been examined in association with pancreatic cancer. According to the 2007 report by WCRF and AICR [2], there is suggestive evidence supporting associations of intakes of total energy, total fat, red meat consumption, animal protein, or fruit intake with risk of pancreatic cancer. The evidence on the role of dietary fiber, vegetables, carbohydrate and sugar, soy products, dairy products, and vitamin C supplement is limited and inconclusive; and coffee consumption is unlikely to have a substantial effect on risk of pancreatic cancer.

4.1   Meat

There is a general consensus that a higher intake of meat and animal product is associated with increased risk of pancreatic cancer. For example, the Multiethnic cohort study [95] including 482 incident pancreatic cancers found a significant association with processed meat; those in the fifth quintile of daily intake had a 68% increased risk compared with those in the lowest quintile (RR, 1.68; 95% CI, 1.35–2.07). The authors also found that intake of total and saturated fat from meat was associated with statistically significant increases in pancreatic cancer risk but that from dairy products was not. Recent studies suggested that the method of meat preparation and subsequent intake of food mutagens might contribute to the development of pancreatic cancer [96–98]. It is known that cooking meat at high temperature, e.g., deep fry, grill or barbeque, could produce potential carcinogens such as heterocyclic amines and polycyclic aromatic hydrocarbons. In a hospital-based case-control study [97] conducted at the University of Texas M. D. Anderson Cancer Center including 626 cases and 530 noncancer controls, Li et al. investigated the dietary exposure to food mutagens and risk of pancreatic cancer. They found that a significantly greater portion of the cases than controls showed a preference to well-done pork, bacon, grilled chicken, and pan-fried chicken. The daily intakes of 2-amino-3,4,8-trimethylimidazo[4,5-f]quinoxaline and benzo(a)pyrene, as well as the mutagenic activity, were the significant predictors for pancreatic cancer with adjustment of other confounders. The NIH-AARP Diet and Health Study [98] including 836 patients with exocrine pancreatic cancer found total, red, and high-temperature cooked meat intake was positively associated with pancreatic cancer among men but not women. Men showed significant 50% increased risks for the highest tertile of grilled/barbecued and broiled meat intake and significant doubling of risk for the highest quintile of overall meat-mutagenic activity. The fifth quintile of the heterocyclic amine, 2-amino-3,4,8-trimethylimidazo[4,5-f] quinoxaline intake showed a significant 29% (P trend = 0.006) increased risk in men and women combined. Interestingly, the M.D. Anderson case-control study reported a significant interaction between NAT1 (N-acetyltransferase 1) genotype and dietary mutagen intake on modifying the risk of pancreatic cancer among men but not women [38]. The OR (95% CI) was 2.23 (1.33–3.72) and 2.54 (1.51–4.25) for men having the NAT1*10 and a higher intake of 2-amino-1-methyl-6 phenylimidazo[4,5-b]pyridine and benzo[a]pyrene, respectively, compared with individuals having no NAT1*10 or a lower intake of these dietary mutagens. These studies support the hypothesis that meat intake, particularly meat cooked at high temperatures and associated mutagens, may play a role in pancreatic cancer development.

4.2   Fruits and Vegetables

Many case-control studies have suggested that higher consumption of fruits and vegetables is associated with a lower risk of pancreatic cancer, whereas cohort studies do not support such an association [99]. A Swedish cohort study with 135 cases [100] and a recent EPIC study [101] with 555 cases did not find an association of overall fruit and vegetable intake, subgroups of vegetables and fruits, and pancreatic cancer risk. The Multiethnic Cohort Study [102] including 526 cases did not find an association between total or specific vegetable intake and risk of pancreatic cancer but high intake of dark green vegetables may exert protective effect among current smokers. The consumption of cruciferous vegetables and pancreatic cancer risk warrants further investigation. In a systematic review including 4 case-control studies and 5 cohort studies, the authors showed that an inverse association in risk of pancreatic caner with intake of citrus fruits [103]. The results varied substantially across studies, and the apparent effect was restricted to case-control studies. In a population-based case-control study in San Francisco Bay area including 532 cases and 1,701 age- and sex-matched controls, inverse associations were found between risk of pancreatic cancer and consumption of total or specific vegetables and fruits such as dark leafy, cruciferous and yellow vegetables, carrots, beans, onions and garlic, and citrus fruits and juice [104]. Compared with less than five servings per day of total vegetables and fruits combined, the risk of pancreatic cancer was 0.49 (95% CI, 0.36–0.68) for more than nine servings per day.

4.3   Flavonoinds, Folate, Lycopene

Fruit and vegetables contain many chemicals with potential anti-cancer properties including carotenoids, vitamins C and E, flavonoids, folate, selenium and plant sterols. Flavonoids, which are found in certain plant foods, are thought to lower cancer risk through their antioxidant, antiestrogenic and antiproliferative properties. In the Multiethnic Cohort Study [105], baseline exposure data were collected in Hawaii and California in 1993–1996. Intake of total flavonols was associated with a reduced pancreatic cancer risk (RR for the highest vs. lowest quintile, 0.77; 95% Cl, 0.58–1.03). Of the three individual flavonols, kaempferol was associated with the largest risk reduction (RR, 0.78; 95% CI, 0.58–1.05). Total flavonols, quercetin, kaempferol, and myricetin were all associated with a significant inverse trend among current smokers but not among never or former smokers. In the ATBC Cancer Prevention Study, the authors found flavonoid-rich diet may decrease pancreatic cancer risk in male smokers not taking supplemental alpha-tocopherol and/or beta-carotene [106]. These two studies provide evidence for a preventive effect of flavonols on pancreatic cancer, particularly for current smokers.

Folate plays an important role in DNA synthesis and repair. A meta-analysis of 1 case-control study and 4 prospective cohort studies found the summary RR for the highest versus the lowest category of dietary folate intake were 0.49 (95% CI, 0.35–0.67) for pancreatic cancer [107]. A Swedish prospective cohort study found increased intake of folate from food sources, but not from supplements, may be associated with a reduced risk of pancreatic cancer [108]. In the ATBC Cancer Prevention Study, serum folate and pyridoxal-5′-phosphate (PLP) concentrations showed statistically significant inverse dose-response relationships with pancreatic cancer risk [109]. In a pooled nested case control analysis, baseline serum concentrations of folate, PLP, vitamin B12, or homocysteine were not associated with risk of pancreatic cancer in general, but a modest inverse trend was observed when the analysis was restricted to nonusers of multivitamins [110]. However, the association of folate intake and risk of pancreatic cancer was not observed in two large studies conducted in the United States [111,112]. The inconsistent observations on the association between folate intake and risk of pancreatic cancer may suggest that the influence of folate consumption may be restricted to populations that are relatively folate deficient, e.g., heavy smokers or heavy alcohol drinkers.

A Canadian case-control study of 462 histologically-confirmed pancreatic cancer cases and 4721 population-based controls found lycopene, provided mainly by tomatoes, was associated with a 31% reduction in pancreatic cancer risk among men [113]. However, the Food and Drug Administration review found very limited evidence to support an association between tomato or lycopene consumption and reduced risk of pancreatic cancer [114]. A meta-analysis on clinical trials could not find evidence that antioxidant supplements can prevent gastrointestinal cancers, including pancreatic cancer [115].

4.4   Carbohydrate, Glycemic Index/Load

A multicenter, population-based case control study of pancreatic cancer showed an increased risk of pancreatic cancer associated with a higher intake of carbohydrate, but not all the associations were statistically significant [116,117]. Some types of carbohydrate increase the level of serum glucose and insulin more than others. Glycemic index and glycemic load are measures designed to take into consideration of these differences. The glycemic index represents the postprandial glucose response of individual food items compared with a reference food. Refined grains, such as white bread or white rice, produce a larger increase in postprandial glucose levels than foods such as whole grain foods. Glycemic load reflects both the quality (i.e., glycemic index) and the quantity of the carbohydrates that are consumed by individuals. A high dietary glycemic index/load could increase the risk of pancreatic cancer due to the adverse effect of high postprandial glucose level and resulting insulin demands. The associations of dietary carbohydrates, refined sugars, and glycemic index/load with pancreatic cancer have been investigated in many studies and the results are inconsistent. However, the seven large-scale prospective studies consistently showed null associations of carbohydrate, glycemic index and glycemic load with risk of pancreatic cancer [118–124]. Six of these studies stratified the analyses by BMI and/or physical activity subgroups, and most of these studies did not report any significant findings, with only one exception [116]. A meta-analysis showed no significant associations between pancreatic cancer risk and either glycemic index or glycemic load in a comparison of the highest with the lowest category of intake [125]. In line with these findings, a recent large cohort study did not show that consumption of added sugar or of sugar-sweetened foods and beverages is associated with overall risk of pancreatic cancer [126].

5   Other Factors

5.1   Infectious Agents

Some data suggest an association between *Helicobacter pylori* or hepatitis B infection and pancreatic cancer [127–129]. *H. pylori* may result in sub-clinical pancreatitis and can increase gastrin levels, which have a trophic effect on the pancreas. In addition, given that the gastric carriage of *H. pylori* is a known risk factor for peptic ulcer formation and gastric cancer, this may explain the association between gastric resection and pancreatic cancer observed in some study [130] but not in others [131]. In a hospital-based case-control study in Austria [127], a serological analysis was performed among 92 patients with histologically confirmed diagnosis of pancreatic adenocarcinoma and controls for the presence of IgG antibodies against *H. pylori*. In pancreatic cancer patients when compared with those suffering from colorectal cancer combined with normal controls, the OR (95% CI) was 2.1 (1.1–4.1). However, microscopic evaluation of human pancreatic cancer specimens showed no evidence for the presence of *H. pylori*. In 2001, a nested case-control study of 121 exocrine pancreatic cancer cases and 226 cancer-free control subjects from a Finnish cohort of older male smokers found that 82% of cases were seropositive for *H. pylori* antibodies, compared with 73% of controls (OR, 1.87; 95% CI, 1.05–3.34) [128]. In this study, CagA$^+$ strains were associated with slightly greater odds of pancreatic cancer than the CagA$^-$ ones (OR, 2.01; 95% CI, 1.09–3.70 and OR, 1.65; 95% CI, 0.82–3.29, respectively). However, a study in Kaiser Permanente Medical Care Program found neither *H. pylori* (OR, 0.85; 95% CI, 0.49–1.48) nor its CagA protein (OR, 0.96; 95% CI, 0.48–1.92) was associated with subsequent development of pancreatic cancer [132]. Similarly, a recent nested case-control study [133] in a Swedish cohort did not find *H. pylori* seropositivity was associated with pancreatic cancer (OR, 1.25; 95% CI, 0.75–2.09). However, a statistically significant association was found in never smokers adjusted for alcohol consumption. These findings should be interpreted cautiously due to the limited number of cases in the subgroup analysis. The role of infection with *H. pylori* is the subject of ongoing research.

A recent case-control study in 476 patients with pathologically confirmed adenocarcinoma of the pancreas and 879 age-, sex-, and race-matched healthy controls found a possible association between past exposure to hepatitis B virus and risk of pancreatic cancer [129]. In this study, anti-HBc was positive in 38 cases (8%) and 35 controls (0.9%). The estimated OR (95% CI) was 1.8 (0.9–3.1) for anti-HBc+/anti-HBs+ and 3.4 (1.3–9.1) for anti-HBc$^+$/anti-HBs$^-$. The proximity of the liver to the pancreas and the fact that the liver and pancreas share common blood vessels and ducts may make the pancreas a potential target organ for hepatitis viruses. In fact, hepatitis B surface antigen (HBsAg), a marker for chronic HBV infection, was detected in pure pancreatic juice and pure bile juice [134] and there was evidence of HBV replication in pancreatic cells and concurrent damage to exocrine and endocrine epithelial cells with an inflammatory response [135,136]. The possibility that viral hepatitis can lead to pancreatic damage was further supported by findings of elevated pancreatic enzyme levels in a substantial percentage of patients with acute and chronic HBV and HCV infection [137,138]. However, de Gonzalez et al. [139] reported in a study of 201,975 Koreans including 664 cases of pancreatic cancer, no association was found between hepatitis B HBsAg positivity and pancreatic cancer (RR, 1.13; 95% CI, 0.84–1.52). The association of hepatitis B infection and pancreatic cancer needs further investigation.

5.2   Occupation

The role of occupational or industrial factors in pancreatic cancer has been investigated extensively. Increased risk of pancreatic cancer has been associated with exposures to some chemicals (e.g., organochlorines, chlorinated hydrocarbons, and formaldehyde), or some specific occupations (e.g., stone miners, cement workers, gardeners, and textile workers). However, the statistical power of most of these studies is quite low because of the rarity of pancreatic cancer. Many of these observations could be by chance alone [5]. A meta-analysis [140,141] reviewed 261 studies published from 1969 through 1998 on pancreatic cancer and job titles including more than 3,799 observed pancreatic cancer cases. The results suggest that occupational exposures to chlorinated hydrocarbon compounds may increase the risk of pancreatic cancer; the summary RR was 2.21 (95% CI: 1.31–3.68). Suggestive weak excess was also found for exposure to insecticides. The summary RR was 1.95 (95% CI: 0.51–7.41). In spite of many investigations, there is no compelling evidence linking occupational exposure to substance to risk of pancreatic cancer. Large studies with refined exposure measurement are required to test the hypothesis generated from the previous studies. The possible interactions between occupational exposure, lifestyle factors, and genetic susceptibility remain to be elucidated.

5.3   Allergy

A number of studies have examined the association of prior allergies with risk of pancreatic cancer. A meta-analysis [142] of 14 population-based studies (4 cohort and 10 case-control studies) with a total of 3,040 pancreatic cancer cases found history of allergy was associated with a reduced risk of pancreatic cancer (RR, 0.82; 95% CI, 0.68–0.99). The risk reduction was stronger for allergies related to atopy (RR, 0.71; 95% CI, 0.64–0.80), but not for asthma (RR, 1.01; 95% CI, 0.77–1.31). There was no association between allergies related to food or drugs and pancreatic cancer (RR, 1.08; 95% CI, 0.74–1.58). In addition, two population-based case control studies based on direct interview consistently demonstrated a 20–30% reduced risk of pancreatic cancer among individuals with any prior history of allergy [143,144]. The hyperactive immune system of allergic individuals may, therefore, in some way lead to increased surveillance and protect against pancreatic cancer development.

5.4   Non-Steroidal Anti-Inflammatory Drugs

Aspirin and other nonsteroidal anti-inflammatory drugs (NSAIDs) have received considerable interest because these agents target cyclooxygenase enzymes, therefore may inhibit tumor growth by enhancing immune responses, modulating cellular proliferation, inhibiting prostaglandin synthesis, influencing apoptosis and tumorigenesis. The Iowa Women's Health Study of 28,283 postmenopausal women including 80 pancreatic cancer cases found a significant lower RR of pancreatic cancer for aspirin user compared to non-user (RR, 0.57; 95% CI, 0.36–0.90) [145]. However, this finding was not confirmed in a later study [146]. A moderate increased risk was reported for women with extended period of regular aspirin use in the Nurses' Health Study including 161 cases [147]. In the Women's Health Initiative study, nearly 40,000 women were randomized to receive either 100 mg aspirin every other day or placebo. No statistically significant difference was noted between tested and placebo group after average 10.1 years of follow-up [148,149]. Larsson et al. reported a meta-analysis of 11 studies conducted from 1966 to October 2006 (3 case-control studies, 7 cohort studies, and 1 randomized trial), involving 6,386 pancreatic cancer cases. Neither use of aspirin, nonaspirin NSAIDs, nor overall NSAIDs were associated with pancreatic cancer risk. In 2007, Capurso et al. [150] conducted a meta-analysis including 8 studies (4 cohort studies, 3 case-control studies, and 1 randomized controlled trial) of 6,301 patients enrolled 1971–2004 and no association was found between use of aspirin or NSAIDs and risk of pancreatic cancer. Whether the negative findings were related to the large baseline exposure in controls in North America needs to be clarified in future study.

5.5   Statins and Metformin

Statins, competitive inhibitors of 3-hydroxy-3-methylglutaryl-coenzyme A (HMG-CoA) reductase, are a class of pharmacologic agents that reduce plasma cholesterol. Statins have been shown to have antitumor activity in various studies on pancreatic cancer cell lines. However, a meta-analysis till December 2007 including 12 studies (5 case–control studies, 4 cohort studies, and 3 randomized placebo-controlled trials) did not support a reduced risk of pancreatic cancer in association with low-dose intake of statins at the population level [151].

6   Conclusion

Pancreatic cancer remains a major cause of cancer-related death. Effective prevention measure depends on well-defined risk factors by epidemiological research. Unlike previous studies that universally impeded by small sample size, survivor bias, and use of proxy respondents for patients, more pooled studies and large prospective studies have emerged to provide epidemiologic evidence on risk factors of pancreatic cancer. Cigarette smoking is a well established risk factor. There is accumulating evidence supporting a role of obesity and diabetes as risk factors for this malignancy. More than 50% of the pancreatic cancer is probably preventable by adapting a healthy lifestyle [152]. The associations of dietary factors, alcohol, pancreatitis, infectious agent, occupational and hormonal factors and risk of pancreatic cancer are inconclusive. The study findings on systematic reviews on exposure and risk of pancreatic cancer should be considered suggestive because there are great between-study heterogeneity due to different assessment tools and study populations. Publication bias is often a concern. Well-designed large prospective studies and consortium studies are required to further define the environmental and host factors contributing to the development of pancreatic cancer. Further research on the genetic susceptibility factors and their interactions with the known risk factors for pancreatic cancer may help better understand the etiology of this disease and offer new tools for identifying high-risk individuals for preventive intervention.

Key Research Points

- The percentage of pancreatic cancer cases attributable to the inherited pancreatic cancer syndromes is small. However, investigations on the molecular mechanisms underlying these inherited syndromes shed light on the pathophysiology of pancreatic tumorigenesis. These individuals may be benefited by close surveillance and screening with imaging modalities.
- Cigarette smoking and obesity may each be responsible for causing as many as 25% of the cases of pancreatic cancer. Therefore, it is possible that as many as 50% of pancreatic cancer

cases are preventable. Avoid smoking and maintaining a healthy body weight offer the best available strategy for reducing the incidence of this disease.

- Diabetes could be the manifestation of pancreatic cancer, but long-standing type II diabetes mellitus has been implicated as a risk factor.
- Other suspected risk factors for pancreatic cancer include heavy alcohol consumption and pancreatitis.
- Consume of a well balanced diet with adequate amounts of fruits and vegetables, limited amounts of alcohol, and limited amounts of red meat, especially high fat or processed meat may also reduce the risk of pancreatic cancer.

Future Scientific Directions

- Effective prevention measure depends on well-defined risk factors by epidemiological research.
- The cause of pancreatic cancer involves multiple factors and complex etiology. Well-designed large prospective studies and consortium studies are required to generate sufficient amount of information on the role of environmental and host factors in pancreatic cancer development.
- Further research on the genetic susceptibility factors and their interactions with the known risk factors for pancreatic cancer may help better understand the etiology of this disease and offer new tools for identifying high-risk individuals for monitoring and screening.
- New molecular techniques, such as genome-wide association scan, microarray analysis of gene expression and proteomic approaches may ultimately help in discovering biomarkers for early diagnosis, which will have a major impact on reducing the mortality of pancreatic cancer.

References

1. Parkin DM, Bray F, Ferlay J, Pisani P: Global cancer statistics, 2002. CA Cancer J Clin 2005;55:74–108.
2. World Cancer Research Fund/American Institute for Cancer Research. Food, Nutrition, Physical Activity, and the Prevention of Cancer: a Global Perspective. Washington DC: AICR, 2007, pp. 271–274.
3. Parkin DM, Muir CS: Cancer incidence in five continents. Comparability and quality of data. IARC Sci Publ 1992;120:45–173.
4. Ries L, Melbert D, Krapcho M, et al.: SEER Cancer Statistics Review, 1975–2005. Bethesda: National Cancer Institute, 2008.
5. Anderson K, Potter JD, Mack TM: Pancreatic cancer. In Cancer Epidemiology and Prevention. Schottenfeld, D Fraumeni, JF Jr., (eds.). New York: Oxford University Press, 2006, pp. 721–762.
6. Parkin DM: International variation. Oncogene 2004;23:6329–6340.
7. Silverman DT, Hoover RN, Brown LM, Swanson GM, Schiffman M, Greenberg RS, Hayes RB, Lillemoe KD, Schoenberg JB, Schwartz AG, Liff J, Pottern LM, Fraumeni JF, Jr: Why do Black Americans have a higher risk of pancreatic cancer than White Americans? Epidemiology 2003;14:45–54.
8. Greer JB, Whitcomb DC, Brand RE: Genetic predisposition to pancreatic cancer: a brief review. Am J Gastroenterol 2007;102:2564–2569.
9. Lynch HT, Lanspa SJ, Fitzgibbons RJ, Jr., Smyrk T, Fitzsimmons ML, McClellan J: Familial pancreatic cancer (Part 1): Genetic pathology review. Nebr Med J 1989;74:109–112.

10. Murphy KM, Brune KA, Griffin C, Sollenberger JE, Petersen GM, Bansal R, Hruban RH: Kern SE.Evaluation of candidate genes MAP2K4, MADH4, ACVR1B, and BRCA2 in familial pancreatic cancer: deleterious BRCA2 mutations in 17%. Cancer Res 2002;62:3789–3793.

11. Goggins M, Schutte M, Lu J, Moskaluk CA, Weinstein CL, Petersen GM, Yeo CJ, Jackson CE, Lynch HT, Hruban RH, Kern SE: Germline BRCA2 gene mutations in patients with apparently sporadic pancreatic carcinomas. Cancer Res 1996;56:5360–5364.

12. Klein AP, Hruban RH, Brune KA, Petersen GM, Goggins M: Familial pancreatic cancer. Cancer J 2001;7:266–273.

13. Goldstein AM, Fraser MC, Struewing JP, Hussussian CJ, Ranade K, Zametkin DP, Fontaine LS, Organic SM, Dracopoli NC, Clark WH, Jr., et al.: Increased risk of pancreatic cancer in melanoma-prone kindreds with p16INK4 mutations. N Engl J Med 1995;333:970–974.

14. Lynch HT, Brand RE, Hogg D, Deters CA, Fusaro RM, Lynch JF, Liu L, Knezetic J, Lassam NJ, Goggins M, Kern S: Phenotypic variation in eight extended CDKN2A germline mutation familial atypical multiple mole melanoma-pancreatic carcinoma-prone families: the familial atypical mole melanoma-pancreatic carcinoma syndrome. Cancer 2002;94:84–96.

15. Hemminki A, Markie D, Tomlinson I, Avizienyte E, Roth S, Loukola A, Bignell G, Warren W, Aminoff M, Hoglund P, Jarvinen H, Kristo P, Pelin K, Ridanpaa M, Salovaara R, Toro T, Bodmer W, Olschwang S, Olsen AS, Stratton MR, de la Chapelle A, Aaltonen LA: A serine/threonine kinase gene defective in Peutz-Jeghers syndrome. Nature 1998; 391(6663):184–187.

16. Giardiello FM, Brensinger JD, Tersmette AC, Goodman SN, Petersen GM, Booker SV, Cruz-Correa M, Offerhaus JA: Very high risk of cancer in familial Peutz-Jeghers syndrome. Gastroenterology 2000;119(6):1447–1453.

17. Su GH, Hruban RH, Bansal RK, Bova GS, Tang DJ, Shekher MC, Westerman AM, Entius MM, Goggins M, Yeo CJ, Kern SE: Germline and somatic mutations of the STK11/LKB1 Peutz-Jeghers gene in pancreatic and biliary cancers. Am J Pathol 1999;154 (6):1835–1840.

18. Lim W, Olschwang S, Keller JJ, Westerman AM, Menko FH, Boardman LA, Scott RJ, Trimbath J, Giardiello FM, Gruber SB, Gille JJ, Offerhaus GJ, de Rooij FW, Wilson JH, Spigelman AD, Phillips RK, Houlston RS: Relative frequency and morphology of cancers in STK11 mutation carriers. Gastroenterology 2004;126:1788–1794.

19. Varley JM: Germline TP53 mutations and Li-Fraumeni syndrome. Hum Mutat 2003;21(3): 313–320.

20. Cowgill SM, Muscarella P: The genetics of pancreatic cancer. Am J Surg 2003;186(3):279–286.

21. Giardiello FM, Offerhaus GJ, Lee DH, Krush AJ, Tersmette AC, Booker SV, Kelley NC, Hamilton SR: Increased risk of thyroid and pancreatic carcinoma in familial adenomatous polyposis. Gut 1993;34 (10):1394–1396.

22. Whitcomb DC, Gorry MC, Preston RA, Furey W, Sossenheimer MJ, Ulrich CD, Martin SP, Gates LK, Jr., Amann ST, Toskes PP, Liddle R, McGrath K, Uomo G, Post JC: Ehrlich GD, Hereditary pancreatitis is caused by a mutation in the cationic trypsinogen gene. Nat Genet 1996;14(2):141–145.

23. Lowenfels AB, Maisonneuve P, DiMagno EP, Elitsur Y, Gates LK, Jr., Perrault J, Whitcomb DC: Hereditary pancreatitis and the risk of pancreatic cancer. International Hereditary Pancreatitis Study Group. J Natl Cancer Inst 1997;89(6):442–446.

24. Keim V: Role of genetic disorders in acute recurrent pancreatitis. World J Gastroenterol 2008;14(7): 1011–1015.

25. Lowenfels AB, Maisonneuve P, Whitcomb DC: Risk factors for cancer in hereditary pancreatitis. International Hereditary Pancreatitis Study Group. Med Clin North Am 2000;84(3):565–573.

26. Tersmette AC, Petersen GM, Offerhaus GJ, Falatko FC, Brune KA, Goggins M, Rozenblum E, Wilentz RE, Yeo CJ, Cameron JL, Kern SE, Hruban RH: Increased risk of incident pancreatic cancer among first-degree relatives of patients with familial pancreatic cancer. Clin Cancer Res 2001;7: 738–744.

27. Permuth-Wey J: Egan KM. Family history is a significant risk factor for pancreatic cancer: results from a systematic review and meta-analysis. Fam Can 2009;8:109–117.

28. Eberle MA, Pfutzer R, Pogue-Geile KL, Bronner MP, Crispin D, Kimmey MB, Duerr RH, Kruglyak L, Whitcomb DC, Brentnall TA: A new susceptibility locus for autosomal dominant pancreatic cancer maps to chromosome 4q32–34. Am J Hum Genet 2002;70:1044–1048.

29. Pogue-Geile KL, Chen R, Bronner MP, Crnogorac-Jurcevic T, Moyes KW, Dowen S, Otey CA, Crispin DA, George RD, Whitcomb DC, Brentnall TA: Palladin mutation causes familial pancreatic cancer and suggests a new cancer mechanism. PLoS Med 3:2006;e516.

30. Slater E, Amrillaeva V, Fendrich V, Bartsch D, Earl J, Vitone LJ, Neoptolemos JP, Greenhalf W: Palladin mutation causes familial pancreatic cancer: absence in European families. PLoS Med 4:2007;e164.

31. Klein AP, de Andrade M, Hruban RH, Bondy M, Schwartz AG, Gallinger S, Lynch HT, Syngal S, Rabe KG, Goggins MG, Petersen GM: Linkage analysis of

chromosome 4 in families with familial pancreatic cancer. Cancer Biol Ther 2007;6:320–323.

32. Iodice S, Gandini S, Maisonneuve P, Lowenfels AB: Tobacco and the risk of pancreatic cancer: a review and meta-analysis. Langenbecks Arch Surg 2008; 393:535–545.

33. Thompson PA, Seyedi F, Lang NP, McLeod SL, Woogen GN, Anderson KE, Tang YM, Coles B, Kadlubar FF: Comparison of DNA adduct levels associated with exogenous and endogenous exposures in human pancreas in relation to metabolic genotype. Mutat Res 1999;424:263–274.

34. Wang M-Y, Abbruzzese JL, Friess H, Hittelman WN, Evans DB, Abbruzzese MC, Chiao PL, Li D: DNA adducts in human pancreatic tissues and their potential role in carcinogenesis. Cancer Res 1998;58:38–41.

35. Prokopczyk B, Hoffmann D, Bologna M, Cunningham AJ, Trushin N, Akerkar S, Boyiri T, Amin S, Desai D, Colosimo S, Pittman B, Ledger G, Ramadani M, Henne-Bruns D, Beger HG, El-Bayoumy K: Identification of tobacco-derived compounds in human pancreatic juice. Chem Res Toxicol 2002;15:677–685.

36. Duell EJ, Wiencke JK, Cheng T-J, Varkonyi A, Zuo ZF, Ashok TD, Mark EJ, Wain JC, Christiani DC, Kelsey KT: Polymorphisms in the DNA repair genes XRCC1 and ERCC2 and biomarkers of DNA damage in human blood mononuclear cells. Carcinogenesis 2000;21:965–971 [published erratum appears in Carcinogenesis (Lond.) 2000;21:1457].

37. Duell EJ, Holly EA, Bracci PM, Liu M, Wiencke JK, Kelsey KT: A population-based, case-control study of polymorphisms in carcinogen-metabolizing genes, smoking, and pancreatic adenocarcinoma risk. J Natl Cancer Inst 2002;4:297–306.

38. Suzuki H, Jiao L, Li Y, Doll MA, Hein DW, Hassan MM, Day RS, Bondy ML, Abbruzzese JL, Li D: Interaction of the Cytochrome P4501A2, SULT1A1 and NAT gene polymorphisms with smoking and dietary mutagen intake in modification of the risk of pancreatic cancer. Carcinogenesis 2008;29(6): 1184–1191.

39. McWilliams RC, Bamlet WR, Cunningham JM, Goode EL, de Andrade M, Boardman LA, Petersen GM: Polymorphisms in DNA Repair Genes, Smoking, and Pancreatic Adenocarcinoma Risk Cancer Res 2008;68(12):4928–4935.

40. Li D, Suzuki H, Liu B, Morris J, Liu J, Okazaki T, Li Y, Chang P, Abbruzzese JL. DNA repair gene polymorphisms and risk of pancreatic cancer. Clin Can Res 2009;15(2):740–746.

41. Hruban RH, van Mansfeld AD, Offerhaus GJ, van Weering DH, Allison DC, Goodman SN, Kensler TW, Bose KK, Cameron JL, Bos JL: K-ras oncogene activation in adenocarcinoma of the human pancreas. A study of 82 carcinomas using a combination of mutant-enriched polymerase chain reaction analysis and allele-specific oligonucleotide hybridization. Am J Pathol 1993;143:545–554.

42. Jiao L, Zhu JJ, Hassan M, Abbruzzese JL, Li D: K-ras mutation and p16 and preproenkephalin promoter hypermethylation in plasma DNA of pancreatic cancer patients in relation to cigarette smoking. Pancreas 2007;34:55–62.

43. Baker F, Ainsworth SR, Dye JT, Crammer C, Thun MJ, Hoffmann D, Repace JL, Henningfield JE, Slade J, Pinney J, Shanks T, Burns DM, Connolly GN, Shopland DR: Health risks associated with cigar smoking. JAMA 2000;284:735–740.

44. Henley SJ, Thun MJ, Chao A, Calle EE: Association between exclusive pipe smoking and mortality from cancer and other diseases. J Natl Cancer Inst 2004;96:853–861.

45. Boffetta P, Aagnes B, Weiderpass E, Andersen A: Smokeless tobacco use and risk of cancer of the pancreas and other organs. Int J Cancer 2005;114:992–995.

46. Shapiro JA, Jacobs EJ, Thun MJ: Cigar smoking in men and risk of death from tobacco-related cancers. J Natl Cancer Inst 2000;92:333–337.

47. Alguacil J, Silverman DT: Smokeless and other non-cigarette tobacco use and pancreatic cancer: a case-control study based on direct interviews. Cancer Epidemiol Biomarkers Prev 2004;13:55–58.

48. Hassan MM, Abbruzzese JL, Bondy ML, Wolff RA, Vauthey J-N, Pisters PW, Evans DB, Khan R, Chou T-H, Lenzi R, Jiao L, Li D: Passive smoking and use of noncigarette tobacco products and risk for pancreatic cancer: case-control study. Cancer 2007;109:2547–2556.

49. Villeneuve PJ, Johnson KC, Mao Y, Hanley AJ: Environmental tobacco smoke and the risk of pancreatic cancer: findings from a Canadian population-based case-control study. Can J Public Health 2004;95: 32–37.

50. Gallicchio L, Kouzis A, Genkinger JM, Burke AE, Hoffman SC, Diener-West M, Helzlsouer KJ, Comstock GW, Alberg AJ: Active cigarette smoking, household passive smoke exposure, and the risk of developing pancreatic cancer. Prev Med 2006;42 (3):200–205.

51. Berrington de Gonzalez A, Sweetland S, Spencer E: A meta-analysis of obesity and the risk of pancreatic cancer. Br J Cancer 2003;89:519–523.

52. Larsson SC, Orsini N, Wolk A: Body mass index and pancreatic cancer risk: A meta-analysis of prospective studies. Int J Cancer 2007;120:1993–1998.

53. Renehan AG, Tyson M, Egger M, Heller RF, Zwahlen M: Body-mass index and incidence of cancer: a systematic review and meta-analysis of prospective observational studies. Lancet 2008;371:569–578.

54. Calle EE, Kaaks R: Overweight, obesity and cancer: epidemiological evidence and proposed mechanisms. Nat Rev Cancer. 2004;8:579–591.

55. Larsson SC, Permert J, Hakansson N, Naslund I, Bergkvist L, Wolk A: Overall obesity, abdominal adiposity, diabetes and cigarette smoking in relation to the risk of pancreatic cancer in two Swedish population-based cohorts. Br J Cancer 2005;93:1310–1315.

56. Patel AV, Rodriguez C, Bernstein L, Chao A, Thun MJ, Calle EE: Obesity, recreational physical activity, and risk of pancreatic cancer in a large U.S. Cohort. Cancer Epidemiol Biomarkers Prev 2005;14:459–466.

57. Berrington de Gonzalez A, Spencer EA, Bueno-de-Mesquita HB, Roddam A, Stolzenberg-Solomon R, Halkjaer J, Tjonneland A, Overvad K, Clavel-Chapelon F, Boutron-Ruault MC, Boeing H, Pischon T, Linseisen J, Rohrmann S, Trichopoulou A, Benetou V, Papadimitriou A, Pala V, Palli D, Panico S, Tumino R, Vineis P, Boshuizen HC, Ocke MC, Peeters PH, Lund E, Gonzalez CA, Larranaga N, Martinez-Garcia C, Mendez M, Navarro C, Quiros JR, Tormo MJ, Hallmans G, Ye W, Bingham SA, Khaw KT, Allen N, Key TJ, Jenab M, Norat T, Ferrari P, Riboli E: Anthropometry, physical activity, and the risk of pancreatic cancer in the European prospective investigation into cancer and nutrition. Cancer Epidemiol Biomarkers Prev 2006;15:879–885.

58. Stolzenberg-Solomon RZ, Adams K, Leitzmann M, Schairer C, Michaud DS, Hollenbeck A, Schatzkin A, Silverman DT: Adiposity, physical activity, and pancreatic cancer in the National Institutes of Health-AARP Diet and Health Cohort. Am J Epidemiol 2008;167:586–597.

59. Luo J, Margolis KL, Adami HO, LaCroix A, Ye W: Obesity and risk of pancreatic cancer among postmenopausal women: the Women's Health Initiative (United States). Br J Cancer 2008;99:527–531.

60. Ansary-Moghaddam A, Huxley R, Barzi F, Lawes C, Ohkubo T, Fang X, Jee SH, Woodward M: The effect of modifiable risk factors on pancreatic cancer mortality in populations of the Asia-Pacific region. Cancer Epidemiol Biomarkers Prev 2006;15:2435–2440.

61. IARC. IARC handbooks on cancer prevention: Weight control and physical activity. Lyon, France: IARC Press, 2002.

62. Michaud DS, Giovannucci E, Willet WC, Colditz GA, Stampfer MJ, Fuchs CS: Physical activity, obesity, height, and the risk of pancreatic cancer. JAMA 2001;286(8):921–929.

63. Fisher WE: Diabetes: risk factor for the development of pancreatic cancer or manifestation of the disease? World J Surg 2001;25:503–508.

64. Gullo L, Pezzilli R, Morselli-Labate AM: Diabetes and the risk of pancreatic cancer. N Engl J Med 1994;331:81–84.

65. Valerio A, Basso D, Brigato L, Ceolotto G, Baldo G, Tiengo A, Plebani M: Glucose metabolic alterations in isolated and perfused rat hepatocytes induced by pancreatic cancer conditioned medium: a low molecular weight factor possibly involved. Biochem Biophys Res Commun 1999;257:622–628.

66. Basso D, Valerio A, Seraglia R, Mazza S, Piva MG, Greco E, Fogar P, Gallo N, Pedrazzoli S, Tiengo A, Plebani M: Putative pancreatic cancer-associated diabetogenic factor: 2030 MW peptide. Pancreas 2002;24:8–14.

67. Chow WH, Gridley G, Nyren O, Linet MS, Ekbom A, Fraumeni JF, Jr., Adami HO: Risk of pancreatic cancer following diabetes mellitus: a nationwide cohort study in Sweden. J Natl Cancer Inst 1995;87:930–931.

68. Everhart J, Wright D: Diabetes mellitus as a risk factor for pancreatic cancer. A meta-analysis. JAMA 1995;273:1605–1609.

69. Huxley RA, Ansary-Moghaddam A, de Gonzalez B, Barzi F, Woodward M: Type-II diabetes and pancreatic cancer: a meta-analysis of 36 studies. Br J Cancer. 2005;92:2076–2083.

70. Chari ST, Leibson CL, Rabe KG, Ransom J, de Andrade M, Petersen GM: Probability of pancreatic cancer following diabetes: a population-based study. Gastroenterology 2005;129:504–511.

71. Chari ST, Leibson CL, Rabe KG, Timmons LJ, Ransom J, de Andrade M, Petersen GM: Pancreatic cancer-associated diabetes mellitus: prevalence and temporal association with diagnosis of cancer. Gastroenterology 2008;134(1):95–101.

72. Pannala R, Leirness JB, Bamlet WR, Basu A, Petersen GM, Chari ST: Prevalence and clinical profile of pancreatic cancer-associated diabetes mellitus. Gastroenterology 2008;134(4):981–987.

73. Stevens RJ, Roddam AW, Beral V: Pancreatic cancer in type 1 and young-onset diabetes: systematic review and meta-analysis. Br J Cancer 2007;96:507–509.

74. Gapstur SM, Gann PH, Lowe W, Liu K, Colangelo L, Dyer A: Abnormal glucose metabolism and pancreatic cancer mortality. JAMA 2000;283:2552–2558.

75. Batty GD, Shipley MJ, Marmot M, Smith GD: Diabetes status and post-load plasma glucose concentration in relation to site-specific cancer mortality: findings from the original Whitehall study. Cancer Cause Control 2004;15:873–881.

76. Stattin P, Bjor O, Ferrari P, Lukanova A, Lenner P, Lindahl B, Hallmans G, Kaaks R: Prospective study of hyperglycemia and cancer risk. Diabetes Care 2007;30:561–567.

77. Stolzenberg-Solomon RZ, Graubard BI, Chari S, Limburg P, Taylor PR, Virtamo J, Albanes D: Insulin, glucose, insulin resistance, and pancreatic cancer in male smokers. JAMA 2005;294(22):2872–2878.

78. Pisani P: Hyper-insulinaemia and cancer, meta-analyses of epidemiological studies. Arch Physiol Biochem 2008;114(1):63–70.

79. Michaud DS, Wolpin B, Giovannucci E, Liu S, Cochrane B, Manson JE, Pollak MN, Ma J, Fuchs CS: Prediagnostic plasma C-peptide and pancreatic cancer risk in men and women. Cancer Epidemiol Biomarkers Prev 2007;16(10):2101–2109.

80. Wolpin BM, Michaud DS, Giovannucci EL, Schernhammer ES, Stampfer MJ, Manson JE, Chochrane BB, Rohan TE, Ma J, Pollak MN, Fuchs CS: Circulating insulin-like growth factor axis and the risk of pancreatic cancer in four prospective cohorts. Br J Cancer 2007;97(1):98–104.

81. Stolzenberg-Solomon RZ, Limburg P, Pollak M, Taylor PR, Virtamo J, Albanes D: Insulin-like growth factor (IGF)-1, IGF-binding protein-3, and pancreatic cancer in male smokers. Cancer Epidemiol Biomarkers Prev 2004;13:438–444.

82. Lin Y, Tamakoshi A, Kikuchi S, Yagyu K, Obata Y, Ishibashi T, Kawamura T, Inaba Y, Kurosawa M, Motohashi Y, Ohno Y: Serum insulin-like growth factor-I, insulin-like growth factor binding protein-3, and the risk of pancreatic cancer death. Int J Cancer 2004;110:584–588.

83. Wolpin BM, Michaud DS, Giovannucci EL, Schernhammer ES, Stampfer MJ, Manson JE, Cochrane BB, Rohan TE, Ma J, Pollak MN, Fuchs CS: Circulating insulin-like growth factor axis and the risk of pancreatic cancer in four prospective cohorts. Br J Cancer 2007;97:98–104.

84. Silverman DT, Brown LM, Hoover RN, Schiffman M, Lillemoe KD, Schoenberg JB, Swanson GM, Hayes RB, Greenberg RS, Benichou J, et al.: Alcohol and pancreatic cancer in blacks and whites in the United States. Cancer Res 1995;55:4899–4905.

85. Hassan MM, Wolff RA, Bondy ML, Abbruzzese JL, Vauthey J-N, Pisters PW, Evans DB, Khan R, Chou T-H, Lenzi R, Jiao L, Li D: Risk factors for pancreatic cancer: case-control study. Am J Gastroenterol 2007;102:2696–2707.

86. Lu XH, Wang L, Li H, Qian JM, Deng RX, Zhou L: Establishment of risk model for pancreatic cancer in Chinese Han population. World J Gastroenterol 2006;12:2229–2234.

87. Olsen GW, Mandel JS, Gibson RW, Wattenberg LW, Schuman LM: A case-control study of pancreatic cancer and cigarettes, alcohol, coffee and diet. Am J Public Health 1989;79:1016–1019.

88. Genkinger JM, Spiegelman D, Anderson KE, Bergkvist L, Bernstein L, Brandt PA, English DR, Freudenheim JL, Fuchs CS, Giles GG, Giovannucci E, Hankinson SE, Horn-Ross PL, Leitzmann M, Mannisto S, Marshall JR, McCullough ML, Miller AB, Douglas J, Reding KR, Rohan TE, Schatzkin A, Stevens, VL, Stolzenberg-Solomon RZ, Verhage BAJ, Wolk A, Ziegler RG, Smith-Warner SA: Alcohol intake and pancreatic cancer risk: a pooled analysis of fourteen cohort studies. Cancer Epidemiol Biomarkers Prev 2009;18:765–776.

89. Rohrmann S, Linseisen J, Vrieling A, Boffetta P, Stolzenberg-Solomon RZ, Lowenfels AB, Jensen MK, Overvad K, Olsen A, Tjonneland A, Boutron-Ruault MC, Clavel-Chapelon F, Fagherazzi G, Misirli G, Lagiou P, Trichopoulou A, Kaaks R, Bergmann MM, Boeing H, Bingham S, Khaw KT, Allen N, Roddam A, Palli D, Pala V, Panico S, Tumino R, Vineis P, Peeters PH, Hjartaker A, Lund E: Cornejo ML, Agudo A, Arriola L, Sanchez MJ, Tormo MJ, Barricarte Gurrea A, Lindkvist B, Manjer J, Johansson I, Ye W, Slimani N, Duell EJ, Jenab M, Michaud DS, Mouw T, Riboli E, Bueno-de-Mesquita HB: Ethanol intake and the risk of pancreatic cancer in the European prospective investigation into cancer and nutrition (EPIC). Cancer Cause Control 2009;20:785–794.

90. Jiao L, Silverman DT, Schairer C, Thiebaut A, Hollenbeck A, Leitzmann M, Schatzkin A, Stolzenberg-Solomon R: Alcohol use and risk of pancreatic cancer - The NIH-AARP Diet and Health Study. Am J Epidemiol 2009;169:1043–1051.

91. Steer ML, Waxman I, Freedman S: Chronic pancreatitis. N Engl J Med 1995;332:1482–1490.

92. Lowenfels AB, Maisonneuve P, Gavallini G, Ammann RW, Lankisch PG, Andersen JR, Dimagno EP, Andren-Sandberg A, Domellof L for The International Pancreatitis Study Group: Pancreatitis and the risk of pancreatic cancer. N Engl J Med 1993;328:1433–1437.

93. Talamini G, Falconi M, Bassi C, Sartori N, Salvia R, Caldiron E, Frulloni L, Di Francesco V, Vaona B, Bovo P, Vantini I, Pederzoli P, Cavallini G: Incidence of cancer in the course of chronic pancreatitis. Am J Gastroenterol 1999;94:1253–1260.

94. Karlson BM, Ekbom A, Josefsson S, McLaughlin JK, Fraumeni JF, Jr., Nyren O: The risk of pancreatic cancer following pancreatitis: an association due to confounding? Gastroenterology 1997;113:587–592.

95. Nothlings U, Wilkens LR, Murphy SP, Hankin JH, Henderson BE, Kolonel LN: Meat and fat intake as risk factors for pancreatic cancer: the multiethnic cohort study. J Natl Cancer Inst 2005;97(19):1458–1465.

96. Anderson KE, Sinha R, Kulldorff M, Gross M, Lang NP, Barber C, Harnack L, DiMagno E, Bliss R, Kadlubar FF: Meat intake and cooking techniques: associations with pancreatic cancer. Mutat Res 2002;506–7:225–231.

97. Li D, Day S, Bondy ML, Sinha R, Nguyen NT, Evans DB, Abbruzzese JL, Hassan M: Dietary mutagen exposure and risk of pancreatic cancer. Cancer Epidemiol Biomarkers Prev 2007;16: 655–661.

98. Stolzenberg-Solomon RZ, Cross AJ, Silverman DT, Schairer C, Thompson FE, Kipnis V, Subar AF, Hellenbeck A, Schatzkin A, Sinha R: Meat and meat-mutagen intake and pancreatic cancer risk in the NIH-AARP cohort. Cancer Epidemiol Biomarkers Prev 2007;16(12):2664–2675.

99. Gold EB, Goldin SB: Epidemiology of and risk factors for pancreatic cancer. Surg Oncol Clin N AM 1998;7:67–91.

100. Larsson SC, Hakansson N, Naslund I, Bergkvist L, Wolk A: Fruit and vegetable consumption in relation to pancreatic cancer risk: a prospective study. Cancer Epidemiol Biomarkers Prev 2006;15:301–305.

101. Vrieling A, Verhage BA, van Duijnhoven FJ, Jenab M, Overvad K, Tjonneland A, Olsen A, Clavel-Chapelon F, Boutron-Ruault MC, Kaaks R, Rohrmann S, Boeing H, Nothlings U, Trichopoulou A, John T, Dimosthenes Z, Palli D, Sieri S, Mattiello A, Tumino R, Vineis P, van Gils CH, Peeters PH, Engeset D, Lund E, Rodriguez Suarez L, Jakszyn P, Larranaga N, Sanchez MJ, Chirlaque MD, Ardanaz E: Manjer J, Lindkvist B, Hallmans G, Ye W, Bingham S, Khaw KT, Roddam A, Key T, Boffetta P, Duell EJ, Michaud DS, Riboli E, Bueno-de-Mesquita HB: Fruit and vegetable consumption and pancreatic cancer risk in the European Prospective Investigation into Cancer and Nutrition. Int J Cancer 2009;124:1926–1934.

102. Nothlings U, Wilkens LR, Murphy SP, Hankin JH, Henderson BE, Kolonel LN: Vegetable intake and pancreatic cancer risk: the multiethnic cohort study. Am J Epidemiol 2007;165:138–147.

103. Bae JM, Lee EJ, Guyatt G: Citrus fruit intake and pancreatic cancer risk: a quantitative systematic review. Pancreas 2009;38:168–174.

104. Chan JM, Wang F, Holly EA: Vegetable and fruit intake and pancreatic cancer in a population-based case-control study in the San Francisco bay area. Cancer Epidemiol Biomarkers Prev 2005;14: 2093–2097.

105. Nothlings U, Murphy SP, Wilkens LR, Henderson BE, Kolonel LN: Flavonols and pancreatic cancer risk: the multiethnic cohort study. Am J Epidemiol 2007;166:924–931.

106. Bobe G, Weinstein SJ, Albanes D, Hirvonen T, Ashby J, Taylor PR, Virtamo J, Stolzenberg-Solomon RZ: Flavonoid intake and risk of pancreatic cancer in male smokers (Finland). Cancer Epidemiol Biomarkers Prev 2008;17:553–562.

107. Larsson SC, Giovannucci E, Wolk A: Folate intake, MTHFR polymorphisms, and risk of esophageal, gastric, and pancreatic cancer: a meta-analysis. Gastroenterology 2006;131:1271–1283.

108. Larsson SC, Hakansson N, Giovannucci E, Wolk A: Folate intake and pancreatic cancer incidence: a prospective study of Swedish women and men. J Natl Cancer Inst 2006;98:407–413.

109. Stolzenberg-Solomon RZ, Albanes D, Nieto FJ, Hartman TJ, Tangrea JA, Rautalahti M, Sehlub J, Virtamo J, Taylor PR: Pancreatic cancer risk and nutrition-related methyl-group availability indicators in male smokers. J Natl Cancer Inst 1999;91:535–541.

110. Schernhammer E, Wolpin B, Rifai N, Cochrane B, Manson JA, Ma J, Giovannucci E, Thomson C, Stampfer MJ, Fuchs C: Plasma folate, vitamin B6, vitamin B12, and homocysteine and pancreatic cancer risk in four large cohorts. Cancer Res 2007;67:5553–5560.

111. Skinner HG, Michaud DS, Giovannucci EL, Rimm EB, Stampfer MJ, Willett WC, Colditz GA, Fuchs CS: A prospective study of folate intake and the risk of pancreatic cancer in men and women. Am J Epidemiol 2004;160(3):248–258.

112. Silverman DT, Swanson CA, Gridley G, Wacholder S, Greenberg RS, Brown LM, Hayes RB, Swanson GM, Schoenberg JB, Pottern LM, Schwartz AG, Fraumeni JF, Jr., Hoover RN: Dietary and nutritional factors and pancreatic cancer: a case-control study based on direct interviews. J Natl Cancer Inst 1998;90:1710–1719.

113. Nkondjock A, Ghadirian P, Johnson KC, Krewski D: Dietary intake of lycopene is associated with reduced pancreatic cancer risk. J Nutr 2005;135: 592–597.

114. Kavanaugh CJ, Trumbo PR, Ellwood KC: The US Food and Drug Administration's evidence-based review for qualified health claims: tomatoes, lycopene, and cancer. J Natl Cancer Inst 2007;99: 1074–1085.

115. Bjelakovic G, Nikolova D, Simonetti RG, Gluud C: Antioxidant supplements for prevention of gastrointestinal cancers: a systematic review and meta-analysis. Lancet 2004;364:1219–1228.

116. Howe GR, Ghadirian P, Bueno de Mesquita HB, Zatonski WA, Baghurst PA, Miller AB, Simard A, Baillargeon J, de Waard F, Przewozniak K, et al.: A collaborative case-control study of nutrient intake and pancreatic cancer within the search programme. Int J Cancer 1992;51(3):365–372.

117. Howe GR Burch JD: Nutrition and pancreatic cancer. Cancer Cause Control 1996;7(1):69–82.

118. Michaud DS, Liu S, Giovannucci E, Willett WC, Colditz GA, Fuchs CS: Dietary sugar, glycemic load, and pancreatic cancer risk in a prospective study. J Natl Cancer Inst 2002;94(17): 1293–1300.

119. Johnson KJ, Anderson KE, Harnack L, Hong CP, Folsom AR: No association between dietary glycemic index or load and pancreatic cancer incidence in postmenopausal women. Cancer Epidemiol Biomarkers Prev 2005;14:1574–1575.

120. Silvera SA, Rohan TE, Jain M, Terry PD, Howe GR, Miller AB: Glycemic index, glycemic load, and pancreatic cancer risk (Canada). Cancer Cause Control 2005;16:431–436.

121. Patel AV, McCullough ML, Pavluck AL, Jacobs EJ, Thun MJ, Calle EE: Glycemic load, glycemic index, and carbohydrate intake in relation to pancreatic cancer risk in a large US cohort. Cancer Cause Control 2007;18:287–294.

122. Nothlings U, Murphy SP, Wilkens LR, Henderson BE, Kolonel LN: Dietary glycemic load, added sugars, and carbohydrates as risk factors for pancreatic cancer: the Multiethnic Cohort Study. Am J Clin Nutr 2007;86:1495–1501.

123. Heinen MM, Verhage BA, Lumey L, Brants HA, Goldbohm RA, van den Brandt PA: Glycemic load, glycemic index, and pancreatic cancer risk in the Netherlands Cohort Study. Am J Clin Nutr 2008;87:970–977.

124. Jiao L, Flood A, Subar AF, Hollenbeck A, Schatzkin A: Stolzenberg-Solomon R. Glycemic index, available carbohydrate, glycemic load and risk of pancreatic cancer in the NIH-AARP Diet and Health Study. Cancer Epidemiol Biomarkers Prev 2009; 18(4):1144–1151.

125. Mulholland HG, Murray LJ, Cardwell CR, Cantwell MM: Glycemic index, glycemic load, and risk of digestive tract neoplasms: a systematic review and meta-analysis. Am J Clin Nutr 2009;89:568–576.

126. Bao Y, Stolzenberg-Solomon R, Jiao L, Silverman DT, Subar AF, Park Y, Leitzmann MF, Hollenbeck A, Schatzkin A, Michaud DS: Added sugar and sugar-sweetened foods and beverages and the risk of pancreatic cancer in the National Institutes of Health-AARP Diet and Health Study. Am J Clin Nutr 2008;88:431–440.

127. Raderer M, Wrba F, Kornek G, et al.: Association between Helicobacter pylori infection and pancreatic cancer. Oncology 1998;55:16–19.

128. Stolzenberg-Solomon RZ, Blaser MJ, Limburg PJ, et al.: Helicobacter pylori seropositivity as a risk factor for pancreatic cancer. J Nat Cancer Inst 2001;93:927–941.

129. Hassan MM, Li D, El-Deeb A, Wolff RA, Bondy ML, Davila M, Abbruzzese JL: Hepatitis B Virus and pancreatic cancer. J Clin Oncol 2008;26 (28):4557–4562.

130. Tersmette AC, Offerhaus GJ, Giardiello FM, et al.: Occurrence of non-gastric cancer in the digestive tract after remote partial gastrectomy: analysis of an Amsterdam cohort. Int J Cancer 1990; 465:792–795.

131. Hedberg M, Ogren M, Janzon L, et al.: Pancreatic carcinoma following gastric resection. Int J Pancreatol 1997;21:219–224.

132. de Martel C, Llosa AE, Friedman GD, Vogelman JH, Orentreich N, Stolzenberg-Solomon RZ, Parsonnet J: Helicobacter pylori infection and development of pancreatic cancer. Cancer Epidemiol Biomarkers Prev 2008;17:1188–1194.

133. Lindkvist B, Johansen D, Borgstrom A, Manjer J: A prospective study of Helicobacter pylori in relation to the risk for pancreatic cancer. BMC Cancer 2008;8:321.

134. Hoefs JC, Renner IG, Askhcavai M, Redeker AG: Hepatitis B surface antigen in pancreatic and biliary secretions. Gastroenterology 1980;79(2):191–194.

135. Yoshimura M, Sakurai I, Shimoda T, Abe K, Okano T, Shikata T: Detection of HBsAg in the pancreas. Acta Pathol Jpn 1981;31(4):711–717.

136. Shimoda T, Shikata T, Karasawa T, Tsukagoshi S, Yoshimura M, Sakurai I: Light microscopic localization of hepatitis B virus antigens in the human pancreas. Possibility of multiplication of hepatitis B virus in the human pancreas. Gastroenterology 1981;81(6):998–1005.

137. Taranto D, Carrato A, Romano M, Maio G, Izzo CM, Del Vecchio BC: Mild pancreatic damage in acute viral hepatitis. Digestion 1989;42(2):93–97.

138. Katakura Y, Yotsuyanagi H, Hashizume K, Okuse C, Okuse N, Nishikawa K et al. Pancreatic involvement in chronic viral hepatitis. World J Gastroenterology 2005;11(23):3508–3513.

139. de Gonzalez AB, Jee SH, Engels EA: No association between hepatitis B and pancreatic cancer in a prospective study in Korea. J Clin Oncol 2009;1:648.

140. Ojajärvi A, Partanen T, Ahlbom A, Boffetta P, Hakulinen T, Jourenkova N, Kauppinen T, Kogevinas M, Vainio H, Weiderpass E, Wesseling C: Risk of pancreatic cancer in workers exposed to chlorinated hydrocarbon solvents and related compounds: a meta-analysis. Am J Epidemiol 2001;153(9):841–850.

141. Ojajärvi A, Partanen T, Ahlbom A, Hakulinen T, Kauppinen T, Weiderpass E, Wesseling C: Estimating the relative risk of pancreatic cancer associated with exposure agents in job title data in a hierarchical Bayesian meta-analysis. Scand J Work Environ Health 2007;33(5):325–335.

142. Gandini S, Lowenfels AB, Jaffee EM, Armstrong TD, Maisonneuve P: Allergies and the risk of pancreatic cancer: a meta-analysis with review of epidemiology and biological mechanisms. Cancer Epidemiol Biomarkers Prev 2005;14(8):1908–1916.

143. Silverman DT, Schiffman M, Everhart J, Goldstein A, Lillemoe KD, Swanson GM, Schwartz AG, Brown LM, Greenberg RS, Schoenberg JB, Pottern LM, Hoover RN, Fraumeni JF, Jr: Diabetes mellitus, other medical conditions and familial history of cancer as risk factors for pancreatic cancer. Brit J Cancer 1999;80(11):1830–1837.

144. Holly EA, Eberle CA, Bracci PM: Prior history of allergies and pancreatic cancer in the San Francisco Bay area. Am J Epidemiology 2003;158(5):432–441.

145. Anderson KE, Johnson TW, Lazovich D, Folsom AR: Association between nonsteroidal anti-inflammatory drug use and the incidence of pancreatic cancer. J Natl Cancer Inst 2002;94(15):1168–1171.

146. Menezes RJ, Huber KR, Mahoney MC, Moysich KB: Regular use of aspirin and pancreatic cancer risk. BMC Public Health 2002;2:18.

147. Schernhammer ES, Kang JH, Chan AT, Michaud DS, Skinner HG, Giovannucci E, Colditz GA, Fuchs CS: A prospective study of aspirin use and the risk of pancreatic cancer in women. J Natl Cancer Inst. 2004;96(1):22–28.

148. Cook NR, Lee IM, Gaziano JM, Gordon D, Ridker PM, Manson JE, Hennekens CH, Buring JE: Low-dose aspirin in the primary prevention of cancer: the Women's Health Study: a randomized controlled trial. JAMA 2005;294(1):47–55.

149. Larsson SC, Giovannucci E, Bergkvist L, Wolk A: Aspirin and nonsteroidal anti-inflammatory drug use and risk of pancreatic cancer: a meta-analysis. Cancer Epidemiol Biomarkers Prev 2006;15(12):2561–2564.

150. Capurso G, Schünemann HJ, Terrenato I, Moretti A, Koch M, Muti P, Capurso L, Delle Fave G: Meta-analysis: the use of non-steroidal anti-inflammatory drugs and pancreatic cancer risk for different exposure categories. Aliment Pharmacol Ther 2007;26(8):1089–1099.

151. Bonovas S, Filioussi K, Sitaras NM: Statins are not associated with a reduced risk of pancreatic cancer at the population level, when taken at low doses for managing hypercholesterolemia: evidence from a meta-analysis of 12 studies. Am J Gastroenterol 2008;103(10):2646–2651.

152. Jiao L, Mitrou PN, Reedy J, Graubard BI, Hollenbeck AR, Schatzkin A, Stolzenberg-Solomon R: A combined healthy lifestyle score and risk of pancreatic cancer in a large cohort study. Arch Intern Med 2009;169(8):764–770.

2 Development and Structure of the Pancreas

Roberto A. Rovasio

1	*Signals Toward the Pancreas Development*	*28*
2	*Microscopic Structure and Functional Activity of the Pancreas*	*31*
2.1	Endocrine Pancreas	32
2.2	Exocrine Pancreas	33
2.2.1	Acini	33
2.3	Ducts System	36
2.4	Blood Vessels and Nerves	36
2.5	Concluding Remarks	36

J. P. Neoptolemos, R. Urrutia, J. L. Abbruzzese, M. W. Büchler (eds.), *Pancreatic Cancer*,
DOI 10.1007/978-0-387-77498-5_2, © Springer Science+Business Media, LLC 2010

Abstract: The goal of this short chapter is to introduce the reader to fundamental concepts on the fine structure of the pancreas and its developmental pattern. This is of paramount importance for any individual that enters the field of pancreatology. In addition, this information is fundamental for understanding issues of histogenesis of pancreatic cancer, animal models, the histopathology of different forms of pancreatitis, pancreatic cysts and pancreatic cancer. The fine structure of the pancreas, as described here, is also essential as a foundation building block where to integrate, at the cellular level, the concepts from cell signaling, transcriptional regulation, secretion, proliferation, apoptosis, and senescence; all cancer-associated mechanisms. Thus, this is a basic, conceptual chapter that will serve as a compass for the reader of this book and in the field.

1 Signals Toward the Pancreas Development

The development of pancreatic gland initiate at week 5 of the human embryo life, starting as dorsal and ventral endodermic evaginations from the most caudal segment of the primitive foregut (❯ *Figs. 2-1* and ❯ *2-3a, b*). When the duodenum grows and rotate around its longitudinal axis in hourly hand sense, the ventral rudiment that will form the uniform process and the lower part of the pancreas head, displaces toward the back and fuses with the dorsal bud during the seventh week of development, forming the pancreas gland (❯ *Fig. 2-3c*). The development of pancreas is largely related to that of the liver. Both of these glands derived from the same endodermal segment of the anterior intestine (❯ *Fig. 2-1*). But, while the molecular signals emitted by the cardiac anlagen induced the liver, the cell communications with the notochord determine the pancreas development [1,2] (❯ *Fig. 2-2*). In fact, notochord repression of Sonic Hedgehog expression in a localized region of the caudal end of the foregut is crucial for the initial stages of pancreatic development [3–5] (❯ *Fig. 2-2*).

◘ Fig. 2-1

Primitive gut in a sagital section of a 4 weeks human embryo. Broken lines: limit between foregut, midgut and hindgut.

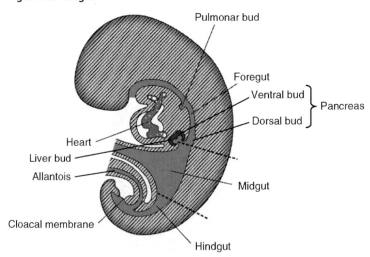

⬛ Fig. 2-2

Molecular signaling in the development of pancreas (see details in the text).

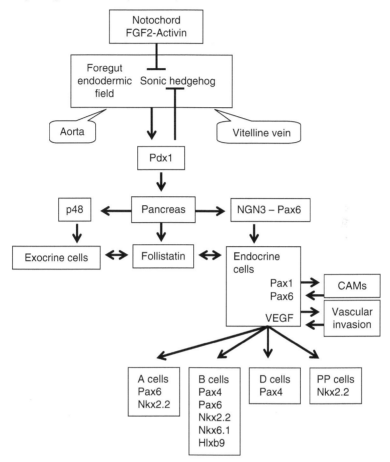

This repression of Sonic Hedgehog allows the endoderm to respond to signals arising from endothelial cells of the next aorta and vitelline vein [6]; consequently, in this segment of the intestine endodermic field, the Pdx1 transcription factor is expressed triggering the formation of the pancreatic bud [7] (⬤ *Fig. 2-2*). Both ventral and dorsal primordia are formed by primitive cords and ducts, from which ends emerges the acinar units, while the islets of Largenhans differentiate from cell groups that segregate from the primitive ducts localizing among the acinus. The evaginations of endodermal foregut epithelium surrounded by mesenchyme become tubular branched structures that about to eighth to tenth weeks of human development originate the endocrine A (glucagon), B (insulin) and D (somatostatin) cells, differentiating also the PP (pancreatic polypeptide) cells at the same time or a pair of weeks later. At the early stage of differentiation, the endocrine cells locate into the primitive endoderm of the emerging diverticulum, then progressively segregate and accumulate forming the pancreatic islets. The topological distribution of endocrine cells is not uniform, being most of the A cells originated from the dorsal bud and the PP cells from the ventral rudiment,

■ Fig. 2-3

Development of the pancreas in human embryos of 5(a), 6(b) and 7(c) weeks. Arrows indicate the sense of primitive intestine rotation around its longitudinal axis. Broken line: limit between foregut and midgut.

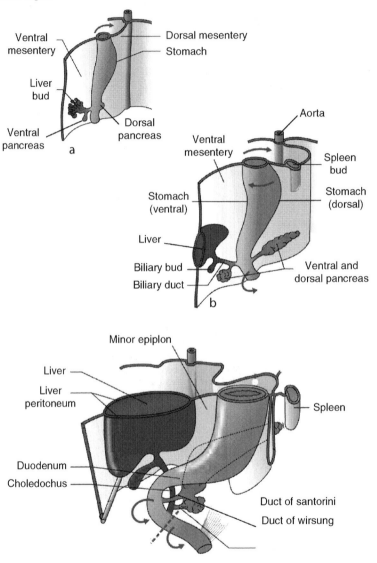

whereas the B cells differentiate from the duct epithelium during the prenatal and early postnatal life. This last characteristic support the notion of the potential capacity of duct cells lineage to differentiate beyond the birth frontier [7]. At the molecular level, while the pancreatic cells acquire different specification, Pdx1 maintains the repression of notochordal Sonic Hedgehog and in coordination with NGN3 [8] and Pax6 transcription factors modulates the induction and determination of the endocrine pancreas (islets of Langerhans) (◉ *Fig. 2-2*). Additional molecules responsible for the morphogenetic and functional induction of each the hormone producing cells are discussed in detail in another chapter (◉ *Fig. 2-2*). Also, Pdx1 functionally interacts with the transcription factor p48 to induce the differentiation of the exocrine pancreas and regulates the early production of amylase and alpha-fetoprotein. The relative proportion of endocrine and exocrine pancreas development is partially modulated by Follistatin expressed in the pancreatic mesenchyme, which inhibits Activin and some members of the BMPs family, promoting the exocrine differentiation. Moreover, Pax1 and Pax6 transcription factors modulate the expression of cell adhesion molecules (CAMs), which maintain the clustering of endocrine cells into islets (◉ *Fig. 2-2*). In turn, the developing islets segregate chemoattractants such as the Vascular Endothelial Growth Factor (VEGF), which induced the spurt and development of blood vessels in close contact with the endocrine cell populations [2].

During the tenth to 15th weeks of human embryo development, cell populations at the lateral and terminal end of the primitive ducts clump together and differentiate into acinar cells, of which zymogen granules, exocrine enzymes activity and/or acinar cell molecular markers are detectable by electron microscopy and immunocytochemical methods. Some cells at the center of the acinar clusters form the blind-ending acini while adjacent cells flattens and organize as centroacinar cells and the wall of intercalated ducts, the first segment of the secretory ducts lacking a peripheric mesenchymal tissue layer. The anastomoses among these thin slender ducts forms the intralobular ducts, which in turn meets with anothers to originate the interlobular ducts, draining then into larger or main ducts. The developing exocrine pancreas may be viewed as a complex network derived from fusion and anastomoses of acinar and duct structures. The main pancreatic duct (duct of Wirsung) derives from the fusion between the ventral bud duct and its homologue duct of the dorsal primordium (◉ *Fig. 2-3c*). The remainder of the dorsal duct, occasionally persist as an accessory pancreatic duct (duct of Santorini) draining either into the duodenum (◉ *Fig. 2-3c*), to the main duct or to the ampulla of Vater. Since only 40% of adults have accessory ducts as compared with 85% of infants, the fusion of the ventral/dorsal system of ducts seems to occur during the postnatal life [9,10]. The choledochus bile duct and the main pancreatic duct also fuses and obliquely cross the second portion of duodenum wall and the sphincter of Oddi to open in the duodenal papilla (◉ *Fig. 2-3c*). Some times, both ducts open separately one next the other; occasionally they fused and form a common expansion ampulla of Vater, which opens into the duodenal papilla. These anatomical variations have particular clinical-surgical importance.

2   Microscopic Structure and Functional Activity of the Pancreas

The pancreas is a retroperitoneal organ, surrounded by a capsule of connective tissue that separates the parenchyma in lobules by means of thin partition walls which contain nerves, lymphatic and blood vessels, and excretory ducts (◉ *Fig. 2-4*). It is a gland of complex secretion, synthesizing, storing and secreting important hormones and digestive enzymes. Daily, the pancreas secretes about 1,200 mL of pancreatic juice, essential for the digestion of carbohydrates, proteins and fats of the foods. The endocrine portion, as a whole, represents only a little proportion of the total volume of the gland and secretes hormones that are mainly

◘ Fig. 2-4

Histologic structure of the adult pancreas: (a) *ac* acini, *iL* islets of langerhans, **(b)** *a* arteria, *v* vein, *n* nerve, **(c)** *ild* interlobular duct, *Arrowheads* ductal cilindric epithelia, *Broken arrows* litle interlobular ducts, *Arrows* basophilic ergastoplasm of acini.

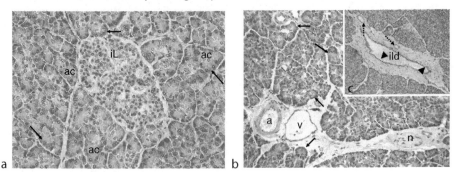

involved in the control of the carbohydrate metabolism. Both, endocrine and exocrine components of the pancreas are independent in their functional characteristics as well as in their's own pathologic alterations [11].

2.1   Endocrine Pancreas

The functional unit of the endocrine pancreas is islet of Langerhans. These spherical structures are formed by tenth to hundreds cells (**◉** *Fig. 2-4*) containing many blood capillar vessels. The islets of Langerhans are scattered into the gland parenchyma surrounded by a thin layer of reticular fibers. In the adult human being, there is more than a million of islets which amounts the 1% of the pancreatic volume. They are mostly in the tail than in the body and head of the pancreas. All the pancreatic endocrine cell types are polarized, with the secretory granules located at the apical domain of the cell, in the vicinity of a fenestrated capillar. As other protein-secreting cells, they have a well-developed rough endoplasmic reticulum and Golgi complex. The cells of the islets are arranged as irregular cords and – with standard hematoxilin-eosin method – has a light staining compared with the surrounding acinar cells (**◉** *Fig. 2-4a*). However, several special stains – as the classic Mallory-Azan – or immunocytochemical techniques can show at least four types of islets cells:

- *Alpha cell* (or A cell), are about 15–20% of the island cells, homogeneously distributed over the gland and mainly around the periphery of the islets. The cytoplasmic granules are relatively large and insoluble in alcohol. These cells – in response to cholecystokinin or insulin – produce glucagon, hyperglycemic hormone that opposes the insulin effect inducing hepatic glycogenolysis and the glucose transport toward the blood.
- *Beta cell* (or B cell), representing the 50–80% of the island cells, the majority are located toward the periphery, and only some of them in the middle of the island. The granules of B cells are smaller than those of the A cells and are soluble in alcohol. They segregate insulin, hypoglycemic hormone that lower the blood glucose level by facilitating its entry into the cell and their conversion to glycogen. Also, insulin participates in the lipid metabolism. The control of insulin secretion is mainly regulated by the level of blood glucose. [11,12].

- *Delta cell* (or D cell), complete the 3–10%; they are scattered by the islets and have small cytoplasmic granules containing somatostatin that suppress the endocrine secretion of insulin and glucagon by means of a paracrine mechanism, modulating the activity of Alpha and Beta cells and maintaining the normal glucose level in blood.
- *F cell* (or PP cell), segregates pancreatic polypeptide, they represent only 1% of the islets cell population, and inhibit the exocrine pancreas.

Besides the secretion of proteic hormones, the cells of the islets of Langerhans also synthesize others molecules similar to those of the APUD system [13].

2.2   Exocrine Pancreas

This portion of pancreas is a typical whole serose, compound, acinous gland, formed by many little lobules delimited by thin connective tissue walls which contain many blood and lymphatic vessels, nerves, and interlobular ducts. At microscopic level, we can clear identify two functional compartments: the acini and duct. [11] (⊗ *Figs. 2-4* and ⊗ *2-5*).

2.2.1   Acini

They are rounded structures formed by 40–50 pyramidal cells resting upon a basal lamina with reticular fibers around a little lumen – which distended during active secretion phase – continued with an intercalated duct (⊗ *Figs. 2-4* and ⊗ *2-5*). The acinar lumen is isolated from the intercellular space by means of zonula occludens (⊗ *Fig. 2-5d*). The gland cells are polarized, having filamentous mitochondria and a significant development of rough endoplasmic reticulum and polyribosomes in the basal-lateral domain (⊗ *Figs. 2-4b* and ⊗ *2-5b, e*). These basophilic components of acinar cells (ergastoplasm = RER + free ribosomes) are more evident after a toluidine blue staining of histologic sections (⊗ *Fig. 2-5b*). At the apical cell domain, a prominent Golgi complex and secretory zymogen granules containing precursors of pancreatic enzymes are seen (⊗ *Fig. 2-5c, d*). These secretory granules are particularly numerous during fasting and diminished after a large meal. After discharge of the zymogen granules, the Golgi complex enlarges as new secretory droplets are forming. The nucleus of the acinar cells, spherical and located at the basal domain, have a prominent nucleolus (⊗ *Figs. 2-4* and ⊗ *2-5b, e*). Toward the inner of the acinus the free surface of the acinar cells exhibited a few short microvilli (⊗ *Fig. 2-5c, d*), as well as the centro-acinar cells with a central nucleous, pale and thin cytoplasm, marking the start of the intercalated duct [11].

The exocrine function of the pancreas follows a cycle of continuous low level of secretion, incremented by meals stimulation through neuro-hormonal signals. This secretory rhytmic cycle is also observed in the number of zymogen granules, showing a higher number during the fasting and scarce ones after the meal-induced liberation. Proteases (trypsin, chymotrypsins, carboxypeptidases, aminopeptidase, elastase, etc.), amylolytic enzymes (amylase), lipases, nucleases (deoxyribonucleases, ribonucleases), are some of the pancreatic hydrolases. After the fusion of a secretory vesicle with the plasma membrane, their proenzymatic content discharges by exocytosis and its membrane becomes part of the plasma membrane of the acinar cell. The amount of vesicle membrane added to the plasma membrane can be temporarily enormous. It was estimated that an acinar cell secreting digestive enzymes, about 900 μm^2 of vesicle membrane is added into the apical cell membrane, whose area is only 30 μm^2 when the cell is

■ Fig. 2-5

(a) Diagram showing the main features of pancreatic acini, (b) histologic section of pancreas (toluidine blue staining). Acini show heavy concentration of ribonucleoproteins (rough endoplasmic reticulum + free ribosomes) at the basal domain of the cells (arrowheads) and vesicular nucleus with prominent nucleolus (arrows), (c) Ultrastructural view of a pancreatic acini showing microvilli (MV) at the apical membrane of glandular cells (arrow), and citoplasm with zymogen secretory granules (Z), (d) the acinar lumen (L) closed with zonula occludens of adjacent cells (ZO, arrows) showing zymogen granules (Z) and rought endoplasmic reticulum (RER), and (e) typical basal domain of acinar cells with dense RER and heterocromatic nucleus with prominent nucleolus (N).

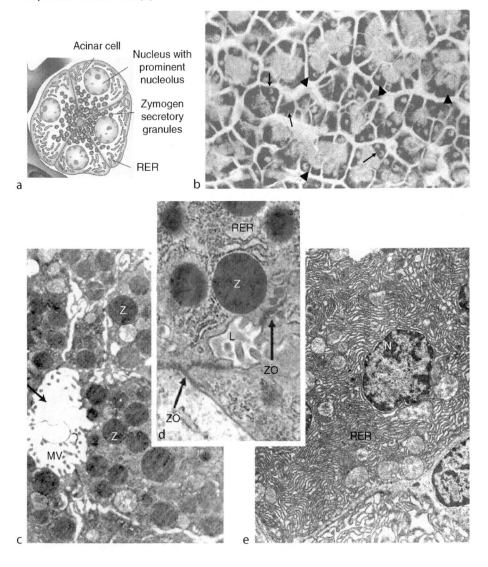

secreting. However, there is not a significant membrane disbalance because the transiently increasing of the plasma membrane is compensate by a simultaneous endocytic mechanism that removes vesicles from the cell surface toward the cytoplasmic domain [14]. It is also known that the membrane proteins surrounding the zymogen granules are involved in the regulation of secretion [15], and recent proteomic studies were undertaken to identify the proteins of the membrane granule related mediating this secretory functions [16]. The pancreatic secretion is regulated by hormones and the autonomic nervous system, being more conspicuous the hormonal control. The presence of foods into the gastric lumen and the traffic of the acid content toward the luminal duodenum, stimulate the secretion of polypeptidic hormones secretin and cholecystokinin (pancreozymin), which are synthesized by the S cells of the intestinal mucosa. In turn, secretin stimulates the secretory cells of the duct systems which secrete pancreatic juice with a high content of bicarbonate and water, but scarce enzymes. The alkaline pH of the pancreatic juice is the main buffer system present in the duodenal lumen neutralizing the acid content coming from the stomach and thus providing the neutral/alkaline millieu required for the pancreatic enzymes activation. On the other hand, the cholecystokinin stimulates the secretion of a high quantity of digestives enzymes without a significant increase of pancreatic juice volume. Other function of the cholecystokinin (pancreozimin) hormone involves the contraction of the gallbladder, which add the tensioactive bile to the duodenal content. The neural regulation is mediated by parasympathetic fibers of the vagus nerve that stimulate the enzyme secretion similarly to the cholecystokinin hormone, and the sympathetic fibers inhibiting the pancreatic secretion.

When specific hormonal stimulus is acting, the granule membrane fuses with the apical cell membrane and exocitosis occurred, liberating the granule contents into the acinar lumen. This enzyme-rich secretory material is then transported along the duct system toward the duodenum lumen where are activated by entero-kinases following a cascade that starts with trypsinogen activation as well as the other pancreatic proteases. The pancreatic proenzymes are activated only after their secretion into the duodenal lumen, participating in the proteins, carbohydrates and lipids digestion, together with other enzymes from the intestinal mucosa. The inactive form of the enzymes and the membrane wrapping of secretory granules protect the pancreatic cells from the potential hydrolytic damage. However, the acute pancreatitis, an inflammatory process comprising pancreatic and peripancreatic tissues, is triggered by improper activation of trypsinogen and the failure of exocitosis of activated secretory granules.

Stellate cells: These are periacinar, perivascular and periductal miofibroblastic cells, having an elongated shape with many cytoplasmic processes surrounding the basal acinus. The name derived from this shape, *stella* in Latin means "a star." This cell population shared structural and functional characteristics with stellate cells in the liver as well as other organs such as kidney and lung. Similar to its hepatic counterpart, pancreatic stellate cells have fat-storing capabilities and express a number of intermediate filaments, such as desmin and glial fibrillary acidic protein. These features are useful to differentiate stellate cells from other mesenchymal cells, e.g., fibroblasts [17,18]. Activation of quiescent stellate cells during an inflammatory process such pancreatitis leads to morphologic changes including nuclear and endoplasmic reticulum, expression α-smooth muscle action and collagen type I. Similarly to changes observed in the hepatic cirrhosis, the sustained activation of the stellate cells is also associated with the fibrosis, vascular changes present in the chronic pancreatitis and cancer of pancreas [19].

Pancreatic stem cells: They are undifferentiated cells with proliferating and multipotent capacity that can replace different cell types of the pancreas. Distinct cell sources were proposed as progenitors, among others, periductal and periisland cells containing nestin, a cytoskeletal intermediate filament, or transcription factors Pdx1 and NGN3, keys molecules during the embryonic development of the pancreas (see above).

2.3 Ducts System

The pancreatic duct system drives the secretion from the acinus to the second portion of duodenum, being also an excretor organ secreting bicarbonate in a concentration 5–6 folds higher than those in the plasma. The lumen of the acinus communicate with the first conducting portion formed by epithelium of low cubic cells, occasionally surrounded by acinar (centroacinar) cells, which in turn form the intercalated duct portion. Centroacinar cells are distinguished in conventional histologic sections because of their pale staining and very low cytoplasmic density, as well as their scarse organelles at the electron microscope level. Several intercalated ducts converge to form an intralobular duct having a wider lumen and limited by a single layer of cubic epithelium, in turn surrounded by acini. These conduction segments form the interlobular ducts that reside among the lobules, and its epithelium is formed by a single layer of cylinder cells (◉ Fig. 2-4c). The main ducts are also formed by a single cylinder epithelium and, next to duodenal wall, occasionally interrupted by goblet cells, and surrounded by a well developed lamina propria. The main terminal duct (duct of Wirsung) usually joins the common bile duct to form the ampulla of Vater that opens through the duodenal papilla and its orifice is encircled by the sphincter of Oddi. In some individuals, there is an accessory pancreatic duct (duct of Santorini) that enters the duodenum more proximally [9]. Both pancreatic ducts of Wirsung and of Santorini develop from each of the two endodermic buds (see above). Cell populations forming the pancreatic ducts comprised more than 10% of the total of pancreatic cells.

2.4 Blood Vessels and Nerves

The pancreatic vascularity is supplied by branches of the celiac and mesenteric superior arteries, besides the splenic and hepatic arteries. The venous drainage is conducted toward the portal hepatic system by the splenic and mesenteric superior veins. The primary lymphatic drainage is produced by a chain of lymphatic ganglia running parallel to the splenic artery; and as secondary or accessory system the pancreatic lymph drain directly to the celiac, aortic, duodenal and subpyloric ganglia. The pancreatic innervation comes from the parasympathetic and sympathetic branches of the autonomic nervous system. The parasympathetic fibers are responsible of the regulation of the pancreatic exocrine secretion, by means of the vagus nerve. The sympathetic fibers arrived from the celiac ganglion and are responsible of the pancreatic vascular innervation and the pain transmission [11].

2.5 Concluding Remarks

The pancreas is a mixed endocrine and exocrine gland that is fundamental to the nutrition and the utilization of nutrients via the secretion of digestive enzymes by the exocrine pancreas and hormones by the endocrine pancreas. During development, an intricate network of signaling and transcriptional regulation events are responsible for forming a gland that is characterized by branching morphogenesis, which surrounds itself with zymogen and secreting hormone cells. The acinar component of the exocrine pancreas secretes enzymes and bicarbonate to the ductal system, which will take it into the duodenum, where digestion occurs. The best characterized diseases of the exocrine pancreas are pancreatitis and cancer. The endocrine pancreas is the origin of diabetes mellitus and neuroendocrine tumors. Therefore, a basic understanding of the structure of the pancreas is a fundamental step for any student in this field.

Key Research Points

- Embryology and histology of the pancreas is of paramount importance as a basis for pancreatic researchers. All the biochemical, biophysical, and pathobiological phenomena are better understood when armed by this knowledge.
- This chapter provides a developmental blueprint that serves to form the pancreas as a mixed exocrine and endocrine gland.
- Studies using animal models or those that focus on pancreatitis and pancreatic cancer are especially dependent upon the knowledge of the normal structural features of the pancreas described in this chapter.

Future Scientific Directions

- Although much is known on the structure and function of both the developing and young adult pancreas, little is known of the aging pancreas. This area offers an opportunity to contribute with the basic structural parameters that define baseline conditions so that better information is gained during diseases in older individuals.
- Cell tracing experiments may help to define how this normal population contributes to specific diseases, such as pancreatic cancer. Cell isolation techniques combined with cell marker development may further inform cell subtypes that might yet be discovered (e.g., different types of ductular cells).
- A better understanding of how different types of cells originate during regeneration is an area of great interest since this knowledge can be applied to tissue engineering, a new frontier in Pancreatology, which has been born with the development of islet transplants.

Clinical Implications

- Many important, but relatively recently described, studies on diseases of the pancreas have been performed by demonstrating the alterations of normal pancreatic structure. Examples include autoimmune pancreatitis and PanIN lesions.
- Ancillary techniques to histology, such as in situ hybridization and immunohistochemistry, are essential for the validation of disease markers and for detecting alterations in molecules that inform the pathobiology of pancreatic diseases.
- There are diseases that alter specific parts of the pancreas, and their structural alterations are better understood by proper knowledge of pancreatic structure, such as ductal changes detected by ERCP. Distinct types of IPMN exist that affect different types of duct systems.

References

1. Gannon M, Wright C: Endodermal patterning and organogenesis. In Cell Lineage and Fate Determination. Moody SA (ed.). San Diego: Academic Press, 1999, pp. 583–615.
2. Gilbert SF: Developmental Biology, 7th ed. Sunderland, MA: nauer Associates, Inc., 2003.
3. Apelqvist A, Ahlgren U, Edlund H: Sonic hedgehog directs specialised mesoderm differentiation in the intestine and pancreas. Curr Biol 1997;7:801–804.
4. Hebrok M, Kim S, Melton DA: Notochord repression of endodermal sonic hedgehog permits pancreas development. Genes Dev 1998;12:1705–1713.
5. Ahlgren U, Jonnson J, Edlund H: The morphogenesis of the pancreatic mesenchyme is uncoupled from that of the pancreatic epithelium in IPF/PDX1-deficient mice. Development 1996;122:1409–1416.
6. Lammert E, Cleaver O, Melton DA: Induction of pancreatic differentiation by signals from blood vessels. Science 2001;294:564–567.
7. Edlund H: Pancreatic organogenesis – developmental mechanisms and implications for therapy. Nat Rev Genet 2002;3(7):524–532.
8. Gu G, Dubauskaite J, Melton DA: Direct evidence for the pancreatic lineage: NGN3 + cells are islet progenitors and are distinct from duct progenitors. Development 2002;129:2447–2457.
9. Githens S: Development of ducts cells, Chapter 32. In Human Gastrointestinal Development. Lebenthal E (ed.). New York: Raven Press, 1989, pp. 669–683.
10. Githens S: Differentiation and development of the pancreas in animals, Chapter 3. In The Pancreas: Biology, Pathobiology, and Disease, 2nd ed. Go VLW et al. (ed.). Raven Press, New York: 1993, pp. 21–55.
11. Eynard AR, Valentich MA, Rovasio RA: Histology and Embryology of the Human Being: Cell and Molecular Bases (in Spanish), 4th ed., Buenos Aires: Editorial Médica Panamericana, 2008, pp. 394–496.
12. Klover PJ, Mooney RA: Hepatocytes: critical for glucose homeostasis. Int J Biochem Cell Biol 2004;36:753–758.
13. Le Douarin NM, Kalcheim C: The Neural Crest. Cambridge: Cambridge University Press, 1999.
14. Alberts B, Bray D, Lewis J, Raff M, Roberts K, Watson JD: Molecular Biology of the Cell, 3rd ed. New York: Galand Publication, Inc., 1994.
15. Braun JE, Fritz BA, Wong SM, Lowe AW: Identification of a vesicle-associated membrane protein (VAMP)-like membrane protein in zymogen granules of the rat exocrine pancreas. J Biol Chem 1994;269:5328–5335.
16. Chen X, Walker AK, Strahler JR, Simon ES, et al.: Organellar proteomics: analysis of pancreatic zymogen granule membranes. Mol Cell Proteomics 2006;5:306–312.
17. Apte MV, Haber PS, Applegate TL, Norton ID, McCaughan GW, Korsten MA, Pirola RC, Wilson JS: Periacinar stellate shaped cells in rat pancreas: identification, isolation, and culture. Gut 1998;43(1):128–133.
18. Bachem MG, Schneider E, Gross H, Weidenbach H, Schmid RM, Menke A, Siech M, Beger H, Grünert A, Adler G: Identification, culture, and characterization of pancreatic stellate cells in rats and humans. Gastroenterology 1998;115:421–432.
19. Vonlaufen A, Phillips PA, Xu Z, Goldstein D, Pirola RC, Wilson JS, Apte MV: Pancreatic stellate cells and pancreatic cancer cells: an unholy alliance. Cancer Res 2008;68(19):7707–7710.

3 Pathologic Classification and Biological Behavior of Pancreatic Neoplasia

Olca Basturk · Ipek Coban · N. Volkan Adsay

1	Introduction	40
2	Pathologic Classification of Pancreatic Neoplasia	41
2.1	Ductal Neoplasia	41
2.1.1	Invasive Ductal Carcinoma	43
2.1.2	Other Invasive Carcinomas of Ductal Lineage	47
2.1.3	Non-Invasive (Preinvasive) Ductal Neoplasia	50
2.1.4	Non-Mucinous Ductal Neoplasia	55
2.2	Endocrine Neoplasia	55
2.2.1	Pancreatic Endocrine Neoplasm	56
2.3	Acinar Neoplasia	58
2.3.1	Acinar Cell Carcinoma	58
2.4	Neoplasms with Multiple Lineages (Pancreatoblastoma and Mixed Acinar-Endocrine Carcinoma)	59
2.5	Neoplasms of Uncertain Histogenesis	61
2.5.1	Solid Pseudopapillary Neoplasm	61
2.6	Miscellaneous Cystic Pancreatic Lesions	62
2.7	Mesenchymal Tumors	62
2.8	Pseudotumors	63
2.9	Secondary Tumors	63
3	Conclusion	64

J. P. Neoptolemos, R. Urrutia, J. L. Abbruzzese, M. W. Büchler (eds.), *Pancreatic Cancer*,
DOI 10.1007/978-0-387-77498-5_3, © Springer Science+Business Media, LLC 2010

Abstract: Pancreatic neoplasms are classified according to which normal cell type of this organ they recapitulate, because the clinicopathologic and biologic characteristics of tumors are determined or manifested mostly by their cellular lineage. Most pancreatic neoplasms are of ductal lineage, characterized by tubular units, cysts, and papilla or mucin formation and expression of mucin-related glycoproteins and oncoproteins. There are also certain genes, molecules and mutations that are fairly specific to ductal neoplasms.

Invasive ductal adenocarcinoma constitutes the vast majority (>85%) of carcinomas of ductal lineage. Ductal adenocarcinoma is characterized by insidious infiltration and rapid dissemination, despite its relatively well-differentiated histologic appearance. The presumed precursors of ductal adenocarcinoma are microscopic intraductal proliferative changes that are now termed pancreatic intraepithelial neoplasia (PanIN). PanINs comprise a neoplastic transformation ranging from early mucinous change (PanIN-1A) to frank *carcinoma in situ* (PanIN-3). A similar neoplastic spectrum also characterizes intraductal papillary mucinous neoplasms and mucinous cystic neoplasms, which are cystic ductal-mucinous tumors with varying degrees of papilla formation, and may be associated with invasive carcinoma. Intraductal papillary mucinous neoplasms are associated with invasive carcinoma of the colloid type, which appears to be a clinicopathologically distinct tumor with indolent behavior. Conversely, mucinous cystic neoplasms are associated with invasive carcinoma of ordinary ductal adenocarcinoma type.

Although most ductal pancreatic neoplasia are characterized by some degree of mucin formation, serous tumors, of which serous cystadenoma is the sole example, lack mucin formation, presumably because they recapitulate centroacinar ducts. These are typically benign tumors.

Among non-ductal tumors of the pancreas, endocrine neoplasms are by far the most common. The vast majority of pancreatic endocrine neoplasia (PENs) is low-intermediate grade malignancies characterized by protracted clinical course. Those that are treated at an early stage are even considered "benign." Poorly differentiated neuroendocrine (small cell) carcinomas are exceedingly uncommon and are highly aggressive tumors.

Pancreatic tumors of predominant acinar lineage, namely acinar cell carcinomas and pancreatoblastomas – the latter mostly a childhood malignancy – are uncommon, and are associated with aggressive clinical course, though not as dismal as that of ductal carcinomas. There is also a tumor in the pancreas which is of undetermined lineage: solid pseudopapillary neoplasm. It typically occurs in young females and follows a benign course in most instances.

Neoplasms may also arise from supportive tissue or may secondarily involve the pancreas. Although these are highly uncommon, they can be problematic in the differential diagnosis.

In conclusion, invasive ductal carcinoma is by far the most common tumor in the pancreas; however, occur in this organ are a plethora of neoplasms of other types with different clinicopathologic, molecular-genetic and biologic characteristics.

1   Introduction

Since the days of Galen of Ephesus, the "physician of physicians" (200 A.D.), who had concluded that pancreas was merely a fat pad serving as a protective cushion to the major vessels lying behind; the pancreas has remained an enigmatic organ, largely neglected by the medical field throughout the history. In Nineteenth century, it began to be appreciated as an organ the failure of which leads to dire consequences. More importantly, it is now widely known that cancers arising from the ductal system of this organ is one of the deadliest of all cancers, and has recently become the fourth leading cause of cancer deaths in the US [1]. This has led the medical field to analyze pancreatic neoplasia more carefully and consequently, in the past two decades, various important developments have taken place in the pathologic classification, terminology and our understanding of various pancreatic tumor types.

2   Pathologic Classification of Pancreatic Neoplasia

Pancreatic neoplasms are classified according to which normal cell type of this organ they recapitulate, because the clinicopathologic and biologic characteristics of tumors are determined or manifested mostly by their cellular lineage (◉ *Table 3-1*, WHO classification).

The cell types that constitute the pancreas form three functionally distinct units:

1. Exocrine pancreas is responsible for the production and delivery of the digestive enzymes such as trypsin, chymotrypsin, amylase and lipase to the duodenum. These enzymes are produced and stored in *acinar cells*. While acinar cells constitute the vast majority of pancreatic tissue (◉ *Fig. 3-1*); neoplasms of acinar lineage are exceedingly uncommon. The second component of the exocrine pancreas is the ducts, the mere function of which is to transport the acinar enzymes to the duodenum. The ductal system begins with the *centroacinar cells* and continues with intralobar and interlobular ductules, and through the main pancreatic duct ultimately opens into the ampulla of Vater. Although the ductal component is not a complex structure when compared with the other components, it is the main source of the vast majority of neoplasms in the pancreas [2]. This propensity for neoplastic transformation may not be very surprising as the ductal system is the only component in pancreas that is exposed to the outside world (mutagens).
2. The second major and physiologically distinct component of this organ is endocrine, which is represented by widely scattered islands of endocrine cells referred as islets of Langerhans, distributed throughout the pancreas in forms of small, distinct nests amidst acinar tissue (◉ *Fig. 3-1*). The islets are responsible for producing a variety of hormones but mostly insulin, glucagon and somatostatin, which play a key regulatory role not only in glucose metabolism but also other systemic metabolic processes as well. Unlike the exocrine component, which releases enzymes locally to the duodenum, the hormones produced by the endocrine component are secreted to a rich capillary network that penetrates into the islets. Endocrine tumors are not uncommon and form an important category, although they occur far less frequently than ductal neoplasia.
3. As in any other organs, there is also supportive tissue including fibroblasts, vessels, nerves and immune cells in the pancreas and these also, on occasion, give rise to pancreatic neoplasia.

There are also tumors in the pancreas that are of undetermined origin and lineage. In the ensuing text, an overview of the clinicopathologic characteristics of pancreatic neoplasia will be discussed based on their lineage. Emphasis will be given to those that are more common.

2.1   Ductal Neoplasia

In order to transport the acinar enzymes to the duodenum, the ductal cells are organized in luminated structures and produce protective and lubricative glycoproteins (the mucins).

◘ Table 3-1

WHO histologic classification of tumors of the pancreas

Epithelial tumors
Benign
Serous cystadenoma
Mucinous cystadenoma
Intraductal papillary-mucinous adenoma
Mature teratoma
Borderline (uncertain malignant potential)
Mucinous cystic neoplasm with moderate dysplasia
Intraductal papillary-mucinous neoplasm with moderate dysplasia
Solid-pseudopapillary neoplasm
Malignant
Ductal adenocarcinoma
Mucinous non-cystic carcinoma
Signet ring cell carcinoma
Adenosquamous.carcinoma
Undifferentiated (anaplastic) carcinoma
Undifferentiated carcinoma with osteoclast-like giant cells
Mixed ductal-endocrine carcinoma
Serous cystadenocarcinoma
Mucinous cystadenocarcinoma
Noninvasive
Invasive
Intraductal papillary-mucinous carcinoma
Noninvasive
Invasive (papillary-mucinous carcinoma)
Acinar cell carcinoma
Acinar cell cystadenocarcinoma
Mixed acinar-endocrine carcinoma
Pancreatoblastoma
Solid-pseudopapillary carcinoma
Others
Non-epithelial tumors
Secondary tumors

Neoplasia of pancreatic ductal lineage recapitulate these characteristics at a variable degree. Tubular (lumen-forming) units, cysts (mega versions of these tubules), and papilla (finger-like projections of the mucosa lining these ducts/cysts) are hallmarks of ductal differentiation in this organ and are incorporated to the names of some of the tumors as well. There are also certain genes, molecules and mutations that are fairly specific to ductal neoplasia.

◘ Fig. 3-1

Normal pancreatic tissue. Acinar cells arranged in lobules constitute the majority of the parenchyma. These cells have apical lightly eosinophilic cytoplasm due to the presence of zymogen granules and basophilia in the basal aspect of the cytoplasm. To aid in their secretory activity, the nuclei are polarized to the periphery and the cells are arranged in round units creating the *acinus*. In the *left middle part* of the field, an islet of Langerhans consisting of round collection of endocrine cells is represented. Endocrine cells have moderate amphophilic cytoplasm and nuclei with finely stippled chromatin pattern. In the *right upper part* of the field an intralobular duct lined by cuboidal-low columnar epithelium is seen.

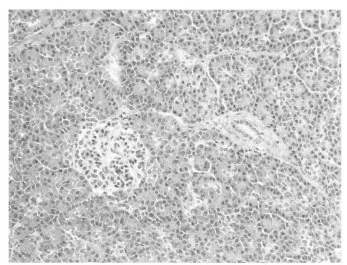

Mucin-related glycoproteins and oncoproteins such as MUC1, CA19-9, CEA, DUPAN are typically detectable by immunohistochemistry in mucinous ductal tumors [3]. Expression of certain subsets of cytokeratin such as CK19 [4], and mutations in *k-ras* oncogene or SMAD4/DPC4 are also fairly specific [5], and are typically lacking in acinar or endocrine tumors with a few exceptions. Moreover, even though rare scattered endocrine cells can be seen in almost any ductal tumor; evidence of acinar differentiation such as enzyme activity is exceedingly uncommon.

2.1.1   Invasive Ductal Carcinoma

More than 85% of pancreatic tumors are invasive ductal adenocarcinoma, also named as pancreatobiliary type, scirrhous, tubular or usual ductal adenocarcinoma [6]. Because it is by far the most common and most important tumor type in the pancreas, ductal adeno-carcinoma has become synonymous with "pancreas cancer," which sometimes leads to erroneous interpretations due to inappropriate inclusion or exclusion of other cancers that occur in this organ but have different clinical, pathologic and behavioral characteristics as discussed below. Patients with ductal adenocarcinoma are usually between 60 and 80-years-old (mean age, 63) and it is very uncommon to see this tumor in patients younger than 40-years-old [7].

Ductal adenocarcinoma grow rapidly, and regardless of the size of the tumor, metastasis to lymph nodes and liver ultimately ensue. They also have very insidious growth pattern, and in fact, along with ovarian cancer, ductal adenocarcinoma is the most common cause of "intraabdominal carcinomatosis," the formation of numerous small tumor nodules throughout the abdomen. It is also one of the most common sources of carcinoma of unknown primary. Only 20% of the cases with ductal adenocarcinoma are resectable at the time of diagnosis [7].

Because of these features (rapid growth, insidious infiltration and early dissemination) cure rate of ductal adenocarcinoma is extremely low; with a 5-year survival still below 2% [7]. In fact, most 5-year survivors of "pancreas cancer" prove to be a tumor type other than ordinary ductal adenocarcinoma after careful reexamination of microscopic features [8].

The diagnosis of invasive ductal adenocarcinoma can be very problematic, both at clinical and microscopic levels. This tumor type is typically associated with abundant host tissue stroma referred as *desmoplastic stroma* (❯ *Fig. 3-2*). This creates a "scirrhous" (scar-like) appearance [9] that can be very difficult to distinguish from true scarring inflammatory lesions of this organ, in particular, autoimmune and paraduodenal types of chronic pancreatitis. This difficulty in the differential diagnosis is also valid for microscopic examination. Injured native ducts of the pancreas can show substantial cytologic atypia that can closely imitate that of carcinoma, and conversely, most ductal adenocarcinoma form well differentiated glandular units that resemble benign ducts [10–12] (❯ *Fig. 3-3*) or cause ductal obstruction and eventually lead to chronic pancreatitis. Consequently, the distinction of ductal adenocarcinoma from pancreatitis is considered one of the most, if not the most, challenging differential diagnosis in diagnostic pathology.

However, ductal adenocarcinoma has some morphologic characteristics that are fairly unique and not seen as much in other common organ cancers. First, despite its highly aggressive behavior, the vast majority of invasive ductal adenocarcinomas are "well or moderately differentiated" (❯ *Figs. 3-3* and ❯ *3-4*); i.e., recapitulate the normal ducts extremely well. They also show a remarkable affinity to spread through the nerves and vessels. Nearly 80% of

❑ Fig. 3-2

(a) Invasive ductal adenocarcinoma, macroscopic findings. A firm, sclerotic, poorly defined mass is seen in the head of the pancreas. The rounded pale structure (arrow) adjacent to the *right lower border* of the specimen represents a lymph node enlarged by metastatic adenocarcinoma. (b) Invasive ductal adenocarcinoma is characterized (and defined) by infiltrating tubular units embedded in desmoplastic stroma.

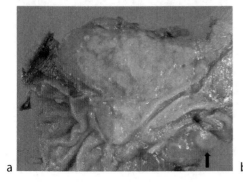
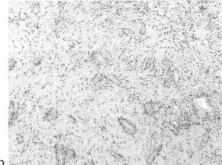

a   b

⬛ Fig. 3-3

Invasive ductal adenocarcinoma, well differentiated. Well formed glandular structures lined by cuboidal cells closely mimic the non-neoplastic ducts.

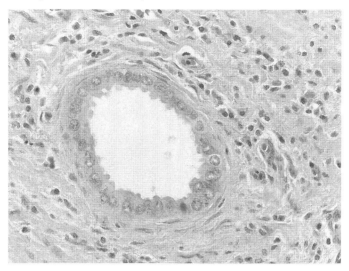

⬛ Fig. 3-4

Invasive ductal adenocarcinoma, moderately differentiated. There is a greater degree of cytologic and nuclear atypia. Loss of polarity can be seen as well.

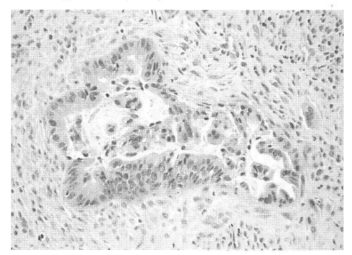

these cases show *perineural invasion* (⬤ *Fig. 3-5*) by microscopic examination, although if the entire tumor is examined this ratio will probably be higher. This feature is thought to be the reason of back pain, one of the more common symptoms of this tumor. *Vascular invasion* is also very common and pancreatic carcinoma cells have this unique ability to form well formed glandular elements in vascular spaces [13] (❯ *Fig. 3-6*). What referred as *isolated solitary ducts,* which are microscopic (grossly invisible) invasive units located away from the main tumor lying individually in peripancreatic fat tissue, is a very common finding (❯ *Fig. 3-7*), and may be responsible for the high recurrence rate of seemingly margin-negative resections [14].

▢ Fig. 3-5

Invasive ductal adenocarcinoma showing perineural invasion.

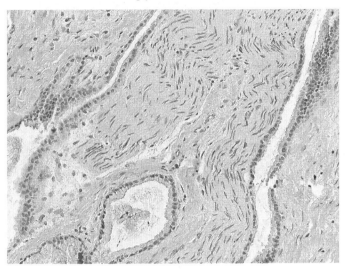

▢ Fig. 3-6

Vascular invasion of infiltrating ductal adenocarcinoma. Carcinoma cells line the luminal surface of vascular walls in such an organized and polarized fashion that they form a well-structured duct-like unit virtually indistinguishable from normal ducts or PanINs.

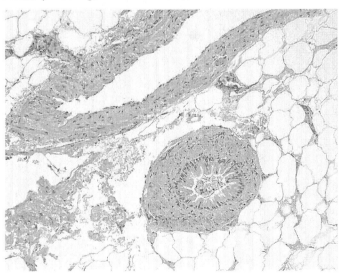

◘ Fig. 3-7

Isolated solitary ducts surrounded entirely by adipocytes without any accompanying islets, acini or other ducts are indicative of invasive carcinoma. This phenomenon of renegade ducts away from the main tumor is a peculiar manifestation of the insidious spread of pancreatic adenocarcinoma.

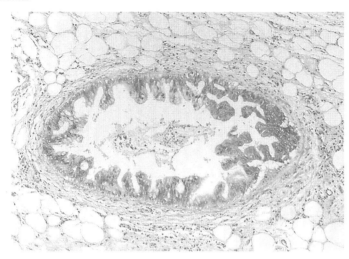

The cells in ductal adenocarcinomas are typically cuboidal shaped with variable amount of cytoplasm that contains mucin and mucin-related glycoproteins, and may occasionally demonstrate predominance of a specific organelle creating distinctive patterns such as "foamy-gland" pattern with swollen, altered mucin, "clear-cell" pattern with abundant glycogen, and "oncocytoid" or "hepatoid" variants with prominent mitochondria or lysosomes, respectively [2].

As discussed earlier, abundant *desmoplastic stroma* (❯ Fig. 3-2) of variable cellularity is a very important feature of this tumor type. Carcinoma cells are somewhat diluted in this desmoplastic stroma and this dilution phenomenon creates major problems for both diagnosticians and researchers. This is an important pitfall, in particular for studies that utilize "global" arrays, which do not discriminate between the different cellular compartments of the specimen, and analyze all pancreatic tissue together. If the intend is to analyze the carcinoma cells, it should be kept in mind that most of the tumor tissue is in fact composed of this desmoplastic stroma not the cancer cells, and further complicating the analysis, normal pancreas is also composed mostly of acini with no relevance to ductal carcinogenesis. Therefore, if a comparison of normal ducts and ductal adenocarcinoma is intended, normal ducts and carcinoma cells need to be dissected out from the background tissue, or alternatively, visual-aided methods of analysis such as immunohistochemistry or in situ hybridization ought to be utilized, preferably by experts who can distinguish between the non-neoplastic and neoplastic elements.

2.1.2 Other Invasive Carcinomas of Ductal Lineage

Various uncommon types of invasive carcinomas of also ductal lineage, classified separately from the conventional ductal adenocarcinomas, have been recognized [2].

Undifferentiated Carcinoma

In some ductal carcinomas of the pancreas, the hallmarks of ductal differentiation, namely the tubule formation, mucin production and others may be lacking. Such cases are classified as "undifferentiated carcinoma." Some can be so undifferentiated that only after adjunct studies such as immunohistochemical studies for keratins or mutation analysis for *k-ras* oncogene, the epithelial and ductal nature of the tumor can be elucidated [15]. In some, epithelial-to-mesenchymal transition can be so complete that the tumor cells may be mostly spindle shaped and resemble sarcomas (i.e., sarcomatoid carcinoma). In fact, some may even show bone and cartilage formation [16]. In others, the undifferentiated cells may form bizarre giant cells. These can be difficult to distinguish from high-grade malignancies like lymphomas or melanomas. Undifferentiated carcinomas are rare and their demographics do not seem to differ from ordinary ductal adenocarcinoma, except that they may have even more aggressive behavior.

Undifferentiated Carcinoma with Osteoclast-Like Giant Cells

Some sarcomatoid carcinomas of the pancreas have a peculiar predilection to attract osteoclast-like giant cells of histiocytic/macrophagic origin [17]. Often, these cells are so abundant that they dominate the picture, and the tumor is referred as "giant cell carcinoma" [18]. Recent molecular studies confirmed what is suspected by morphologic observations that these osteoclasts are in fact reactive in nature and that the malignant cells are actually the smaller, ovoid to spindle cells in the background (⊙ *Fig. 3-8*). Once inspected carefully, a more conventional adenocarcinoma component composed of invasive tubular elements is identified in most cases.

⬛ Fig. 3-8

Undifferentiated carcinoma with osteoclast-like giant cells. Non-neoplasic multinucleated giant cells of histiocytic origin are mixed with neoplastic mononuclear spindle shaped epitheloid cells. The mononuclear cells have hyperchromatic, occasionally bizarre nuclei.

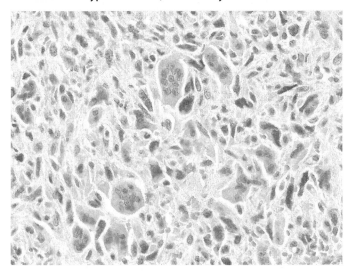

Adenosquamous and Squamous Carcinoma

In the normal pancreas, squamous cells are found only rarely in injured ductal epithelium as a result of a metaplastic process. Same metaplastic phenomenon also seems to take place focally in some examples of ductal adenocarcinoma. When this finding is prominent (arbitrarily defined as >25% of the tumor), the tumor is classified as adenosquamous carcinoma, and if the tumor is exclusively squamous, then squamous cell carcinoma [19]. One may observe keratinization in various degrees in these tumors [20]. They constitute <2% of all invasive cancers of pancreas and appear to be as aggressive as ordinary ductal adenocarcinoma, if not more.

Colloid Carcinoma (Pure Mucinous or Mucinous Non-Cystic Carcinoma)

Colloid carcinoma has been a well established tumor type in other exocrine organs such as the breast where pure examples of this entity are associated with an excellent prognosis. In the pancreas, this tumor type has come to attention only after the delineation of intraductal papillary mucinous neoplasia (discussed below) as a distinct entity in mid-1990s, because colloid carcinomas often seen in association with these tumors. It is characterized by extensive extracellular mucin deposition [21], which is responsible for its soft, gelatinous appearance grossly. By microscopic examination, there are mucin lakes that contain scanty clusters of carcinoma cells floating within this mucin (◉ Fig. 3-9).

The prevailing theory is such that the mucin of colloid carcinoma is biochemically and biologically different than the mucins of other ductal cancers, made up of the "gel-forming mucin," the MUC2 glycoprotein [22]. It is speculated that, with its tumor suppressor

◘ Fig. 3-9

Colloid carcinoma (mucinous non-cystic carcinoma) characterized by large amounts of mucin pools. Detached fragments of tumor cells can be observed in these pools.

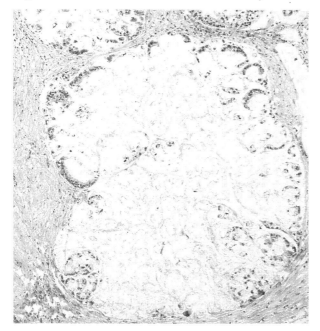

properties, and its physical distribution around the cells, this mucin acts as a containing factor, limiting the growth, and thus culminating in the more protracted clinical course observed in many studies [23].

Medullary Carcinoma

This is an exceedingly uncommon tumor type as a primary in the pancreas [24], although it can occur in the periampullary region. The term medullary is adopted from similar tumors that occur in the GI tract and are often associated with a defect in DNA mismatch-repair genes (genes that are responsible for correcting the mismatches that occur routinely in the DNA), which in turn leads to microsatellite instability. Medullary carcinomas are characterized by nodular pattern and sheet-like growth of poorly differentiated epithelioid cells without any intervening stroma, as opposed to ordinary ductal adenocarcinoma, which have widely scattered well formed tubular units with abundant stroma. In addition, there is often dense lymphoplasmacytic immune cell participation associated with medullary carcinomas. In one study, a subset of these tumors were found to have more protracted clinical course [25], but further data are necessary to elucidate the behavior of these rare tumors.

Signet-Ring Cell Carcinoma

Signet-ring cell carcinoma is a tumor type that is well characterized in the stomach, and is featured by a distinctive infiltration pattern referred as "diffuse-infiltrative." The carcinoma cells form small cords or chains of cells or invade as individual cells without any tubule formation. Commonly, this pattern is also associated with abundant intracytoplasmic mucin accumulation that pushes the nucleus to the periphery of the cell, which in turn creates the signet-ring like morphology.

Defined as such, signet-ring cell carcinoma with all these characteristics is exceedingly uncommon in the pancreas [26,27]. Many authors believe that those that are reported in the pancreas may very well represent secondary invasion from the stomach. Focal signet-ring like formations does occur in otherwise classical ductal adenocarcinoma of the pancreas; however, most authors feel that these should not be classified as signet-ring carcinomas. Similarly, signet-ring morphology may also be seen in colloid carcinomas of the pancreas, but in the absence of other characteristic features, these are not classified as signet ring carcinomas.

2.1.3   Non-Invasive (Preinvasive) Ductal Neoplasia

Pancreatic Intraepithelial Neoplasia

It has long been recognized that there are abnormal *intraductal* proliferations that often accompany invasive ductal adenocarcinoma, and may occasionally also be seen in the absence of ductal adenocarcinoma. For decades these were termed variably as hyperplasia, metaplasia or dysplasia [28]. In 1999, a group of pathologists interested in pancreatic neoplasia were brought together by National Cancer Institute in a Think Tank that took place in Park City, Utah, and during that meeting it was proposed to refer these lesions as *pancreatic intraepithelial neoplasia (PanIN)* [29]. Included in this neoplastic category as PanIN-1A (mucinous duct lesion) were changes that used to be called mucinous hypertrophy or mucinous metaplasia, based on the fact that although these mucinous changes seem perfectly innocuous and do not show classical morphologic attributes of neoplasia, they nevertheless exhibit some molecular alterations that are considered hallmarks of neoplastic change such mutation in *k-ras* oncogene [30]. It is believed that starting with these earliest forms of neoplastic transformation, the process advances to accumulate more genetic abnormalities including p53 gene mutations. These genetic abnormalities are manifested microscopically as nuclear enlargement and hyperchromasia (deposition of abnormal nuclear material). Altered cellular metabolism leads to accumulation of different types of glycoproteins (mucins) as well as disorganization of cells, manifested as loss of polarity of the cells. Furthermore, loss of "guardians of genetic stability" leads to uncontrolled cellular proliferation that is reflected as increased mitotic activity. The spectrum of changes is graded into three as, PanINs 1, 2 and 3 (❯ *Fig. 3-10*). PanIN-3 is also regarded synonymous as *carcinoma in situ*, the last step before invasive cancer develops [31].

Mass-Forming Preinvasive Neoplasia

These lesions are in some ways similar to PanIN in the sense that, they arise from the ductal system, they are noninvasive neoplasia with potential for cancerous transformation. Unlike PanINs, however, they present clinically with mass formation, usually as a cystic

❑ Fig. 3-10

(a) PanIN-1B. In PanIN-1, the normal cuboidal to low columnar ductal epithelial cells are replaced by tall columnar cells containing abundant apical mucin. The nuclei are basally located. The epithelium can be relatively flat in PanIN-1A but papilla formation is well established in the PanIN-1B stage. (b) PanIN-2 usually is papillary. Cytologically, there is nuclear crowding, pseudo-stratification, loss of polarity, and enlarged nuclei. Mitoses are rare, but when present are not atypical. (c) PanIN-3 is characterized by severe cytologic atypia that is seen in full-blown carcinoma. Loss of polarity, nuclear irregularities and prominent (macro) nucleoli (inset) and mitoses, which may occasionally be abnormal, are usually prominent.

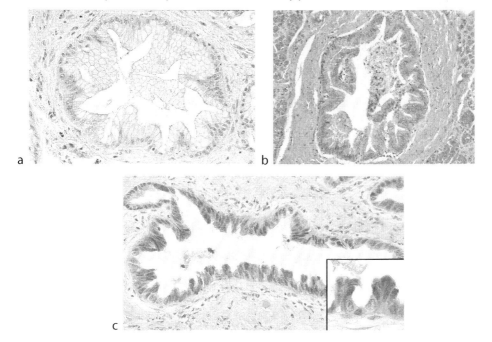

a   b

c

tumor [32–34], and this obviously raises possibility of curative intervention. There are essentially three tumor types that can be included in this category of mass-forming preinvasive neoplasia: *mucinous cystic neoplasms, intraductal papillary mucinous neoplasms and intraductal oncocytic papillary neoplasms*, the latter regarded as subtype of IPMN by some authors [22,35,36].

These lesions are being encountered with increasing frequency and constitute >10% of pancreatic resections in some institutions [37,38], especially because they are often resectable tumors. The incidence of invasive carcinoma in these tumors is about 25%. Conversely, the estimated ratio for invasive pancreatic adenocarcinomas to arise in association with these lesions is about 1%. Even though there are controversies regarding their management, it is certain that these tumors are potentially curable and because of this, the differential features of the lesions under this category and recognizing their clinicopathologic characteristics is important.

Intraductal Papillary Mucinous Neoplasms Intraductal papillary mucinous neoplasms (IPMNs) are characterized by intraductal proliferation of mucin-producing neoplastic cells that often form papillary configuration and lead to cystic dilatation of the ducts [39–49] (◑ *Fig. 3-11*). This process is reflected in imaging studies as dilatation of the ductal system with cyst formation and thus used to be called "ductectatic mucinous cystic neoplasm," and endoscopically, they are often associated with mucin extrusion from ampulla of Vater, thus the previous name, "mucin-producing tumor."

There is a spectrum of neoplastic transformation in IPMNs representing *adenoma-carcinoma sequence*. Those with no cytoarchitectural atypia are classified by the WHO as *adenoma* [50] (or *low-grade dysplasia* by the recent AFIP proposal [51]). Included in this group are those that are so innocuous that they used to be called "hyperplasia" in the Japanese literature. These are composed of relatively simple papillary units lined by well-polarized,

◘ Fig. 3-11

Intraductal papillary mucinous neoplasm (IPMN). Tall, exuberant papillary structures lined by columnar cells with abundant mucin and cigar-shaped nuclei filling and dilating the ducts (cystic transformation). The overall picture of the process is highly similar to that of villous adenomas of the colon.

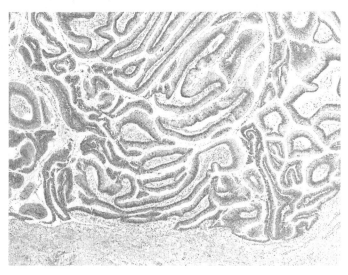

tall columnar cells with basally oriented non-atypical nuclei and abundant apical cytoplasm with mucin. As the neoplasm progresses, presumably with accumulation of other molecular-genetic alterations, the cells begin to show morphologic alterations including hyperchromatism, pleomorphism (variably sized and shaped nuclei), along with loss of organization. Proliferation of cells lead to complex papillary elements and irregular clustering of cells, and mitotic figures become evident. Altogether, these are reflections of cancerous transformation of the epithelium, and termed *high-grade dysplasia or carcinoma in situ.* [42,43,52,53]. The wide spectrum in between the adenoma and CIS is classified as *borderline* or *intermediate grade.* The cancerous transformation within an IPMN culminates in invasive carcinoma in many patients. There are two types of invasive carcinomas that occur: (1) ductal (tubular) type [40,41], which is virtually indistinguishable from conventional ductal adenocarcinoma of the pancreas discussed previously, and often behaves like one as well (with rapid recurrences, metastasis and fatality [54] and (2) colloid type [21], characterized by abundant extracellular mucin in which the carcinoma cells "float" (◉ *Fig. 3-9*). Presumably due to the containing effect of this stromal mucin, the spread of colloid carcinoma cells is much slower and prognosis is significantly better than that of the ductal type [23].

Despite the earlier concerns and contentions, it has become clear in the past few years that if these tumors are carefully evaluated by experts, and the possibility of in situ and invasive carcinoma is excluded definitively, this classification of IPMNs as adenoma, *carcinoma in situ* or invasive is highly predictive of clinical outcome [54]. The important issue is that it is difficult to ascertain the absence of carcinoma without thorough pathologic examination of the tumors because foci of carcinoma can be focal and well hidden [55], not only from the eyes of the imagers on radiologic/endoscopic examination, but even naked eyes inspecting the resected tumors in the pathology gross rooms; thus the mandate for complete microscopic examination of these lesions. There are, however, surrogate findings that seem to be very helpful in preoperative classification of most (unfortunately not all) patients with IPMN. Most IPMNs confined to the *branch ducts* in the uncinate process tend to be small and less complex and prove to be adenomas (i.e., without carcinoma) by pathologic examination [56,57]. The cell type of these "branch-duct type IPMNs" also tends to be of gastric-foveolar type [58]. Studies have shown that if a branch-duct IPMN is asymptomatic, smaller than 3 cm, without mural nodularities (lack of complex papillary nodules) and EUS-guided cytologic examination fails to show any suspicious cells, the case can be managed conservatively because most of these prove to be adenomas [37,38,57,59]. In contrast, branch-duct IPMNs that are larger and more complex with suspicious findings have a higher incidence of malignancy, which appears to justify surgery. IPMNs that also involve the main duct is referred as *main-duct* type. These have a high propensity to contain or evolve into frank carcinoma and for this reason they typically warrant resection [37,38,57]. Interestingly, these commonly show villous-intestinal pattern virtually indistinguishable from colonic villous adenomas [58]; in fact, some were previously reported as villous adenoma of Wirsung duct. This metaplastic intestinal differentiation, which is also reflected at molecular level by expression of markers of intestinal programming, namely MUC2 and CDX2 [58], is an intriguing and unique aspect of IPMNs. The problem is that these main-duct type IPMNs are also often diffuse, involving a large portion of or the entire pancreas, thus their complete removal often mean total pancreatectomy [54], which is an operation with relatively high complication rate, and it is difficult to balance the risk-benefit ratio in such patients, especially considering most IPMN patients are relatively old (mean age, 68) with other comorbid conditions. Interestingly, many patients with IPMNs also have other neoplasms [41].

Mucinous Cystic Neoplasms Mucinous cystic neoplasms (MCNs) are seen almost exclusively in perimenopausal women (mean age 48; >95% of the patients are female). They typically form a thick-walled multilocular cyst in the body or the tail of pancreas [60–66]. Some examples may become infected and mimic pseudocysts. In most, there is no obvious communication with the ductal system, which distinguishes MCNs from IPMNs. Cyst fluid is often rich in mucin-related glycoproteins and oncoproteins such as CEA, which may help differentiate these tumors from serous adenomas (see below) preoperatively. The cysts are lined by a mucinous epithelium, which, similar to IPMNs, may exhibit various degrees of cytologic and architectural atypia that have been traditionally graded as adenoma, borderline or *carcinoma in situ*, and currently also classified as low-, intermediate-, and high-grade/CIS [9,50–52]. Typically, small (<3 cm) and less complex lesions tend to be adenomas, whereas larger, more complex lesions with abundant intracystic papillary nodules may harbor carcinoma (in situ or invasive). As happened for IPMNs, although some studies have questioned the validity of grading MCNs, it has become evident in the past few years that if these tumors are examined thoroughly and the presence of in situ and invasive carcinoma excluded, the grade does accurately predict the clinical outcome [61,62,64,65], and that the cases classified as adenoma or borderline (low- or intermediate-grade dysplasia) are typically cured by complete removal. One caveat, however, is that both in situ and invasive carcinoma may be very focal and easily missed if the tumor is not thoroughly examined, and for this reason some authors advocate the total submission of these tumors for microscopic evaluation. Most authors agree that these tumors ought to be resected completely.

A microscopic feature that has become a requirement for the diagnosis of MCN is the presence of an "ovarian-type" stroma (◗ *Fig. 3-12*) [37,38]. This stroma is not only similar to

◘ Fig. 3-12

Mucinous cystadenoma (MCN). The cyst lining is composed of tall columnar mucinous epithelium, surrounded by a cuff of distinctive hypercellular stroma, which shows all the characteristics of ovarian stroma.

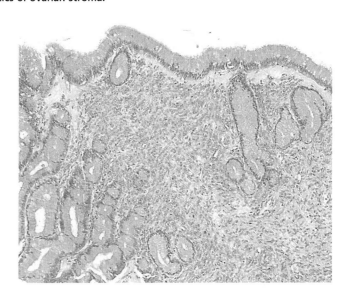

that of the ovarian cortex, but also expresses estrogen and progesterone receptors that are detectable by immunohistochemistry, suggesting that hormones may have a role on initiation and progression of these tumors. This distinctive mesenchyme also helps distinguish MCN from other similar neoplasms, especially IPMNs.

Invasive carcinoma is seen in 5–35% of the MCNs resected [63–66]. In a recent study, invasive carcinomas arising in association with MCNs were found to be predominantly of the tubular type [67]. Interestingly, none of the cases had pure colloid type invasion, which is the predominant type of invasion in IPMNs.

2.1.4   Non-Mucinous Ductal Neoplasia

Serous Cystadenoma

Serous cystadenomas (SCA), also called glycogen rich or microcystic adenomas, are seen predominantly in elderly females (mean age 63; female/male = 3/1) [68,69]. They appear to recapitulate centroacinar cells and although they are of ductal lineage, they lack the features of mucinous differentiation. Grossly they form well-demarcated, relatively large lesions (mean size, 9 cm; some up to 25 cm) with a central satellite scar. SCAs are typically composed of innumerable small cysts (microcysts) each measuring a few millimeters, which leads to the characteristic spongy appearance of the lesion by macroscopic examination, thus the name microcystic adenoma. Oligocystic and solid variants have been described but are uncommon. Microscopically the microcysts correspond to variably sized gland-like structures lined by a single layer of non-mucinous cuboidal epithelium that contains intracytoplasmic glycogen that is responsible for the distinctive clear cytoplasm in the tumor cells (◉ *Fig. 3-13*). The cysts contain watery, clear fluid that is devoid of mucin-related gycoproteins and oncoproteins in contrast with mucinous ductal tumors described above. This feature may be helpful in preoperative diagnosis. Similar cysts may be observed in von Hippel–Lindau (VHL) disease [70] and some SCAs show *VHL* gene alterations [71,72]. Concurrent ductal adenocarcinomas, pancreatic endocrine neoplasms and congenital pathologic conditions can be observed in association with SCAs.

Even though SCAs are invariably benign, it appears that a subset has a rapid doubling rate [73], which may be responsible for their large size in some patients. There are also a few serous cystadenocarcinomas of dubious nature reported in the literature [74,75]. Many are histologically identical to their benign counterparts. The only difference reported is that they recur, metastasize or show angioinvasive growth. For those that are reported to recur or metastasize, the question of multifocality rather than true metastatic spread has been raised.

2.2   Endocrine Neoplasia

Aberrant endocrine differentiation (presence of scattered endocrine cells or a small endocrine component) is not uncommon in tumors with ductal differentiation (discussed above) and in acinar tumors (discussed later). However, if a tumor is predominantly composed of cells with endocrine lineage, it is classified as "endocrine." For practical purposes, in the pancreas, the terms endocrine and neuroendocrine are used interchangeably referring to the same process.

□ Fig. 3-13

Serous cystadenoma. Typical honeycomb (microcystic) pattern due to innumerable cysts of various sizes. The lining of these cysts compose of low cuboidal epithelial cells with clear (glycogen-rich) cytoplasm showing distinctive uniform, round, small nuclei with homogenous, dense chromatin (inset).

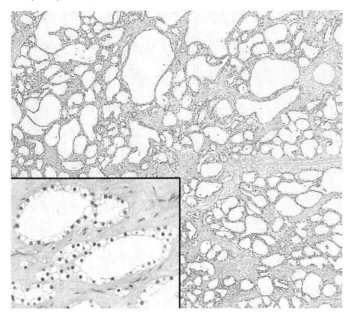

2.2.1 Pancreatic Endocrine Neoplasm

Pancreatic endocrine neoplasms (PENs; previously referred as islet cell tumors) are the majority of the endocrine neoplasms in the pancreas [76]. They recapitulate the islets of Langerhans to variable degrees. Macroscopically they form solid, circumscribed, fleshy lesions that appear significantly different than the scirrhous ductal adenocarcinomas. They can sometimes be multinodular. The tumor cells mimic the islet cells by forming nests, trabecular and gyriform patterns, and show the typical endocrine cytologic features including round monotonous nuclei, salt and pepper chromatin, and moderate amount of cytoplasm (❯ *Fig. 3-14*).

Those that are associated with increased serum levels of hormones and lead to corresponding symptoms are referred as "functional." These constitute nearly half of the PENs and are named according to which hormone they secrete (insulinoma, glucagonoma, gastrinoma, somatostatinoma, VIPoma, and others). Depending on the type and level of hormone secreted, the patients may suffer from a variety of symptoms or "syndromes." For example, insulinoma patients may present with symptoms related to excessive and erratic insulin secretion by the tumor that leads to "Whipple triad": (1) symptoms of hypoglycemia including confusion, convulsion, fatigue and weakness, (2) serum fasting glucose level <50 mg/dL (3) relief of symptoms after intravenous glucose administration. Patients with "glucagonoma syndrome" have weight loss, diabetes mellitus anemia, painful glossitis (sore and red tongue), venous thrombosis and necrolytic migratory erythema. Excessive gastrin production may lead to Zollinger–Ellison syndrome characterized by multiple gastric

◘ Fig. 3-14
Pancreatic endocrine neoplasm. Uniform cells are arranged in nests and nuclear features show the characteristic clumped, "salt and pepper" chromatin pattern.

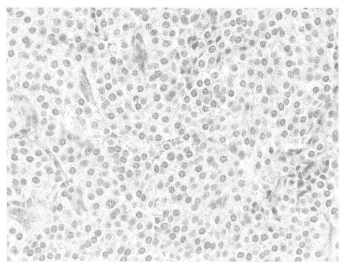

and duodenal ulcers. Interestingly, the amount of hormone detected immunohistochemically in the tumor cells does not necessarily correlate with the functionality status.

There are different approaches in classifying PENs based on the potential behavior of these tumors. According to the WHO-2004 [77], which is not widely used in the United States, PENs are classified into three categories: Category 1 ("well-differentiated endocrine tumor") is reserved for PENs that are confined to the pancreas at the time of diagnosis. This category is further subdivided into two categories as "benign behavior" (Category "1A"), for those that display none of the indicators of aggressive behavior (i.e., tumor size <2 cm, no vascular or perineural invasion, mitotic activity <2/10 high power fields of a microscope, and low proliferation index; i.e., Ki-67 immunolabeling less than 2%) versus "uncertain behavior" (Category "IB") for those that exhibit one of these adverse signs. Category 2 is referred as "well differentiated endocrine *carcinoma*" and is applied to those with extrapancreatic spread or metastasis at the time of diagnosis. This complex terminology can be problematic at times. Moreover, studies have shown that even the ones that are referred as "benign behavior" may occasionally recur or metastasize during long-term follow up, and those of "uncertain behavior" have recurrences and metastasis in 40% of the cases in long-term (10-year) follow up [78].

The other approach by the group at Memorial Sloan–Kettering [79] regards all PENs as potentially malignant, and divides them into *low-grade* and *intermediate-grade* groups according to presence of necrosis and their mitotic rate (≥2 per 50 high power fields of the microscope). It is believed that this approach reflects the biologic behavior more accurately and also has strong predictive value. This approach also avoids using terms such as "benign" and "uncertain" for tumors that clearly have malignant behavior in a substantial number of cases.

Additionally, insulinomas also often follow a benign course since they are highly symptomatic even when they are small, thus detected in an early phase. PENs associated with multiple endocrine neoplasia, type 1 (MEN-1) tend to be multifocal and less aggressive as well.

MEN-1 patients also often have multiple microscopic (<0.5 cm) nodules (dysplasia), which can be regarded as precursors of fully developed PENs.

As discussed above, PENs are low-grade malignancies. Those that are diagnosed at an early stage are often (but not always) curable, and on the other hand, even those that are advanced with metastases may have a relatively protracted clinical course that may stretch up to decades. It should be noted here though that poorly differentiated counterpart of these tumors ("poorly differentiated neuroendocrine carcinomas," also called small cell carcinomas) are highly aggressive and rapidly fatal tumors. Thankfully, these are exceedingly uncommon.

2.3 Acinar Neoplasia

Focal acinar differentiation can occasionally be observed as a small component of PENs and is also present as an important constituent of pancreatoblastomas (see below); however, most pancreatic tumors with predominant acinar differentiation are acinar cell carcinomas. With the exception of the recently described acinar cell cystadenoma, which is probably not a neoplasm (also called cystic acinar transformation) [80], acinar differentiation is seen essentially only in malignant neoplasms in this organ.

2.3.1 Acinar Cell Carcinoma

Acinar cell carcinomas (ACCs) are rare neoplasms constituting <1% of all pancreatic carcinomas [81,82]. Occasionally, the neoplastic cells may secrete lipase and other digestive enzymes to the serum which may lead to the so-called lipase hypersecretion syndrome characterized by fat necrosis, polyarthopathy, occasional eosinophilia and non bacterial thrombotic endocarditis. Elevated levels of AFP in serum may also be observed.

Most ACCs are large (mean, 10 cm) at diagnosis, and patients often present with early metastasis to liver and lymph nodes. Macroscopically they form a well-delineated, nodular, fleshy, yellow-tan tumor. Dense fibrotic appearance created by desmoplastic stroma characteristic of ductal adenocarcinoma is not a feature of ACCs. Microscopically these are highly cellular tumors with solid sheets of cells that may form nests or rosette-like (acinar) patterns (◉ Fig. 3-15). Many examples maintain production of digestive enzymes, which is represented as a distinctive eosinophilic granularity in the apical portions of their cytoplasms. These zymogenic granules are positive immunohistochemically by antibodies targeting specific enzymes trypsin, chymotrypsin, and lipase. Nuclei of acinar cell carcinomas are fairly round and relatively uniform. The most distinctive histologic feature of this tumor type is the presence of single prominent eosinophilic nucleolus (◉ Fig. 3-15), recapitulating the normal acinar cells. K-ras mutation, which is positive in more than 90% of ductal adenocarcinoma, is negative in ACCs; in contrast, ACCs show beta-catenin expression.

Aberrant and mixed differentiation, especially endocrine, is quite common in acinar tumors (see below) [83]. Also some ACCs exhibit prominent intraductal growth associated with papillary and papillocystic patterns [84]. Such cases can be mistaken as other intraductal neoplasia including intraductal papillary mucinous neoplasms or intraductal tubular carcinomas. On occasion, ACCs may present as cystic tumors.

Acinar cell carcinomas are fairly aggressive neoplasms. Liver metastases are seen in more than half of the cases, and are mostly present at the time of diagnosis. However, the overall

■ Fig. 3-15

Acinar cell carcinoma. The tumor cells are highly atypical but at the same time fairly monotonous and round. They display markedly chromopholic cytoplasm, mostly reflecting the enzymatic granules and cytoplasmic organelles involved in their production. Single prominent nucleoli are also among the most distinctive histologic features of this tumor type.

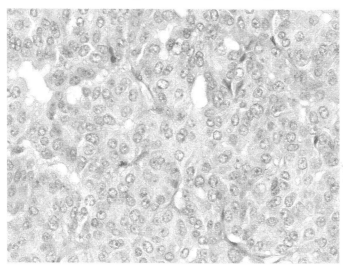

prognosis seems to be better than that of ductal adenocarcinoma. Recent studies have documented a 5-year survival of more than 40% (as opposed to <5% for ductal adenocarcinoma) [85,86].

2.4   Neoplasms with Multiple Lineages (Pancreatoblastoma and Mixed Acinar-Endocrine Carcinoma)

Aberrant differentiation is exceedingly rare in the ductal adenocarcinoma whereas it is rather common in non-ductal tumors.

Pancreatoblastoma is the principle example of the tumors with polyphenotypic differentiation; all three main constituents of normal pancreas, namely acinar, ductal and endocrine are represented in pancreatoblastomas, the acinar elements being the most consistent. In many ways, pancreatoblastoma can be regarded as pancreatic counterpart of other childhood "blastic" tumors such as Wilms (nephroblastoma), which is also a multi-lineage neoplasm. Pancreatoblastomas are very rare; however, they are the most frequent pancreatic tumor of early childhood (mean age 4). There appears to be a second peak in adults of 1930s [87]. Elevated serum levels of AFP can be observed and the tumors might be associated with Beckwith-Widemann [88] or familial adenomatous polyposis (FAP) syndromes.

Grossly they form large (7–18 cm), well-demarcated, solitary, solid, multilobulated tumors that can extend outside of the pancreas. Microscopically, solid sheets, nests, trabecula and strands of neoplastic cells are divided by variable amount of stroma, which on occasion may contain heterologous elements such as osteoid. Necrosis may be present. Squamoid corpuscles composed of large, spindled squamoid cells that form small morular arrangements, occasionally with keratinization, are a pathognomonic finding of pancreatoblastoma (❯ *Fig. 3-16*), not seen in other tumor types of the pancreas. Acinar ductal and endocrine elements can be highlighted by the markers discussed in the corresponding sections. Genetic alterations are similar to those of ACC's and starkly different from the ones seen in ductal adenocarcinomas [89].

As in other "blastic" tumors of childhood, pancreatoblastomas also appear to be chemotherapy-sensitive, and is even curable if detected at an early stage [87]. It is typically fatal in adults. Although experience is rather limited, 5-year survival is generally considered to be about 25%.

In addition to pancreatoblastoma, prominent multi-lineage differentiation is also seen in tumors that are classified as "*mixed*." While acinar carcinomas often show focal aberrant endocrine differentiation in forms of microfoci or scattered individual cells, in some cases, there is a well-established, prominent endocrine component. If this component constitutes more than 25% of the tumor, the designation of "mixed acinar-endocrine" carcinoma is given [83]. Similarly, on occasion, acinar carcinomas may have a significant ductal component, and if this component is more than 25% of the tumor, the diagnosis of "mixed acinar-ductal" carcinoma is rendered. It may be important to note that in these "mixed" carcinomas, invariably the dominant component is acinar. Mixed carcinomas are very rare, thus their clinical behavior is difficult to ascertain, but most appear to behave like acinar carcinomas (discussed above).

⬛ Fig. 3-16

Pancreatoblastoma. The acinar component predominates in most pancreatoblastomas as seen here. The most distinctive and characteristic finding in this tumor type is the *squamoid corpuscles,* which are well defined nests of plump to spindle-shaped cells that form a vague fascicular or whorled pattern highly similar to the "morules" seen in other malignant tumors related to beta-catenin pathway alterations.

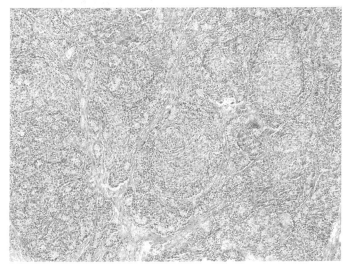

2.5   Neoplasms of Uncertain Histogenesis

2.5.1   Solid Pseudopapillary Neoplasm

Solid pseudopapillary neoplasm (SPN) is a peculiar tumor of indeterminate lineage. This is reflected in the various descriptive names previously used for this tumor: "papillary-cystic," "cystic and papillary," "solid and cystic," and "solid and papillary" [90]. It is also known as Frantz or Hamoudi tumor, crediting the observers that recognized this as a distinct category.

Clinically, SPNs are significantly more common in women (male/female = 1/9). They have been described in all age groups, but the mean age is 30 [91]. Symptoms are nonspecific, and some cases are detected incidentally following trauma or during gynecologic or obstetrical exams. As experience with these relatively uncommon tumors developed, it became clear that these are essentially solid tumors, which often undergo cystic degeneration [91,92]. Unlike in other cystic tumors, the cysts are not lined by an epithelium. Grossly, their appearances vary from beige-tan to brown-hemorrhagic depending on the degree of hemorrhage and degeneration. Histomorphologically, SPNs typically show diffuse cellular proliferation of relatively bland appearing cells admixed with variable degree of stroma ranging from dense collagen, to myxoid, to hemorrhagic (❱ Fig. 3-17). The cells can also be arranged in vague nests, intervened by fairly dense but relatively inconspicuous microvasculature. The preferential dyscohesiveness of the cells away from the microvasculature, presumably related to the alterations in cell adhesion molecules (catenins and cadherins) [93,94], lead to the highly distinctive arrangement of cells that is referred as "pseudopapillary," which was recently incorporated to the name of this entity, although it is not present in all cases. Other characteristic and rather specific findings include nuclear grooves and the eosinophilic cytoplasmic globules.

◻ Fig. 3-17

Solid pseudopapillary tumor. Prominent pseudopapillary growth pattern is seen most cases, and is a characteristic feature of this enigmatic tumor.

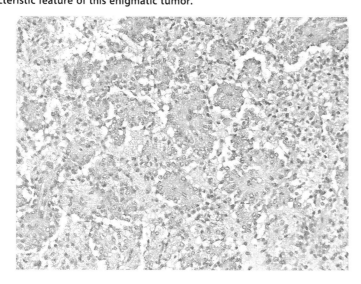

Despite intensive study, the line of differentiation of these neoplasms remains uncertain [91,92]. Although some cases appear to exhibit some endocrine differentiation, chromogranin is never expressed. Both acinar and ductal markers are also consistently negative. In fact, the weak expression of keratin casts doubt on even epithelial nature of these tumors, although some authors classify them as "carcinoma." There are various markers expressed by this neoplasm that were thought could be helpful in its diagnosis, and also in establishing its lineage; however, none are specific. These include vimentin, alpha-1-antitrypsin, progesteron receptors, beta-catenin, CD10 and CD56. Among these, beta-catenin expression appears to be most helpful because it is not seen in endocrine tumors, which is the main differential. Furthermore, its presence suggests a role of beta-catenin pathway in the pathogenesis of these tumors.

SPNs are considered malignant, but metastases occur in only 10–15% of cases [91]. In almost every instance, metastases are either in the liver or peritoneum; nodal metastases are rare. Interestingly, even patients with metastatic disease often survive for many years (even decades) with few symptoms. In fact, only rare deaths have been attributed to direct effects of SPNs. None of the pathologic findings, with the exception of anaplastic/sarcomatoid differentiation, have been proven of value in determining which rare cases will have metastasis [95,96].

2.6   Miscellaneous Cystic Pancreatic Lesions

In contrast to the ones seen in salivary glands, *lymphoepithelial cysts* (LEC) of the pancreas [97] do not show any association with immunosupressive, autoimmune or malignant diseases. They are mainly seen in adult men (mean age: 52, male/female = 3/1) [97,98] and usually are asymptomatic and incidental lesions, which can locate within the pancreas or protrude from the pancreas and present as a peripancreatic mass. Gross examination reveals a well demarcated, often encapsulated, uni/multilocular cystic lesion with semisolid, caseous keratinaceous or sometimes watery luminal contents. Histologically, the cysts lined by mature stratified squamous epithelium with variable keratinization are surrounded by a band of dense lymphoid tissue, which may show lymphoid follicle formation. Lymphoepithelial islands can also be seen in some cases. Leakage of the cyst content might cause inflammatory reaction and granuloma formation in the surrounding tissue. Cholesterol clefts, fat necrosis can be seen as well. LEC-like epidermoid cysts may evolve in intrapancreatic accessory spleens.

Other entities that may form cystic lesions are the following: *Dermoid cysts* [97,98] are similar to LECs but lack of lymphoid tissue and have skin adnexal elements including sebaceous glands. *Lymphangiomas* [99] are seen in young females (mean age 29, male/female = 1/3) and form endothelial-lined cysts surrounded by a rim of lymphocytes and foamy histiocytes. *Squamoid cyst of pancreatic ducts* is a recently described entity that is probably reactive in nature but may produce high CEA levels [100]. *Congenital cysts* [101] and *intestinal duplications* may also form cystic lesions in the vicinity of the pancreas and periampullary region. These may have variable lining including respiratory-type, intestinal, squamous or transitional.

2.7   Mesenchymal Tumors

Mesenchymal tumors including fibromatosis (desmoid tumor), solitary fibrous tumor, leiomyoma, schwannoma, primary sarcomas such as primitive neuroectodermal tumor, synovial sarcoma, desmoplastic small round cell tumor, leiomyosarcoma, malignant fibrous histiocytoma, and others may rarely arise primarily in pancreas [102–104].

2.8   Pseudotumors

In the pancreas, a variety of non-neoplastic conditions may form solid masses that may mimic cancer. Up to 5% of pancreatectomies performed with the preoperative clinical diagnosis of carcinoma prove to be non-neoplastic by pathologic examination, although this figure has been on a steep decline in the past few years with improved preoperative diagnostic modalities and the experience in their usage. Chronic inflammatory lesions are the leading cause of pseudotumor formation, and among these, two entities remain highly problematic as close mimickers of cancer: (1) Lymphoplasmacytic sclerosing variant of autoimmune pancreatitis is characterized by a pseudotumor composed of dense lymphoplasmacytic infiltrates, in particular IgG4-positive plasma cells, which concentrate around the ducts ("duct-centric pancreatitis") as well as medium sized venules (periphlebitis), and is associated with prominent proliferation of fibroblasts. The process may be associated with diffuse enlargement of pancreatic tissue or may form a localized lesion. Autoimmune disorders are evident in only 25% of the cases at the time of diagnosis, but serum IgG4 levels are fairly high in most cases, which can be very helpful in distinguishing it from carcinoma [105–107]. (2) Paraduodenal pancreatitis, previously also referred as cystic dystrophy of heterotopic pancreas, paraduodenal wall cyst, or groove pancreatitis, typically forms thickening, nodularities and stricture of duodenal wall at the region of accessory ampulla and resembles periampullary cancers. The lesion is characterized by dense myoid proliferation of stroma admixed with pancreatic ducts, rounded acinar lobules, extravasated acinar secretions that illicit stromal and inflammatory reaction rich in eosinophils, as well as Brunner's gland hyperplasia. Most patients are middle aged and have history of alcohol abuse. It is hypothesized that paraduodenal pancreatitis forms as a result of localized alcoholic pancreatitis differentially involving the region drained by the accessory duct.

Other lesions that may form pseudotumor and mimic cancer are the following [107]: *Adenomyomatous hyperplasia of ampulla of Vater* is a subtle lesion that is difficult to define; larger examples (>5 mm) have been found to be the cause of obstructive jaundice. *Accessory (heterotopic) spleen* may also form a well-defined nodule within the tail of the pancreas and is typically mistaken for endocrine neoplasm. *Lipomatous hypertrophy* is the replacement of pancreatic tissue with mature adipose tissue that occasionally leads to moderate to marked enlargement of the pancreas. *Hamartomas* are very rare if the entity is defined strictly. They are characterized by irregularly arranged mature pancreatic elements admixed with stromal tissue. A cellular, spindle-cell variant with c-kit (CD117) expression is recognized. *Pseudolymphomas* form well-defined nodules composed of hyperplastic lymphoid tissue. Rarely, foreign-body deposits, granulomatous inflammations (such as sarcoidosis or tuberculosis), and congenital lesions may form tumoral lesions.

2.9   Secondary Tumors

Secondary tumors involving the pancreas can be listed according to the decreased frequency as: pulmonary tumors, lymphomas, gastrointestinal tract carcinomas, renal cell carcinomas and breast carcinomas [108]. Majority are detected only at autopsy [2]. Tumors arising in retroperitoneum, nearby lymph nodes or gastrointestinal system may also show direct extension to the pancreas. Lymphomas and renal cell carcinomas involving the pancreas are more prone to mimic primary cancers [108]. Renal cell carcinomas may even form polypoid ampullary lesions and may grow within ducts.

3   Conclusion

The vast majority of pancreatic neoplasms are of ductal lineage rather than endocrine or acinar; thus most research focuses on the ductal tumors. Consequently, significant developments have taken place in the classification and in our understanding of ductal neoplasia in the recent years.

A major recent development was the more unified terminology and grading of precursor lesions, namely pancreatic intraepithelial neoplasia (PanIN) 1A, 1B, 2, and 3 comprising a neoplastic transformation ranging from early mucinous change (PanIN-1A) to frank *carcinoma in situ* (PanIN-3).

Also, it is now well known that even the different types of ductal neoplasia vary greatly in their clinicopathologic characteristics and prognoses. Although invasive ductal adenocarcinoma, the most common carcinoma occurring in the pancreas, is one of the deadliest of all cancers; cystic lesions are often either benign or low-grade indolent neoplasia. Better characterization of cystic ductal tumors such as intraductal papillary mucinous neoplasms and mucinous cystic neoplasms has been a major step not only from the standpoint of patient care but also for cancer researchers, because they serve as an interesting model of carcinogenesis. They have well-established malignant potential, representing an *adenoma-carcinoma sequence* that often culminates in invasive carcinoma. Invasive carcinomas in intraductal papillary mucinous neoplasms are predominantly colloid type, which is now regarded as clinicopathologically distinct type of pancreas cancer with indolent behavior.

Among non-ductal tumors of the pancreas, endocrine neoplasms are by far the most common and form an important category. Majority of these are low-intermediate grade malignancies and their behavior is far better than that of invasive ductal adenocarcinoma. Those that are treated at an early stage are even considered "benign." However, it should be noted that high grade neuroendocrine carcinomas are highly aggressive and rapidly fatal tumors.

Key Practice Points

- Pancreatic neoplasms are classified according to which normal cell type of this organ they recapitulate (ductal, acinar, endocrine), because the clinicopathologic and biologic characteristics of tumors are determined or manifested mostly by their cellular lineage.
- Most pancreatic neoplasms are of ductal lineage. Invasive ductal adenocarcinoma constitutes the vast majority (>85%) of carcinomas of ductal lineage. These are rapidly progressive and highly aggressive solid tumors despite their relatively well-differentiated appearance. They have a tendency to illicit abundant desmoplastic stroma, and high propensity for perineural invasion and vascular spread.
- In contrast with solid tumors, cystic lesions of the pancreas are often either benign or low-grade indolent neoplasia. However, those that are mucinous, namely intraductal papillary

mucinous neoplasms (IPMNs) and mucinous cystic neoplasms (MCNs), constitute an important category, because they have well-established malignant potential, representing an *adenoma-carcinoma sequence*. Approximately one third of IPMNs and MCNs have an associated invasive carcinoma. Invasive carcinoma in IPMNs is predominantly colloid type, and those associated with MCNs are almost exclusively of the ordinary ductal type.

- Among non-ductal tumors, pancreatic endocrine neoplasms (PENs) are by far the most common. These are much more indolent tumors than ductal adenocarcinomas and can be associated with multiple endocrine neoplasia, type 1 (MEN-1). They form solid, circumscribed, fleshy lesions. Microscopically the tumor cells mimic the islet cells.

Future Scientific Directions

- Most of the ductal adenocarcinoma tissue is composed of desmoplastic stroma not the cancer cells. Therefore, if the intend is to analyze the carcinoma cells, carcinoma cells need to be dissected out from the background tissue, or alternatively, visual-aided methods of analysis such as immunohistochemistry or in situ hybridization ought to be utilized.
- *Preinvasive* neoplasms (PanINs, IPMNs and MCNs) constitute a very important category not only because they are early cancers and thus catching in early stage often leads to cure but also they offer an invaluable model of carcinogenesis to analyze. They all show a spectrum of cytoarchitectural atypia. It is now known that starting with the earliest forms of neoplastic transformation, the process advances to accumulate genetic abnormalities. Some of these abnormalities are well documented in the literature but a lot more awaits to be elucidated.
- A major subset of IPMNs appears to represent a "metaplastic" intestinal differentiation. The mechanisms of carcinogenesis of this metaplastic pathway might shed new light to pancreatic tumorigenesis in general.
- On the cyst wall and septae of MCNs, a distinctive ovarian-type stroma that regularly expresses progesterone receptors, and sometimes estrogen receptors is seen. This stroma is an entity-defining feature of these neoplasms, to an extent that it has become a requirement for the diagnosis. Moreover, some MCNs are reported to be associated with ovarian thecomas. Efforts should be made to further elucidate the nature of this stroma, and hormone influence in the pathogenesis of these neoplasms.
- Despite intensive study, the line of differentiation of solid pseudopapillary neoplasm remains uncertain.
- Currently, it is difficult to determine which PENs will have recurrences and metastasis. More studies are needed to more accurately estimate the malignant potential of a given PEN.

Clinical Implications

- Invasive ductal adenocarcinoma cases have highly insidious infiltrative patterns, and often the carcinoma cells are spread far beyond the seemingly confines of the main tumor. Perineural invasion is common and is thought to be the reason of back pain, one of the more common symptoms of this tumor.

- It has become clear in the past few years that if IPMNs are carefully evaluated, and the possibility of in situ and invasive carcinoma is excluded definitively, classification of IPMNs as adenoma, *carcinoma in situ* or invasive is highly predictive of clinical outcome. This is also valid for MCNs.
- There are surrogate findings that seem to be very helpful in preoperative classification of most patients with IPMN. Most IPMNs confined to the *branch ducts* in the uncinate process tend to be small and less complex and prove to be adenomas by pathologic examination. In contrast, IPMNs involving main ducts are usually larger and more complex with suspicious findings and have a higher incidence of malignancy.
- Pancreatic endocrine neoplasms are low-grade malignancies. Those that are diagnosed at an early stage are often curable. Even those that are advanced with metastases may have a relatively protracted clinical course. It should be noted here though those poorly differentiated counterparts of these tumors (poorly differentiated neuroendocrine carcinomas) are highly aggressive and rapidly fatal tumors.
- Nearly half of the PENs are associated with increased serum levels of hormones and are named according to which hormone they secrete (insulinoma, glucagonoma, gastrinoma, somatostatinoma, VIPoma, etc). Depending on the type and level of hormone secreted, the patients may suffer from a variety of symptoms or "syndromes."

References

1. Jemal A, Siegel R, Ward E, et al.: Cancer statistics, 2006. CA Cancer J Clin 2006;56(2):106–130.
2. Klimstra DS, Adsay NV: Benign and malignant tumors of the pancreas. In Surgical Pathology of the GI Tract, Liver, Biliary Tract and Pancreas. RD Odze, JR Goldblum, JM Crawford (eds.). Philadelphia: Saunders, 2004, pp. 699–731.
3. Klimstra DS: Cell lineage in pancreatic neoplasms. In Pancreatic Cancer: Advances in Molecular Pathology, Diagnosis and Clinical Management. F Sarkar, MC Dugan (eds.). Natick: Biotechniques, 1998.
4. Chen J, Baithun SI: Morphological study of 391 cases of exocrine pancreatic tumours with special reference to the classification of exocrine pancreatic carcinoma. J Pathol 1985;146(1):17–29.
5. Hruban RH, Iacobuzio-Donahue C, Wilentz RE, Goggins M, Kern SE: Molecular pathology of pancreatic cancer. Cancer J 2001;7(4):251–258.
6. VonHoff DD, Evans DB, Hruban RH (eds.): Pancreatic Cancer. Boston: Jones & Bartlett, 2005.
7. Evans DB, Abruzzese JL, Rich TA: Cancer of the pancreas. In Cancer: Principles and Practice of Oncology, 6th ed. VT Devita, S Hellman, SA Rosenberg (eds.). Philadelphia: Lippincott-Raven, 2001, pp. 1126–1161.
8. Jorgensen MT, Fenger C, Kloppel G, Luttges J: Long-term survivors among Danish patients after resection for ductal adenocarcinoma of the pancreas. Scand J Gastroenterol 2008;43(5):581–583.
9. Klöppel G, Hruban RH, Longnecker DS, et al.: Tumours of the exocrine pancreas. In World Health Organization Classification of Tumours-Pathology and Genetics of Tumours of the Digestive System. S Hamilton, LA Aaltonen (eds.). Lyon: IARC Press. 2000, pp. 219–305.
10. Adsay N, Basturk O, Klimstra D, Klöppel G: Pancreatic pseudotumors: non-neoplastic solid lesions of the pancreas that clinically mimic pancreas cancer Semin Diagn Pathol 2005;21(4):260–267.
11. Adsay N, Zamboni G: Paraduodenal pancreatitis: a clinico-pathologically distinct entity unifying "cystic dystrophy of heterotopic pancreas", "para-duodenal wall cyst" and "groove pancreatitis". Semin Diagn Pathol 2005;24(4): 247–254.
12. Adsay NV, Klimstra DS, Klöppel G: Inflammatory conditions and pseudotumors of the pancreas and ampulla. Semin Diagn Pathol 2005; 21(4):260–267.
13. Basturk O, Bandyopadhyay S, Feng J, et al.: Predilection of pancreatic ductal adenocarcinoma cells to form duct-like structures in vascular and perineural spaces, mimicking normal ducts and PanIN: a peculiar form of tumor-stroma interaction. Mod Pathol 2008;20(1):1486A.
14. Bandyopadhyay S, Basturk O, Coban I, et al.: Isolated solitary ducts (naked ducts) in adipose tissue: a specific but underappreciated finding of pancreatic adenocarcinoma and one of the potential reasons of under-staging and high recurrence rate. Am J Surg Pathol 2009;33(3):425–429.

15. Westra WH, Sturm P, Drillenburg P, et al.: K-ras oncogene mutations in osteoclast-like giant cell tumors of the pancreas and liver: genetic evidence to support origin from the duct epithelium. Am J Surg Pathol 1998;22(10):1247–1254.

16. Alguacil-Garcia A, Weiland LH: The histologic spectrum, prognosis, and histogenesis of the sarcomatoid carcinoma of the pancreas. Cancer 1977;39 (3):1181–1189.

17. Dhall D, Klimstra DS: The cellular composition of osteoclastlike giant cell-containing tumors of the pancreatobiliary tree. Am J Surg Pathol 2008;32 (2):335–337.

18. Dworak O, Wittekind C, Koerfgen HP, Gall FP: Osteoclastic giant cell tumor of the pancreas. An immunohistological study and review of the literature. Pathol Res Pract 1993;189(2):228–231.

19. Kardon DE, Thompson LD, Przygodzki RM, Heffess CS: Adenosquamous carcinoma of the pancreas: a clinicopathologic series of 25 cases. Mod Pathol 2001;14(5):443–451.

20. Adsay V, Sarkar F, Vaitkevicius V, Cheng J, Klimstra D: Squamous cell and adenosquamous carcinomas of the pancreas: a clinicopathologic analysis of 11 cases (abstract). Mod Pathol 2000;13(1):179A.

21. Adsay NV, Pierson C, Sarkar F, et al.: Colloid (mucinous noncystic) carcinoma of the pancreas. Am J Surg Pathol 2001;25(1):26–42.

22. Adsay NV, Merati K, Andea A, et al.: The dichotomy in the preinvasive neoplasia to invasive carcinoma sequence in the pancreas: differential MUC1 and MUC2 expression supports the existence of two separate pathways of carcinogenesis. Mod Pathol 2002;15(10):1087–1095.

23. Adsay NV, Merati K, Nassar H, et al.: Pathogenesis of colloid (pure mucinous) carcinoma of exocrine organs: coupling of gel-forming mucin (MUC2) production with altered cell polarity and abnormal cell-stroma interaction may be the key factor in the morphogenesis and indolent behavior of colloid carcinoma in the breast and pancreas. Am J Surg Pathol 2003;27(5):571–578.

24. Wilentz RE, Goggins M, Redston M, et al.: Genetic, immunohistochemical, and clinical features of medullary carcinoma of the pancreas: a newly described and characterized entity. Am J Pathol 2000;156 (5):1641–1651.

25. Goggins M, Offerhaus GJ, Hilgers W, et al.: Pancreatic adenocarcinomas with DNA replication errors (RER+) are associated with wild-type K-ras and characteristic histopathology. Poor differentiation, a syncytial growth pattern, and pushing borders suggest RER+. Am J Pathol 1998;152(6):1501–1507.

26. Chow LT, Chow WH: Signet-ring mucinous adenocarcinoma of the pancreas. Chin Med Sci J 1994;9 (3):176–178.

27. McArthur CP, Fiorella R, Saran BM: Rare primary signet ring carcinoma of the pancreas. Mo Med 1995;92(6):298–302.

28. Klöppel G, Bommer G, Ruckert K, Seifert G: Intraductal proliferation in the pancreas and its relationship to human and experimental carcinogenesis. Virchows Arch A Pathol Anat Histol 1980;387 (2):221–233.

29. Hruban RH, Adsay NV, Albores-Saavedra J, et al.: Pancreatic intraepithelial neoplasia: a new nomenclature and classification system for pancreatic duct lesions. Am J Surg Pathol 2001;25(5):579–586.

30. Klimstra DS, Longnecker DS: K-ras mutations in pancreatic ductal proliferative lesions. Am J Pathol 1994;145(6):1547–1550.

31. Brat DJ, Lillemoe KD, Yeo CJ, Warfield PB, Hruban RH: Progression of pancreatic intraductal neoplasias to infiltrating adenocarcinoma of the pancreas. Am J Surg Pathol 1998;22(2):163–169.

32. Furukawa T, Kloppel G, Volkan Adsay N, et al.: Classification of types of intraductal papillary-mucinous neoplasm of the pancreas: a consensus study. Virchows Arch 2005;447(5):794–799.

33. Kosmahl M, Pauser U, Peters K, et al.: Cystic neoplasms of the pancreas and tumor-like lesions with cystic features: a review of 418 cases and a classification proposal. Virchows Arch 2004;445 (2):168–178.

34. Adsay NV: Cystic lesions of the pancreas. Mod Pathol 2007;20:71–93.

35. Hruban RH, Takaori K, Klimstra DS, et al.: An illustrated consensus on the classification of pancreatic intraepithelial neoplasia and intraductal papillary mucinous neoplasms. Am J Surg Pathol 2004;28 (8):977–987.

36. Adsay NV, Adair CF, Heffess CS, Klimstra DS: Intraductal oncocytic papillary neoplasms of the pancreas. Am J Surg Pathol 1996;20(8):980–994.

37. Tanaka M: International consensus guidelines for the management of IPMN and MCN of the pancreas. Nippon Shokakibyo Gakkai Zasshi 2007;104 (9):1338–1343.

38. Tanaka M, Chari S, Adsay V, et al.: International consensus guidelines for management of intraductal papillary mucinous neoplasms and mucinous cystic neoplasms of the pancreas. Pancreatology 2006;6(1–2):17–32.

39. Furukawa T, Kloppel G, Volkan Adsay N, et al.: Classification of types of intraductal papillary-mucinous neoplasm of the pancreas: a consensus study. Virchows Arch 2005;447(5):794–799.

40. Adsay NV, Longnecker DS, Klimstra DS: Pancreatic tumors with cystic dilatation of the ducts: intraductal papillary mucinous neoplasms and intraductal oncocytic papillary neoplasms. Semin Diagn Pathol 2000;17(1):16–30.

41. Adsay NV, Conlon KC, Zee SY, Brennan MF, Klimstra DS: Intraductal papillary-mucinous neoplasms of the pancreas: an analysis of in situ and invasive carcinomas in 28 patients. Cancer 2002;94 (1):62–77.

42. Adsay NV: The "new kid on the block": intraductal papillary mucinous neoplasms of the pancreas: current concepts and controversies. Surgery 2003;133 (5):459–463.

43. Klöppel G: Clinicopathologic view of intraductal papillary-mucinous tumor of the pancreas. Hepatogastroenterology 1998;45(24):1981–1985.

44. Longnecker DS: Observations on the etiology and pathogenesis of intraductal papillary-mucinous neoplasms of the pancreas. Hepatogastroenterology 1998;45(24):1973–1980.

45. Fukishima N, Mukai K, Kanai Y, et al.: Intraductal papillary tumors and mucinous cystic tumors of the pancreas: clinicopathologic study of 38 cases. Hum Pathol 1997;28:1010–1017.

46. Sessa F, Solcia E, Capella C, et al.: Intraductal papillary-mucinous tumours represent a distinct group of pancreatic neoplasms: an investigation of tumour cell differentiation and K-ras, p53 and c-erbB-2 abnormalities in 26 patients. Virchows Arch 1994;425(4):357–367.

47. Falconi M, Salvia R, Bassi C, et al.: Clinicopathological features and treatment of intraductal papillary mucinous tumour of the pancreas. Br J Surg 2001;88 (3):376–381.

48. Salvia R, Fernandez-del Castillo C, Bassi C, et al.: Main-duct intraductal papillary mucinous neoplasms of the pancreas: clinical predictors of malignancy and long-term survival following resection. Ann Surg 2004;239(5):678–685; discussion 85–87.

49. Sarr MG, Murr M, Smyrk TC, et al.: Primary cystic neoplasms of the pancreas. Neoplastic disorders of emerging importance-current state-of-the-art and unanswered questions. J Gastrointest Surg 2003;7 (3):417–428.

50. Zamboni G, Kloppel G, Hruban RH, Longnecker DS, Adler G: Mucinous Cystic Neoplasms of the Pancreas, Lyon: IARC Press, 2000.

51. Hruban RH, Pitman MB, Klimsra DS: Tumors of the Pancreas, Vol. 6. Washington: ARP Press, 2007.

52. Klöppel G, Lüttges J: WHO-classification 2000: exocrine pancreatic tumors. Verh Dtsch Ges Pathol 2001;85:219–228.

53. Klöppel G, Hruban RH, Longnecker DS, et al.: Pathology and Genetics of Tumours of the Digestive System. Lyon: IARC Press, 2000.

54. Chari ST, Yadav D, Smyrk TC, et al.: Study of recurrence after surgical resection of intraductal papillary mucinous neoplasm of the pancreas. Gastroenterology 2002;123(5):1500–1507.

55. Yamaguchi K, Ohuchida J, Ohtsuka T, Nakano K, Tanaka M: Intraductal papillary-mucinous tumor of the pancreas concomitant with ductal carcinoma of the pancreas. Pancreatology 2002;2(5):484–490.

56. Sohn TA, Yeo CJ, Cameron JL, et al.: Intraductal papillary mucinous neoplasms of the pancreas: an updated experience. Ann Surg 2004;239(6):788–797; discussion 97–99.

57. Sugiyama M, Izumisato Y, Abe N, et al.: Predictive factors for malignancy in intraductal papillary-mucinous tumours of the pancreas. Br J Surg 2003;90(10):1244–1249.

58. Adsay NV, Merati K, Basturk O, et al.: Pathologically and biologically distinct types of epithelium in intraductal papillary mucinous neoplasms: delineation of an "intestinal" pathway of carcinogenesis in the pancreas. Am J Surg Pathol 2004;28(7):839–848.

59. Crippa S, Fernandez-del Castillo C: Management of intraductal papillary mucinous neoplasms. Curr Gastroenterol Rep 2008;10(2):136–143.

60. Compagno J, Oertel JE: Mucinous cystic neoplasms of the pancreas with overt and latent malignancy (cystadenocarcinoma and cystadenoma). A clinicopathologic study of 41 cases. Am J Clin Pathol 1978;69(6):573–580.

61. Wilentz RE, Albores-Saavedra J, Hruban RH: Mucinous cystic neoplasms of the pancreas. Semin Diagn Pathol 2000;17(1):31–43.

62. Wilentz RE, Talamani MA, Albores-Saavedra J, Hruban RH: Morphology accurately predicts behavior of mucinous cystic neoplasms of the pancreas. Am J Surg Pathol 1999;23(11):1320–1327.

63. Thompson LDR, Becker RC, Pryzgodski RM, Adair CF, Heffess C: Mucinous cystic neoplasm (mucinous cystadenocarcinoma of low malignant potential) of the pancreas: a clinicopathologic study of 130 cases. Am J Surg Pathol 1999; 23(1):1–16.

64. Zamboni G, Scarpa A, Bogina G, et al.: Mucinous cystic tumors of the pancreas: clinicopathological features, prognosis, and relationship to other mucinous cystic tumors. Am J Surg Pathol 1999;23 (4):410–422.

65. Sarr MG, Carpenter HA, Prabhakar LP, et al.: Clinical and pathologic correlation of 84 mucinous cystic neoplasms of the pancreas: can one reliably differentiate benign from malignant (or premalignant) neoplasms? Ann Surg 2000;231(2):205–212.

66. Reddy RP, Smyrk TC, Zapiach M, et al.: Pancreatic mucinous cystic neoplasm defined by ovarian stroma: demographics, clinical features, and prevalence of cancer. Clin Gastroenterol Hepatol 2004;2 (11):1026–1031.

67. Khalifeh I, Qureshi F, Jacques S, et al.: The nature of "ovarian-like" mesenchyme of pancreatic and hepatic mucinous cystic neoplasms: a recapitulation

of the periductal fetal mesenchme? (abstract). Mod Pathol 2004;17(1):304A.

68. Compagno J, Oertel JE: Microcystic adenomas of the pancreas (glycogen-rich cystadenomas): a clinicopathologic study of 34 cases. Am J Clin Pathol 1978;69(3):289–298.

69. Compton CC: Serous cystic tumors of the pancreas. Semin Diagn Pathol 2000;17(1):43–56.

70. Thirabanjasak D, Basturk O, Altinel D, Cheng JD, Adsay NV: Is serous cystadenoma of pancreas a model of clear cell associated angiogenesis and tumorigenesis? Pancreatology 2008; 9:182–188.

71. Kosmahl M, Wagner J, Peters K, Sipos B, Kloppel G: Serous cystic neoplasms of the pancreas: an immunohistochemical analysis revealing alpha-inhibin, neuron-specific enolase, and MUC6 as new markers. Am J Surg Pathol 2004;28(3):339–346.

72. Mohr VH, Vortmeyer AO, Zhuang Z, et al.: Histopathology and molecular genetics of multiple cysts and microcystic (serous) adenomas of the pancreas in von Hippel-Lindau patients. Am J Pathol 2000;157(5):1615–1621.

73. Tseng JF, Warshaw AL, Sahani DV, et al.: Serous cystadenoma of the pancreas: tumor growth rates and recommendations for treatment. Ann Surg 2005;242(3):413–419.

74. Matsumoto T, Hirano S, Yada K, et al.: Malignant serous cystic neoplasm of the pancreas: report of a case and review of the literature. J Clin Gastroenterol 2005;39(3):253–256.

75. Strobel O, Z'Graggen K, Schmitz-Winnenthal FH, et al.: Risk of malignancy in serous cystic neoplasms of the pancreas. Digestion 2003;68(1):24–33.

76. Heitz PU, Kasper M, Polak JM, Kloppel G: Pancreatic endocrine tumors. Hum Pathol 1982; 13:263–271.

77. Heitz PU, Komminoth P, Perren A, et al.: Pancreatic Endocrine Tumors: Introduction. Lyon: IARC Press, 2004.

78. Schmitt AM, Anlauf M, Rousson V, et al.: WHO 2004 criteria and CK19 are reliable prognostic markers in pancreatic endocrine tumors. Am J Surg Pathol 2007;31(11):1677–1682.

79. Hochwald SN, Zee S, Conlon KC, et al.: Prognostic factors in pancreatic endocrine neoplasms: an analysis of 136 cases with a proposal for low-grade and intermediate-grade groups. J Clin Oncol 2002;20 (11):2633–2642.

80. Zamboni G, Terris B, Scarpa A, et al.: Acinar cell cystadenoma of the pancreas: a new entity? Am J Surg Pathol 2002;26(6):698–704.

81. Klimstra DS, Heffess CS, Oertel JE, Rosai J: Acinar cell carcinoma of the pancreas. A clinicopathologic study of 28 cases. Am J Surg Pathol 1992;16 (9):815–837.

82. Holen KD, Klimstra DS, Hummer A, et al.: Clinical characteristics and outcomes from an institutional series of acinar cell carcinoma of the pancreas and related tumors. J Clin Oncol 2002;20(24): 4673–4678.

83. Ohike N, Kosmahl M, Klöppel G: Mixed acinarendocrine carcinoma of the pancreas. A clinicopathological study and comparison with acinar-cell carcinoma. Virchows Arch 2004;445(3):231–235.

84. Basturk O, Zamboni G, Klimstra DS, et al.: Intraductal and papillary variants of acinar cell carcinomas: a new addition to the challenging differential diagnosis of intraductal neoplasms. Am J Surg Pathol 2007;31(3):363–370.

85. Wisnoski NC, Townsend CM, Jr., Nealon WH, Freeman JL, Riall TS: 672 patients with acinar cell carcinoma of the pancreas: a population-based comparison to pancreatic adenocarcinoma. Surgery 2008;144(2):141–148.

86. Kitagami H, Kondo S, Hirano S, et al.: Acinar cell carcinoma of the pancreas: clinical analysis of 115 patients from Pancreatic Cancer Registry of Japan Pancreas Society. Pancreas 2007;35(1):42–46.

87. Klimstra DS, Wenig BM, Adair CF, Heffess CS: Pancreatoblastoma. A clinicopathologic study and review of the literature. Am J Surg Pathol 1995;19 (12):1371–1389.

88. Kerr NJ, Fukuzawa R, Reeve AE, Sullivan MJ: Beckwith-Wiedemann syndrome, pancreatoblastoma, and the wnt signaling pathway. Am J Pathol 2002;160(4):1541–1542; author reply 1542.

89. Cao D, Maitra A, Saavedra JA, et al.: Expression of novel markers of pancreatic ductal adenocarcinoma in pancreatic nonductal neoplasms: additional evidence of different genetic pathways. Mod Pathol 2005;18(6):752–761.

90. Basturk O, Coban I, Adsay NV: Cystic neoplasms of the pancreas. Arch Lab Med 2009;133 (3):438–443.

91. Klimstra DS, Wenig BM, Heffess CS: Solidpseudopapillary tumor of the pancreas: a typically cystic tumor of low malignant potential. Semin Diagn Pathol 2000;17(1):66–81.

92. Solcia E, Capella C, Klöppel G: Tumors of the Pancreas, 3rd ed., Vol. 20. Washington: American Registry of Pathology, 1997.

93. Tiemann K, Heitling U, Kosmahl M, Kloppel G: Solid pseudopapillary neoplasms of the pancreas show an interruption of the Wnt-signaling pathway and express gene products of 11q. Mod Pathol 2007;20(9):955–960.

94. Chetty R, Jain D, Serra S: p120 catenin reduction and cytoplasmic relocalization leads to dysregulation of E-cadherin in solid pseudopapillary tumors of the pancreas. Am J Clin Pathol 2008;130 (1):71–76.

95. Tang LH, Aydin H, Brennan MF, Klimstra DS: Clinically aggressive solid pseudopapillary tumors of the pancreas: a report of two cases with components of undifferentiated carcinoma and a comparative clinicopathologic analysis of 34 conventional cases. Am J Surg Pathol 2005;29 (4):512–519.

96. Nishihara K, Nagoshi M, Tsuneyoshi M, Yamaguchi K, Hayashi I: Papillary cystic tumors of the pancreas. Assessment of their malignant potential. Cancer 1993;71(1):82–92.

97. Adsay NV, Hasteh F, Cheng JD, et al.: Lymphoepithelial cysts of the pancreas: a report of 12 cases and a review of the literature. Mod Pathol 2002;15 (5):492–501.

98. Adsay NV, Hasteh F, Cheng JD, Klimstra DS: Squamous-lined cysts of the pancreas: lymphoepithelial cysts, dermoid cysts (teratomas) and accessory-splenic epidermoid cysts. Semin Diagn Pathol 2000;17(1):56–66.

99. Paal E, Thompson LD, Heffess CS: A clinicopathologic and immunohistochemical study of ten pancreatic lymphangiomas and a review of the literature [published erratum appears in Cancer 1998;83(4):824]. Cancer 1998;82(11):2150–2158.

100. Othman M, Basturk O, Groisman G, Krasinskas A, Adsay NV: Squamoid cyst of pancreatic ducts: a distinct type of cystic lesion in the pancreas. Am J Surg Pathol 2007;31(2):291–297.

101. Martin DF, Haboubi NY, Tweedle DE: Enteric cyst of the pancreas. Gastrointest Radiol 1987;12 (1):35–36.

102. Bismar TA, Basturk O, Gerald WL, Schwarz K, Adsay NV: Desmoplastic small cell tumor in the pancreas. Am J Surg Pathol 2004;28(6):808–812.

103. Khanani F, Kilinc N, Nassar H, et al.: Mesenchymal lesions involving the pancreas (abstract). Mod Pathol 2003;16(1):279A.

104. Lüttges J, Pierre E, Zamboni G, et al.: [Malignant non-epithelial tumors of the pancreas]. Pathologe 1997;18(3):233–237.

105. Zamboni G, Lüttges J, Capelli P, et al.: Histopathological features of diagnostic and clinical relevance in autoimmune pancreatitis: a study on 53 resection specimens and 9 biopsy specimens. Virchows Arch 2004;445(6):552–563.

106. Klimstra DS, Adsay NV: Lymphoplasmacytic sclerosing (autoimmune) pancreatitis. Semin Diagn Pathol 2004;21(4):237–246.

107. Adsay NV, Basturk O, Klimstra DS, Kloppel G: Pancreatic pseudotumors: non-neoplastic solid lesions of the pancreas that clinically mimic pancreas cancer. Semin Diagn Pathol 2004;21(4):260–267.

108. Adsay NV, Andea A, Basturk O, et al.: Secondary tumors of the pancreas: an analysis of a surgical and autopsy database and review of the literature. Virchows Arch 2004;444(6):527–535.

4 Developmental Molecular Biology of the Pancreas

Ondine Cleaver · Raymond J. MacDonald

1	Overview of Pancreatic Development	72
2	Overview of Extrinsic and Intrinsic Developmental Factors	75
2.1	Extrinsic Factors: Cell-Cell Signals	77
2.2	Intrinsic Factors: DNA-Binding Transcription Factors	81
3	The Roles of Extrinsic and Intrinsic Factors During Pancreatic Development	83
3.1	Specification of Endodermal Domains to Pancreatic Fate (6.5–9 dpc)	83
3.1.1	Early Endoderm and Gut Tube Formation	83
3.1.2	Anteroposterior Patterning of the Endoderm	84
3.1.3	Dorsoventral Patterning of the Prepancreatic Endoderm	85
3.1.4	Initiation of Pancreatic Budding	86
3.2	Initial Growth of Pancreatic Buds and the Primary Developmental Transition (9–12 dpc)	88
3.2.1	Growth and Elaboration of Pancreatic Buds	88
3.2.2	Epithelial Lobulation and Branching	89
3.2.3	The Primary Transition	89
3.2.4	The "Proto-Differentiated" State (9.5–12 dpc)	91
3.2.5	Epithelial-Mesenchymal Crosstalk: Control of the "Protodifferentiated" state	91
3.3	Onset of Islet and Acinar Development by the Secondary Developmental Transition (12.5–15.5 dpc)	94
3.3.1	The Secondary Transition	94
3.3.2	Ductal Development	100
3.3.3	The Second Wave of Endocrine Cells – Formation of Primitive Islets	101
3.3.4	Comparison of First and Second Waves of Endocrine Cells	105
3.3.5	Dorsal and Ventral Bud Fusion	106
3.4	Perinatal Growth and Differentiation (16 dpc to Neonate)	106
3.4.1	Isletogenesis	107
4	End Note	107

J. P. Neoptolemos, R. Urrutia, J. L. Abbruzzese, M. W. Büchler (eds.), *Pancreatic Cancer*,
DOI 10.1007/978-0-387-77498-5_4, © Springer Science+Business Media, LLC 2010

Abstract: Pancreatic organogenesis is a complex and coordinated process that generates a compound gland of exocrine tissue composed of acini and ducts, and endocrine tissue organized in islets of Langerhans. Both tissues originate from the same early endodermal epithelium through cell-cell signaling exchanges with associated mesenchyme that direct a cascade of transcriptional regulatory events. Current research is aimed at elucidating the formation of pancreatic cell types and the molecular mechanisms that shape the anatomy and physiology of the pancreas. A number of intrinsic factors, such as transcriptional regulators, and extrinsic signaling factors, such as secreted growth factors, morphogens and cell-surface ligands, have been shown to be determinants of cell-fate decisions, proliferation, or differentiation. The interplay between organ-restricted intrinsic factors and widely used extrinsic factors guides the step-wise process of pancreatic development from early endodermal patterning and specification of the initial pancreatic field, to expansion of pools of progenitors, resolution of individual cell-types, and the differentiation of mature exocrine and endocrine cells. A better understanding of pancreatic development is proving useful for comprehending the regulatory defects that drive pancreatic carcinogenesis and for devising effective therapies to correct those defects.

1   Overview of Pancreatic Development

The mammalian pancreas is a compound gland of exocrine and endocrine epithelia. In adults, the exocrine compartment is composed of ducts and acini and comprises ~90% of the mass of the gland. The endocrine compartment is organized as islets of Langerhans and comprises ~2% [1]. These two tissues serve two distinct functions: (1) the production of digestive enzymes, which are secreted from the exocrine acinar cells and channeled to the duodenum via the ducts; and (2) the regulation of blood sugar levels by the endocrine cells of the islets of Langerhans via the islet vasculature. A description of the embryonic formation of the pancreas must include the genesis of both exocrine and endocrine tissues and the mechanisms that distinguish these two developmental programs and balance the proportion of precursor cells committed to each. Although the organogenesis of the pancreas has been well characterized for mouse, rat, rabbit and chicken, it is much less studied for human. We largely restrict this review to mouse development due to the depth of understanding of the developmental programs in this model system, a direct result of the use of mouse genetics and manipulation of the mouse genome. When known, we note similarities or differences between mouse and human pancreatic development.

The exocrine and endocrine tissues of the pancreas derive from common precursor cells that arise from a dorsal and a ventral domain along the posterior foregut endoderm at the end of gastrulation. The endoderm evaginates (◉ *Fig. 4-1a*) at these two sites to form two epithelial buds encased in mesenchyme (◉ *Fig. 4-1a*; mouse 9.5–10 dpc; human 25–30 dpc). The dorsal bud receives important inductive signals first from the overlying notochord, then from the dorsal aorta and finally from the surrounding mesoderm. The ventral bud receives signals from adjacent splanchnic and procardial mesoderms, as well as from the septum transversum. All epithelial tissues of the pancreas derive from these two endodermal buds, which develop further via a dynamic signaling dialog between the epithelium and the overlying mesenchymes. The dorsal bud generates the gastric and splenic lobes of the murine pancreas, while the ventral bud forms the extensive lobe that runs along the proximal duodenum. In the more compact human pancreas, the dorsal bud forms the head, body and tail, and the ventral bud forms the uncinate process and inferior part of the head.

Shortly after budding (about 10.5 dpc), the pancreatic epithelium initiates dramatic morphogenetic changes including dense branching [2] or epithelial stratification and microlumen formation [3] or both (● Fig. 4-1b). In rodents (but not in humans), the first differentiated endocrine cells appear at this time in the early dorsal bud. The period of bud formation with this early wave of endocrine cells (9.5–10.5 dpc) has been termed the "primary transition" [2]. Slightly later, around 11.5 dpc (35–37 dpc human), both buds have grown and extended, the gut tube turns, and the organ primordia along its axis change their positions relative to each other. At this time, the ventral bud migrates with the bile duct dorsally around the duodenum, resulting in the fusion of the ducts of the dorsal and ventral buds. Whereas the dorsal and ventral pancreases of rodents retain their major ducts, the principal ducts in humans generally fuse to form a main pancreatic duct (of Wirsung) that connects through the ventral pancreas to the common bile duct, while a vestigial accessory duct (of Santorini) maintains its connection to the duodenum through the dorsal pancreas.

By embryonic day 12.5 (40–45 dpc human) cell division has created a densely packed epithelium (● Fig. 4-1c) containing mostly progenitor cells for the islets, acini and ducts. The dynamics of the epithelium are not yet fully understood: either microlumen formation [3] or dense branching [4] generates the tree-like branching pancreas that is evident later (● Fig. 4-1c). The number of progenitor cells in the epithelium at this stage determines the eventual size of the mature pancreas [5]. Detailed three-dimensional rotating views of the development of the mouse pancreatic rudiment up to the secondary transition are invaluable for understanding the first stages of pancreatic morphogenesis [6].

Beginning about 12.5–13 dpc, the epithelium undergoes a striking morphogenesis termed the "secondary transition" [2]. This transformation begins as newly forming branches emerge from specialized multipotent precursor cells at epithelial "tips" [7] and resolves into a dynamic epithelium of branching tubules with acini forming around the organ periphery and islets forming centrally (● Fig. 4-1d). As acini form and begin cellular differentiation, the epithelium continues to grow outward and initiate new acini. Thus, acinar differentiation

● Fig. 4-1

Overview of pancreatic organogenesis. Schematics and photographs of embryonic pancreas depict development at stages indicated, from (a) bud evagination from the endoderm, (b) initiation of stratification or branching, (c) onset of the secondary transition, (d) exocrine and endocrine differentiation, and (e) the maturing anatomy of acinar, ductal and endocrine tissues and associated vasculature just prior to birth. Left panels depict the pancreatic epithelium at each stage (mesenchyme not shown). Note the alternative models for dense branching (left) versus stratification and microlumen formation (right) of the epithelium at 10.5 (B1) and 12.5 dpc (C1). Yellow, pancreatic epithelium; orange, multipotent precursor cells (MPCs); red, differentiating acini; light blue, newly emerged endocrine cells; dark blue, maturing endocrine cells. Middle panels show whole mount views of Pdx1-expressing (blue stain) dorsal and ventral pancreatic buds. At 12.5–15.5 dpc, the pancreas is associated with underlying stomach and duodenum. Right panels show sections through Pdx1-expressing epithelium (blue stain) surrounded by pancreatic mesenchyme (pink eosin staining). a, aorta; ac, acini; d, duodenum; dp, dorsal pancreas; du, duct; ec, endocrine cord; m, mesenchyme; p, portal vein; pa, proacinus; st, stomach; te, tubular precursor epithelium; vp, ventral pancreas.

4

■ Fig. 4-1 (continued)

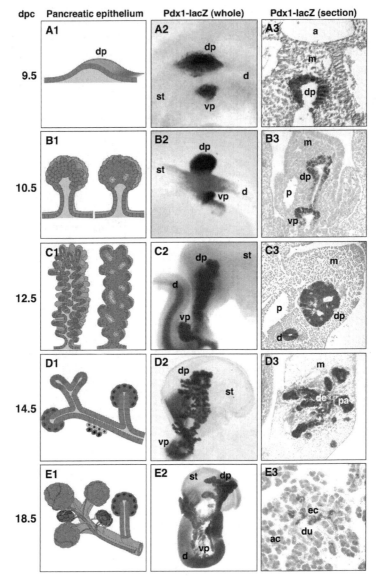

appears as a wave from the interior outward. Pancreatic acini have their own peculiar morphogenesis that is unique among mammalian exocrine glands. The simple tips of the growing epithelium thicken, enlarge, then engulf and extend over the ends of the tubules, which become intra-acinar intercalated ducts (❯ Fig. 4-1d). Consequently, the termini of intercalated ducts extend into the center of the mature acinus [8]. These intra-acinar inter-calated duct cells have been called centroacinar cells and have been postulated to possess stem-cell like qualities [9,10].

Select cells within the interior tubular epithelium commit to islet-cell fate and then escape through a process involving either an epithelial-to-mesenchymal transition (EMT) [11] or a reorientation of the axis of cell division orthogonal to the circumference of the epithelial tubes [2]. The new islet precursor cells associate along the main pancreatic ducts and in close association with the major pancreatic blood vessels. Thus, whereas acini and ducts remain within the topological integrity of the tubular epithelium, individual islet precursor cells delaminate from the epithelium (❯ *Fig. 4-1d*). After a short migration and likely still in contact with the underlying epithelium, these islet precursors coalesce into small amorphous cell clusters, reform epithelial contacts, and then differentiate into one of five major cell types, each of which expresses one of the major pancreatic polypeptide hormones (insulin, glucagon, somatostatin, pancreatic polypeptide, or ghrelin).

Prenatal development continues the expansion of the tree-like ductal and acinar tissues and the maturation of islets (❯ *Fig. 4-1e*). After the secondary transition (in mouse, after ~E15.5), expansion of acinar tissue is predominantly through acinar cell replication rather than de novo formation of acini. Extensive acinar cell cytodifferentiation occurs during this period and is marked by the polarization of cells with basal nuclei surrounded by extensive rough endoplasmic reticulum, a highly active Golgi apparatus, and the accumulation of dense secretory (zymogen) granules that fill the entire apical region of the cells. mRNAs encoding approximately 25 digestive enzymes rise to very high levels and dominate the total mRNA population [12].

Maturation of the islet cell clusters of rodents occurs progressively, starting with the genesis of endocrine cells at the secondary transition and lasting until their gradual coalescence in late gestation and in the weeks after birth. Maturation is characterized by the formation of an α-(glucagon) cell mantle, with interspersed δ- (somatostatin), ε- (ghrelin) and PP- (pancreatic polypeptide) cells surrounding a predominantly β- (insulin) cell core. Prenatal replication of differentiated endocrine cells is infrequent, and the increase of endocrine tissue during embryogenesis is due almost exclusively to de novo formation from precursor cells in the tubules [13].

Postnatal growth and tissue maintenance occurs principally through proliferation of differentiated endocrine and exocrine cells. Replication of insulin-expressing β-cells begins shortly after birth, and gradually decreases until weaning. Dividing β-cells are subsequently uncommon, but are sufficient to maintain β-cell mass [14–16]. Similarly, acinar cell proliferation decreases postnatally [17,18], but appears to be the sole source of acinar cell replacement in mature animals [19].

The common origins of islets, ducts and acini from the duct-like epithelium of the embryonic pancreas, underlies an intimate relationship between islets, ducts and acini in the mature gland [20]. A greater understanding of the development of the endocrine and exocrine compartments, including their structural and physiologic relationships and the principal intrinsic and extrinsic molecular regulators that drive their formation, is important to our growing understanding of the origin and nature of diseases that affect them.

2   Overview of Extrinsic and Intrinsic Developmental Factors

The embryonic formation of all organs is regulated through the step-wise interplay between extracellular developmental signals (generally diffusible extrinsic growth factors, acting as inducers and/or morphogens; see ❯ *Box 4-1*) and intracellular mediators of developmental programs (e.g., transcription factors that bind and control specific target genes see ❯ *Box 4-2*). Extrinsic factors (EFs) alter the interacting network of intrinsic transcription factors (TFs), which in turn adjust the developmental state of a cell by changing its pattern of gene expression. The induction of new regulatory proteins and the loss of others determine the developmental potential of the cell and its response to subsequent signals. Successive signals during a developmental program transform the transcriptional network of precursor cells in a stepwise manner, increasing cellular differentiation and limiting the developmental options in response to later signals. The program-specific response of a certain cell type to a common signal is dictated by the nature of the signal and the developmental history of the cell – i.e., its lineage. The record of a cell's lineage is embodied in a particular collection of TFs and the interacting network they create; this network establishes the competence of the cell to respond to a signal and the type of response that is elicited. This chapter will focus on the nature of the extrinsic (intercellular signals) and intrinsic (mostly transcriptional regulatory proteins) factors for pancreatic organogenesis and the developmental processes they control.

Remarkably, the genesis of the great diversity of cell-types, their integration into distinct complex tissues, and the assembly of tissues into unique organs are directed by a few signaling pathways, each of which is used in the formation of most if not all organs (❯ *Box 4-1*). Usually, a single DNA-binding TF (although sometimes a few related factors) specific to a pathway binds target gene promoters and alters their activity in response to the activation of that pathway. There are six principal developmental signaling pathways, each with their specific transcriptional mediators (❯ *Fig. 4-2*).

1. The Transforming Growth Factor β family (TGFβ/activin/BMP/GDF)-pathway with Smad TFs. The TGFβ pathway is generally subdivided into two: TGFβ/Activin/Nodal using Smads 2 & 3 and BMP using Smads 1, 5 & 8.
2. The Hedgehog (Hh)-pathway with Gli TFs.
3. The Wnt-pathway with Lef/Tcf TFs.
4. The Notch-pathway with Rbpj.
5. Nuclear hormones with intracellular hybrid receptors.
6. Receptor tyrosine kinase (RTK) pathways with a wide variety of extracellular ligand families (such as fibroblast growth factors (FGFs), epidermal growth factor (EGF), Eph-ephrins, and many more) and downstream transcriptional mediators.

All of these pathways are critical to proper pancreatic development.

Box 1 Extrinsic Developmental Factors (EFs): Cell-Cell Signaling Molecules

Cells and tissues send signals across extracellular space via extrinsic factors. The principal signaling pathways that control organogenesis include: TGFbeta/BMP, Notch, Wnt, hedgehog, receptor tyrosine kinase of FGF, EGF, IGF and Eph signaling, nuclear hormone, and JAK/STAT (❯ *Fig. 4-2*). Each pathway regulates developmental decisions through the binding of an extracellular factor (e.g., a Wnt ligand) to a transmembrane receptor (e.g., Frizzled) on a recipient cell. Binding to the receptor transduces an intracellular response into the recipient cell. The response is then propagated as an intracellular signaling event that activates pathway-specific TFs to change gene expression patterns by binding and altering the transcription of a battery of downstream target genes. Myriad extrinsic factors have been demonstrated to control developmental programs. Many of these cell-cell signaling factors have been termed 'morphogens', which are secreted into the extracellular space and that transmit their developmental effects to nearby cells in a concentration-dependent manner. Cells near a source are exposed to high levels of the morphogen and respond in one way, while cells farther away are exposed to lower levels and may respond in a different way. Extrinsic developmental factors can also act in a 'relay' fashion. For example, a cell that secretes an extrinsic factor may induce a transcriptional response in a nearby responding cell, which reacts by secreting a second extrinsic factor that influences other neighboring cells or the initiating cell, and so on, in a signaling dialogue that alters either the fate of responding cells or their own signaling potential.

Extracellular (or extrinsic) signaling molecules are 'cell non-autonomous' factors. In other words, they generally regulate genes/responses in recipient cells, rather than in the cells that produce them. 'Cell non-autonomy' is a genetic designation indicating that mutations in these genes affect neighboring cells rather than the cells in which they are expressed.

Box 2 Intrinsic Developmental Factors: DNA-binding transcription factors (TFs)

Gene regulatory proteins with the ability to recognize and bind short DNA sequences play the central role in controlling the spatial and temporal transcription of developmentally regulated genes. Once bound to a regulatory site in a promoter or enhancer, these proteins recruit chromatin modifying enzyme complexes or additional TF-complexes that initiate or maintain transcription, or, in some instances, do both of these in a stepwise fashion. TFs are often composed of discrete structural domains with specialized functions. A simple DNA-binding TF usually contains a DNA-binding domain, a dimerization domain (TFs often function as homo- or heterodimers), and a transactivation domain (which interacts with the general transcriptional machinery). Approximately 1300 genes in a typical mammalian genome encode DNA-binding TFs. Based on the structural homologies among DNA-binding domains, approximately 30 families of factors are recognized. The major families are classified as zinc finger (ZF), basic helix-loop-helix (bHLH), homeodomain (HD), basic leucine zipper (bZip), nuclear receptor (NHR), high mobility group (HMG-box), Tbox, ETS/IRF, and Forkhead factors. Members of each of these families play prominent regulatory roles in organ development through the genes they bind and control. Many establish the developmental status of cells and determine stage-specific changes in gene expression in response to extrinsic signaling molecules. Others are the transcriptional effectors of extrinsic signaling pathways.

2.1   Extrinsic Factors: Cell-Cell Signals

Extrinsic signaling cues are essential for much of pancreatic organogenesis, and yet the molecular mechanisms by which they control development are just beginning to be unraveled. Although the signaling pathways and principal signaling molecules are known, the precise timing of their actions, the source of these signals, the developmental status of the cells they affect, and the complexity of the cellular response, including the spectrum of induced genes, are still obscure. Filling these gaps of knowledge is a next major undertaking for understanding the molecular bases of pancreatic development. In addition, given the step-wise process of

■ Fig. 4-2

Major developmental signaling pathways. The key to a unique cell-specific outcome (e.g., activation of Gene X) of signaling by a commonly used pathway lies in the developmental history of the responding cell, which is embodied by a specific collection of lineage-specific and spatially restricted transcription factors, such as members of the ETS, bHLH, and homeodomain transcription factor families. Although all pathways discussed in the text are shown, all are not likely to act on the promoter of a single gene.

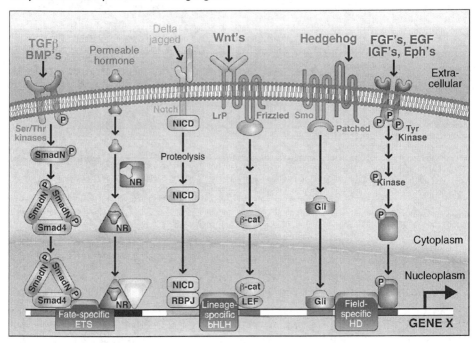

pancreatic development, the responses of pancreatic cells to an EF change with developmental time. Therefore, generalizations regarding a specific EF or an EF family are difficult to make. Extrinsic signals must be considered in the context of the developmental history of a cell and its changing competence to respond to those signals. Knowledge of the roles of EFs is also critical to understanding pancreatic neoplasia, as most cancers of the pancreas are associated with the dysregulation of these bioactive molecules [21–25].

Here we introduce those EFs signaling pathways known to control pancreatic organogenesis. We briefly describe the molecular components that constitute the canonical pathways leading to transcriptional changes in responding cells (❖ Fig. 4-2) and provide a specific example for each pathway in pancreatic development.

1. Transforming Growth Factor β (TGFβ) signaling is based on the binding of secreted extracellular ligands to single-pass transmembrane serine/threonine kinase receptors on responding cells [21,26]. Ligands in this large family include subfamilies of TGFβs, activins, bone morphogenetic proteins (BMPs) and growth and differentiation factors (GDFs). Ligand-binding induces the heterodimerization of type I and type II receptors. Upon heterodimer formation, the type II receptor phosphorylates and activates the type I

receptor, which then transduces the signal by phosphorylating a member of the Smad family of transcription factors. Three types of Smad proteins mediate the transcriptional effects of TGFβ signaling within the responding cell: the receptor-regulated Smads (R-Smads), the common mediator Smads (co-Smads) and the inhibitory Smads (I-Smads). During pancreas specification, TGFβ produced by the notochord induces pancreatic identity in cells of the underlying endoderm by limiting hedgehog signaling within the pre-pancreatic domain of the early patterned endoderm [27,28]. Similarly, BMP and activin from the splanchnic mesoderm are required for proper specification of the early ventral pancreas [29]. Later, as the pancreas branches and grows, TGFβ-signaling via ActRIIA and ActRIIB is required for proper endocrine and exocrine expansion, and for endocrine function (insulin secretion and glucose metabolism) [30,31].

2. Hedgehogs (Hhs) compose a family of secreted signaling peptides that includes Sonic (Shh), Indian (Ihh) and Desert (Dhh) hedgehogs, all of which bind a 12-pass receptor subunit called Patched 1 (Ptc 1) [32]. The binding relieves Ptc1-mediated repression of Smoothened (Smo), which is a G-protein-like membrane-associated signaling molecule that transduces intracellular signaling to the nucleus via the Gli family of TFs. During pancreatic specification, Hedgehog produced throughout much of the endoderm restricts the pancreatic domain to hedgehog-free islands [27,33]. The suppression of Hh in the endoderm by signals from the notochord is required for endodermal acquisition of pancreatic cell fate, as Hh inhibits early Pdx1 expression and the formation of the pancreas [27,34,35].

3. The Wnts (Wingless/int) are a family of secreted glycoproteins that control cell proliferation, asymmetric cell division and cell-fate [36,37]. Wnts transduce signaling to responsive cells by binding Frizzled receptors and a variety of co-receptors, such as LRP5/6, RORs1/2, or Ryks. Signaling downstream of the receptor is transduced via two alternative pathways, roughly categorized as either "canonical" or "non-canonical." The latter includes both the Ca^{2+} signaling pathway (Ca/G-protein/PKC pathway) and the planar cell polarity (or PCP) pathway (frizzled/Rho/JNK). Pathway specificity of individual ligands appears to depend on cellular context, including presence or absence of co-receptors and intercellular mediators. Complex crosstalk and overlap between these branches of the pathway determine the overall cellular readout of Wnt signaling. For the canonical pathway, the absence of Wnt-activation of the receptor permits the degradation of the downstream cytoplasmic molecule β-catenin by a "destruction complex" that includes the proteins APC, axin and the serine/threonine kinase GSK3. In the absence of signaling, GSK3 phosphorylates β-catenin and targets it for ubiquitin-mediated degradation, and thereby keeps the intracellular level of β-catenin low. The binding of a Wnt to its receptor activates the intracellular protein Disheveled (Dsh), which disrupts the destruction complex, thus allowing cytoplasmic β-catenin to accumulate, enter the nucleus, associate with the DNA binding proteins LEF/TCF, and activate target genes. Whereas Wnt signaling must be inhibited in the early endoderm for pancreas specification [38,39], it must be activated later for the development of the acinar cell lineage [40–42]. These properties of Wnt signaling are an illustration of the dynamic roles of signaling pathways. It is likely that the canonical and noncanonical branches of the pathway function during pancreas development; however, only a role for the canonical branch has been uncovered.

4. The Notch family of receptors mediate short-range signaling [43]. The Notch signaling pathway is unusual in two ways. First, its single transmembrane receptors (the Notches) and most of its ligands are transmembrane proteins (Deltas and Jaggeds), which limits signaling to adjacent cells. Second, intracellular signal transduction is very simple because

there is no separate second messenger (❯ *Fig. 4-2*). Upon binding a ligand, the Notch receptor is cleaved to release an intracellular portion, which migrates into the nucleus, binds the Notch transcriptional mediator Rbpj, and converts it from a repressor to an activator. Key target genes include the Hes subfamily of bHLH repressor factors, which bind and suppress the transcription of pro-differentiation genes. Notch signaling acts as a binary switch to control two general functions critical to many developmental programs [3]. In some instances, it promotes the expansion of a precursor cell population by suppressing the decision to begin differentiation; in others, it controls the decision of cells in a population to choose one of two possible differentiation programs. During pancreatic development, Notch signaling performs both developmental functions: it controls the size of the progenitor population prior to the secondary transition by suppressing differentiation and determines the allocation of endocrine cells during the secondary transition [44–48].

5. Retinoic Acid (RA), the active metabolite of Vitamin A, binds two types of nuclear receptors, the RARs (Retinoic Acid Receptors) and the RXRs (Retinoid X Receptors, or co-receptors), which form heterodimers that translocate to the nucleus to control the transcription of genes containing RAREs (RA Responsive Elements) [49]. RA is the simplest signaling pathway; its receptor is also the DNA-binding TF that mediates transcriptional control. RA is synthesized from circulating retinol (Vitamin A), via an enzymatic pathway including retinaldehyde dehydrogenases (Raldh). Raldh2 is present early and widely during embryonic development [50] and is critical to the development of many organs and tissues, including the pancreas [51,52]. RA from the dorsomedial splanchnic mesoderm promotes the outgrowth of the dorsal pancreatic bud and the formation of the early endocrine cells. In addition to promoting pancreatic development, RA signaling also is critical to early endodermal patterning [51]. These roles for RA are evolutionarily conserved in frogs and fish [53–55].

6. Receptor Tyrosine Kinases (RTKs) mediate signaling from numerous families of growth factors, such as FGFs, EGFs, insulin-like growth factors (IGFs), vascular endothelial growth factors (VEGFs), platelet derived growth factor (PDGF) ephrins, and many others. The cellular outcomes of RTK signaling span a wide range of cell behaviors, including cell proliferation, migration, morphogenesis, cell fate choices and regulation of cell survival. RTKs are single pass transmembrane receptors, which often hetero- or homo-dimerize, usually cross phosphorylate each other, and then transduce signaling within the responding cell via either the extracellular signal-regulated kinase (ERK) or the mitogen-activated protein kinase (MAPK) signaling cascades. Critical roles have been identified for members of many different RTK families in pancreatic development. Fgf10, for instance, is required for proliferation of pancreatic epithelial progenitor cells [56]. EGF receptor signaling is required for the proliferation and maintenance of proper β-cell mass [57]. Also, tight regulation of VEGF within the pancreas is required, as increased levels alter pancreatic vasculature, which indirectly leads to disruption in both exocrine and endocrine differentiation and abnormalities in insulin secretion [58,59].

Extrinsic signaling is thus a critical and often initiating catalyst for the development of most embryonic organs, including regulatory roles in pancreatic development. In this chapter, we review experimental evidence that elucidated these roles and place them in the context of the landmarks of pancreatic development.

2.2   Intrinsic Factors: DNA-Binding Transcription Factors

The key transcription factors (TFs) that pattern the endoderm, specify and maintain pancreatic fate, and resolve the individual pancreatic cell lineages are known. A model for the pancreatic lineage with associated TFs is shown in ⊘ *Fig. 4-3*. For example, the Forkhead factor Hepatocyte nuclear factor 3b (Hnf3b/FoxA3) controls the formation of the anterior endoderm during gastrulation; the HD protein Hlxb9 participates in endoderm patterning and cell-lineage specification within the pancreatic domain; the bHLH factor Neurogenin3 (Ngn3) specifies endocrine cell identity; the HMG factor Sry-box9 (Sox9) maintains the undifferentiated state of precursor cells during the primary and secondary transition; and the bZip proteins MafA and MafB control the final stages of β-cell differentiation. It is important to note that some of these intrinsic factors play critical roles

◘ Fig. 4-3

Primary transcriptional regulators of pancreatic development. Regulatory TFs discussed in the text are listed in association with the progression of cellular commitment and differentiation. Key TFs that appear at a particular stage and likely control the transition to that stage are in *red*. The multipotent precursor cell (MPC) state is highlighted with a grey background. The TFs for the first wave endocrine cells are not listed, but are similar to those for the second wave α- and β-cells. The list of factors is not comprehensive; for example, not all the TFs that distinguish the islet cell types are listed, and some assignments to intermediate cell-types are tentative and need confirmation.

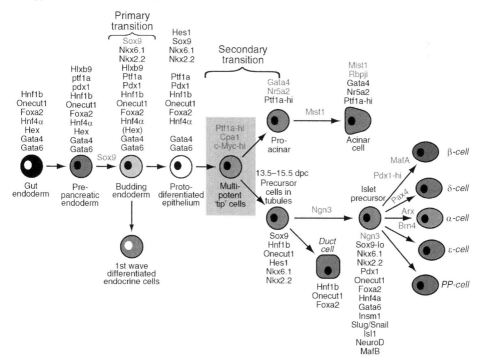

at more than one developmental stage. In this regard, two stage- and lineage-specific TFs merit special mention. The HD factor Pancreas duodenal homeobox (Pdx1) and the bHLH protein Pancreas transcription factor 1a (Ptf1a) perform distinct regulatory functions at early, middle and late stages of development. Murine embryos and human fetuses homozygous deficient for *Pdx1* [60–62] or *Ptf1a* [63–65] do not form a pancreas. Although neither Pdx1 nor Ptf1a is required for the formation of the initial pancreatic buds at 9.5 dpc, both are necessary for the growth, branching morphogenesis and the transition to the protodifferentiated state. Pdx1 controls the formation and growth of the protodifferentiated cell population, is required at the secondary transition for the formation of the acinar, ductal and islet cell lineages, and later controls the differentiation and maintenance of β-cells. Ptf1a maintains pancreatic identity in the nascent buds, sustains precursor cell growth of the early epithelium, defines the multipotent precursor population that initiates the secondary transition, and later controls the differentiation of acinar cells.

The TFs at the end of signal transduction pathways (❯ *Fig. 4-2*) are the intrinsic mediators of transcriptional control by extrinsic signaling factors. The signaling pathway TFs are thought to interact with stage- and lineage-specific TFs in two related ways. One is by binding and activating the promoter of a gene encoding a stage- or lineage-specific TF to produce that factor at a specific time and place. The other way is to activate transcription by cooperating with stage- and lineage-specific factors by binding together on the promoter of a developmentally regulated gene (❯ *Fig. 4-2*). This cooperation is the basis for the ability of a signal for a widely used transduction pathway to activate a particular gene in a developmentally unique context (see Side ❯ *Box 4-3*). In general, gene promoters require the binding and cooperation of several DNA-binding TFs to be activated. The binding of the transcriptional mediator of a signaling pathway alone is insufficient to active the promoter. This makes sense: otherwise activation of a pathway would induce in a cell the expression of all possible genes regulated by that pathway for all developmental programs. In a complementary fashion, the binding of stage/lineage-specific transcriptional activators alone is also insufficient. Otherwise, developmental programs would initiate and continue in the absence of extrinsic control without regard to correct timing and position in the embryo. Thus, to activate a particular developmentally regulated gene properly, a cell must have the correct history embodied in the presence of the pathway receptor and the appropriate stage/lineage-specific TFs. The cell also must be in the correct position to receive an effective concentration of the extrinsic signaling molecule released from nearby cells. To regulate this particular gene, it must have a promoter with the nucleotide sequences for binding the appropriate stage/lineage-specific TFs of that program and the transcriptional mediator of the signaling pathway(s).

Although the critical signaling pathways and stage/lineage-specific TFs have been identified for pancreatic organogenesis, little is known of their direct cooperation. Much of what is known derives from studies of the development of model organisms such as the fruit fly (Drosophila melanogaster) and the soil nematode (Caenorhabditis elegans) (*http://stke.sciencemag.org/cm/*). However, these studies cannot address their interplay during pancreatic development. The following sections outline the roles of intrinsic and extrinsic factors that direct specific processes during discrete developmental windows of pancreatic organogenesis. Relationships, when known for pancreatic development, are discussed.

3   The Roles of Extrinsic and Intrinsic Factors During Pancreatic Development

Here we divide embryonic pancreatic development into four temporal stages and review the roles of extrinsic and intrinsic factors in distinct cellular or morphogenetic events that occur during these stages:

1. Specification of endodermal domains to pancreatic fate (mouse 6.5–9 dpc).
2. Initial growth of pancreatic buds and the primary developmental transition (9–12 dpc).
3. Onset of acinar, ductal and islet development by the secondary developmental transition (12.5–15.5 dpc).
4. Perinatal growth and differentiation (16 dpc to neonate).

3.1   Specification of Endodermal Domains to Pancreatic Fate (6.5–9 dpc)

3.1.1   Early Endoderm and Gut Tube Formation

The pancreas forms from the embryonic definitive endoderm. The definitive endoderm is one of three germ layers (ectoderm and mesoderm are the others) that emerge during gastrulation.

The ectoderm gives rise to the nervous system and the epidermis; the mesoderm to muscle, heart, kidney, blood, vasculature and gut mesenchyme; and the endoderm to the lining of the entire gastrointestinal system, including most organs along its length, such as the pharynx, thyroid, lungs, liver, stomach, pancreas and intestine. The mouse endoderm emerges from the primitive streak and forms a single epithelial sheet of approximately 500–1,000 cells [66]. As the embryo takes shape, the epithelial sheet rolls up into a primitive gut tube, which runs along the anterior to posterior axis of the embryo. A thick layer of splanchnic mesoderm adheres to the gut tube endoderm during this early phase of morphogenesis, inducing and supporting endodermal proliferation, morphogenesis and differentiation.

Broad patterning of the definitive endoderm begins as it forms during gastrulation and is based on the timing of the movement of the pre-endodermal epiblast cells through the primitive streak [67,68]. The first presumptive endodermal cells exiting the primitive streak become the most-anterior and most-posterior endoderm, followed by cells that form the middle endoderm and the rest of the posterior endoderm. During this passage of cells through the primitive streak, signaling by nodal (a member of the extended TGFβ/BMP family of morphogens) preferentially establishes the anterior foregut endoderm through, in part, induction of FoxA2, a Forkhead TF also important for subsequent endodermal organogenesis. Embryos deficient in Smad2, a TF mediator specific to the TGFβ/activin/nodal subfamily of extrinsic signals, fail to generate endoderm properly [69].

Additional extrinsic signaling factors (EFs) are required for regionalization of the gut tube [70]. Wnt signaling, for instance, displays a clear anteroposterior gradient, with signaling repressed anteriorly and actively transmitted posteriorly. Wnt activity must be suppressed for proper foregut development in fish [71] and frog [72,73], as repression of canonical Wnt signaling is critical for both liver and pancreas specification. Experimentally enhancing Wnt signaling in the pancreatic endoderm ablates the formation of the exocrine and endocrine pancreas [71]. Conversely, inhibiting Wnt signaling induces liver and pancreatic buds at ectopic sites in the endoderm [72]. Similarly, constitutive activation of Wnt signaling in prepancreatic mouse endoderm by the forced expression of Wnt1 [39] or activated β-catenin [38] greatly reduces pancreas formation.

3.1.2   Anteroposterior Patterning of the Endoderm

The broad developmental domains of the early definitive endoderm resolve progressively to form the pharynx, esophagus, stomach, intestine and colon and the glands that bud off the tube during organogenesis (the submandibular and sublingual glands, thyroid, parathyroids, trachea, lungs, liver and pancreas). Although the early endoderm appears morphologically homogeneous prior to the onset of organogenesis, it is in fact patterned along its anteroposterior axis.

Several transcription factors with restricted expression cooperate with developmental signaling to control regional identity along the endoderm. The foregut endoderm expresses several regulators of anterior developmental programs not found in posterior endoderm, such as the HMG-box factor Sox2 and the HD proteins Six, Nkx2.1, and Hex. Six and its coactivator Eya1 pattern a subregion of the pharyngeal endoderm for thyroid and parathyroid formation [74]. Sox2 plays multiple roles in the patterning and differentiation of the anterior foregut endoderm [75]. Sox2 and the HD factor Nkx2.1 play reciprocal roles in resolving the esophagus and trachea: Sox2-deficient esophageal endoderm acquires a tracheal phenotype including ectopic Nkx2.1 expression and Nkx2.1-deficient tracheal endoderm initiates a partial esophageal developmental program, including ectopic Sox2 expression [75,76]. The HD factor Pdx1 is first restricted to the initial domains of the prepancreatic buds and then expands to include the proximal duodenum and the distal stomach [61]. The HD factors Cdx1 and Cdx2 establish the intestinal region of the gut tube distinct from the stomach and more anterior regions, and are excluded from the pancreatic domain [77]. In the absence of Cdx2, cells of the intestine form gastric mucosa similar to the stomach epithelium [78]; conversely, ectopic expression of a Cdx2 transgene in developing mouse stomach causes the replacement of gastric mucosal cells with intestinal goblet, absorptive and enteroendocrine cells [79,80].

How is the broad anteroposterior regionalization of the nascent endoderm refined? The regional expression of lineage-specific intrinsic factors is established through complex extrinsic signaling from the mesoderm to the underlying endoderm and back again [81,82]. However, only fragments of the complete story are known. For example, the dorsal pancreas domain is initiated by signals of the TGFβ family (see below) from the notochord ($\bullet$ Fig. 4-4), and posterior endoderm is patterned in a concentration dependent manner by FGF4 produced by adjacent mesoderm ($\bullet$ Fig. 4-4) [83]. Exposure of chick endoderm explants to high levels of FGF4 promotes a more posterior or intestinal fate, whereas lower levels allow more anterior cell fates, as shown by an anterior shift in Pdx1 and CdxB expression domains and a concomitant repression of anterior markers such as Hex1 and Nkx2.1 [84]. This extrinsic FGF signal acts directly on cells of the endoderm (rather than indirectly via the mesoderm), as expression of a constitutively active FGF receptor (FGFR1) in the endoderm also leads to the same anterior expansion of Pdx1 expression.

3.1.3 Dorsoventral Patterning of the Prepancreatic Endoderm

The gut tube endoderm is also patterned dorsoventrally. This is evident morphologically by the positioning of some organs either dorsally (such as the dorsal pancreas) or ventrally (such as the lung, ventral pancreas, gall bladder and liver). However, it is also evident molecularly, prior to onset of organogenesis by the dorsoventral distribution of developmental factors within the early endoderm. The regionalization of the gut tube into distinct organ fields is defined by overlapping anteroposterior and dorsoventral pre-patterning of the endoderm.

The positioning of the dorsal and ventral pancreatic buds is partly understood. Early during gut tube formation, the presence of the HD transcription factor TGIF2 in the dorsal endoderm antagonizes the ventralizing action of TGFβ signaling by binding the TGFβ transcriptional effector Smads and repressing TGFβ target genes [85]. Suppression of TGFβ signaling by TGIF2 in the dorsal endoderm prevents the activation of Hex, a HD transcription factor that favors liver development, and allows the activation of Pdx1, and thereby the induction of pancreatic development [86].

Conversely for the ventral pancreatic bud, intense BMP/TGFβ signaling from the immediately adjacent septum transversum mesenchyme appears to overcome TGIF2-mediated repression to induce Hex and thereby hepatic fate, rather than pancreatic fate, in the ventral endoderm. Hex also promotes the posterior movement of the ventral prepancreatic endodermal ridge beyond the reach of high BMP/TGFβ from the cardiogenic mesenchyme [87]; exposed to lower levels of BMP/TGFβ signals, the cells within the ridge retain TGIF2-repression of Hex, are able to activate Pdx1, and so acquire pancreatic rather than hepatic fate [88]. In Hex-deficient embryos, that region remains within the influence of BMP/TGFβ

◘ Fig. 4-4

Cell-cell signaling during pancreatic development. Developmental signaling depends on the proper spatiotemporal communication between embryonic tissues. Multiple sequential inductions between adjacent developing tissues are mediated by secreted or cell-tethered factors. During pancreatic bud development, sequential signals are produced by (1) the primitive streak during gastrulation (prior to the stage shown), which patterns the endoderm with a gradient of FGF4; (2) the notochord, which sends permissive signals (such as Fgf2 and activin-βB) that promote the pancreas domain; (3) the aorta, which provides endothelial signals (EC factors) required for *Ptf1a* induction, *Pdx1* maintenance and first wave insulin expression; and (4) the lateral plate mesoderm, which produces Fgf10 and retinoic acid (RA) required for bud outgrowth. Reciprocally, structures such as the gut endoderm and somites produce VEGF, which is required for patterning the dorsal aorta.

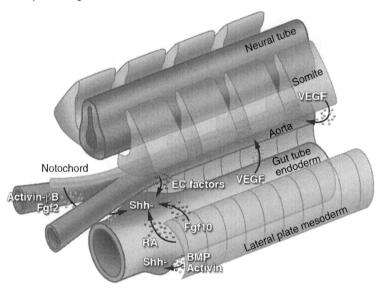

signals from the cardiogenic mesenchyme, fails to form the ventral pancreatic bud, and initiates the hepatic developmental program instead. A proper balance of BMP signaling is required, because its absence also disrupts development of the ventral pancreatic bud [29]. This ventral region of the endoderm has an interesting triple potential: strong signaling from the cardiogenic mesenchyme induces hepatic fate; lower levels of that signaling permits the pancreatic fate; and in the complete absence of that signaling or *Ptf1a* (a field-specific bHLH factor for pancreatic development), the region assumes intestinal fate (see below) [63].

3.1.4   Initiation of Pancreatic Budding

Soon after early endodermal gut tube formation, the first morphological sign of pancreatic development is a local thickening and evagination of the dorsal midline endoderm at about E8.75 in the mouse and during the fourth week of gestation in humans. Cells within the thickening epithelium change from cuboidal to columnar, which drives the growth of a small fin-like evagination. Approximately 12 h later, as the anterior intestinal portal closes over the pancreatic domain, the ventral pancreatic evagination becomes evident. The dorsal pancreatic bud emerges just caudal to the developing stomach, and the ventral bud appears just caudal to the developing liver, near the base of the primordium of the common bile duct. Some mammals are thought to form a single ventral bud (rat and human), whereas others have two clear ventral buds (frogs and chick). In mouse, a second ventral bud is present transiently [27,58].

A number of transcription factors are critical to proper pancreatic specification and early budding. *Hlxb9* expression, for example, foretells the position of the dorsal evagination and is required for the subsequent activation of *Pdx1* in the dorsal epithelium [89]. Conversely, *Pdx1* foretells the position of the ventral evagination, and is required for the activation of *Hlxb9* in the ventral epithelium [89]. Whereas *Hlxb9* is required for the onset of dorsal (but not ventral) budding, *Pdx1* is not required for either [61]. However, *Pdx1* is necessary for the subsequent growth of both buds. *Ngn3* is also expressed specifically in the pre-pancreatic endoderm prior to budding, and is necessary later for the differentiation of all pancreatic endocrine cell types [90,91].

Gata4 and Gata6 are stage/lineage-specific TFs required for pancreatic development. Both are potent inducers of endoderm and its pre-pancreatic regionalization by controlling the expression of *Pdx1* and other fate-specifying TFs [86, 92]. Gata4 and Gata6 are expressed broadly in the early mouse foregut endoderm and later throughout the nascent dorsal and ventral pancreatic buds [93, 94]. In the absence of Gata4, the ventral bud does not form, although the dorsal bud does. Without *Gata4*, the expression of *Hlxb9* and *Pdx1* does not begin in the region of the ventral bud, but does appear in the dorsal bud. Thus, the inductive sequence among these TFs for the ventral bud is *Gata4* → budding/*Hlxb9* → *Pdx1*; and the critical role for *Gata4* is the induction of *Hlxb9* expression. The absence of *Gata6*, a closely related TF, causes a similar, though less complete, loss of the ventral bud and also no discernible effect on growth of the dorsal bud. The differential dependence for *Gata4* and *Gata6* by the ventral versus the dorsal pancreas reflects the different tissue interactions and growth factor requirements described previously.

Cell extrinsic factors secreted by tissues adjacent to the endoderm establish the early pre-pancreatic domain of the endoderm. The notochord, which initially lies in contact with the midline endoderm, produces activin-βB, Nodal (TGFβ family members) and FGF2. These secreted morphogens promote pancreatic cell fate by suppressing Shh expression in pre-patterned regions of the endoderm [27,30,95]. This effect was demonstrated experimentally by the inhibition of Shh expression in dorsal pancreatic endoderm explants upon exposure to activin-βB or FGF2 [95]. Conversely, disruption of TGFβ signaling in mice also lacking the activin receptors (ActRIIA−/−; ActRIIB−/−) led to Shh expression in the pancreatic domain and the disruption of pancreatic development [27]. Indeed, hedgehog signaling must be specifically excluded from the early pancreatic domain for normal development. During normal development, Pdx1 expression is restricted to the hedgehog-free regions of the posterior foregut endoderm. Experimental manipulations that change the size of the hedgehog-free regions alter the size of the Pdx1-expression domain and the amount of the pancreatic tissue that forms. For instance, cyclopamine, a steroidal alkaloid that blocks hedgehog signaling, expands the region of endoderm that forms pancreatic tissue [33]. A related effect is observed in Shh- and Ihh-deficient mouse embryos, which form more extensive pancreatic tissue, in some cases annular, with increased numbers of acinar as well as endocrine cells [27]. Thus, the expression pattern of hedgehog factors, such as Sonic (Shh) and Indian (Ihh), in the endoderm establishes the boundaries of the early pancreatic field.

Retinoic acid (RA) is another signaling molecule required after general endodermal patterning for the specification of the pancreatic lineage (◉ *Fig. 4-4*). A role for RA was originally suggested by observations in fish, frog and avian embryos [29,54,55,71,96]. Recent work with mouse embryos has shown that Raldh2, an enzyme of RA biosynthesis, is expressed in the splanchnic mesoderm that surrounds the early budding pancreatic epithelium [51,52]. Raldh2 mutant embryos fail to express Pdx1 in the dorsal pancreatic epithelium (but ventral expression continues) and have reduced expression of Isl1 and Hlxb9; this effect can be reversed by maternal RA administration. In contrast to Pdx1-deficient embryos, the initial formation of the first wave endocrine cells is greatly decreased in the Raldh2 mutants, indicating that RA has a role beyond its regulation of *Pdx1* [51]. RA is thus an extrinsic cue from the mesoderm to the dorsal pancreatic endoderm that is critical to normal pancreatic development.

Interplay between extrinsic and intrinsic signaling is illustrated by the action of the Hnf1b/Tcf2 transcription factor. Hnf1b is required for proper patterning of the prepancreatic domain of the posterior foregut through its suppression of hedgehog expression in the endoderm [97]. The absence of Hnf1b in the gut endoderm allows expansion of the hedgehog-expression domains, which constricts the hedgehog-free island of Pdx1-expression to a very narrow region; in addition, the expression of Ptf1a and Hlx1b is never activated. As a consequence, the ventral bud does not develop and the dorsal bud is greatly reduced in size, fails to thrive, and disappears prior to the time of the secondary transition.

3.2   Initial Growth of Pancreatic Buds and the Primary Developmental Transition (9–12 dpc)

The early phase of pancreatic development involves growth of the epithelium, the appearance of a few differentiated "first wave" endocrine cells in rodents, and initial branching morphogenesis. The result of these initial events is a complex, stratified epithelium containing a common pool of progenitor cells (in a "protodifferentiated state") of sufficient size to allow the proper transformation of the pancreas into a tubular tree-like organ at the "secondary transition," containing islet, ductal and acinar tissues. We describe the developmental progress of the dorsal pancreatic epithelium during this early phase. A review by Jorgensen and colleagues is a unique source of rotating 3-D views of mouse pancreatic development up to the secondary transition and is an invaluable learning tool [6].

3.2.1   Growth and Elaboration of Pancreatic Buds

Prior to budding, the endoderm destined for dorsal pancreas is a flat, thin and simple cuboidal epithelium (◉ *Fig. 4-1a*). As growth of the dorsal bud proceeds, the neck of the bud constricts and the bud takes on a "fist-like" appearance containing a compact epithelium surrounded by mesenchyme. It is unclear whether this compact epithelium is stratified, with multiple cell layers [3], or whether it is in fact simply the beginning of dense branching within a confined space that creates an extremely narrow, convoluted and branched lumen, as described by Pictet et al. [4]. The presence of multiple, separate "microlumens" in this complex epithelium has recently been suggested as an initial event in the formation of branches [3]. Support for this mechanism comes from an elegant analysis of the development of the exocrine pancreas in zebrafish [98]. In this species, the branched ductal epithelium arises from the formation of short microlumens in a stratified precursor epithelium and the subsequent fusion of the microlumens in a manner that creates the branching ductal tree. Although not yet proven, a mechanism involving microlumen fusion may initiate pancreatic branching in mammals as well.

3.2.2 Epithelial Lobulation and Branching

Following the initial budding and branching of the early pancreatic epithelium, the growing bud begins additional morphogenetic changes. As the gut tube undergoes "turning," a process that breaks bilateral symmetry of the alimentary tract and changes the relative position of digestive organs relative to one another, the dorsal epithelium extends from a "fist-like" to a "bat-like" shape while extending numerous lateral (90° from the main axis) branches along its proximo-distal axis. Small lobulations form along each lateral branch. Here, we define "lobulation" as the formation of multiple short blunt branches, or "lobules" [99,100], while we refer to "branching" as the extension of longer, definitive epithelial branches that display multiple lobulations, more predictable organization, and generate the main branches of the maturing organ (A. Villasenor and O. C., unpublished observations).

It has long been hypothesized that pancreatic branching occurs as a result of random folding and buckling of the endodermal epithelium [2], and it is clear that branching of the pancreatic epithelium occurs by very different mechanisms than the well characterized terminal bifid (bifurcation) branching of lung and kidney development [101,102]. Recent observations using high resolution live microscopy confirm lateral branching in pancreatic epithelium, in which only about 20% of branching events are bifid [103]. It will be of great interest to understand branching more completely, as branching has been closely associated with allocation of progenitors to the different pancreatic cell lineages [7].

3.2.3 The Primary Transition

The epithelial cells of the nascent buds are specified to begin the pancreatic program, but can be considered "predifferentiated" (⊙ Fig. 4-5) [2]. Although specified to pancreatic fate, they are not yet irreversibly committed to do so. A "primary developmental transition" then occurs in which the majority of cells within the pancreatic epithelium acquire this commitment – the "protodifferentiated" state. The primary transition was originally recognized by the detection of low levels of some acinar enzymes and the appearance of early differentiated endocrine cells expressing glucagon [2]. These "first wave" endocrine cells in rodents are distinct from the "second wave" endocrine cells, which form during the secondary transition and participate directly in the formation of islets. We define these first "early" endocrine cells below.

3.2.3.1 First Wave Endocrine Cells – Glucagon Cells Bud from the Epithelium

The endocrine cells of the primary transition appear at 9 dpc either as single cells integrated in the epithelium or clusters of cells that remain attached to the pancreatic epithelium. Initially all of these early endocrine cells express the glucagon gene, and as the number increases, a few cells co-express glucagon and insulin, and later some only insulin, although the majority express glucagon only. These observations suggest that the early insulin-expressing cells derive from glucagon-expressing cells through an intermediate co-expressing both hormone genes.

■ Fig. 4-5

The primary and secondary transitions of pancreatic development. The primary and secondary transitions were originally defined by William Rutter, Raymond Pictet and their colleagues on morphologic criteria [4] and biochemical quantification of the products made by differentiated endocrine and exocrine cells [104–106]. The primary developmental transition marks the appearance of very low levels of acinar digestive enzymes (principally Cpa1) and the first wave glucagon-gene and subsequently insulin-gene expressing cells. The secondary developmental transition spans the geometric increase of acinar digestive enzymes and insulin. Human pancreatic development has a primary transition that forms a protodifferentiated epithelium, but not first wave endocrine cells. Human development also has a secondary transition stage, but it does not begin at the same time in all regions of the larger pancreatic rudiment and so appears much less concerted than the rodent transition [107]. The first endocrine cells appear in the primary transition at 9 dpc in mouse embryos (red M) and at about 50 dpc during the extended secondary transition in human fetuses (red H).

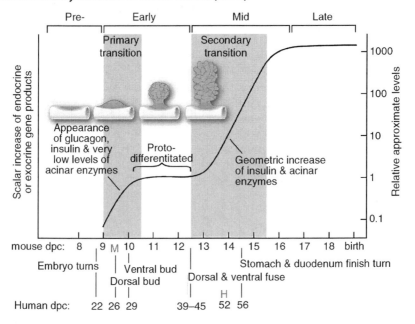

This peculiarity of the early endocrine cells and the lack of understanding that first and second wave endocrine cells are developmentally distinct led to the confounding notion that islet β-cells were derived from glucagon-expressing precursors.

There remains an interesting controversy and uncertainty regarding the precise fate and potential function of these first endocrine cells. It has been argued that the majority of early insulin-expressing and the insulin/glucagon co-expressing cells do not contribute to the mature endocrine pancreas [108]. However, lineage analysis of these cells demonstrates that at least a portion contributes to the mature pancreas [109]. Indeed, the early endocrine cell clusters appear to fuse with immature islets formed during the secondary transition and may contribute the α-cell mantle in mature islets [110,111]. It should be noted that the absence of first wave endocrine cells in human fetal pancreas [112,113] makes their relevance to human pancreatic development unlikely.

3.2.4 The "Proto-Differentiated" State (9.5–12 dpc)

The vast majority of cells remain protodifferentiated following the first transition (● *Fig. 4-5*). Indeed they contain transcription factors that suppress further differentiation and promote the proliferation necessary to expand the progenitor cell pool to the size needed at the secondary transition to generate the proper number of differentiated acinar, ductal and islet cells. The final size of the pancreatic gland is established by cell-signaling and transcription factor control of the expansion of the protodifferentiated cell population [5]. Experimental ablation of a fraction of pancreatic progenitor cells prior to 9.5 dpc has little or no effect on final organ size. In contrast, ablation of progenitors during the phase of protodifferentiated cell expansion (9.5–12.5 dpc) limits the size of the pancreas at birth and in adulthood in proportion to the fraction of lost progenitors. The smaller proportion affects both endocrine and exocrine cells. Thus, pancreatic size is dependent on the number of progenitor cells established prior to the secondary transition, and is largely independent of regulatory influences that might modulate this population during subsequent growth and development. This intrinsic determination of size is in contrast to the well known "regulative growth" of other organs such as liver, blood and nervous tissue, in which the depletion of precursors can be compensated by extending cell proliferation or limiting programmed cell death. The relative regenerative abilities of liver (high) and pancreas (low) in adult animals may reflect this developmental difference. It is unknown whether this developmental strategy of controlling organ size contributes to particular nuances of the initiation, nature or severity of pancreatic adenocarcinoma.

3.2.5 Epithelial-Mesenchymal Crosstalk: Control of the "Protodifferentiated" state

Growth of the pancreatic epithelium requires critical signals from the surrounding mesoderm. This was demonstrated decades ago in elegant embryological recombination experiments [114,115]. Epithelial cell differentiation was profoundly affected by altering the normal mesenchymal/epithelial ratio of cultured explants. Removal of the mesenchyme accelerated differentiation at the expense of epithelial growth [115] and biased differentiation toward endocrine [116,117]. The nature of the cell-cell signaling molecules that emanate from the mesenchyme remained elusive until recently [118]. Many of them, including EGF, HGF, TGFβ and various FGFs, are powerful regulators of pancreatic growth, survival and differentiation [3,35,70,119]. The control of proliferation versus differentiation in the protodifferentiated epithelium requires multiple rounds of signaling between the epithelium and mesenchyme involving Wnt, FGF and Notch pathways.

FGF signaling is critical to proper pancreatic development through its regulation of the expansion of the protodifferentiated cell population. Mouse embryos lacking the FGF receptor 2b (FGFR2b) or expressing a dominant negative form develop acute hypoplasia affecting both exocrine and endocrine lineages [120,121]. FGF10, a ligand for FGFR2b, is expressed by pancreatic mesenchyme and required early (10.0–12.5 dpc) for proper pancreatic budding and growth. Loss of *Fgf10* function eliminates the expansion of the progenitor cell pool, but not the specification of the first wave endocrine cells [56]. Conversely, Fgf10 over-expression in the pancreatic endoderm leads to marked hyperplasia, prolonged maintenance of *Pdx1* expression, and suppression of pancreatic endocrine and exocrine differentiation [122,123]. This effect appears to be partly due to the dysregulation of the Notch pathway.

Notch signaling is known principally for its regulation of binary cell fate decisions, a process termed "lateral specification," in tissues as diverse as the epithelium of the fly wing to stem cells of the vertebrate neural tube [3]. Notch control of cell fate is based on reciprocal signaling between adjacent cells in an epithelium and is active in the early pancreatic epithelium. In this process, a ligand (e.g., Delta or Jagged) produced under the direction of a transcriptional regulator (e.g., Ngn3) binds and activates a cell-surface Notch receptor on a neighboring cell, which, in turn, initiates an intracellular signal that activates a transcriptional response in the receiving cell through the Notch-pathway transcription factor Rbpj (◉ *Fig. 4-2*). The key element of the response is the induction of *Hes1* or related members of the *Hes* gene family within the cell bearing Notch receptors. In mutant mouse embryos lacking Rbpj or Hes1 in the pancreatic epithelium, the protodifferentiated cell population is not maintained [44–46,48]. The Hes TFs are transcriptional repressors that inhibit the expression of pro-endocrine factors such as Ngn3 in receiving cells. In the pancreatic epithelium prior to 12.5 dpc, this suppression of differentiation promotes the expansion of the protodifferentiated cell population. Meanwhile, the signaling cell undergoes progressive strengthening of its endocrine character and likely begins differentiation into a bona fide endocrine precursor cell. Loss of function of Notch pathway genes at this stage of development leads to the uncontested expression of *Ngn3* and to the premature differentiation of protodifferentiated progenitors [44,46]. Because the only active differentiation program at this stage is the formation of first wave endocrine cells, unabated *Ngn3* expression in the *Rbpj* or *Hes1* mutants drives unchecked the formation of excessive glucagon-expressing cells, thereby depleting the progenitor population and preventing further pancreatic development.

As mentioned above, the control of endocrine cell fate by Notch signaling is itself affected by extrinsic factors, such as Fgf10, from the mesenchyme. Forced expression of Fgf10 in the early pancreatic epithelium causes the inappropriate high-level expression of the Notch ligands Jagged 1 and 2, which leads to the persistent induction of Notch receptors and Hes1 [122,123]. The super-induction of Hes1 and possibly other Hes-family members suppresses differentiation, at least in part, by repressing *Ngn3* expression, and promotes cell proliferation. This cascade of effects suggests that pancreatic mesenchyme normally promotes acinar and beta cell development indirectly by extending the window of epithelial Notch signaling via Fgf10, thus allowing the protodifferentiated progenitor pool of the epithelium to expand [56]. Mesenchyme thus drives a required delay in progenitor cell differentiation, allowing the proper proportion of endocrine versus exocrine cell development [124].

It is likely that Wnt signaling plays a reciprocal role in the regulation of mesenchymal Fgf10 signaling. Constitutive activation of the Wnt-pathway by the forced expression of activated β-catenin in the early pancreatic epithelium causes a surprising cell-nonautonomous loss of Fgf10 expression in the mesenchyme [38]. Thus, alteration of normal Wnt signaling in pancreas epithelium before E11.5 disrupts an important component of the signaling crosstalk that occurs between epithelium and its associated mesenchyme. This loss of mesenchymal Fgf10 predictably results in severe abrogation of pancreatic growth and ultimate mass, as well as early postnatal lethality.

Many similar regulatory relationships exist between extrinsic signaling pathways and intrinsic transcriptional regulators during early pancreatic development. Four additional key transcriptional regulators – Sox9, Pdx1, Ptf1a, and Hnf1b – of the precursor cell pool are co-expressed in the protodifferentiated epithelium (◉ *Fig. 4-3*). Although a regulatory link between Fgf10 signaling and the maintenance of these transcription factors is likely, no direct evidence has been reported. The HMG-box transcription factor Sox9 sustains the precursor cell population by deferring differentiation while promoting cell-proliferation and survival [9]. Developmental abnormalities in Sox9-haploinsufficient human fetuses are consistent with an inability to sustain a proper pancreatic progenitor population during pancreatic organogenesis [125]. Other members of the Sox-subfamily play similar roles in other developing tissues. Elimination of Sox9 in the developing pancreas causes failure to maintain the pool of protodifferentiated precursor cells due to decreased cell proliferation, increased apoptosis, and diversion of cells to differentiation to the early endocrine lineage of glucagon-expressing cell) [9]. Interestingly, Sox9 expression in the mature murine and human glands is restricted to centroacinar cells [9], which is consistent with proposals that centroacinar cells may retain stem/progenitor cell characteristics with regenerative and oncogenic potential [10,126].

Experimental manipulation of embryonic *Pdx1* expression in utero was used to show that *Pdx1* is also required for the expansion of the protodifferentiated epithelium and its subsequent differentiation [127]. Depletion of Pdx1 during the protodifferentiated stage (9.5–12.5 dpc) inhibited cell proliferation (M. Hale and R.J.M, unpublished). Depletion at progressively later developmental times allowed incremental expansion of the protodifferentiated epithelium and thereby further pancreatic growth and development. For example, the depletion of Pdx1 after 12.5 dpc allows some acinar and islet development.

As for Pdx1, the expression of the bHLH factor Ptf1a begins in the epithelium of the nascent pancreatic bud, expands throughout exocrine and endocrine cell progenitors of the primary transition, and slowly wanes during the protodifferentiated state [47,63,128]. Ptf1a is necessary for the formation of the ventral pancreatic bud and for the proper growth and development of the dorsal bud [47,63,64]. In the absence of Ptf1a, the protodifferentiated cell population does not expand; consequently, the secondary transition does not occur and only an incomplete main pancreatic duct forms.

bHLH transcription factors like Ptf1a generally act as homo- or heterodimers that bind a 6-base pair DNA recognition sequence. Ptf1a is the only bHLH factor known that requires a third DNA-binding subunit (either Rbpj or Rbpjl), which extends its functional binding site to 21-base pairs [129]. A single tryptophan-to-alanine substitution near the carboxyl terminus of Ptf1a disrupts the ability of Ptf1a to recruit Rbpj (but not Rbpjl) into the trimeric complex. The extensive developmental defects of Ptf1a-null embryos are recapitulated in embryos homozygous for this single amino acid change [47]. Thus, the biochemical form of Ptf1a required for the early stages of pancreatic development is the trimeric complex including Rbpj, PTF1-J. This developmental role for Rbpj is distinct from its role in Notch signaling. Whereas its function as part of the Notch-pathway is to prolong the protodifferentiated state by preventing cellular differentiation, its function as a subunit of the PTF1-J complex is to sustain the developmental program of the early epithelium [47].

Hnf1b is another intrinsic factor required for the protodifferentiated state and the expansion of pancreatic progenitors. The ventral pancreatic bud does not form in the absence of Hnf1b; however, the dorsal bud forms, begins normal growth, then fails to expand the protodifferentiated cell population effectively, even though Pdx1 expression is maintained [97]. This developmental phenotype is strikingly similar to that of Ptf1a-deficient embryos [47,63]. Indeed, this defect is due, at least in part, to the loss of *Ptf1a* expression during the early stages of development of Hnf1b-deficient pancreatic rudiments. The presence of an Hnf1b binding site in the *Ptf1a* gene promoter suggests that Hnf1b may regulate *Ptf1a* transcription directly [97].

3.3   Onset of Islet and Acinar Development by the Secondary Developmental Transition (12.5–15.5 dpc)

The next stage of pancreatic organogenesis converts the protodifferentiated epithelium of expanding progenitor cells into a dynamic epithelium that generates acinar cells, differentiated ductal cells, and the second (principal) wave of endocrine cells that form the islets. This dramatic and critical conversion period is termed the "secondary transition" (● *Fig. 4-5*). It was recognized initially by the sudden appearance of large numbers of insulin-producing β-cells [2], the expansion of the glucagon-producing α-cell population [130], and the appearance of pro-acini coincident with a massive increase in the synthesis of acinar digestive enzymes [105]. Highly proliferative cells in epithelial tips around the periphery of the pancreatic rudiment form a domain of rapid outward growth [131]. As the tips forge outward, progeny left behind differentiate. By the end of the secondary transition, a greatly expanded and highly branched tubular epithelium has formed from the protodifferentiated epithelium (● *Fig. 4-6*). Acini form at the tips of the branches and islets form near the center of the epithelium. In this section, we describe the developmental processes that occur during the secondary transition and the extrinsic and intrinsic factors that control these processes.

3.3.1   The Secondary Transition

The secondary transition is initiated at about 12 dpc by the formation of multipotent precursor cells (MPCs) at the tips of young branches around the periphery of the epithelium (● *Fig. 4-7*) [7]. The MPCs were identified from the restricted expression of four developmental markers: (1) a high level of Ptf1a, whereas other cells of the epithelium have lost Ptf1a; (2) Pdx1; (3) low carboxypeptidase A1 (Cpa1) and the absence of the acinar markers amylase and elastase; and (4) high c-Myc, consistent with high replication rate of these cells and the requirement for Myc to attain normal acinar cell mass [132]. Genetic lineage-tracing experiments of cells expressing *Cpa1* at 12.5 dpc showed that acinar, ductal and islet cells all derive from the MPC population [7]. Cpa1 is used routinely as a specific marker of differentiated acinar cells. Its presence in progenitor cells with the potential to generate duct and islet cells, as well as acinar cells, afforded a surprising and fortuitous readout of an intermediate developmental state. The absence of other acinar digestive enzymes (e.g., elastase and amylase) is a further indication that the MPCs are not merely pre-acinar cells. A critical role for *Cpa1* in the formation or maintenance of MPCs is excluded by the absence of developmental defects in embryos homozygous null for *Cpa1* [7].

The MPCs constitute the majority of replicating epithelial cells during the secondary transition, and their rapid reproduction drives the remodeling of the epithelium (● *Fig. 4-7*). The high rate of cell division propels the epithelial tips outward and leaves behind partly differentiated progeny with slower rates of cell division. Branching of the epithelium begins in the MPC-containing tips by the formation of a "cleft" of differentiating tubule cells within the cluster of MPCs at a tip, which separates the MPC domain into two tips [7]. Both tips continue the epithelial extension outward and each may create further branches with further iterations of cleft formation. Growth and branching continues in this fashion for several days, until the MPC population becomes depleted. Genetic lineage-tracing of the descendants of cells expressing *Cpa1* after 14.5 dpc detected differentiated acinar cells, but not ductal or islet cells. Thus,

Fig. 4-6

The branched pancreatic epithelium in the middle of the secondary transition of an embryonic mouse pancreas. A section through the dorsal pancreas at late 14.5 dpc with immunolocalization of the transcription factor Pdx1 (*green*) displays the pancreatic epithelium during the secondary transition. At this stage, most of the cells of the epithelial tubules containing islet and ductal precursors (yellow outlines) and pro-acini (white indicators around the periphery) have nuclear Pdx1.

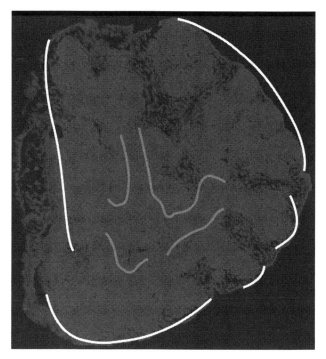

after about 14.5 dpc, *Cpa1*-expression no longer represents transient MPCs, but rather cells now committed to the acinar fate.

After 14.5 dpc, the progeny left in the wake of the replicating tips form epithelial tubules, while those cells remaining at the tips become proacini, which begin terminal acinar differentiation at the ends of short branches (◉ *Fig. 4-7*). The proacinar cells begin the synthesis of the other secretory digestive enzymes in addition to Cpa1, and their rate of cell replication decreases. Thus, as development proceeds, acinar differentiation appears as a gradient from the center toward the periphery of the epithelium, with an overlapping but inverse gradient of cellular replication [131].

Ductal and islet cells derive from the MPC-progeny deposited in the tubule epithelium. MPC daughter cells that enter this developmental compartment initially may be bipotent for the ductal and islet lineages, although this has not been tested directly. Cell replication continues in the tubules, though at a lower level than in MPCs (M. Hale & R.J.M, unpublished). Scattered within the tubule epithelium are precursor cells that then initiate expression of the TF Ngn3 to a high level and commit to the islet cell fate [3,109,133,134]. To date, an analogous transcriptional regulatory factor that commits precursor cells to the

⬛ Fig. 4-7

Multipotent precursors for acinar, ductal and islet cells initiate the secondary transition at epithelial tips. Yellow, precursors in the tubules for duct and islet cells. Orange, multipotent precursor cells (MPCs) [7]. Burnt orange, proacinar cells at the ends of branched tubules that have lost multipotency and committed to acinar differentiation. Red, differentiating acini that have revised their relationship with the terminal tubule cells, which will become centroacinar cells. Brown, domains in the tubules initiate ductal cell differentiation. Green nuclei, scattered cells in the tubules initiate Ngn3 expression. Green cells have escaped the epithelium and begun the islet cell developmental program. Light blue, differentiating endocrine cells that have initiated the synthesis of an islet hormone. Blue, clusters of differentiated islet cells. Arrows indicate the outward growth of the epithelia. Although the drawing depicts a uniform population of bipotent precursor cells (yellow, islet and duct potential), it is also possible that two discrete precursor populations are present, one for islet cells and one for ductal cells.

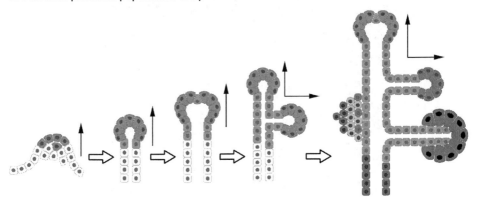

ductal lineage has not been identified;. ductal development may be the default option for the cells of the tubular epithelium that do not activate Ngn3 expression. Alternatively, bipotent MPC progeny may resolve quickly to more stable progenitors specified to either ductal or islet fate, which await further developmental cues. For the islet lineage, this is Notch signaling, which induces Ngn3 gene activation in a controlled temporal and spatial manner leading to the proper formation of islets.

The extrinsic signaling that induces the formation of MPCs is unknown, although Notch signaling has been proposed to maintain the localized concentration of MPCs in epithelial tips by suppressing differentiation [7]. The retention and elevation of Ptf1a restricted to MPCs suggest that Ptf1a plays an important role at this stage. The predominant form of Ptf1a at this stage is in the trimeric PTF1-J complex [135]. The requirement for Pdx1 in order for the secondary transition to begin [127] is due to an as yet unappreciated function in MPCs. Little else is known of the transcriptional regulators of this important developmental intermediate from which the acinar, ductal and islet lineages directly arise.

Thus, the MPCs are a multipotent replicating progenitor population that creates the branching epithelial network during the secondary transition. This progenitor population resolves into committed acinar precursor cells and what appear to be bipotent precursors for islet and ductal cells (portrayed in the pancreatic lineage diagram of ◗ Fig. 4-3). This developmental path links the embryonic ductal lineage more closely to the islet lineage than to the acinar cell lineage. This is an important notion because the favored historical model has been an initial separation of the endocrine lineage from a common ductal and acinar one, followed by the formation of acini from ductal precursors.

In sum, the morphogenetic processes of the secondary transition generate a greatly expanded and branched tubular epithelium (❯ Fig. 4-6) with regions specialized for the formation of islet cells near the center and acinar cell clusters toward the periphery. After this transition, the pancreatic epithelium has undergone three transformations: predifferentiated →1→ protodifferentiated →2→ tubular epithelium of ductal and endocrine progenitor cells with MPCs and differentiating acini at the tips →3→ differentiated ductal epithelium linking acini and separated from the delaminated endocrine cells. We consider next some of the developmental processes, both cellular and molecular, that create the acini, ducts and islets.

3.3.1.1   Formation of Acini from the Multipotent Precursor Cells (MPCs)

As the epithelial expansion of the secondary transition runs its course, MPCs at the ends of branches decrease their rate of replication, commit to the acinar lineage and differentiate to proacinar cell clusters. To form acini, the pro-acinar cells at the ends of the precursor tubules may alter their cell-cell contacts and extend back over the tubule to form an acinar cell "cap" (❯ Fig. 4-8). This process is consistent with a developmental intermediate of a mature acinus with the terminus of the intercalated duct (aka centroacinar cells) inserting deep into the acinus [8]. Although much is known of the transcriptional regulators for islet formation and for the early stage of pancreatic development common to islet and acinar cells, relatively little is known about the control of acinar formation. No extrinsic signal or transcriptional regulator has yet been shown directly to initiate acinar development.

The expression of *Hes1* in the precursor epithelium of the secondary transition implicates the presence of active Notch-signaling [137]. *Hes1* expression in the precursor tubules extends up to but does not include the pro-acinar cells [138], suggesting that Notch-signaling may control this developmental boundary. Indeed, in zebrafish proper allocation of precursors to acinar and ductal lineages requires functional Notch-signaling [98,139]. In reconstitution experiments, Hes1 can interfere with Ptf1a activity directly [138]. If Notch-ligands regulate both islet and acinar developmental programs, additional positional cues must be necessary to specify one or the other program.

Wnt signaling has been implicated directly in acinar development, and may provide the second extrinsic cue to direct cells released from Notch-suppression to the acinar rather than islet or ductal fate. Cell-autonomous β-catenin function is required for the formation of acinar cells as part of the canonical Wnt signaling pathway rather than cellular architecture or planar cell polarity [40–42,140]. In particular, the increase of Ptf1a at the secondary transition does not occur in β-catenin-deficient pancreatic tissue. Although the Wnt induction of *Ptf1a* directly through β-catenin-LEF/TCF binding to *Ptf1a* gene control sequences has not been proven, a LEF/TCF binding site is conserved among mammals in the acinar specific enhancer for Ptf1a [135].

Proacinar cells derived from MPCs lose the transcriptional regulators that maintain the progenitor status of the epithelium. Hes1 is not detected in cells expressing amylase, and the TFs Sox9 and Hnf1b rapidly disappear from these cells [2,138,141]. However, *Ptf1a* expression continues at a high level in proacini, whereas it is shut off in the tubules containing the ductal and islet precursors. In this new context, Ptf1a acquires a new developmental function, which is to direct the differentiation of acinar cells. The active form of Ptf1a during early development is the trimeric PTF1-J complex (Section 3.2), which is necessary to initiate the formation

⬛ Fig. 4-8

A stereotypic model for the morphogenetic processes that generate islets centrally and acini peripherally. (a): A close-up view of the structure of Pdx1-expressing tubules, peritubular cords, and proacini from a section nearby that of ❯ *Fig. 4-6*. Note the subset of cells located in the cell cords or the tubules in contact with the cords that have very high Pdx1; these may be cells committed selectively to the β-cell differentiation program [136]. Green, Pdx1; red, glucagon, which marks the majority of the differentiated endocrine cells at this stage (E14.5). (b): Diagram of the proposed developmental compartments of the post-MPC epithelium. Yellow, progenitors of islet and ductal cells retain the capacity for cell proliferation. Beige, committed ductal cell precursors. Orange (left), committed pro-acinar cells retain cell-proliferation and continuity with the tubular epithelium and have begun the synthesis of other digestive enzymes in addition to Cpa1. Red (right), differentiating acinar cells with low cell-replication capacity, ongoing cytodifferentiation and accumulation of secretory (zymogen) granules. The acinar cells have formed a cap engulfing the tubule end cells, which become the centroacinar cells of the mature acinus. Green-to-blue, islet precursors initiate the islet program via Ngn3 expression (green nuclei) and release from the tubule epithelium. The disposition of cell-cell junctions is not confirmed. Orthogonal/Asymmetric division model (upper): Parallel cell divisions are symmetric and generate equivalent daughter cells that remain in the epithelium. Orthogonal divisions (green) are asymmetric and retain one daughter in the epithelium with intracellular junctions intact and release the other. EMT model (lower): Pre-endocrine cells in the epithelium break intracellular junctions, acquire transient mesenchymal properties, migrate from the epithelium, congregate in clusters, re-establish epithelial cell properties, and differentiate. Inset left: pro-acinus with connecting tubule. Inset right: differentiating acinus with cap structure.

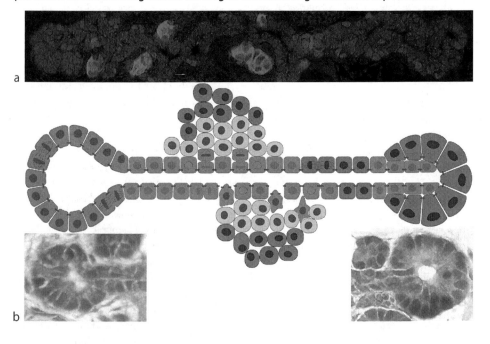

of acini. Ptf1a, as part of the PTF1 complex, sits near the top of a transcription factor network that directs acinar development.

An early step in acinar differentiation is the synthesis of Rbpj-like (Rbpjl), the product of an Rbpj gene that was duplicated sometime during vertebrate evolution and since diverged. Whereas Rbpj is the transcriptional mediator for Notch, Rbpjl has lost the ability to participate in the Notch signaling pathway [142]. Rbpjl expression is largely limited to acinar cells of the pancreas and discrete regions of the forebrain. Transcription of the *Rbpjl* gene is activated in proacinar cells by the PTF1-J complex bound to the *Rbpjl* promoter [47]. As Rbpjl protein accumulates, it replaces the Rbpj subunit in the PTF1 complex. It is the Rbpjl form (PTF1-L) that binds and drives the promoters of most if not all the secretory digestive enzymes of differentiated acinar cells. PTF1-L also replaces PTF1-J on the Rbpjl promoter and creates a positive regulatory loop that ensures the continued production of Rbpjl in acinar cells. In a complementary fashion, the Ptf1a gene has a transcriptional enhancer with a PTF1-binding site that requires the presence of a trimeric PTF1 complex for activity [135]. Consequently, the genes for both pancreas-restricted subunits of the complex are auto-activated in acinar cells by PTF1-L. Similar transcriptional positive feedback loops are commonly found near the top of a regulatory hierarchy in developing systems and serve to first drive development toward a particular state and then to stabilize that state [143]. It is likely that the PTF1-J complex helps establish the MPC population and a developmental signal such as Wnt (see above) pushes some MPCs toward acinar development by activating Rbpjl and other regulatory genes. The requirement for Rbpj during acinar development [45,48] is most likely due to its role in the PTF1-J complex of the MPCs and not its role in Notch-signaling. Ensuring the continued transcription of Ptf1a and Rbpjl through their autoregulatory loops may then drive acinar differentiation and stabilize the phenotype of mature acinar cells.

The PTF1-L complex resides on the promoters of all the genes encoding the secretory zymogens tested: amylase (*Amy1*), elastases 1 & 2 (*Ela1, Ela2*), carboxypeptidase A1 (*Cpa1*), chymotrypsin B (*Ctrb*) and trypsin (*Prss3*) [47,129]. Potential PTF1-L binding sites are present near the start of the genes of fourteen other acinar secretory enzymes. It is likely that the PTF1-L complex coordinately controls the entire collection of acinar secretory proteins.

The bHLH TF Mist1 is expressed selectively in the serous-type secretory cells of many exocrine glands [144]. During pancreatic development, Mist1 is required to establish proper apical-basal cell polarity and complete acinar differentiation [145]. Mist1 acts downstream of Ptf1a, because Mist1-deficient embryos initiate acinar development normally, but acinar cells do not acquire proper cytoarchitecture or the pathway for regulated exocytosis. In the absence of Mist1, acinar cells lose intercellular communication because gap junctions do not form properly [146], have mitochondria with compromised Ca++ uptake and Golgi positioned incorrectly [147], and have defective regulated exocytosis [148]. The loss of functional gap junctions is due to greatly reduced expression of connexin32, which normally pairs with connexin26 to form the intracellular channels of the junctions. The gene encoding Connexin32 is a direct target of Mist1 [148]. As a consequence of these defects in gene expression and cellular or-ganization, normal acinar cell polarity is not established, Ca++ signaling is abnormal, packaging the secretory enzymes is defective, intracellular zymogens are activated, and genes characteristic of duct cells are expressed aberrantly [146–148]. Mist1 also limits acinar cell replication by controlling the expression of the cell cycle regulator p21 [18]. Thus, Mist1 controls the final stage of differentiation that establishes the functional and stable acinar cell phenotype.

The Zinc-finger TF Gata4 is present throughout the early pancreatic epithelium, becomes restricted in the tips of epithelial branches during the secondary transition, and is present exclusively in the acinar cells of the mature gland [93,149]. Because Gata4 null embryos die at 9.5dpc, it is not known whether Gata4 plays the important role in acinar development its expression pattern suggests.

Lrh1/Nr5a2 is a member of the family of nuclear hormone receptors and is required for proper gastrulation [150] and regulation of bile acid metabolism in adult liver [151,152]. It is present at high levels in pancreatic acinar cells and regulated at least in part by the action of Pdx1 on its promoter [153]. Preliminary evidence indicates that Lrh1 is super-induced directly by PTF1 at the onset of acinar development and is required for most of the acinar developmental program (M. Hale, Y.K. Lee, G.H. Swift, S. Kliewer and R.J.M., unpublished observations).

The homeodomain protein Prox1 is required for the proper allocation of progenitor cells to the endocrine versus exocrine lineage. *Prox1*-deficient embryos have precocious acinar development and diminished total acinar and islet tissue formation [154]. These developmental defects suggest that Prox1 might help maintain the multipotent progenitor cell population by delaying acinar development. Because Prox1 can interact with and inhibit the transcriptional activity of Lrh1 in other contexts [155], it may govern the orderly formation of acini by restraining Lrh1 function during pancreatic development. Indeed, Prox1 and Lrh1 are expressed in complementary patterns during the secondary transition. Just as eliminating the restraining effects of Notch signaling on Ngn3 activity causes progenitor cell-depletion by allowing precocious endocrine development, so too might the absence of Prox1 allow unrestrained Lrh1 activity and the premature induction of acinar development.

The crucial next steps in understanding further the nature of acinar cells and their formation are to identify the extrinsic signal(s) that resolves the acinar lineage from the multipotent precursor cells and to define the interacting transcription factor network that includes PTF1, Mist1, Lrh1, Prox1 and Gata4.

3.3.2   Ductal Development

The ductal system of the mature pancreas comprises the two main pancreatic ducts that drain into the intestine, small interlobular ducts that link the lobules to the main drainage, smaller intralobular ducts, and even finer intercalating ducts (IDs) that connect to individual acini [156,157]. In addition, the pancreas is the only exocrine gland in which the connecting ducts (here intercalated ducts) insert into the acinus. These extensions of the intercalated duct have been designated "centroacinar cells," a term that obscures their function, origin and relationship with the ductal tree, and we suggest instead the designation intra-acinar duct cells (IAD cells). The ductal nature of the IAD cells is indicated by their expression of Muc-1, an O-glycosylated transmembrane protein present at the apical pole of all ductal cells [158], and their specific binding to Dolicus biflurous agglutinin (DBA) [126,159]. The evidence that the IDs derive from a developmental program distinct from that of large ducts is several-fold. The two programs can be resolved by the gestational times at which each requires PDX1 [127]: depleting Pdx1 experimentally just prior to the secondary transition at E12.5 allows the formation of the large ducts, but not IDs or IAD cells. The ductal structure that forms upon Pdx1-depletion at sequential time-points appears to represent incomplete main ducts (one from each bud), primary branches from the main ducts (the interlobular ducts), and the beginning of secondary branches distally (intralobular ducts). In a similar fashion, the directed germline inactivation of *Ptf1a* allows the formation of the large but not the small ducts [47,63,64].

The large pancreatic ducts are similar and developmentally related to the common bile duct [61,160]. Indeed, the biliary epithelium has the potential for pancreatic development. *Hes1* normally is expressed throughout the extrahepatic biliary epithelium during bile duct development. In mice that are homozygous-deficient for *Hes1*, the developing biliary epithelium inappropriately expresses *Ngn3* and *Ptf1a*. This ectopic *Ngn3*-expession leads to aberrant formation of islet-like structures, and *Ptf1a*-expression to acini [61, 160]. Simply freeing embryonic extrahepatic biliary duct explants from in vivo constraints by dissection permits activation of *Sox9, Pdx1, Hnf6/Onecut1, Hes1* and *Ngn3* transiently, and the formation of β-like endocrine cells during tissue culture [161]. In other studies, the HD factor Hnf6/Onecut1 was shown to be required for proper development of the biliary tract [162] and the large pancreatic ducts [158]. The development of the large pancreatic ducts is disrupted in *Hnf6*-deficient embryos, but IDs form normally [158]. Thus, different regulatory programs appear to control the formation of the two subsets of pancreatic ducts. This is further illustrated molecularly, as two classes of ducts can be distinguished in the adult pancreas: *Tcf2* expression is maintained in differentiated large ducts, but not in IDs and IAD cells [163].

Hnf6 and other TFs that it controls are critical regulators of ductal development. The absence of Hnf6 causes extensive developmental defects of the pancreas [164]. Whereas the extent and morphology of acinar tissue is near normal and the first wave endocrine cells form, the second wave lineage does not appear and dilated cystic duct structures appear in the epithelium. The cystic ductal phenotype appears at 15 dpc, which may mark the onset of duct-specific differentiation. The cystic ducts express the differentiation marker Muc1, but are devoid of the primary cilia normally present throughout the mature large ductal tree [158]. Mutations in the genes for the structural proteins of the cilium cause similar defects in ductal differentiation, but the second wave endocrine cells form [165]. These observations suggest that ductal precursors form but do not differentiate properly, in part due to the absence of primary cilia. Because the second wave endocrine cells form in the absence of cilia, they evidently require *Hnf6* for a different (or additional) purpose, possibly the formation of the immediate second wave precursor cells.

Hnf6 controls the formation of the cilia, and thereby ductal development, via Hnf1b, another key pancreatic TF. Hnf6 is needed for the expression of Hnf1b during liver and pancreatic development [163], and Hnf1b is known to control the expression of genes for cilium function in the kidney [162]. The absence of Hnf1b in the cells of the cystic ducts of Hnf6-deficient embryonic pancreas [158, 165] indicates that the cilium defect is due to the loss of Hnf1b. To understand the control of ductal development further, it will be important to identify the extrinsic signals that initiate the ductal program and additional TFs that control it.

3.3.3   The Second Wave of Endocrine Cells – Formation of Primitive Islets

A new population of endocrine cells, distinct from the first wave of the early pancreatic bud, arises during the secondary transition from a population of progenitors left behind by the advancing MPCs in the epithelial tips (see ❯ *Fig. 4-7*). The transient intense expression of *Ngn3* in scattered cells of the tubular precursor tubule epithelium directs these cells to begin the endocrine developmental program by inducing pro-endocrine TFs that include Snail2/Slug, NeuroD1, Pax4, Arx and Nkx2.2. The activation of *Ngn3* appears to be promoted by the binding of TFs Hnf1, Hnf6 and Hnf3b to a distal regulatory region of the *Ngn3* gene [166]. These factors are present throughout the interior region of the precursor epithelium, but *Ngn3* transcription is repressed in all but a few scattered cells at any one instant by Notch signaling, resulting in the binding of Hes1 or other members of the Hes1 repressor family to the proximal promoter region of *Ngn3* [166]. Limited *Ngn3* expression provides a measured induction of endocrine development without exhausting the progenitor population prematurely and without preempting ductal cell development from the same population. By the time islet precursors become committed and leave the epithelial tubule, *Ngn3* expression has been abruptly shut off. The transient nature of *Ngn3* transcription appears to be due, at least in part, to direct feedback repression by Ngn3 [167].

Ngn3 initiates a developmental cascade by activating the promoters of genes for TFs with roles in endocrine differentiation. Two members of the Zn-finger family of repressor TFs (Snail2 and Insm1) are induced shortly after the transient appearance of high Ngn3. In other developmental contexts, Snail2 initiates an epithelial-to-mesenchymal transition that releases cells from the confines of epithelial sheets and so may also program the release of endocrine precursor cells from the tubular epithelium (see below). Other target genes control the endocrine differentiation program directly. NeuroD1 sits just below Ngn3 in a regulatory hierarchy. Indeed, the forced expression of either Ngn3 or NeuroD1 in pancreatic ductal cell lines induces the endocrine differentiation program [168], consistent with the close relationship between pancreatic ductal and islet lineages (⊙ *Fig. 4-3*). The two sets of genes induced by Ngn3 or NeuroD1 are similar, but not completely overlapping; thus, both are necessary and each has specific functions. A primary function of Ngn3 is the induction of NeuroD1 by binding and activating the *NeuroD1* promoter [169] and NeuroD1 then continues the endocrine differentiation program after Ngn3 expression stops.

Genes encoding intrinsic factors that resolve the α, β, δ, and ε, and PP sub-lineages of islet cells are among the set of endocrine regulatory genes induced by Ngn3. In this regard, Ngn3 cooperates with Hnf3b to activate the promoter of *Pax4* [167], which commits cells to β- and δ-cell fates and subsequently directs completion of β-cell differentiation through the genes it controls [170,171]. As a complement to Pax4, the HD factor Arx directs β/δ precursors toward δ-cell differentiation [171]. Pax4 and Arx are initially present together in an intermediate endocrine precursor cell and mutually antagonize the expression of the other by binding and inhibiting the transcription of the other's gene [172]. Unknown influences that give the upper hand to one or the other determine the relative ratio of β- and δ-cells.

Although Pdx1 is expressed in the progenitor cells for all islet cell-types, its presence at distinctly higher levels in scattered cells within the precursor epithelium is thought to be instructive for the β-cell fate (⊙ *Fig. 4-8a*). Deletion of the transcriptional enhancer required specifically for the superinduction of *Pdx1* in the epithelium of the secondary transition greatly decreased the formation of β-cells and complementarily increased in α-, δ- and PP-cells [136], suggesting that preferential allocation of precursor cells to the β-lineage requires a higher threshold level of Pdx1. The bZIP factor MafA is required to complete the final stages of β- cell differentiation by activating genes important to β-cell function, including insulin [173,174]. Pdx1, Nkx2.2 and Hnf3b cooperate to activate *MafA* preferentially in differentiating β-cells [175]; MafA in turn binds a regulatory region of *Pdx1* to help maintain high levels of Pdx1 in β-cells [176].

These few examples of competing and reinforcing regulatory loops linking transcription factors and their genes illustrate common mechanisms that resolve similar cellular lineages and stabilize the differentiation process and the final differentiated cell phenotypes. More complete descriptions of the TFs that control islet cell differentiation are presented in several excellent reviews [6,119,141,170,177].

Extrinsic factors also regulate the second wave of endocrine differentiation. The control of the commitment to endocrine fate by Notch-signaling has been well characterized by experimental manipulation. Driving Notch1-ICD expression in precursors to both endocrine and exocrine lineages prevents the differentiation of both compartments and leaves an incompletely differentiated ductal epithelium [178]. The in vivo over-expression of constitutively active Notch (Notch1-ICD) selectively in the Ngn3+ precursor population also suppresses endocrine differentiation [59].

TGFβ signaling helps fashion islet structure and function. Components of the TGFβ pathway are present in the precursor epithelium and mesenchyme. In particular, activin receptors (ActRIIa and ActRIIb) are found in the pancreatic epithelium and later in islets. Null or dominant-negative mutations of these receptors or their downstream mediator Smad2 in the pancreatic precursor epithelium or in differentiating endocrine cells results in decreased islet hormone expression and islet hypoplasia [30,31,179]. Similarly, over-expression of the inhibitory Smad7 within the *Pdx1* domain greatly decreases β-cell development. Importantly, the TGFβ inhibitor follistatin is in the mesenchyme following the second transition and later in islets at E18.5. Explant studies suggest that follistatin inhibits endocrine differentiation and promotes exocrine differentiation, and may also play an active role in isletogenesis by regulating the matrix metalloproteinase MMP-2 [117]. Together, these results support a role for TGFβ and activin during endocrine differentiation. Regulation by follistatin is likely to be required for both the initial allocation of progenitors to the exocrine or endocrine lineages and the proper morphogenesis of islets.

The TGFβ family member GDF11 is required for β-cell differentiation and maturation [180,181]. Mice lacking GDF11 have more Ngn3 expressing precursor cells late in gestation, suggesting that GDF11 suppresses endocrine maturation. This role appears to be restricted to embryogenesis, because the final number of endocrine cells in adult mutant mice is smaller than normal. The exocrine compartment of the GDF11 null mice is also smaller than normal, indicating that GDF11 may control the choice of progenitors between endocrine and exocrine fates [180]. It is thought that GDF11 plays a parallel role to Notch signaling, because both are required for proper expansion of endocrine progenitors by suppressing their differentiation during a defined window of time, thereby regulating the total number of differentiated endocrine cells. The need for tight regulation of TGFβ signaling in pancreatic tissue is reflected by the many pancreatic cancers with elevated levels of both TGFβ and Smad2 [182].

3.3.3.1 Formation of Islet Precursor Cells by Delamination

Whereas acini form at the ends of precursor tubules and maintain topological continuity of with the ductal system, islets form from cells that escape the continuum of the epithelial tubules. The escaped islet precursor cells coalesce into cords that remain intimately associated with and within the basal lamina of the single-cell layer tubules [2]. The endocrine cell cords grow by continued recruitment of precursors from the epithelial tubules, rather than by replication of the differentiating endocrine cells.

The endocrine cell cords are thus endocrine cells early in their differentiation process and these can be distinguished from the tubules by the presence of synaptophysin (L. Shi, M.A. Hale & R.J.M., unpublished), a component of the microvesicle secretory process and an early differentiation marker of neuroendocrine cells [13]. Cord cells with synaptophysin, but without any of the five principal islet hormones, appear to constitute the less differentiated cells most recently released from the tubules. Approximately half of the synaptophysin-expressing cells at 14.5–15.5 dpc are pre-hormone precursors, while the remainder have endocrine hormones and are therefore more differentiated. As the endocrine cords mature, increase in size, and form spherical structures, the basal lamina surrounding the forming islet eventually pinches off near its association with the differentiating duct and thereby separates the extracellular spaces of the endocrine and exocrine tissues.

Two cellular processes have been proposed for the release of islet precursors from the tubular epithelium (❯ *Fig. 4-8*). One, a classical epithelial-to-mesenchymal transition or EMT, is a common developmental process for generating motile mesenchymal cells from cells in an epithelial sheet. During EMT, epithelial cells escape their epithelial neighbors by acquiring mesenchymal cell properties. For this process to be a viable option for islet cell derivation, reversion from a transient mesenchymal state back to an epithelial state must occur prior to endocrine differentiation within the endocrine cell cords. The other process is orthogonal or asymmetric cell division, which releases cells from the epithelium by a reorientation of the cell division plane in a manner that frees one daughter from the junctional complexes that tether cells in the epithelial sheet. We discuss the evidence for each.

The Epithelial-Mesenchymal Transition (EMT)   The release of islet precursor cells from the embryonic pancreatic epithelium has been proposed many times to involve a process related to EMT, but as yet there has been no proof that it occurs. During gastrulation, the involution of mesodermal precursor cells through the primitive streak occurs by an EMT. In addition, migrating neural crest cells arise via delamination of cells from the dorsolateral neural tube by an EMT.

Instances of EMTs share a number of similar properties that are relatively well understood at the cellular level [183]. Individual cells escape from an epithelial sheet and begin EMT by breaking the tight junction complexes with their neighbors and degrading junctional proteins. Changes in the cytoarchitecture of the delaminating cell drive a basal retraction of the newly untethered apical domain. These cells generally lose their polarized epithelial character, become motile and develop a fibroblastic appearance. In some instances ruffling of the basal cell boundary by actin filaments initiates movement of the cell out of the epithelial sheet.

An EMT is often initiated by TGFβ, FGF or Wnt signaling by inducing TFs that repress epithelial maintenance genes and others that promote the mesenchymal phenotype. Signaling through these pathways induces the master EMT regulators Snail1 or its close paralog Snail2. In some experimental settings, the forced expression of Snail1/2 is sufficient to repress epithelial cell characteristics and induce mesenchymal characteristics [184]. The Snail factors repress E-cadherin gene transcription and induce accelerated degradation of E-cadherin [185]. Wnt and FGF signaling can cooperate to induce, stabilize and increase the nuclear concentration of Snail1 and Snail2 and repress the E-cadherin gene directly via LEF/TCF factors [185]. Most cells beginning an EMT have increased GSK-3β activity (an important regulatory node of Wnt and FGF signaling pathways) coincident with increased nuclear accumulation of β-catenin. Each of these signaling pathways is important to pancreatic development, and they may well control an EMT process for the release endocrine precursors from the tubular precursor epithelium.

The only evidence thus far that an EMT process occurs during the endocrine development of the secondary transition is the presence of Snail2 in scattered cells of the tubular precursor epithelium [11]. Snail2 is often (80%) coincident with Ngn3 [11], suggesting that Snail2 is an early gene induced by Ngn3. The appearance of Snail2 thus occurs at the appropriate time for initiating EMT shortly after precursor cells commit to endocrine fate, and is a tantalizing suggestion pointing to the involvement of EMT during endocrine differentiation.

Orthogonal Cell Division Pictet and Rutter [2] proposed that islet precursors escape from the epithelium by a change from the normal axis of cell division, parallel to the epithelial lumen, to one that is orthogonal to the lumen (◐ *Fig. 4-8*). This process is similar to that for the development of the embryonic neuroepithelia of the brain, spinal cord and retina [186]. These epithelia are composed of a single layer of cells with a strong apical-basal polarity and linked by tight junctions and adherens junctions. Cell divisions parallel to the epithelial lumen maintain the progenitor cell population, by generating equivalent daughter progenitor cells, whereas divisions perpendicular to the lumen (orthogonal) retain one progenitor daughter in the epithelium and release the other to begin neuronal development. The cleavage plane in a parallel division bisects the apical plasma membrane and segregates apical and basal cell constituents equally to both daughter cells. The equivalent daughters retain junctional complexes with their neighbors and form a new one with each other, so that the fidelity of the epithelium remains intact.

A cleavage plane off the perpendicular that bypasses the apical membrane creates one daughter cell that inherits apical cell constituents (including the apical plasma membrane and the adherens junctions) and another that inherits basal constituents. This cell division generates two cells with distinctly different composition of apical and basal protein content, including regulatory molecules with biased apical or basal distribution. If islet cells form by asymmetric division of cells in the tubular epithelium of the secondary transition, the "basal" daughter cells would be specified to begin the islet developmental program and release from the epithelium, whereas the "apical" daughters would remain within the epithelium and either retain progenitor status or become a ductal cell.

It is surprising that investigations to distinguish between an EMT and asymmetric division have not been performed in the pancreatic epithelium, as they have in other epithelial derived organs such as the kidney [187]. These two mechanisms can be distinguished through their very different cellular processes, use of cytoplasmic components and regulators, manipulation of the cytoarchitecture, and segregation of basal and apical markers.

3.3.4 Comparison of First and Second Waves of Endocrine Cells

The precise developmental relationship between the first and second wave endocrine cells is unknown; however, differences between them suggest that they represent different cellular lineages [35].

1. Although both first and second wave endocrine cells require *Ngn3* [90], the formation of the first wave cells does not require *Pdx1* [61, 188] or *Ptf1a* [63], which are critical to the formation of the second wave lineage. Indeed, only a few of the first wave cells express *Pdx1* and none express *Ptf1a*; the absence of *Pdx1* and/or *Ptf1a* distinguishes the differentiated first wave endocrine cells distinct from the remainder of the proto-differentiated epithelium at this stage [127].
2. Many more β-cells than α-cells are made during the secondary transition. In addition, glucagon and insulin co-expressing endocrine cells are not observed following the secondary transition. The ratio of β- and α-cells seems to be an inherent property of the two lineages, because experimental manipulation by super-induction of Ngn3 to high levels

during the primary transition leads to overproduction of glucagon-cells and during the secondary transition leads to overproduction of β-cells [133].

3. Clusters of first wave endocrine cells are invariably connected to the precursor epithelium by a cellular bridge, and appear to separate from the proto-differentiated endoderm by a completing a budding process [110], rather than the delamination that occurs during the secondary transition.

Whereas the α-cells that form during the secondary transition use prohormone convertase 2 (PC2) to process the proglucagon polypeptide precursor to active glucagon, the early cells have PC1/3 rather than PC2 and cleave the precursor to GLP1 and GLP2 [189]. Because the glucagon-expressing first wave cells have PC1/3 and produce the GLP peptides, they are not strictly α-cells. If these cells contribute to the α-cell population of neonatal islets, as proposed, they must switch to PC2 from PC1/3 to produce glucagon. Processing proglucagon to GLP1 and GLP2 by PC1/3 is a characteristic of the enteroendocrine L-cells of the intestine and stomach. Thus, the early endocrine cells may be closely related to an enteroendocrine lineage, which also requires Ngn3.

The developmental origins and fates of the first and second wave cells are notable in two respects. First, the cells of the first wave are not the progenitors of the second [3,108]. Consequently, two separate endocrine programs occur rather than a single, continuous one. Second, an equivalent, predominately glucagon-expressing, first wave endocrine cell population does not occur during human pancreatic development [112]. During human development, insulin cells appear first and are always prevalent, followed shortly by the appearance of glucagon and somatostatin cells. These earliest human endocrine cells form during a period of morphogenesis that appears related to the murine second transition, rather than an earlier primary transition. For comparisons with the developmental processes of human islet formation, it is important to distinguish the first and second waves of murine endocrine cells.

3.3.5 Dorsal and Ventral Bud Fusion

As the dorsal and ventral buds grow, branch and extend, they are brought into contact at the base of their primary ducts by the movements of gut turning. The primary ducts fuse at around 11.5 dpc while their distal portions remain largely separate. In humans, fusion of the dorsal and ventral buds creates a more integrated organ than in rodents. The dorsal bud forms the upper part of the head of the human pancreas, as well as the main body and tail (or splenic portion). The ventral bud forms the lower part of the head of pancreas – the uncinate process. The compositions of the dorsal and ventral portions differ. The dorsal pancreas forms more abundant large islets, with a higher number of β- and α-cells and a smaller number of PP-cells. In contrast, the ventral pancreas gives is interspersed with smaller islets, which have been shown to contain proportionally more PP-cells [190]. However, the relative density of islets within the two sections of the pancreas are comparable [191].

3.4 Perinatal Growth and Differentiation (16 dpc to Neonate)

Following the secondary transition and the acquisition of acinar, ductal or endocrine cell fates, the pancreas continues growth in parallel with most other embryonic organs. The pancreas expands by cell proliferation with exocrine tissue added at the periphery and endocrine cells coalescing into progressively larger and more mature clusters. The proportion of endocrine cells declines due to the massive expansion of maturing exocrine tissue. During the first few weeks after birth, the first mature islets become distinguishable with the recognizable architecture of a β-cell core surrounded by a mantle of α, ε and recently emerged δ and PP cells (which begin to appear at 15.5 dpc).

3.4.1 Isletogenesis

Islet morphogenesis begins at the secondary transition with the endocrine cell precursors released from the tubular pancreatic epithelium. Unlike the first wave cells, these pre-endocrine cells aggregate into ribbon-like cords that remain in close association with the precursor epithelium. The cells migrate along rather than away from the underlying epithelium, and not far from their origin. Shortly before birth glucagon-expressing α-cells begin to envelop the β-cell cords [110], initiating the formation of a peripheral mantle in mature islets. The cords of mixed endocrine cells are proposed to be broken up by the growth of acinar tissue, which intercedes and divides the cords into segments, like beads-on-a-string [3]. Shortly before birth, the forming islets acquire a characteristic spherical shape, lose their tight association with the ductal epithelium, and organize nearby within the acinar parenchyma [2]. An important aspect of islet morphogenesis is the internal organization of β-cells into tightly bundled and polarized epithelial sheaths surrounding blood vessels [192]. Although isletogenesis is readily observed in the developing pancreas, and the term widely used, it has been almost completely ignored by researchers, with only a few exceptions outlined below.

   Mutations in a number of key developmental extrinsic and intrinsic factors disrupt the morphogenesis of normal islets. The defects fall into two main categories – disruption of intra-islet organization or aberrant islet growth – which have been observed in mouse models of diabetes [193–196]. Disruption of BMP signaling via deletion of the BMP receptor 1a gene, for instance, disrupts the segregated distribution of α-cells to the mantle and β-cells to the interior, and impairs glucose stimulated insulin secretion [197]. Proper control of the matrix metalloproteinase MMP-2 by TGF-β1 also is required for normal islet morphogenesis [117]. Persistent expression of HNF6 beyond 18.5 dpc causes failure of islet architecture and β-cell dysfunction [198]. When Nkx2.2 is experimentally converted into a repressor (via fusion with the engrailed repressor domain) and expressed in the perinatal endocrine compartment, α-cells form within the islet core and the affected mice become overtly diabetic after birth [199]. These are only a few of many similar examples of mutations that cause aberrant islet anatomy. It is likely that much of the control of islet architecture by EF and TF pathways occurs via their regulation of cell-surface adhesion molecules or components of the extracellular matrix, which direct many aspects of tissue morphogenesis. Indeed, integrins and cell adhesion molecules, such as E-cadherin and NCAM, have been implicated in guiding the migration and organization of endocrine cells into islets.

4   End Note

A complex and dynamic interplay of extrinsic and intrinsic signaling pathways create the great cell diversity, anatomy, and finely tuned physiologic functions of the adult pancreas. Because each signaling pathway is used broadly during embryogenesis, pathway defects often cause early embryonic lethality, prior to the onset of pancreatic organogenesis, and consequently pancreatic defects generally cannot be distinguished. In contrast, because most of the key pancreatic TFs discussed in this review have functions largely restricted to pancreatic development or function, many are directly linked to heritable human pancreatic maladies including endocrine cell defects in diabetes [200] and exocrine agenesis [62,65].

On the other hand, defects in signaling pathways are common in human pancreatic cancers. Aberrations in Notch, TGFβ, Hedgehog and Wnt pathways occur in adenocarcinoma [25,182,201], and are discussed in other chapters of this Handbook. To our knowledge, however, mutations in genes encoding key pancreatic TFs that control development are not commonly associated with pancreatic carcinogenesis. Nonetheless, it is to be expected that signaling defects must lead to suppression of pancreatic TFs that promote differentiation over proliferation (for example, Mist1) or activation of TFs that promote the inverse (such as c-Myc).

Understanding the complex relationships between these factors and how they influence pancreatic cell growth, proliferation and/or differentiation, will be critical to developing therapeutic approaches diseases affecting a wide range of conditions from metabolic defects to pancreatic cancer. One striking example is the recent demonstration that insulin gene expression can be induced in vivo by directed transdifferentiation of adult acinar cells through the forced expression of just three endocrine transcription factors, Pdx1, Ngn3 and MafA [202]. Refinement of this process may lead to a therapeutic approach to replace lost β-cell function in diabetics. It is imaginable that similar approaches may someday provide the option of inducing acinar function to reverse exocrine pancreatic insufficiency.

Key Research Points

- The acinar, ductal and endocrine cells of the pancreas derive from a common progenitor cell population that evaginates from the posterior foregut endoderm.
- The budding pancreatic epithelium, encased in mesenchyme, first stratifies and then resolves into a branched epithelium of early pancreatic progenitors.
- A primary developmental transition forms an epithelium of sufficient progenitor cells to sustain subsequent development and establish the final size of the pancreas.
- A secondary transition converts the early progenitor cells to more developmentally restricted multipotent precursor cells (MPCs) that initiate the formation of acini, ducts and islets.
- Proliferation of the MPCs at the tips of epithelial branches propel the tips outward, leaving behind precursors for duct and islet cells and forming acini at the tips as proliferation wanes.
- Islet precursor cells delaminate from central regions of the epithelium, begin endocrine differentiation, and progressively aggregate to form islets.
- The pancreatic program of organogenesis is coordinated by a repeating interplay between extrinsic signals and intrinsic transcriptional regulators.
- Hedgehog, FGF, retinoic acid, Wnt, TGFb, BMP4 and Notch cell-cell signaling pathways all contribute to the extrinsic control of pancreatic development.
- Known pancreas-restricted transcription factors, in intrinsic regulatory networks, specify a pancreatic response to the widely used extrinsic signals.
- In turn, temporal changes in extracellular signals reformulate the transcription factor network in a stepwise manner to resolve cell-lineages and control lineage-specific differentiation programs.

Future Scientific Directions

- Define the morphogenetic events that form the early branching pancreatic epithelium.
- Identify signals from vasculature and mesoderm that control pancreatic growth and differentiation.
- Define the cellular and molecular processes that underlie the formation of islet cell precursors by the delamination of cells from the pancreatic epithelium.
- Determine the lineage relationships between ductal, centroacinar and acinar cells.
- Define the plasticity of exocrine and endocrine cell phenotypes that allows transdifferentiation.
- Understand molecular and cellular consequences of defects in the extrinsic signaling pathways that control pancreatic organogenesis.

Clinical Implications

- Apply our understanding of the developmental programs that resolve ductal, centroacinar and acinar cells to identify the cell-type of origin of adenocarcinoma.
- An understanding of developmental factors involved in growth and differentiation lays the foundations for developing clinically relevant therapies for pancreatic exocrine cancer.
- Understanding the key developmental factors has already led to the in vitro generation of beta-cells for potential replacement therapy for diabetics.
- Apply an emerging understanding of the development of ducts and acini to design regeneration strategies for exocrine tissue destroyed by disease.

Acknowledgments

We thank Chris Wright for the Pdx1-lacZ mice used for ⊙ *Fig. 4-1*. We are indebted to Galvin Swift for critical readings of the manuscript, helpful discussions and invaluable comments; to Jose Cabrera for the tireless creation of beautiful schematics illustrating complex pancreatic processes and developmental anatomy; to Alethia Villasenor, Diana Chong, Ling Shi and Mike Hale for contributing unpublished data and images. This work was supported by NIH R01 grant DK79862-01, JDRF Award 99-2007-472 and a Basil O'Connor March of Dimes Award to O.C., and NIH DK61220 and an American Pancreatic Foundation award to R.J.M.

References

1. Githens S: The pancreatic duct cell: proliferative capabilities, specific characteristics, metaplasia, isolation and culture. J Ped Gastroent Nutr 1988;7:486–506.
2. Pictet R, Rutter WJ: Development of the embryonic endocrine pancreas. In Handbook of Physiology. Section 7: Endocrinology, Vol. I. Endocrine Pancreas.

DF Steiner, N Freinkel (ed.). Baltimore: Williams and Wilkins, 1972, pp. 25–66.
3. Jensen J: Gene regulatory factors in pancreatic development. Dev Dyn 2004;229:176–200.
4. Pictet RL, Clark WR, Williams RH, Rutter WJ: An ultrastructural analysis of the developing embryonic pancreas. Dev Biol 1972;29:436–467.

5. Stanger BZ, Tanaka AJ, Melton D: Organ size is limited by the number of embryonic progenitor cells in the pancreas but not the liver. Nature 2007;445:886–891.

6. Jorgensen MC, Ahnfelt-Ronne J, Hald J, Madsen OD, Serup P, Hecksher-Sorensen J: An illustrated review of early pancreas development in the mouse. Endo Rev 2007;28:685–705.

7. Zhou Q, Law AC, Rajagopal J, Anderson WJ, Gray PA, Melton DA: A multipotent progenitor domain guides pancreatic organogenesis. Dev Cell 2007;13:103–114.

8. Motta PM, Macchiaraelli G, Nottola SA, Correr S: Histology of the exocrine pancreas. Microsc Res Tech 1997;37:384–398.

9. Seymour PA, Freude KK, Tran MN, Mayes EE, Jensen J, Kist R, Scherer G, Sander M: SOX9 is required for maintenance of the pancreatic progenitor cell pool. Proc Natl Acad Sci USA 2007;104:1865–1870.

10. Stanger BZ, Stiles B, Lauwers GY, Bardeesy N, Mendoza M, Wang Y, Greenwood A, Chen K-h, McLaughlin M, Brown D, DePinho RA, Wu H, Melton DA, Dor Y: Pten constrains centroacinar cell expansion and malignant transformation in the pancreas. Cancer Cell 2005;8:185–195.

11. Rukstalis JM, Habener JF: Snail2, a mediator of epitheliall-mesenchymal transitions, expressed in progenitor cells of the developing endocrine pancreas. Gene Expr Patterns 2007;7:471–479.

12. Harding JD, MacDonald RJ, Przybyla AE, Chirgwin JM, Pictet RL, Rutter WJ: Changes in the frequency of specific transcripts during development of the pancreas. J Biol Chem 1977;252:7391–7397.

13. Bouwens L, Lu WG, Krijger R: Proliferation and differentiation in the human fetal endocrine pancreas. Diabetologia 1997;40:398–404.

14. Dor Y, Brown J, Martinez OI, Melton DA: Adult pancreatic beta-cells are formed by self-duplication rather than stem-cell differentiation. Nature 2004; 429:41–46.

15. Finegood DT, Scaglia L, Bonner-Weir S: Dynamics of beta-cell mass in the growing rat pancreas. Estimation with a simple mathematical model. Diabetes 1995;44:249–256.

16. Teta M, Rankin MM, Long SY, Stein GM, Kushner JA: Growth and regeneration of adult beta cells does not involve specialized progenitors. Dev Cell 2007; 12:817–826.

17. Githens S: Differentiation and development of the pancreas in animals. In The Pancreas: Biology, Pathobiology and Disease. VLE Go (ed.). New York: Raven Press, 1993, pp. 21–55.

18. Jia D, Sun Y, Konieczny SF: Mist1 Regulates Pancreatic Acinar Cell Proliferation Through p21(CIP1/ WAF1). Gastroenterology 2008;135:1687–1697. doi:10.1053/j.gastro.2008.07.026.

19. Desai BM, Oliver-Krasinski J, De Leon D, Farzad C, Hong N, Leach SD, Stoffers DA: Preexisting pancreatic acinar cells contribute to acinar cell, but not islet beta cell, regeneration. J Clin Invest 2007; 117:971–977.

20. Bertelli E, Bendayan M: Association between endocrine pancreas and ductal system. More than an epiphenomenon of endocrine differentiation and development? J Histochem Cytochem 2005; 53:1071–1086.

21. Attisano L, Labbe E: Tgfbeta and Wnt pathway cross-talk. Cancer metastasis rev 2004;23:53–61.

22. Berman DM, Karhadkar SS, Maitra A, Montes De Oca R, Gerstenblith MR, Briggs K, Parker AR, Shimada Y, Eshleman JR, Watkins DN, Beachy PA: Widespread requirement for Hedgehog ligand stimulation in growth of digestive tract tumours. Nature 2003;425:846–851.

23. Miyamoto Y, Maitra A, Ghosh B, Zechner U, Argani P, Iacobuzio-Donahue CA, Sriuranpong V, Iso T, Meszoely IM, Wolfe MS, Hruban RH, Ball DW, Schmid RM, Leach SD: Motch mediates TGF alpha-induced changes in epithelial differentiation during pancreatic tumorigenesis. Cancer Cell 2003; 3:565–676.

24. Moustakas A, Heldin CH: Signaling networks guiding epithelial-mesenchymal transitions during embryogenesis and cancer progression. Cancer sci 2007; 98:1512–1520.

25. Pasca di Magliano M, Biankin AV, Heiser PW, Cano DA, Gutierrez PJ, Deramaudt T, Segara D, Dawson AC, Kench JG, Henshall SM, Sutherland RL, Dlugosz A, Rustgi AK, Hebrok M: Common activation of canonical Wnt signaling in pancreatic adenocarcinoma. PLoS ONE 2007;2:e1155.

26. Guo X, Wang XF: Signaling cross-talk between TGF-beta/BMP and other pathways. Cell Res 2008;19:17–88. epub. doi:10.1038/cr.2008.302.

27. Hebrok M, Kim SK, Melton DA: Notochord repression of endodermal Sonic hedgehog permits pancreas development. Genes Dev 1998;12:1705–1713.

28. Hebrok M, Kim SK, St-Jacques B, McMahon AP, Melton DA: Regulation of pancreas development by hedgehog signaling. Development 2000;127: 4905–4913.

29. Kumar M, Jordan N, Melton D, Grapin-Botton A: Signals from lateral plate mesoderm instruct endoderm toward a pancreatic fate. Dev Biol 2003; 259:109–122.

30. Kim SK, Hebrok M, Li E, Oh SP, Schrewe H, Harmon EB, Lee JS, Melton DA: Activin receptor patterning of foregut organogenesis. Genes Dev 2000;14:1866–1871.

31. Yamaoka T, Idehara C, Yano M, Matsushita T, Yamada T, Ii S, Moritani M, Hata J, Sugino H, Noji S, Itakura M: Hypoplasia of pancreatic islets in transgenic mice expressing activin receptor mutants. J Clin Invest 1998;102:294–301.

32. Varjosalo M, Taipale J: Hedgehog: functions and mechanisms. Genes Dev 2008;22:2454–2472.

33. Kim SK, Melton DA: Pancreas development is promoted by cyclopamine, a Hedgehog signaling inhibitor. Proc Natl Acad Sci USA 1998;95:13036–13041.

34. Apelqvist A, Ahlgren U, Edlund H: Sonic hedgehog directs specialised mesoderm differentiation in the intestine and pancreas. Curr Biol 1997;7:801–804.

35. Kim SK, MacDonald RJ: Signaling and transcriptional control of pancreatic organogenesis. Curr Opin Genet Dev 2002;12:540–547.

36. Murtaugh LC: The what, where, when and how of Wnt/beta-catenin signaling in pancreas development. Organogenesis 2008;4:81–86.

37. Nelson WJ, Nusse R: Convergence of Wnt, beta-catenin, and cadherin pathways. Science 2004; 303:1483–1487.

38. Heiser PW, Lau J, Taketo MM, Herrera PL, Hebrok M: Stabilization of beta-catenin impacts pancreas growth. Development 2006;133:2023–2032.

39. Heller RS, Dichmann DS, Jensen J, Miller C, Wong G, Madsen OD, Serup P: Expression patterns of Wnts, Frizzleds, sfrps, and misexpression in transgenic mice suggesting a role for Wnts in pancreas and foregut pattern formation. Dev Dyn 2002; 225:260–270.

40. Dessimoz J, Bonnard C, Huelsken J, Grapin-Botton A: Pancreas-specific deletion of beta-catenin reveals Wnt-dependent and wnt-independent functions during development. Curr Biol 2005;15:1677–1683.

41. Murtaugh LC, Law AC, Dor Y, Melton DA: B-catenin is essential or pancreatic acinar but not islet development. Development 2005;132:4663–4674.

42. Wells JM, Esni F, Boivin GP, Aronow BJ, tuart W, Combs C, Sklenka A, Leach SD, Lowy AM: Wnt/beta-catenin signaling is required for development of the exocrine pancreas. BMC Dev Biol 2007;7:4.

43. Fiuza UM, Arias AM: Cell and molecular biology of Notch. J Endocrinol 2007;194:459–474.

44. Apelqvist A, Li H, Sommer L, Beatus P, Anderson DJ, Honjo T, Hrabe de Angelis M, Lendahl U, Edlund H: Notch signalling controls pancreatic cell differentiation. Nature 1999;400:877–881.

45. Fujikura J, Hosoda K, Iwakura H, Tomita T, Noguchi M, Masuzaki H, Tanigaki K, Yabe D, Honjo T, Nakao K: Notch/Rbp-j signaling prevents premature endocrine and ductal cell differentiation in the pancreas. Cell Metab 2006;3:59–65.

46. Jensen J, Pedersen EE, Galante P, Hald J, Heller RS, Ishibashi M, Kageyama R, Guillemot F, Serup P, Madsen OD: Control of endodermal endocrine development by Hes-1. Nat Genet 2000;24:36–44.

47. Masui T, Long Q, Beres TM, Magnuson MA, MacDonald RJ: Early pancreatic development requires the vertebrate Suppressor of Hairless (RBPJ) in the PTF1 bhlh complex. Genes Dev 2007;21:2629–2643.

48. Nakhai H, Siveke JT, Klein B, Mendoza-Torres L, Mazur PK, Algul H, Radtke F, Strobl L, Zimber-Strobl U, Schmid RM: Conditional ablation of Notch signaling in pancreatic development. Development 2008;135:2757–2765.

49. Ross SA, McCaffery PJ, Drager UC, De Luca LM: Retinoids in embryonal development. Physiol Rev 2000;80:1021–1054.

50. Niederreither K, McCaffery P, Drager UC, Chambon P, Dolle P: Restricted expression and retinoic acid-induced downregulation of the retinaldehyde dehydrogenase type 2 (RALDH-2) gene during mouse development. Mech Dev 1997;62:67–78.

51. Martin M, Gallego-Llamas J, Ribes V, Kedinger M, Niederreither K, Chambon P, Dolle P, Gradwohl G: Dorsal pancreas agenesis in retinoic acid-deficient Raldh2 mutant mice. Dev Biol 2005;284:399–411.

52. Molotkov A, Molotkova N, Duester G: Retinoic acid generated by Raldh2 in mesoderm is required for mouse dorsal endodermal pancreas development. Dev Dyn 2005;232:950–957.

53. Pan FC, Chen Y, Bayha E, Pieler T: Retinoic acid-mediated patterning of the pre-pancreatic endoderm in Xenopus operates via direct and indirect mechanisms. Mech Dev 2007;124:518–531.

54. Stafford D, Hornbruch A, Mueller PR, Prince VE: A conserved role for retinoid signaling in vertebrate pancreas development. Dev Genes Evol 2004; 214:432–441.

55. Stafford D, Prince VE: Retinoic acid signaling is required for a critical early step in zebrafish pancreatic development. Curr Biol 2002;12:1215–1220.

56. Bhushan A, Itoh N, Kato S, Thiery JP, Czernichow P, Bellusci S, Scharfmann R: Fgf10 is essential for maintaining the proliferative capacity of epithelial progenitor cells during early pancreatic organogenesis. Development 2001;128:5109–5117.

57. Miettinen P, Ormio P, Hakonen E, Banerjee M, Otonkoski T: EGF receptor in pancreatic beta-cell mass regulation. Biochem Soc Trans 2008; 36:280–285.

58. Lammert E, Cleaver O, Melton D: Induction of pancreatic differentiation by signals from blood vessels. Science 2002;294:564–567.

59. Lammert E, Gu G, McLaughlin M, Brown D, Brekken R, Murtaugh LC, Gerber HP, Ferrara N, Melton DA: Role of VEGF-A in vascularization of pancreatic islets. Curr Biol 2003;13:1070–1074.

60. Jonsson J, Carlsson L, Edlund T, Edlund H: Insulin-promoter-factor 1 is required for pancreas development in mice. Nature 1994;371:606–609.

61. Offield MF, Jetton JL, Labosky PA, Ray M, Stein RW, Magnuson MA, Hogan BLM, Wright CVE: PDX-1 is required for pancreatic outgrowth and differentiation of the rostral duodenum. Development 1996; 122:983–995.

62. Stoffers DA, Zinkin NT, Stanojevic V, Clarke WL, Habener JF: Pancreatic agenesis attributable to a single nucleotide deletion in the human IPF1 gene coding sequence. Nat Genet 1997;15:106–110.

63. Kawaguchi Y, Cooper B, Gannon M, Ray M, MacDonald RJ, Wright CVE: The role of the transcriptional regulator PTF1a in converting intestinal to pancreatic progenitors. Nat Genet 2002; 32:128–134.

64. Krapp A, Knofler M, Ledermann B, Burki K, Berney C, Zoerkler N, Hagenbuchle O, Wellauer PK: The bhlh protein PTF1-p48 is essential for the formation of the exocrine and the correct spatial organization of the endocrine pancreas. Genes Dev 1998;12:3752–3763.

65. Sellick GS, Barker KT, Stolte-Dijkstra I, Fleischmann C, Coleman RJ, Garrett C, Gloyn AL, Edghill EL, Hattersley AT, Wellauer PK, Goodwin G, Houlston RS: Mutations in PTF1A cause pancreatic and cerebellar agenesis. Nat Genet 2004;36:1301–1305.

66. Wells JM, Melton DA: Vertebrate endoderm development. Ann Rev Cell Dev Biol 1999;15:393–410.

67. Lewis SL, Tam PP: Definitive endoderm of the mouse embryo: formation, cell fates, and morphogenetic function. Dev Dyn 2006;235:2315–2329.

68. Tam PP, Khoo PL, Lewis SL, Bildsoe H, Wong N, Tsang TE, Gad JM, Robb L: Sequential allocation and global pattern of movement of the definitive endoderm in the mouse embryo during gastrulation. Development 2007;134:251–260.

69. Tremblay KD, Hoodless PA, Bikoff EK, Robertson EJ: Formation of the definitive endoderm in mouse is a Smad2-dependent process. Development 2000; 127:3079–3090.

70. Kumar M, Melton D: Pancreas specification: a budding question. Curr Opin Genet Dev 2003;13:401–407.

71. Nadauld LD, Sandoval IT, Chidester S, Yost HJ, Jones DA: Adenomatous polyposis coli control of retinoic acid biosynthesis is critical for zebrafish intestinal development and differentiation. J Biol Chem 2004;279:51581–51589.

72. McLin VA, Rankin SA, Zorn AM: Repression of Wnt/beta-catenin signaling in the anterior endoderm is essential for liver and pancreas development. Development 2007;134:2207–2217.

73. Zorn AM, Butler K, Gurdon JB: Anterior endomesoderm specification in Xenopus by Wnt/beta-catenin and TGF-beta signalling pathways. Dev Biol 1999; 209:282–297.

74. Zou D, Silvius D, Davenport J, Grifone R, Maire P, Xu PX: Patterning of the third pharyngeal pouch into thymus/parathyroid by Six and Eya1. Dev Biol 2006;293:499–512.

75. Que J, Okubo T, Goldenring JR, Nam KT, Kurotani R, Morrisey EE, Taranova O, Pevny LH, Hogan BL: Multiple dose-dependent roles for Sox2 in the patterning and differentiation of anterior foregut endoderm. Development 2007;134: 2521–2531.

76. Minoo P, Su G, Drum H, Bringas P, Kimura S: Defects in tracheoesophageal and lung morphogenesis in Nkx2.1(−/−) mouse embryos. Dev Biol 1999;209:60–71.

77. Beck F, Erler T, Russell A, James R: Expression of Cdx-2 in the mouse embryo and placenta: possible role in patterning of the extra-embryonic membranes. Dev Dyn 1995;204:219–227.

78. Beck F, Chawengsaksophak K, Luckett J, Giblett S, Tucci J, Brown J, Poulsom R, Jeffery R, Wright NA: A study of regional gut endoderm potency by analysis of Cdx2 null mutant chimaeric mice. Dev Biol 2003;255:399–406.

79. Mutoh H, Hakamata Y, Sato K, Eda A, Yanaka I, Honda S, Osawa H, Kaneko Y, Sugano K: Conversion of gastric mucosa to intestinal metaplasia in Cdx2-expressing transgenic mice. Biochem Biophys Res Commun 2002;294:470–479.

80. Silberg DG, Sullivan J, Kang E, Swain GP, Moffett J, Sund NJ, Sackett SD, Kaestner KH: Cdx2 ectopic expression induces gastric intestinal metaplasia in transgenic mice. Gastroenterology 2002;122: 689–696.

81. Fukuda K, Yasugi S: The molecular mechanisms of stomach development in vertebrates. Dev Growth Differ 2005;47:375–382.

82. Roberts DJ: Molecular mechanisms of development of the gastrointestinal tract. Dev Dyn 2000; 219:109–120.

83. Wells JM, Melton DA: Early mouse endoderm is patterned by soluble factors from adjacent germ layers. Development 2000;127:1563–1572.

84. Dessimoz J, Opoka R, Kordich JJ, Grapin-Botton A, Wells JM: FGF signaling is necessary for establishing gut tube domains along the anterior-posterior axis in vivo. Mech Dev 2006;123:42–55.

85. Melhuish TA, Gallo CM, Wotton D: TGIF2 interacts with histone deacetylase 1 and represses transcription. J Biol Chem 2001;276:32109–32114.

86. Spagnoli FM, Brivanlou AH: The Gata5 target, TGIF2, defines the pancreatic region by modulating BMP signals within the endoderm. Development 2008;135:451–461.

87. Bort R, Martinez-Barbera JP, Beddington RS, Zaret KS: Hex homeobox gene-dependent tissue positioning is required for organogenesis of the ventral pancreas. Development 2004;131:797–806.

88. Rossi JM, Dunn NR, Hogan BLM, Zaret KS: Distinct mesodermal signals, including bmps from the septum transversum mesenchyme, are required in combination for hepatogenesis from the endoderm. Genes Dev 2001;15:1998–2009.

89. Li H, Arber S, Jessell TM, Edlund H: Selective agenesis of the dorsal pancreas in mice lacking homeobox gene Hlxb9. Nat Genet 1999;23:67–70.

90. Gradwohl G, Dierich A, LeMeur M, Guillemot F: Neurogenin3 is required for the development of the four endocrine cell lineages of the pancreas. Proc Natl Acad Sci USA 2000;97:1607–1611.

91. Villasenor A, Chong DC, Cleaver O: Biphasic Ngn3 expression in the developing pancreas. Dev Dyn 2008;237:3270–3279.

92. Afouda BA, Ciau-Uitz A, Patient R: GATA4, 5 and 6 mediate tgfbeta maintenance of endodermal gene expression in Xenopus embryos. Development 2005;132:763–774.

93. Decker K, Goldman DC, Grasch CL, Sussel L: Gata6 is an important regulator of mouse pancreas development. Dev Biol 2006;298:415–429.

94. Watt AJ, Zhao R, Li J, Duncan SA: Development of the mammalian liver and ventral pancreas is dependent on GATA4. BMC Dev Biol 2007;7:37.

95. Kim SK, Hebrok M, Melton DA: Notochord to endoderm signaling is required for pancreas development. Development 1997;124:4243–4252.

96. Chen Y, Pan FC, Brandes N, Afelik S, Solter M, Pieler T: Retinoic acid signaling is essential for pancreas development and promotes endocrine at the expense of exocrine cell differentiation in Xenopus. Dev Biol 2004;271:144–160.

97. Haumaitre C, Barbacci E, Jenny M, Ott MO, Gradwohl G, Cereghini S: Lack of TCF2/vhnf1 in mice leads to pancreas agenesis. Proc Natl Acad Sci USA 2005;102:1490–1495.

98. Yee NS, Lorent K, Pack MA: Exocrine pancreas development in zebrafish. Devel Biol 2005; 284:84–101.

99. Metzger RJ, Klein OD, Martin GR, Krasnow MA: The branching programme of mouse lung development. Nature 2008;453:745–750.

100. Ritvos O, Tuuri T, Eramaa M, Sainio K, Hilden K, Saxen L, Gilbert SF: Activin disrupts epithelial branching morphogenesis in developing glandular organs of the mouse. Mech Dev 1995;50: 229–245.

101. Costantini F: Renal branching morphogenesis: concepts, questions, and recent advances. Differentiation 2006;74:402–421.

102. Warburton D, Bellusci S, De Langhe S, Del Moral PM, Fleury V, Mailleux A, Tefft D, Unbekandt M, Wang K, Shi W: Molecular mechanisms of early lung specification and branching morphogenesis. Pediatr Res 2005;57:26R–37R.

103. Puri S, Hebrok M: Dynamics of embryonic pancreas development using real-time imaging. Dev Biol 2007;306:82–93.

104. Clark WR, Rutter WJ: Synthesis and accumulation of insulin in the fetal rat pancreas. Dev Biol 1972;29:468–481.

105. Kemp JD, Walther BT, Rutter WJ: Protein synthesis during the secondary developmental transition of the embryonic rat pancreas. J Biol Chem 1972;247:3941–3952.

106. Rutter WJ, Kemp JD, Bradshaw WS, Clark WR, Ronzio RA, Sanders TG: Regulation of specific protein synthesis in cytodifferentiation. J Cell Physiol 1968;72:1–18.

107. Sarkar SA, Kobberup S, Wong R, Lopez AD, Quayum N, Still T, Kutchma A, Jensen JN, Gianani R, Beattie GM, Jensen J, Hayek A, Hutton JC: Global gene expression profiling and histochemical analysis of the developing human fetal pancreas. Diabetologia 2008;51:285–297.

108. Herrera PL: Adult insulin- and glucagon-producing cells differentiate from two independent cell lineages. Development 2000;127:2317–2322.

109. Gu G, Dubauskaite J, Melton DA: Direct evidence for the pancreatic lineage: NGN3 + cells are islet progenitors and are distinct from duct progenitors. Development 2002;129:2447–2457.

110. Hara A, Kadoya Y, Kojima I, Yamashina S: Rat pancreatic islet is formed by unification of multiple endocrine cell clusters. Dev Dyn 2007;236: 3451–3458.

111. Larsson LI: On the development of the islets of Langerhans. Microsc Res Tech 1998;43:284–291.

112. Piper K, Brickwood S, Turnpenny LW, Cameron IT, Ball SG, Wilson DI, Hanley NA: Beta cell differentiation during early human pancreas development. J Endocr 2004;181:11–23.

113. Polak M, Bouchareb-Banaei L, Scharfmann R, Czernichow P: Early pattern of differentiation in the human pancreas. Diabetes 2000;49:225–232.

114. Golosow N, Grobstein C: Epitheliomesenchymal interaction in pancreatic morphogenesis. Devel Biol 1962;4:242–255.

115. Wessells NK, Cohen JH: Early pancreas organogenesis: Morphogenesis, tissue interactions, and mass effects. Devel Biol 1967;15:237–270.

116. Gittes GK, Galante PE, Hanahan D, Rutter WJ, Debas HT: Lineage-specific morphogenesis in the developing pancreas: role of mesenchymal factors. Development 1996;122:439–447.

117. Miralles F, Czernichow P, Scharfmann R: Follistatin regulates the relative proportions of endocrine versus exocrine tissue during pancreatic development. Development 1998;125:1017–1024.

118. Ronzio RA, Rutter WJ: Effects of a partially purified factor from chick embryos on macromolecular synthesis of embryonic pancreatic epithelia. Devel Biol 1971;30:307–320.

119. Oliver-Krasinski JM, Stoffers DA: On the origin of the beta cell. Genes Dev 2008;22:1998–2021.

120. Celli G, LaRochelle WJ, Mackem S, Sharp R, Merlino G: Soluble dominant-negative receptor uncovers essential roles for fibroblast growth factors in multi-organ induction and patterning. EMBO J 1998;17:1642–1655.

121. Revest JM, Spencer-Dene B, Kerr K, De Moerlooze L, Rosewell I, Dickson C: Fibroblast growth factor receptor 2-iiib acts upstream of Shh and Fgf4 and is required for limb bud maintenance but not for the induction of Fgf8, Fgf10, Msx1, or Bmp4. Dev Biol 2001;231:47–62.

122. Hart A, Papadopoulou S, Edlund H: Fgf10 maintains notch activation, stimulates proliferation, and blocks differentiation of pancreatic epithelial cells. Dev Dyn 2003;228:185–193.

123. Norgaard GA, Jensen JN, Jensen J: FGF10 signaling maintains the pancreatic progenitor cell state revealing a novel role of Notch in organ development. Dev Biol 2003;264:323–338.

124. Duvillie B, Attali M, Bounacer A, Ravassard P, Basmaciogullari A, Scharfmann R: The mesenchyme controls the timing of pancreatic beta-cell differentiation. Diabetes 2006;55:582–589.

125. Piper K, Ball SG, Keeling JW, Mansoor S, Wilson DI, Hanley NA: Novel SOX9 expression during human pancreas development correlates to abnormalities in Campomelic dysplasia. Mech Dev 2002;116:223–226.

126. Jensen JN, Cameron E, Garay MV, Starkey TW, Gianani R, Jensen J: Recapitulation of elements of embryonic development in adult mouse pancreatic regeneration. Gastroenterology 2005;128:728–741.

127. Hale MA, Kagami H, Shi L, Holland AM, Elsasser HP, Hammer RE, MacDonald RJ: The homeodomain protein PDX1 is required at mid-pancreatic development for the formation of the exocrine pancreas. Devel Biol 2005;286:225–237.

128. Esni F, Stoffers DA, Takeuchi T, Leach SD: Origin of exocrine pancreatic cells from nestin-positive precursors in developing mouse pancreas. Mech Dev 2004;121:15–25.

129. Beres TM, Masui T, Swift GH, Shi L, Henke RM, MacDonald RJ: PTF1 is an organ-specific and Notch-independent basic helix-loop-helix complex containing the mammalian Suppressor of Hairless (RBP-J) or its paralogue, RBP-L. Mol Cell Biol 2006;26:117–130.

130. Rall LB, Pictet RL, Williams RH, Rutter WJ: Early differentiation of glucagon-producing cells in embryonic pancreas: a possible developmental role for glucagon. Proc Natl Acad Sci USA 1973;70: 3478–3482.

131. Wessells NK: DNA synthesis, mitosis and differentiation in pancreatic acinar cells in vitro. J Cell Biol 1964;20:415–433.

132. Nakhai H, Siveke JT, Mendoza-Torres L, Schmid RM: Conditional inactivation of Myc impairs development of the exocrine pancreas. Development 2008;135:3191–3196.

133. Johansson KA, Dursun U, Jordan N, Gu G, Beermann F, Gradwohl G, Grapin-Botton A: Temporal control of neurogenin3 activity in pancreas progenitors reveals competence windows for the generation of different endocrine cell types. Dev Cell 2007;12:457–465.

134. Schwitzgebel VM, Scheel DW, Conners JR, Kalamaras J, Lee JE, Anderson DJ, Sussel L, Johnson JD, German MS: Expression of neurogenin3 reveals an islet cell precursor population in the pancreas. Development 2000;127:3533–3542.

135. Masui M, Swift GH, Hale MA, Meredith D, Johnson JE, MacDonald RJ: Transcriptional autoregulation controls pancreatic Ptf1a expression during development and adulthood. Mol Cell Biol 2008;28:5458–5468, Accepted for publication.

136. Fujitani Y, Fujitani S, Boyer DF, Gannon M, Kawaguchi Y, Ray M, Shiota M, Stein RW, Magnuson MA, Wright CVE: Targeted deletion of a cis-regulatory region reveals differential gene dosage requirements for Pdx1 in foregut organ differentiation and pancreas formation. Genes Dev 2006;20:253–266.

137. Hald J, Hjorth P, German MS, Madsen OD, Serup P, Jensen J: Activated Notch1 prevents differentiation of pancreatic acinar cells and attenuate endocrine development. Devel Biol 2003; 260:426–437.

138. Esni F, Ghosh B, Biankin AV, Lin JW, Albert MA, Yu X, MacDonald RJ, Civin CI, Real FX, Pack MA, Ball DW, Leach SD: Notch inhibits Ptf1a function and acinar cell differentiation in developing mouse and zebrafish pancreas. Development 2004; 131:4213–4224.

139. Lorent K, Yeo SY, Oda T, Chandrasekharappa S, Chitnis A, Mathews RP, Pack MA: Inhibition of Jagged-mediated Notch signaling disrupts zebrafish biliary development and generates multiorgan defects compatible with an Alagille syndrome phenocopy. Development 2004;131:5753–5766.

140. Goessling W, North TE, Lord AM, Ceol C, Lee S, Weidinger G, Bourque C, Strijbosch R, Haramis AP, Puder M, Clevers H, Moon RT, Zon LI: APC mutant zebrafish uncover a changing temporal requirement for wnt signaling in liver development. Devel Biol 2008;305:epub. doi:10.1016/j.ydbio.2008.05.526.

141. Servitja JM, Ferrer J: Transcriptional networks controlling pancreatic development and beta cell function. Diabetologia 2004;47:597–613.

142. Minoguchi S, Taniguchi Y, Kato H, Okazaki T, Strobl LJ, Zimber-Strobl U, Bornkamm GW, Honjo T: RBP-L, a transcription factor related to RBP-Jk. Mol Cell Biol 1997;17:2679–2687.

143. Stathopoulos A, Levine M: Genomic regulatory networks and animal development. Dev Cell 2005;9:449–462.

144. Pin CL, Bonvissuto AC, Konieczny SF: Mist1 expression is a common link among serous exocrine cells exhibiting regulated exocytosis. Anat Rec 2000;259:157–167.

145. Pin CL, Rukstalis JM, Johnson C, Konieczny SF: The bhlh transcription factor Mist1 is required to maintain exocrine pancreas cell organization and acinar cell identity. J Cell Biol 2001; 155:519–530.

146. Zhu L, Tran T, Rukstalis JM, Sun P, Damsz B, Konieczny SF: Inhibition of Mist1 homodimer formation induces pancreatic acinar-to-ductal metaplasia. Mol Cell Biol 2004;24:2673–2681.

147. Luo X, Shin DM, Wang X, Konieczny SF, Muallem S: Aberrant localization of intracellular organelles, Ca2 + signaling, and exocytosis in Mist1 null mice. J Biol Chem 2005;280:12668–12675.

148. Rukstalis JM, Kowalik A, Zhu L, Lidington D, Pin CL, Konieczny SF: Exocrine specific expression of Connexin32 is dependent on the basic helix-loop-helix transcription factor Mist1. J Cell Sci 2003;116:3315–3325.

149. Ketola I, Otonkoski T, Pulkkinen MA, Niemi H, Palgi J, Jacobsen CM, Wilson DB, Heikinheimo M: Transcription factor GATA-6 is expressed in the endocrine and GATA-4 in the exocrine pancreas. Mol Cell Endocrinol 2004;226:51–57.

150. Labelle-Dumais C, Jacob-Wagner M, Pare JF, Belanger L, Dufort D: Nuclear receptor NR5A2 is required for proper primitive streak morphogenesis. Dev Dyn 2006;235:3359–3369.

151. Fayard E, Auwerx J, Schoonjans K: LRH-1: an orphan nuclear receptor involved in development, metabolism and steroidogenesis. Trends Cell Biol 2004;14:250–260.

152. Lee YK, Schmidt DR, Cummins CL, Choi M, Peng L, Zhang Y, Goodwin B, Hammer RE, Mangelsdorf DJ, Kliewer SA: Liver receptor homolog-1 regulates bile acid homeostasis but is not essential for feedback regulation of bile acid synthesis. Mol Endocrinol 2008;22:1345–1356.

153. Annicotte JS, Fayard E, Swift GH, Selander L, Edlund H, Tanaka T, Kodama T, Schoonjans K, Auwerx J: Pancreatic-duodenal homeobox 1 regulates expression of liver receptor homolog 1 during pancreas development. Mol Cell Biol 2003;23.

154. Wang J, Kilic G, Aydin M, Burke Z, Oliver G, Sosa-Pineda B: Prox1 activity controls pancreas morphogenesis and participates in the production of "secondary transition" pancreatic endocrine cells. Devel Biol 2005;286:182–194.

155. Liu YW, Gao W, Teh HL, Tan JH, Chan WK: Prox1 is a novel coregulator of Ff1b and is involved in the embryonic development of the zebra fish interrenal primordium. Mol Cell Biol 2003;23:7243–7255.

156. Ashizawa N, Endoh H, Hidaka K, Watanabe M, Fukumoto S: Three-dimensional structure of the rat pancreatic duct in normal and inflamed pancreas. Microsc Res Tech 1997;37:543–556.

157. Githens S: Development and differentiation of pancreatic duct epithelium. In Lebenthal (ed.). E Gastrointestinal Development. New York: Raven Press, 1989, pp.669–683.

158. Pierreux CE, Poll AV, Kemp CR, Clotman F, Maestro MA, Cordi S, Ferrer J, Leyns L, Rousseau GG, Lemaigre FP: The transcription factor hepatocyte nuclear factor-6 controls the development of pancreatic ducts in the mouse. Gastroenterology 2006;130:532–541.

159. Watanabe M, Muramatsu T, Shirane H, Ugai K: Discrete Distribution of binding sites for Dolichos biflorus agglutinin (DBA) and for peanut agglutinin (PNA) in mouse organ tissues. J Histochem Cytochem 1981;29:779–780.

160. Sumazaki R, NShiojiri N, Isoyama S, Masu M, Keino-Masu K, Osawa M, Nakauchi H, Kageyama R, Matsui A: Conversion of biliary system to pancreatic tissue in Hes1-deficient mice. Nat Genet 2004;36:83–87.

161. Eberhard D, Tosh D, Slack JM: Origin of pancreatic endocrine cells from biliary duct epithelium. Cell Mol Life Sci 2008;65:3467–3480.

162. Clotman F, Lannoy VJ, Reber M, Cereghini S, Cassiman D, Jacquemin P, Roskams T, Rousseau GG, Lemaigre FP: The onecut transcription factor HNF6 is required for normal development of the biliary tract. Development 2002;129:1819–1828.

163. Maestro MA, Boj SF, Luco RF, Pierreux CE, Cabedo J, Servitja JM, German MS, Rousseau GG, Lemaigre FP, Ferrer J: Hnf6 and Tcf2 (MODY5) are linked in a gene network operating in a precursor cell domain of the embryonic pancreas. Human Mol Gen 2003;12:3307–3314.

164. Jacquemin P, Durviaux SM, Jensen J, Godfraind C, Gradwohl G, Guillemot F, Madsen OD, Carmeliet P, Dewerchin M, Collen D, Rousseau GG, Lemaigre FP: Transcription factor hepatocyte nuclear factor 6 regulates pancreatic endocrine cell differentiation and controls expression of the proendocrine gene ngn3. Mol Cell Biol 2000;20:4445–4454.

165. Cano DA, Murcia NS, Pazour GJ, Hebrok M: Orpk mouse model of polycystic kidney disease reveals essential role of primary cilia in pancreatic tissue organization. Development 2004;131: 3457–3467.

166. Lee JC, Smith SB, Watada H, Lin J, Scheel D, Wang J, Mirmira RG, German MS: Regulation of the pancreatic pro-endocrine gene neurogenin3. Diabetes 2001;50:928–936.

167. Smith SB, Gasa R, Watada H, Wang J, Griffen SC, German MS: Neurogenin3 and hepatic nuclear factor 1 cooperate in activating pancreatic expression of Pax4. J Biol Chem 2003;278:38254–38259.

168. Gasa R, Mrejen C, Leachman N, Otten M, Barnes M, Wang J, Chakrabarti S, Mirmira R, German M: Proendocrine genes coordinate the pancreatic islet differentiation program in vitro. Proc Natl Acad Sci USA 2004;101:13245–13250.

169. Huang HP, Liu M, El-Hodiri HM, Chu K, Jamrich M, Tsai MJ: Regulation of the pancreatic islet-specific gene BETA2 (neurod) by neurogenin 3. Mol Cell Biol 2000;20:3292–3307.

170. Collombat P, Hecksher-Sorensen J, Serup P, Mansouri A: Specifying pancreatic endocrine cell fates. Mech Dev 2006;123:501–512.

171. Collombat P, Mansouri A, Hecksher-Sorensen J, Serup P, Krull J, Gradwohl G, Gruss P: Opposing actions of Arx and Pax4 in endocrine pancreas development. Genes Dev 2003;17:2591–3603.

172. Collombat P, Hecksher-Sorensen J, Broccoli V, Krull J, Ponte I, Mundiger T, Smith J, Gruss P, Serup P, Mansouri A: The simultaneous loss of Arx and Pax4 genes promotes a somatostatin-producing cell fate specification at the expense of the alpha- and beta-cell lineages in the mouse endocrine pancreas. Development 2005; 132:2969–2980.

173. Artner I, Hang Y, Guo M, Gu G, Stein R: Mafa is a dedicated activator of the insulin gene in vivo. J Endocrinol 2008;198:271–279.

174. Tweedie E, Artner I, Crawford L, Poffenberger G, Thorens B, Stein R, Powers AC, Gannon M: Maintenance of hepatic nuclear factor 6 in postnatal islets impairs terminal differentiation and function of beta-cells. Diabetes 2006;55:3264–3270.

175. Raum JC, Gerrish K, Artner I, Henderson E, Guo M, Sussel L, Schisler JC, Newgard CB, Stein R: Foxa2, Nkx2.2, and PDX-1 regulate islet beta-cell-specific mafa expression through conserved sequences located between base pairs -8118 and -7750 upstream from the transcription start site. Mol Cell Biol 2006;26:5735–5743.

176. Vanhoose AM, Samaras S, Artner I, Henderson E, Hang Y, Stein R: Mafa and mafb regulate Pdx1 transcription through the Area II control region in pancreatic beta cells. J Biol Chem 2008;283:22612–22619.

177. Wilson ME, Scheel D, German MS: Gene expression cascades in pancreatic development. Mech Dev 2003;120:65–80.

178. Murtaugh LC, Stanger BZ, Kwan DM, Melton DA: Notch signaling controls multiple steps of pancreatic differentiation. Proc Natl Acad Sci USA 2003;100:14920–14925.

179. Shiozaki S, Tajima T, Zhang YQ, Furukawa M, Nakazato Y, Kojima I: Impaired differentiation of endocrine and exocrine cells of the pancreas in transgenic mouse expressing the truncated type II activin receptor. Biochimica et biophysica acta 1999;1450:1–11.

180. Dichmann DS, Yassin H, Serup P: Analysis of pancreatic endocrine development in GDF11-deficient mice. Dev Dyn 2006;235:3016–3025.

181. Harmon EB, Apelqvist AA, Smart NG, Gu X, Osborne DH, Kim SK: GDF11 modulates NGN3 + islet progenitor cell number and promotes beta-cell differentiation in pancreas development. Development 2004;131:6163–6174.

182. Kleeff J, Friess H, Simon P, Susmallian S, Buchler P, Zimmermann A, Buchler MW, Korc M: Overexpression of Smad2 and colocalization with TGF-beta1 in human pancreatic cancer. Dig Dis Sci 1999;44:1793–1802.

183. Shook D, Keller R: Mechanisms, mechanics and function of epithelial-mesenchymal transitions in early development. Mech Dev 2003;120: 1351–1383.

184. del Barrio MG, Nieto MA: Overexpression of Snail family members highlights their ability to promote chick neural crest formation. Development 2002; 129:1583–1593.

185. Katoh M, Katoh M: Cross-talk of WNT and FGF signaling pathways at GSK3beta to regulate beta-catenin and SNAIL signaling cascades. Cancer Biol Ther 2006;5:1059–1064.

186. Gotz M, Huttner WB: The cell biology of neurogenesis. Nature Rev 2005;6:777–788.

187. Fischer EG, Lager DJ: Anti-glomerular basement membrane glomerulonephritis: a morphologic study of 80 cases. Am J Clin Pathol 2006;125:445–450.

188. Ahlgren U, Jonsson J, Edlund H: The morphogenesis of the pancreatic mesenchyme is uncoupled from that of the pancreatic epithelium in IPF1/PDX1-deficient mice. Development 1996; 122:1409–1416.

189. Wilson ME, Kalamaras JA, German MS: Expression pattern of IAPP and prohormone convertase 1/3 reveals a distinctive set of endocrine cells in the embryonic pancreas. Mech Dev 2002;115:171–176.

190. Stefan Y, Grasso S, Perrelet A, Orci L: The pancreatic polypeptide-rich lobe of the human pancreas: definitive identification of its derivation from the ventral pancreatic primordium. Diabetologia 1982;23:141–142.

191. Orci L: Macro- and micro-domains in the endocrine pancreas. Diabetes 1982;31:538–565.

192. Bonner-Weir S: Islets of Langerhans: morphology and postnatal growth. In Joslin's Diabetes Mellitus, 14th edn. CR Kahn, RJ Smith, AM Jacobson, GC Weir, EL King (ed.). Philadelphia, PA: Lippincott Willilams & Wilkins, 2004, pp. 41–52.

193. Ahlgren U, Jonsson J, Jonsson L, Simu K, Edlund H: Beta-cell specific inactivation of the mouse Ipf1/Pdx1 gene results in impaired glucose transporter expression and late onset diabetes. Genes Dev 1998;12:1763–1768.

194. Hart AW, Baeza N, Apelqvist A, Edlund H: Attenuation of FGF signalling in mouse beta-cells leads to diabetes. Nature 2000;408:864–868.

195. Steneberg P, Rubins N, Bartoov-Shifman R, Walker MD, Edlund H: The FFA receptor GPR40 links hyperinsulinemia, hepatic steatosis, and impaired glucose homeostasis in mouse. Cell Metab 2005;1:245–258.

196. Yamagata K, Nammo T, Moriwaki M, Ihara A, Iizuka K, Yang Q, Satoh T, Li M, Uenaka R, Okita K, Iwahashi H, Zhu Q, Cao Y, Imagawa A, Tochino Y, Hanafusa T, Miyagawa J, Matsuzawa Y: Overexpression of dominant-negative mutant hepatocyte nuclear fctor-1 alpha in pancreatic beta-cells causes abnormal islet architecture with decreased expression of E-cadherin, reduced beta-cell proliferation, and diabetes. Diabetes 2002;51:114–123.

197. Goulley J, Dahl U, Baeza N, Mishina Y, Edlund H: BMP4-BMPR1A signaling in beta cells is required for and augments glucose-stimulated insulin secretion. Cell Metab 2007;5:207–219.

198. Gannon M, Ray MK, Van Zee K, Rausa F, Costa RH, Wright CV: Persistent expression of HNF6 in islet endocrine cells causes disrupted islet architecture and loss of beta cell function. Development 2000;127:2883–2895.

199. Doyle MJ, Loomis ZL, Sussel L: Nkx2.2-repressor activity is sufficient to specify alpha-cells and a small number of beta-cells in the pancreatic islet. Development 2007;134:515–523.

200. Mitchell SM, Frayling TM: The role of transcription factors in maturity-onset diabetes of the young. Mol Genet Metab 2002;77:35–43.

201. Ghaneh P, Costello E, Neoptolemos JP: Biology and management of pancreatic cancer. Gut 2007;56:1134–1152.

202. Zhou Q, Brown J, Kanarek A, Rajagopal J, Melton DA: In vivo reprogramming of adult pancreatic exocrine cells to beta-cells. Nature 2008;455:627–632.

203. Barolo S, Posakony JW: Three habits of highly effective signaling pathways: principles of transcriptional control by developmental cell signaling. Genes Dev 2002;16:1167–1181.

5 Molecular Pathology of Precursor Lesions of Pancreatic Cancer

Georg Feldmann · Anirban Maitra

1	*Introduction*	*120*
2	*Pancreatic Intraepithelial Neoplasia (PANIN)*	*120*
2.1	Clinical and Histopathological Features of PanINs	120
2.2	Molecular Genetics of PanINs	121
2.2.1	Oncogene Mutations in PanIN Lesions	122
2.2.2	Tumor Suppressor Gene Mutations in PanIN Lesions	124
2.2.3	Caretaker Gene Mutations in PanIN Lesions	125
2.2.4	Genomic Instability and Telomere Length Alterations in PanIN Lesions	126
2.2.5	Epigenetic Alterations in PanIN Lesions	126
2.2.6	Transcriptomic Abnormalities in PanIN Lesions	127
2.2.7	Cell Cycle and Proliferation Abnormalities in PanIN Lesions	127
2.2.8	Aberrantly Activated Growth Factor Signaling Pathways in PanIN Lesions	128
2.2.9	Aberrantly Activated Embryonic Signaling Pathways in PanIN Lesions	128
2.2.10	Genetically Engineered Mouse Models and Murine PanINs (mPanINs)	129
2.3	Therapeutic Implications of Isolated PanIN Lesions	130
3	*Intraductal Papillary Mucinous Neoplasms (IPMN)*	*130*
3.1	Clinical Features of IPMNs	130
3.2	Histopathological Features of IPMNs	131
3.3	Molecular Features of IPMNs	132
3.4	Genetically Engineered Mouse Model of IPMNs	132
3.4.1	Therapeutic Considerations regarding IPMNs	133
4	*Mucinous Cystic Neoplasms (MCN)*	*133*
4.1	Clinical Features of MCNs	133
4.2	Histopathology of MCNs	134
4.3	Molecular Genetics of MCNs	134
4.4	Genetically Engineered Mouse Models of MCN	135
4.5	Therapeutic Implications of MCNs	135

J. P. Neoptolemos, R. Urrutia, J. L. Abbruzzese, M. W. Büchler (eds.), *Pancreatic Cancer*,
DOI 10.1007/978-0-387-77498-5_5, © Springer Science+Business Media, LLC 2010

Abstract: It has become evident over the past decade that pancreatic ductal adenocarcinoma (a.k.a. pancreatic cancer) does not originate de novo, but rather, through a multistep progression that involves histologically defined precursor lesions. Three major subtypes of precursor lesions of pancreatic cancer have been identified to date, including pancreatic intraepithelial neoplasia (PanIN), intraductal papillary mucinous neoplasm (IPMN) and mucinous cystic neoplasm (MCN). PanINs constitute by far the most common precursor lesions, and are, by definition, microscopic in nature, while IPMNs and MCNs occur less frequently and are macroscopic (i.e., radiologically detectable) precursor lesions. In addition to the development of consensus histopathological criteria for the identification and classification of pancreatic cancer precursors, there has also been considerable progress made in characterizing the genetic abnormalities underlying these lesions. Elucidating the molecular pathology of precursor lesions has enabled a better understanding of the pathogenesis of early pancreatic neoplasia, and provided a seedbed for developing tools for early detection and chemoprevention of pancreatic cancer prior to onset of invasion. Histopathology, molecular genetics as well as clinical implications and possible directions for future research of PanINs, IPMNs and MCNs will be discussed in this chapter.

1 Introduction

The first example linking the progression from a non-invasive precursor lesion to invasive cancer with a cumulative sequence of genetic aberrations was established for the adenoma-carcinoma sequence in colon cancer [1]. This concept has since been extrapolated many solid cancers, including pancreatic cancer [2]. In fact, there is now increasing evidence to suggest, that almost all of the major epithelial malignancies might be associated with discrete non-invasive precursor lesions, and that histological progression in such lesions is paralleled by an underlying genetic progression [3].

The general concept that invasive adenocarcinomas of the pancreas do not arise de novo, but rather originate from tangible non-invasive precursor lesions, was first proposed over a century ago [4]. However, only over the last decade has the identity of these precursor lesions been concretized through meticulous histopathological and molecular biological analysis, and through introduction of a consensus nomenclature [5, 6] (see also http://pathology.jhu.edu/pancreas_panin). Three different types of precursor lesions to pancreatic cancer are recognized: Pancreatic intraepithelial neoplasia (PanIN), by far the most common, as well as the less common intraductal papillary mucinous neoplasms (IPMN) and mucinous cystic neoplasms (MCN). The key features of these three neoplasms are listed in ◉ *Table 5-1*, and each will be discussed independently in the text.

2 Pancreatic Intraepithelial Neoplasia (PANIN)

2.1 Clinical and Histopathological Features of PanINs

PanIN lesions are microscopic non-invasive precursor lesions with varying degrees of cytologic and architectural atypia, which are located in interlobular ducts of <5 mm in diameter [5, 6]. Based on the degree of atypia, PanINs are divided into three grades. PanIN-1 lesions

◘ Table 5-1

Precursor lesions to pancreatic cancer, key clinical features (reproduced with minor modifications from [7])

	MCN	IPMN	PanIN
Predominant age	40–50 years	60–70 years	Prevalence increases with age
Female: male ratio	20:1	2:3	1:1
Predominant intrapancreatic localization	Body/tail	Head	Head > body/tail
Relation of cysts to large ducts	Usually not connected	Always connected	N/A
Cyst contents	Mucoid	Mucoid	N/A
Mucin oozing from ampulla	No	Yes	No
Stroma	Ovarian-type	Collagen-rich	Collagen-rich
Multifocal disease	Very rare	In ~20–30%	Often
Typical ERCP findings	Displaced or compressed pancreatic duct	Dilated pancreatic duct and filling defects	Normal

N/A: = not applicable

show only minimal atypia, PanIN-2 lesions show moderate atypia, and lesions with marked atypia are designated PanIN-3 (carcinoma-in-situ). PanIN-1 lesions are further subdivided into flat PanIN-1A and papillary PanIN-1B lesions [5, 6]. ◑ *Figure 5-1a,b* show representative examples of PanIN-1 and -2 lesions.

The overall prevalence of PanINs increases with age, and low-grade PanINs are found in over half of the population above the age of 65 years. An increased prevalence of PanINs is not only observed in pancreatic cancer, but also in the setting of chronic pancreatitis [8]. In one series, Andea and collegues found PanIN lesions in 67/82 pancreata (82%) from patients with invasive adenocarcinomas and in 54/86 (63%) of cases with chronic pancreatitis, but only in 10/36 (28%) of otherwise normal cases. Interestingly, PanINs are also frequently found adjacent to other periampullary neoplasms, including ampullary adenomas and adenocarcinomas, acinar cell carcinomas, well-differentiated pancreatic endocrine neoplasms, serous cystadenomas and solid-pseudopapillary neoplasms [9, 10].

2.2 Molecular Genetics of PanINs

The histological progression of PanIN lesions has been linked to progressive accumulation of genetic aberrations that are shared with invasive pancreatic cancer. These aberrations do not occur in a random manner, but rather in a well-described sequence of early and later events (◑ *Fig. 5-2*), as depicted in the PanIN progression model ("PanIN-gram").

■ Fig. 5-1

Representative histologies of low-grade (a) and high-grade (b) PanINs, low-grade (c) and high-grade (d) IPMNs and low-grad (e) and high-grade (f) MCNs (H&E stainings). Note the prominent ovarian-type stroma beneath the epithelial layer in f.

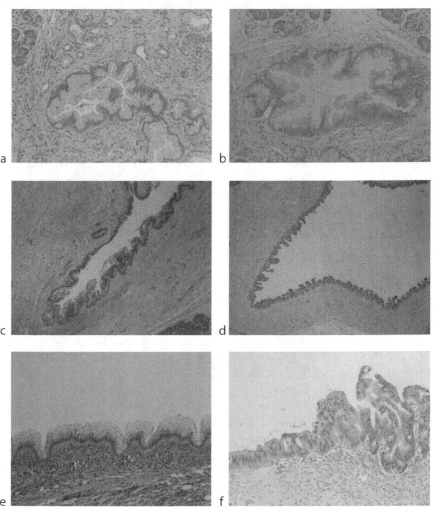

2.2.1   Oncogene Mutations in PanIN Lesions

A growing number of oncogenes have been identified that contribute to pancreatic carcinogenesis upon activation, usually through intragenic mutations or copy number alterations. The most commonly observed activating point mutations in pancreatic cancer, as well as in PanINs, are found in the *KRAS2* oncogene on chromosome 12p. These mutations, that are also among the earliest genetic alterations observed during pancreatic carcinogenesis, can be detected in up to 90% of pancreatic cancers and most often occur on codons 12, 13 or 61

Fig. 5-2

Schematic illustration of some of the key molecular alterations observed during the multistep progression towards pancreatic cancer in the form of a "PanIN-gram." The alterations shown here are not comprehensive and are discussed in the text in more detail. (Reproduced from [11] with permission.)

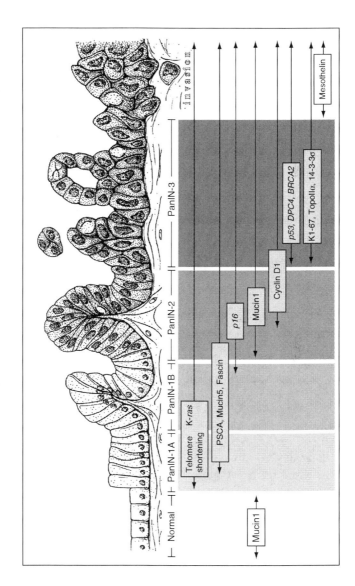

[12, 13]. In one series, oncogenic *KRAS2* mutations were found in 36% of PanIN-1A, 44% of PanIN-1B and 87% of PanIN 2/3 lesions, respectively, suggesting that this oncogene plays a critical role in pancreatic cancer initiation. The importance of constitutively activated *KRAS2* gene product in pancreatic cancer initiation is further underscored by recently developed genetically engineered mouse models of pancreatic cancer, wherein a mutant *Kras* allele is sufficient for the development of murine PanIN (mPanIN) lesions [14, 15]. Activating mutations impair the intrinsic GTPase activity of the *KRAS2* gene product, leading to constitutive activation of downstream intracellular signaling cascades. Three major downstream Ras effector cascades have been identified that are involved in mediating the oncogenic properties conferred by constitutively active *KRAS2*, namely the RAF/MEK/ERK, the PI3K/AKT and the RalGDS/Ral pathways. Of note, oncogenic Ras signaling seems to be involved not only in pancreatic cancer initiation, but is also required for tumor maintenance in established cancers [16, 17]. Interestingly, in a proportion of pancreatic cancers more than one distinct mutation within the *KRAS2* gene can be detected, suggesting that within the same organ, multi-focal precursor lesions can develop independently from the one that eventually culminates in invasive neoplasia.

2.2.2 Tumor Suppressor Gene Mutations in PanIN Lesions

Three tumor suppressor genes frequently inactivated in PanIN lesions, mirroring their common loss of function in invasive pancreatic cancers, are *CDKN2A/p16*, *TP53*, and *DPC4/SMAD4/MADH4*. The *CDKN2A/p16* gene on chromosome 9p21 encodes for a cell-cycle checkpoint protein, which binds to the cyclin-dependent kinases CDK4 and CDK6, thereby inhibiting cyclin D1-binding and causing cell-cycle arrest in G1-S [18]. The *CDKN2A/p16* gene is inactivated in virtually all pancreatic cancers; in approximately 40% of cases, this is due to homozygous deletion, another 40% carry intragenic mutations and show loss of the second allele, and 15% demonstrate epigenetic inactivation [19]. Loss of p16 expression, which can be exploited as reliable surrogate marker of the *CDKN2A/p16* genetic status, correlates with PanIN progression and is observed in 30% of PanIN-1A and -1B, 55% of PanIN-2 and 71% of PanIN-3 lesions, respectively [20]. Interestingly, frequencies of *CDKN2A/p16* inactivation appear to be lower in PanIN lesions associated with chronic pancreatitis. In a subset of cases, homozygous deletions of *CDKN2A/p16* at 9p21 can also include homozygous deletion of the *methylthioadenosine phosphorylase* (*MTAP*) gene, whose product is required for the salvage pathway of purine synthesis. Co-deletion of *MTAP* and *CDKN2A/p16* is observed in approximately one third of pancreatic cancers, and 10% of high-grade PanIN lesions [21].

The tumor suppressor gene *TP53* on the short arm of chromosome 17 encodes the protein p53, which plays a key role in mediating several important physiological functions, including regulation of the G1/S cell-cycle checkpoint, maintenance of G2/M arrest and induction of apoptosis. Therefore, inactivation of p53 in the majority of pancreatic cancers affects two major mechanisms controlling cell number – cell proliferation and apoptosis. Moreover, recent findings suggest that p53 abrogation may contribute to genomic instability observed in pancreatic cancers [22]. Loss of *TP53* function is observed in 50–75% of pancreatic cancers, almost exclusively through intragenic mutations and loss of the second allele. Nuclear accumulation of p53 using immunohistochemistry largely correlates with the mutational status of *TP53* [23] and can therefore be used as a surrogate marker of *TP53* mutations in PanIN lesions. Immunohistochemistry reveals intranuclear p53 accumulation mostly in advanced PanIN-3 lesions, suggesting that TP53 mutations constitute rather late events in the multistep pancreatic cancer progression cascade [11].

DPC4/SMAD4/MADH4 on chromosome 18q is inactivated in approximately 55% of pancreatic cancers, i.e., through homozygous deletion in 30% of cases, or through intragenic mutation and loss of the second allele in another 25% [24]. *DPC4/SMAD4/MADH4* encodes the protein Smad4, which is involved in transforming growth factor (TGF)-beta signaling. Activation of the TGF-beta signaling pathway leads to binding of Smad4 to a phosphorylated Smad2/3 protein complex and its translocation to the nucleus, where it binds to specific promoter regions and induces expression of respective target genes. Therefore, loss of Smad4 function interferes with the intracellular signaling cascade downstream of TGF-beta and leads to reduced growth inhibition through loss of pro-apoptotic stimuli and inappropriate G1/S transition [25]. A potential alternative mechanism was recently unmasked in an elegant study showing that selective loss of Smad4-dependent signaling in T-cells leads to development of epithelial cancers of the gastrointestinal tract in mice, while no tumor development was observed in mice with epithelial-specific deletion of SMAD4. These observations suggest that in addition to the above-mentioned cell functions, Smad4 might also be crucially involved in interactions between cancer cells and the microenvironment and/or modulation of immune surveillance [26]. As described above for p53, immunohistochemical labeling for Smad4 can be used as a surrogate marker of the *DPC4/SMAD4/MADH4* mutational status. Loss of Smad4 expression is observed in about one third of high-grade PanIN-3 lesions, while it is preserved in normal ducts and low-grade PanIN-1 and -2 lesions [11, 27]. Therefore, *DPC4/SMAD4/MADH4* mutations, like mutations of *TP53*, represent a relatively late event in the multistep progression model.

2.2.3   Caretaker Gene Mutations in PanIN Lesions

Caretaker genes comprise a third class of cancer-related genes, which are not directly involved in controlling cell growth or apoptosis, but rather help to maintain DNA integrity, e.g., by means of mismatch repair, nucleotide-excision repair and base-excision repair [28]. By repairing subtle changes in the genomic DNA sequence that occur due to polymerase errors or as a result of exposure to mutagens, as well as gross chromosomal aberrations, caretaker genes prevent accumulation of mutations within a cell that might provide a selective advantage leading towards a malignant phenotype.

The Fanconi anemia gene family is a group of caretaker genes known to be involved in pancreatic carcinogenesis. The Fanconi anemia gene family is involved in homologous recombination repair in response to DNA damage, e.g. by cross-linking agents or radiation [29]. One member of this family, the breast and ovarian cancer susceptibility gene *BRCA2* on chromosome 13q, is of particular interest in the setting of familial pancreatic cancer, since germline *BRCA2* mutations are found in 5–10% of familial cases, especially in individuals of Ashkenazi Jewish heritage [30]. In addition, pancreatic cancers harboring Fanconi anemia mutations are exquisitely sensitive to DNA cross-linking agents, presenting an avenue for synthetic lethal therapy [31]. In patients with germline *BRCA2* mutations, loss of the second allele is observed in PanIN-3 lesions, suggesting that akin to p53 and Smad4, inactivation of Brca2 function also constitutes a late event during pancreatic carcinogenesis.

2.2.4   Genomic Instability and Telomere Length Alterations in PanIN Lesions

Telomeres consist of hexameric TTAGGG repeats at the ends of chromosomal DNA strands, which confer chromosomal stability during cell division by preventing the ends from becoming sticky. Decrease in telomere length is among the earliest and most common molecular alterations observed in PanIN lesions. Significant telomere shortening as compared to normal pancreatic ductal cells is observed in over 90% of even low-grade PanIN lesions. It has been speculated that telomeres conduct functions similar to those of caretaker genes in pancreatic carcinogenesis, such that telomere dysfunction facilitates progressive accumulation of additional chromosomal abnormalities that culminates in development of a fully malignant phenotype.

Reflecting their inherent genomic instability, structural and numerical chromosomal aberrations can be found in almost all cases of pancreatic cancer and often involve loss of significant proportions or the entirety of chromosomal arms. Chromosomal regions frequently involved in loss of one allele (designated loss of heterozygosity (LOH)) in PanINs include 9p, 18q and 17p [32, 33]. Of note, the frequency of LOH observed at a given locus commonly increases from lower to higher grade PanINs [33]. It has been proposed that LOH might in many cases be the first event in the "two-hit" cascade leading to inactivation of tumor suppressor genes [32]. This concept is in line with the hypothesis of genomic instability beginning early in the multistep PanIN progression model.

2.2.5   Epigenetic Alterations in PanIN Lesions

The most common form of epigenetic alterations found in pancreatic cancer cells, and also in PanIN lesions, consists of methylation of CpG islands within promoter regions, leading to transcriptional silencing of the regulated gene [34]. Over recent years, epigenetic gene silencing – in addition to genetic alterations such as deletions and intragenic mutations – has increasingly been recognized as one of the most ubiquitous mechanisms exploited by cancer cells to alter their inherent transcriptomic programs in favor of more rapid cell growth, invasiveness and resistance to apoptosis [35].

In a recent study, Goggins and co-workers determined the methylation status of eight genes (*ST14, CDH3, CLDN5, LHX1, NPTX2, SARP2, SPARC, Reprimo*), which had previously been found to be aberrantly methylated in pancreatic cancers, in a series of 65 PanIN lesions [36]. The authors were able to demonstrate aberrant methylation in at least one of the eight gene loci in 12/17 (71%) PanIN-1A lesions, suggesting that aberrant DNA methylation is an early event during the multistep progression towards pancreatic cancer. Moreover, the average number of methylated loci was significantly higher in high-grade (PanIN-3) than in low-intermediate (PanIN-1 and -2) lesions, raising the possibility that aberrant methylation might be causally involved in the progression from lower to higher grades of PanIN lesions. Previously, Peng et al. had examined promoter methylation patterns of 12 cancer related genes (*p14, p15, p16, p73, APC, hMLH1, MGMT, BRCA1, GSTP1, TIMP-3, CDH1* and *DAPK-1*) in 40 microdissected PanIN lesions and 147 discrete areas sampled from ductal adenocarcinomas [37]. The frequency of at least one methylated gene locus increased significantly from normal ductal epithelium lacking signs of inflammation to PanINs, and from PanINs to ductal adenocarcinomas, respectively, further underscoring that epigenetic progression is also a feature of the traditional "PanIN-gram" model. Determination of aberrantly methylated gene promoters in pancreatic juice samples has emerged as a potential diagnostic tool for pancreatic cancer and precursor lesions, with a suggestion that it might be more specific than detection of mutated or differentially expressed genes [38]. In particular, certain promoter sequences like that of the *TSLC1* gene are methylated only in higher-grade PanIN lesions and therefore, might identify those lesions that pose a greater relative risk of progression to invasive neoplasia.

2.2.6   Transcriptomic Abnormalities in PanIN Lesions

With the advent and increasingly widespread deployment of global gene expression profiling techniques, including serial analysis of gene expression (SAGE) and various forms of oligonucleotide and cDNA microarrays, there has been a dramatic increase in our knowledge of differential gene expression patterns in pancreatic cancer tissues in recent years. A few compelling examples of differentially expressed genes with translational potential will be discussed here. Although initially discovered in the context of invasive cancer, the differential expression of these genes has since been validated in varying grades of PanIN lesions as well.

Prostate stem cell antigen (PSCA) is overexpressed in 30% of PanIN-1, 40% of PanIN-2 and 60% of PanIN-3 lesions, in line with PSCA up-regulation being an early event in the PanIN progression model [11]. Of note, recent pilot studies showed that PSCA overexpression might be a suitable target for the development of novel diagnostic tools for pancreatic cancer [39, 40]. Another example is mesothelin, a membrane-bound GPI-anchored protein known to play a role in cell adhesion. Unlike PSCA, mesothelin expression was detected only in 1/16 (6%) of PanIN-1, 2/14 (14%) of PanIN-2 and 1/7 (14%) of PanIN-3 lesions, but close to 100% of invasive ductal adenocarcinomas, suggesting that mesothelin overexpression is a late event [11, 41]. Recent studies have examined mesothelin as an antigen for cancer cell-specific drug delivery and for cancer immunotherapy [42, 43]. A study by Sutherland and colleagues using oligonucleotide microarrays described the up-regulation of several components of the retinoic acid signaling pathway, including RAR-alpha, HOXB6 and HOXB2 in pancreatic cancer, as compared to normal pancreas [44]. In particular, HOXB2 expression was identified as prognostic marker in pancreatic cancer that correlated with survival, surgical resection and tumor stage at the time of diagnosis. Nuclear immunostaining for HOXB2 was observed in 48/128 (38%) of pancreatic cancer tissues, but also in 2/26 (8%) of histologically normal ducts, 1/24 (4%) of PanIN-1A, 3/20 (15%) of PanIN-1B, 3/10 (30%) of PanIN-2 and 1/4 (25%) of PanIN-3 lesions, suggesting that HOXB2 overexpression increases during the multistep progression towards pancreatic cancer.

2.2.7   Cell Cycle and Proliferation Abnormalities in PanIN Lesions

Much like pancreatic cancer, PanIN lesions also demonstrate aberrations in cell cycle checkpoint control and proliferation. While low-grade PanIN lesions are minimally proliferative, this index significantly increases in higher-grade PanIN lesions, as assessed by nuclear expression of the proliferation antigen Ki67/MIB-1. For example, one study described nuclear Ki67/MIB-1 labeling indices as 0.7% for PanIN-1A, 2.3% for PanIN-1B, 14.1% for PanIN-2 and 22.0% for PanIN-3 lesions. The average labeling index for ductal adenocarcinomas was 37.0%, reflecting the progressive increase in proliferative potential during the multistep progression towards more advanced PanIN lesions and pancreatic cancer [45]. Cyclin D1 is involved in regulating cell cycle progression by acting as a co-factor in phosphorylating and inactivating the retinoblastoma (Rb) protein, and its expression has been linked to poor prognosis and decreased survival in pancreatic cancer. Overexpression of cyclin D1 represents an intermediate to late event during pancreatic carcinogenesis, being observed in 29% of PanIN-2, 57% of PanIN-3 lesions and in up to 60–85% of adenocarcinomas, but not in PanIN-1 lesions, [11]. $p21^{WAF/CIP1}$ acts as cyclin-dependent kinase inhibitor that inhibits cyclin E/CDK2 complexes and prevents phosphorylation of Rb. Overexpression of $p21^{WAF/CIP1}$ is an early event and is already observed in 16% of PanIN-1A, 32% of PanIN-1B, 56% of PanIN-2 and 80% of PanIN-3 lesions [46].

2.2.8 Aberrantly Activated Growth Factor Signaling Pathways in PanIN Lesions

Cyclooxygenase-2 (COX-2) is upregulated in pancreatic cancer, possibly secondary to activation of nuclear factor kappa B signaling, and is postulated to be involved in cell proliferation and tumor angiogenesis. In PanINs, COX-2 is generally found to be overexpressed in late PanIN-2/3 lesions as compared to early PanIN1 lesions, and in PanIN-1 lesions as compared to normal ducts, respectively. COX-2 inhibitors have been suggested as potential chemopreventive agents against pancreatic cancer, but initial clinical efficacy data have been equivocal so far [47, 48]. Members of the matrix metalloproteinase (MMP) family of zinc-dependent extracellular proteinases are involved in enabling pancreatic cancer cell invasion and metastasis [49]. Overexpression of MMP-7 is observed in the majority of pancreatic cancers, as well as in greater than half of low-grade PanIN lesions [50]. Urinary plasminogen activator (uPA) converts plasminogen into plasmin, which in turn activates MMP precursors. In addition, uPA induces upregulation of various downstream signaling molecules, including fibroblast growth factor 2 (FGF2) and angiostatin. In one study, uPA immunolabeling was observed not only in the majority pancreatic cancer tissues, but also in 19/27 PanIN-2 and 12/27 PanIN-3 lesions [51].

2.2.9 Aberrantly Activated Embryonic Signaling Pathways in PanIN Lesions

Embryonic signaling pathways, including Hedgehog, Notch and Wnt, which are usually inactive in differentiated tissues of the adult pancreas, have recently been found to be aberrantly re-activated in pancreatic cancers as well as in a variety of other epithelial human cancers [52]. This finding is of particular interest, since these signaling networks might contribute to maintain specific subpopulations of cancer cells with enhanced tumor-initiating properties, often referred to as "cancer stem cells." This concept has direct translational implications, since all of the three above mentioned embryonic signaling pathways represent candidate drug targets. The phenotype of the putative cancer stem cell compartment in pancreatic cancer has recently been elucidated by multiple groups. For example, Simeone and collegues have demonstrated that a subpopulation of CD44 + /CD24 + /ESA + cells, which represent less than 1% of pancreatic cancer cells within a "bulk" isolate, harbor more than 100-fold increased tumorigenic potential in immunodeficient mice, as compared to non-tumorigenic cells. Of note, in this population they also observed a ~10-fold over-expression of the Hedgehog ligand sonic hedgehog (Shh) as compared to bulk tumor tissues [53]. Similarly, Feldmann et al. found that inhibition of Hedgehog signaling by means of small molecule inhibitors diminished tumor initiation and metastasis in orthotopic xenograft models of pancreatic cancer, mirrored by significant reduction of a subpopulation of cancer cells with high aldehyde dehydrogenase (ALDH) activity in vivo and in vitro [54, 55]. The concept of Hedgehog signaling being involved in maintaining a "pancreatic cancer stem cell niche" would imply, that Hedgehog pathway reactivation occurs very early during the carcinogenic cascade, and indeed overexpression of Shh has been observed by immunohistochemistry in the earliest PanIN-1 lesions, but not in normal pancreatic ductal epithelia [56]. Further evidence came from another study by Leach et al. demonstrating that human PanIN-1 and -2 lesions express a cluster of "foregut-specific" markers, including pepsinogen C, MUC6, KLF4, GATA6, Sox-2, Forkhead-6 and TFF1, which is very similar to differential gene expression patterns observed in immortalized human pancreatic ductal epithelial cells upon transfection with the Hedgehog transcription factor Gli1 [57].

Analogous to the aberrant expression of Hedgehog pathway components, murine and human PanINs and pancreatic cancers also express multiple Notch components. As observed for Hedgehog signaling, Notch pathway activation during pancreatic carcinogenesis is most likely to be due to endogenous ligand overexpression, rather than mutational events. For example, the activating Notch ligand Jagged-1 is overexpressed in PanINs 1 and 2 [57]. Activation of Wnt signaling in cancer tissues usually occurs due to intragenic mutations, i.e., either activating beta-catenin mutations or loss-of-function mutations within the APC gene, resulting in nuclear translocation of beta-catenin and subsequent transcription of wnt target genes. In pancreatic cancer, however, canonical pathway activation is more often ligand-dependent, than through mutational events [58]. Immunohistochemical detection of nuclear beta-catenin can be used as a surrogate marker of Wnt pathway activation. One paper reported nuclear overexpression of beta-catenin in a small proportion of high-grade PanIN-2/3 lesions [59], but observations regarding pancreatic ductal adenocarcinomas have been conflicting [60].

2.2.10 Genetically Engineered Mouse Models and Murine PanINs (mPanINs)

A remarkable advance achieved in the last few years in the pancreatic cancer research arena has been the development of genetically engineered mouse models, which resemble cognate properties of the human disease, such as a multistep progression involving non-invasive precursor lesions culminating in lethal disseminated malignancy [14, 15, 22]. In order to distinguish the precursor lesions in mice from those arising in human pancreata, the former have been designated as murine PanIN (mPanIN) [61]. Interestingly, mPanIN lesions observed in these models also harbor many of the molecular aberrations found in humans, including activation of the Notch and Hedgehog signaling pathways [14, 22, 62]. These mouse models represent a unique platform for discovery of early pancreatic neoplasia-associated biomarkers in serum, as recently demonstrated by Hanash and colleagues [63]. In this study, the investigators identified a large panel of abnormally expressed proteins in sera of mice from both early and late stage disease. Of note, when five of these proteins were examined in human sera obtained from pancreatic cancer patients, they were able to predict the diagnosis of malignancy as much as 7–13 months prior to onset of clinical symptoms, underscoring the commonalities between mouse and human disease models. Genetically engineered mouse models of mPanINs and pancreatic cancer have also begun to be utilized as in vivo platforms for assessment of novel chemoprevention and treatment modalities. For example, it has been recently demonstrated that the COX-2 inhibitor nimesulide can slow down mPanIN formation in genetically predisposed mice [64], a not unexpected finding given that mPanINs (as well as their human counterparts) overexpress COX-2 [14].

2.3 Therapeutic Implications of Isolated PanIN Lesions

Currently, detection of PanIN lesions is hampered by the lack of sensitive non-invasive diagnostic tools. Due to their microscopic size, PanIN lesions are usually not diagnosed by standard clinical imaging techniques. Recent data from the Johns Hopkins Hospital suggest that a combinatorial approach using endoscopic ultrasound (EUS) and computer tomography might enable the detection of morphological changes associated with PanIN lesions in the adjacent pancreatic parenchyma, especially in patients with multi-focal PanIN lesions [65, 66]. In particular, Brune et al. showed that PanINs can be associated with a lobulocentric form of atrophy in the adjacent parenchyma, and a diffuse distribution of this atrophy observed in patients with multi-focal PanIN lesions confers a diagnostic pattern on EUS [65]. Even if further improvements in imaging techniques and other diagnostic tools will provide the means to reliably and non-invasively screen for the presence of PanIN lesions, the therapeutic implications of such findings are largely unknown. While the pathophysiological concept of a multistep progression of PanINs culminating in pancreatic cancer has become acceptable, the appropriate clinical management of non-invasively diagnosed PanIN lesions in an individual patient still needs to be defined. In an effort to estimate the approximate probability of a single PanIN to progress to cancer, Terhune et al. applied a mathematical model, assuming that PanIN lesions can be found in 37.5% of cases in a normal population with an average of 5 foci per affected pancreas, and that 0.8% of pancreata develop pancreatic cancer [67]. The authors argued that based on these assumptions only about 1% on PanIN lesions progress to pancreatic cancer. These considerations underscore the caution mandated in drawing therapeutic conclusions based on the identification of PanIN lesions alone, in the absence of a discernible malignancy.

3 Intraductal Papillary Mucinous Neoplasms (IPMN)

3.1 Clinical Features of IPMNs

Intraductal papillary mucinous neoplasms (IPMN) are cystic neoplasms that arise in the main pancreatic duct or one of its branches. IPMNs usually form finger-like papillae and produce abundant extracellular mucin [5]. The mean age at the time of diagnosis is approximately 65, with men being affected slightly more often than women (see ◉ *Table 5-1*). Patients that harbor IPMNs with mild dysplasia tend to be several years younger at the time of diagnosis than those with IPMNs associated with an invasive carcinoma (mean ages 63 vs. 68 years, respectively, in one report) [68, 69]. Presenting complaints include abdominal pain, chronic obstructive pancreatitis, nausea, vomiting, steatorrhea, diabetes mellitus, weight loss, jaundice and back pain. Many patients report symptoms long (often months to several years) before an IPMN is diagnosed, which suggests that there may be a tangible window of opportunity for detection and surgical resection of these lesions while they are still non-invasive and hence curable. Common CT findings include a dilated main pancreatic duct or an accumulation of cysts representing dilated branch ducts [70]. A finding often observed during upper endoscopy is mucin extruding from a patulous ampulla of Vater. Endoscopic retrograde cholangiopancreatography (ERCP) often reveals a dilated pancreatic duct and filling defects, caused by intraluminal mucin plugs or papillary projections of the neoplasm itself. An increasing proportion of IMPNs is being diagnosed as an incidental pancreatic cyst by computed tomography (CT) or ultrasound imaging performed for an unrelated indication. Such asymptomatic neoplastic cysts (incidentalomas) represent a viable opportunity for detection and surgical resection of these lesions while they are still non-invasive and hence curable.

3.2   Histopathological Features of IPMNs

IPMNs can be subdivided into two groups: main duct type and branch duct type IPMNs. As suggested by the name, the former predominantly involve the main pancreatic duct, while the latter involve a side branch of the main duct. Examples that involve both the main duct as well as a side branch exist. ◉ *Table 5-2* lists some key features that are useful in differentiating between these two forms of IPMNs. Depending on the degree of architectural and cellular atypia, noninvasive IPMNs are graded into IPMN with low-grade dysplasia (IPMN adenoma), moderate dysplasia and high-grade dysplasia (carcinoma in situ), respectively. Representative histology of the lesions is shown in ◉ *Figs. 5-1c,d*. Main duct IPMNs tend to have higher degrees of dysplasia and are more often associated with an invasive carcinoma than those arising in branch ducts [70, 74]. The epithelium lining the papillae can resemble intestinal adenomas (intestinal-type), gastric foveolar epithelium (gastric type), or be comprised of higher grade epithelium seen in pancredato-biliary malignancies (pancreato-bilary type). The intestinal and pancreato-biliary types of IPMN more commonly arise in the main duct, while the gastric type of IPMN is usually a branch duct lesion. The histological subtypes also demonstrate different patterns of apomucin labeling, with the intestinal-type IPMNs expressing MUC2, the pancreato-biliary type expressing MUC1, and the gastric type IPMN expressing MUC5AC, but usually lacking MUC1 and MUC2 [75]. A rare histological variant of

◨ Table 5-2
Features distinguishing main from branch duct IMPNs [71–73]

	Main duct IPMN	Branch duct IPMN
Age peak	55 years	65 years
Location in pancreas	57% in head	93% in head
Dysplasia		
Adenoma	43%	85%
Carcinoma in situ	20%	15%
Invasive	37%	0%

IMPNs is referred to as intraductal oncocytic papillary neoplasm (IOPN). The neoplastic cells found within IOPNs show abundant eosinophilic cytoplasm, due to the high number of mitochondria in these cells.

IPMNs are associated with invasive adenocarcinomas, which can be either colloid (mucinous non-cystic) carcinoma, or demonstrate more garden variety ductal features [76, 77]. Distinguishing the subtypes of invasive cancer is clinically important, since colloid carcinomas carry a significantly better prognosis [78]. Great care should be taken not to overlook an associated focal carcinoma, particularly because the neoplastic epithelium in an IPMN can extend intraductally for several centimeters beyond the grossly dilated duct. Of note, patients with IPMN show an increased risk for extrapancreatic malignancies. In particular, higher rates of colorectal, gastric, esophageal and lung malignomas have been reported.

3.3   Molecular Features of IPMNs

Activating mutations in the *KRAS2* oncogene occur early in the development of IPMNs. They are already observed in low-grade IPMNs, and the frequency increases in higher-grade IPMN lesions. Inactivation of *CDKN2A* and *TP53* gene function represent late events, while DPC4/MADH4/SMAD4 gene mutations seem to be less frequent in IPMNs [79, 80]. Of note, *STK1/LKB1*, a serine/threonine kinase gene associated with Peutz-Jeghers syndrome, is inactivated in about 30% of IPMNs. Mutations of the gene encoding for one of the subunits of PI-3 kinase, *PIK3CA*, have been reported in approximately 10% of cases [81].

Epigenetic silencing by aberrant promoter methylation has been described for a number of candidate tumor suppressor genes in IPMNs, including *SOCS1, ppENK, CDKN1C* and *CDKN2A*. In recent years several studies have uncovered a plethora of differentially expressed genes in IPMNs. Transcripts found to be overexpressed in IPMNs that represent candidate biomarkers, and which might also potentially be involved in IPMN progression, include *lipocalin-2, galactin-3, cathepsin-E, claudin-4, TFF-1, TFF-2, TFF-3, CXCR-4, S100A4, matrix metalloproteinase 7 (MMP-7)*, and *sonic hedgehog (SHH)* [82–85]. The recent availability of technologies that can enable mass spectrometric based approaches on microdissected tissues has enabled one of the first global proteomic analysis of a non-invasive IPMN [86]. This study, using microdissected material from an archival IPMN, identified tissue transgluaminase-2 (TG-2) and deleted in malignant brain tumor 1 (DMBT1) as candidate biomarkers in these precursor lesions.

3.4   Genetically Engineered Mouse Model of IPMNs

In a recent elegant study, Schmidt and co-workers described that concomitant pancreas-specific expression of an oncogenic Kras allele and transforming growth factor-alpha (TGF-alpha) led to formation of acinar-ductal metaplasia, accelerated progression of Kras-induced mPanINs, as compared to Kras expression alone, and to the development of cystic lesions resembling key features observed in human IPMNS starting at 2–3 months after birth [87]. Histologically, these cystic lesions were characterized by papillary proliferations which had formed in branches of the main pancreatic duct. In line with findings in humans, the observed murine IPMNs were shown to express CK-19, MUC1 and MUC5AC.

3.4.1 Therapeutic Considerations regarding IPMNs

The most important prognostic factor in IPMNs is the presence, size and histological classification of an associated invasive carcinoma. Therefore, the term "intraductal papillary mucinous carcinoma" should be avoided, since it really confuses a benign, potentially curable lesion (IPMN with high-grade dysplasia) and a malignant carcinoma arising in association with an IPMN [88]. While the overall 5-year survival rate is below 50% in cases of IPMN associated with an invasive carcinoma [68], patients with a fully resected benign IMPN generally have an excellent prognosis. However, since IPMNs can occur in a multifocal distribution, patients with partial pancreatic resection cannot necessarily be considered as completely cured. For example, in one series of 73 patients in which a non-invasive IPMN was resected, 8.3% suffered from recurrence later on [68]. Because of the risk of multifocal disease and metachronous relapse even patients with resected benign IPMNs should be continuously followed clinically. In addition, clinicians should keep in mind the possibility of accompanying extrapancreatic malignancies, as mentioned earlier.

While there is general consensus that an IPMN should be surgically resected if it is more than 3 cm in diameter, becomes symptomatic, is associated with dilation of the pancreatic duct or contains a mural nodule [89], the appropriate management of the incidentally discovered smaller IPMN lesions is less clearly defined. In these cases elimination of the risk of an IPMN progressing to an invasive carcinoma through resection must be weighed against the potential risks of the surgical procedure and impact on quality of life. Moreover, it has to be taken into account that most intra-pancreatic cysts less than 3 cm in diameter usually do not show significant dysplasia histologically (only 3 of 83 surgically removed cysts <3 cm harbored high-grade dysplasia in one reported series) [90, 91]. On the other hand, in another recent study, Tada and collegues argued that simple follow-up observation of these small lesions could also pose a significant risk for a subset of patients. In that series, 7 of 197 patients carrying pancreatic cysts that were followed finally developed pancreatic cancer, representing an incidence rate of 0.95% per year, which was more than 22 times higher than expected for the general population [92]. Considering these observations, prospective studies and clearly defined, evidence-based criteria for individual risk-estimation and management of cystic pancreatic lesions are highly desirable. It is likely that molecular studies on cyst fluid or other clinical specimens will be incorporated in therapeutic decision making in the future.

4 Mucinous Cystic Neoplasms (MCN)

4.1 Clinical Features of MCNs

Mucinous cystic neoplasms are cyst-forming, mucin-producing neoplasms of the pancreas with a distinctive ovarian-type stroma. Most commonly they are located in the body or tail of the pancreas (⊙ *Table 5-1*). Over 90% of MCNs are diagnosed in females, and the mean age at diagnosis is between 40 and 50 years, with a wide range described in the literature (14–95 years). Not surprisingly, patients presenting with non-invasive MCNs tend to be 5–10 years younger on average as compared to those carrying MCNs with associated invasive carcinoma, in line with the concept of MCN being a precursor lesion eventually progressing to invasive pancreatic cancer. Clinical symptoms are often unspecific and include epigastric pain, a sense of abdominal fullness and abdominal mass. Carcinoembryonic antigen 19-9 (CA19-9) blood concentrations are usually normal in non-invasive MCN patients and elevated only in cases that are associated with an invasive carcinoma. Of note, MCNs, like IPMNs, can be discovered as incidental cystic lesions of the pancreas. Computed tomography typically reveals a relatively large (up to 10 cm) intrapancreatic cystic mass. Intramural nodules are more common in MCNs with associated carcinoma. The cysts themselves are usually 1–3 cm in diameter and divided by fibrous septa, cyst contents vary from mucoid to hemorrhagic fluid [88]. The cysts do not communicate with the pancreatic duct, and this feature is often exploited to differentiate MCNs from IPMNs in the clinical setting.

4.2   Histopathology of MCNs

The cysts of MCNs are lined by a columnar mucin-producing epithelium, associated with a spectrum of architectural and nuclear atypia, akin to what is observed in IPMNs. Areas with significant dysplasia are often found directly adjacent to entirely benign epithelium. MCNs with low-grade dysplasia consist of uniform columnar cells with abundant supranuclear mucin. The nuclei are uniformly small and located basally (⊙ *Fig. 5-1e*). MCNs with moderate dysplasia demonstrate slight variation of nuclei in size and shape as well as beginning loss of nuclear polarity. In MCN with high-grade dysplasia ("carcinoma in situ") there is a significant degree of architectural and cytologic atypia, similar to what is seen in invasive cancers (⊙ *Fig. 5-1f*). However, these lesions are also non-invasive per definition [7]. In addition to neoplastic epithelium, MCNs comprise a distinct "ovarian-type" stroma. This ovarian-type stroma consists of densely packed spindle-shaped cells, which can in some cases even show luteinization, and that form a band directly underneath the neoplastic epithelium. Per the current consensus definition, the ovarian-type stroma is an essential prerequisite for the diagnosis of an MCN. Therefore, a proportion of lesions previously referred to as MCNs are now categorized as IPMNs, and the ratio of MCNs relative to IPMNs tends to decrease in newer reports [71]. Diagnostically, ovarian-type stroma can be particularly useful for MCN samples where the neoplastic epithelium is focally denuded.

Around one third of resected MCNs are found to be associated with invasive adenocarcinoma, usually of the tubular or ductal type [88, 93]. These carcinomas may arise focally in an MCN, and depth of invasion has been shown to be one of the most important prognostic factors. Therefore, in those cases the sizes both of the invasive and the non-invasive portions of a resected MCN should be clearly described separately in the pathology report.

4.3   Molecular Genetics of MCNs

Activating point mutations of the *KRAS2* gene have been described as early events in the development of MCNs. Mutational inactivation of the tumor suppressor genes *TP53* and *DPC4/SMAD4/MADH4* occur comparatively later, usually at the invasive stage. Aberrant methylation patterns of the *CDKN2A* gene have been observed in a minority of MCNs. Immunohistochemistry can be used to demonstrate overexpression of alpha-inhibin (in approximately 90% of cases), progesterone receptors (60–90%) and estrogen receptors (30%) by ovarian-type stroma cells of MCNs. Likewise, neoplastic epithelial cells show positive immunolabeling for keratins (AE1/AE3, CAM5.2), epithelial membrane antigen, carcinoembryonic antigen (CEA) and mucin 5AC (MUC5AC). Scattered intraepithelial cells can frequently by identified by labeling for endocrine markers such as chromogranin [94, 95]. Moreover, recent studies on global expression profiling of MCNs have uncovered tissue specific overexpression of a variety of proteins. Among others, c-met, S100P, prostate stem cell antigen (PSCA), jagged-1, c-myc, cathepsin E and pepsinogen C were found to be over-expressed by neoplastic epithelial cells, and steroidogenic acute regulatory protein (STAR) and estrogen receptor-1 (ESR-1) by ovarian-type stroma cells, respectively [96, 97].

4.4   Genetically Engineered Mouse Models of MCN

In recent years, at least two genetically engineered mouse models have been described, closely resembling key features of human MCNs. In 2006 Andrew McMahon's group reported that activation of the Hedgehog signaling pathway through overexpression of a mutationally activated smoothened allele (R26-Smo-M2) under the control of ubiquitously expressed inducible Cre transgene (CAGGS-CreER) in mice led to the rapid development of rhabdo-myosarcomas, basal cell carcinomas and medulloblastomas. Of interest, they also observed development of a novel form of pancreatic lesions resembling low-grade MCNs in approximately half of tamoxifen-induced mice. These lesions were characterized by cyst formation of varying size, lined by cuboidal epithelium with foci of columnar metaplasia and by a supporting proliferative ovarian-like stroma. Moreover, PAS and Alcian blue stains indicated mucin expression by the epithelial cells within these lesions [98]. The following year, Hingorani and colleagues described that pancreas-specific expression of oncogenic Kras^{G12D} in combination with SMAD4 haploinsufficiency, achieved by expression of a floxed SMAD4$^{flox/+}$ allele under control of a p48$^{Cre/+}$ construct led to the formation of macroscopically visible cystic lesions in the body and tail of murine pancreata. Histopathological examination revealed formation of low-grade mPanINs as well as cystic lesions resembling histological features of human MCNs, including lining by a neoplastic epithelium consisting of columnar, mucin-filled, CK-19 positive epithelial cells displaying focal areas of low to high-grade dysplasia, as well as a surrounding stroma that was frequently very cellular and contained spindle-shaped cells with distinctive "wavy" nuclei. Interestingly, the cysts did not seem to communicate with the duct system. Again, mucin expression was confirmed by Alcian blue stain [99].

4.5   Therapeutic Implications of MCNs

The prognosis of MCNs depends largely on whether or not they are associated with a focally invasive carcinoma component. If an invasive carcinoma is not diagnosed after thorough histopathological evaluation of a surgically completely resected MCN, the patient has an excellent prognosis and can be considered as cured. If, on the other hand, a resected MCN is found to be associated with an invasive carcinoma, patients show a much worse overall 5-year survival of only about 60%, which is, nevertheless, still considerably better than survival rates observed for ductal adenocarcinomas of the pancreas not associated with an MCN.

At least three clinically relevant conclusions can be drawn from these observations: Firstly, the striking difference in prognosis between MCN with and without accompanying carcinoma underscores the importance and potential of early detection and resection of these precursor lesions. Unlike non-invasive IPMNs, MCNs are typically unifocal, and represent surgically curable lesions even if they are associated with high-grade dysplasia at the time of diagnosis. The observed age difference of patients with and without associated carcinoma further indicates that there is probably a sufficient time window of probably several years in a given patient, before an existing MCN develops an invasive carcinoma, and during which early detection and curative resection are possible. Secondly, these findings indicate that the generic term "mucinous cystic carcinoma" should be avoided, because one must distinguish between lesions of distinct biological potential. While non-invasive MCNs themselves are curable lesions, they may eventually give rise to adenocarcinomas with metastatic potential and significantly worse prognosis. Thirdly, pathologists need to sample MCNs for histological review as extensively as possible, since the invasive component can be quite focal, and be underdiagnosed upon selective sampling. In this context it should also be mentioned that reports of "metastasizing non-invasive MCNs" almost certainly represent examples where lesions were misdiagnosed as benign MCNs without a carcinoma component, because the focus of invasion was missed due to incomplete histological sampling.

Key Research Points

- Three types of precursor lesions are recognized that can progress to invasive adenocarcinoma of the pancreas – pancreatic intraepithelial neoplasia (PanIN), intraductal papillary mucinous neoplasm (IPMN) and mucinous cystic neoplasm (MCN).
- Over the past decade consensus histopathological criteria have been established that facilitate the accurate diagnosis and classification of these precursors, and permit comparable data to be generated between different institutions.
- The multistep progression from early to later stages of these precursor lesions is mirrored by a series of accumulating genetic alterations.

Future Scientific Directions

- While potent therapeutic options for established pancreatic cancer are lacking accounting for ts overall dismal prognosis, the precursor lesions of pancreatic cancer (i.e., PanINs, IPMNs or MCNs) represent a unique therapeutic opportunity for curative intervention.
- Future research should be aimed at developing diagnostic and imaging tools which allow for reliable early detection of these precursor lesions in a clinical setting.
- This is particularly desirable for PanINs, which are by far the most frequently observed precursor lesions and are difficult or impossible to detect with current clinically available imaging techniques.
- Moreover, prospective studies should address individual risk estimation of diagnosed precursor lesions in order to enable evidence-based guidelines for the appropriate clinical management in individual cases.

Clinical Implications

- Early detection of precursor lesions of pancreatic cancer has the potential to identify high-risk patients and treat a pancreatic lesion before it progresses into a frank malignancy.
- The clinical implications for some precursor lesions are more obvious than others. MCNs should always be resected and thoroughly evaluated histopathologically for the presence of an associated carcinoma.

- The same holds true for IPMNs, if they are bigger than 3 cm, are asymptomatic, contain a mural nodule or cause dilation of the pancreatic duct.
- There are currently opposing opinions as to whether the smaller, typically branch duct IPMNs should also be surgically resected, or followed conservatively.
- PanINs are a common finding in the elderly population, but to date appropriate tools to reliably diagnose isolated PanINs in a clinical setting are lacking.
- Recently, endoscopic ultrasound has enabled the diagnosis of multifocal PanIN lesions in patients at risk for developing pancreatic cancer (for example, individuals in familial pancreatic cancer kindred).
- Improvements in imaging strategy and the incorporation of molecular techniques in the diagnosis and workup of precursor lesions should facilitate improved therapeutic decision making.

References

1. Vogelstein B, Fearon ER, Hamilton SR, Kern SE, Preisinger AC, Leppert M, Nakamura Y, White R, Smits AM, Bos JL: Genetic alterations during colorectal-tumor development. N Engl J Med 1988; 319:525–532.

2. Hruban RH, Wilentz RE, Maitra A: Identification and analysis of precursors to invasive pancreatic cancer. Methods Mol Med 2005;103:1–13.

3. Berman JJ, Albores-Saavedra J, Bostwick D, Delellis R, Eble J, Hamilton SR, Hruban RH, Mutter GL, Page D, Rohan T, Travis W, Henson DE: Precancer: a conceptual working definition – results of a consensus conference. Cancer Detect Prev 2006;30:387–394.

4. Hulst SLP: Zur kenntnis der genese des adenokarzinoms und karzinoms des pankreas. Virchows Archiv 1905;180:288–316.

5. Hruban RH, Takaori K, Klimstra DS, Adsay NV, Albores-Saavedra J, Biankin AV, Biankin SA, Compton C, Fukushima N, Furukawa T, Goggins M, Kato Y, Kloppel G, Longnecker DS, Luttges J, Maitra A, Offerhaus GJ, Shimizu M, Yonezawa S: An illustrated consensus on the classification of pancreatic intraepithelial neoplasia and intraductal papillary mucinous neoplasms. Am J Surg Pathol 2004;28:977–987.

6. Hruban RH, Adsay NV, Albores-Saavedra J, Compton C, Garrett ES, Goodman SN, Kern SE, Klimstra DS, Kloppel G, Longnecker DS, Luttges J, Offerhaus GJ: Pancreatic intraepithelial neoplasia: a new nomenclature and classification system for pancreatic duct lesions. Am J Surg Pathol 2001;25:579–586.

7. Hruban RH, Maitra A, Kern SE, Goggins M: Precursors to pancreatic cancer. Gastroenterol Clin North Am 2007;36:831–849.

8. Andea A, Sarkar F, Adsay VN: Clinicopathological correlates of pancreatic intraepithelial neoplasia: a comparative analysis of 82 cases with and 152 cases

9. Agoff SN, Crispin DA, Bronner MP, Dail DH, Hawes SE, Haggitt RC: Neoplasms of the ampulla of vater with concurrent pancreatic intraductal neoplasia: a histological and molecular study. Mod Pathol 2001;14:139–146.

10. Stelow EB, Adams RB, Moskaluk CA: The prevalence of pancreatic intraepithelial neoplasia in pancreata with uncommon types of primary neoplasms. Am J Surg Pathol 2006;30:36–41.

11. Maitra A, Adsay NV, Argani P, Iacobuzio-Donahue C, De Marzo A, Cameron JL, Yeo CJ, Hruban RH: Multicomponent analysis of the pancreatic adenocarcinoma progression model using a pancreatic intraepithelial neoplasia tissue microarray. Mod Pathol 2003;16:902–912.

12. Almoguera C, Shibata D, Forrester K, Martin J, Arnheim N, Perucho M: Most human carcinomas of the exocrine pancreas contain mutant c-k-ras genes. Cell 1988;53:549–554.

13. Hruban RH, van Mansfeld AD, Offerhaus GJ, van Weering DH, Allison DC, Goodman SN, Kensler TW, Bose KK, Cameron JL, Bos JL: K-ras oncogene activation in adenocarcinoma of the human pancreas. A study of 82 carcinomas using a combination of mutant-enriched polymerase chain reaction analysis and allele-specific oligonucleotide hybridization. Am J Pathol 1993;143:545–554.

14. Hingorani SR, Petricoin EF, Maitra A, Rajapakse V, King C, Jacobetz MA, Ross S, Conrads TP, Veenstra TD, Hitt BA, Kawaguchi Y, Johann D, Liotta LA, Crawford HC, Putt ME, Jacks T, Wright CV, Hruban RH, Lowy AM, Tuveson DA: Preinvasive and invasive ductal pancreatic cancer and its early detection in the mouse. Cancer Cell 2003;4:437–450.

15. Aguirre AJ, Bardeesy N, Sinha M, Lopez L, Tuveson DA, Horner J, Redston MS, DePinho RA: Activated

without pancreatic ductal adenocarcinoma. Mod Pathol 2003;16:996–1006.

kras and ink4a/arf deficiency cooperate to produce metastatic pancreatic ductal adenocarcinoma. Genes Dev 2003;17:3112–3126.

16. Baines AT, Lim KH, Shields JM, Lambert JM, Counter CM, Der CJ, Cox AD: Use of retrovirus expression of interfering rna to determine the contribution of activated k-ras and ras effector expression to human tumor cell growth. Methods Enzymol 2006;407:556–574.

17. Brummelkamp TR, Bernards R, Agami R: Stable suppression of tumorigenicity by virus-mediated rna interference. Cancer Cell 2002;2:243–247.

18. Sherr CJ: Cell cycle control and cancer. Harvey Lect 2000;96:73–92.

19. Caldas C, Hahn SA, da Costa LT, Redston MS, Schutte M, Seymour AB, Weinstein CL, Hruban RH, Yeo CJ, Kern SE: Frequent somatic mutations and homozygous deletions of the p16 (mts1) gene in pancreatic adenocarcinoma. Nat Genet 1994; 8:27–32.

20. Wilentz RE, Geradts J, Maynard R, Offerhaus GJ, Kang M, Goggins M, Yeo CJ, Kern SE, Hruban RH: Inactivation of the p16 (ink4a) tumor-suppressor gene in pancreatic duct lesions: loss of intranuclear expression. Cancer Res 1998;58:4740–4744.

21. Hustinx SR, Leoni LM, Yeo CJ, Brown PN, Goggins M, Kern SE, Hruban RH, Maitra A: Concordant loss of mtap and p16/cdkn2a expression in pancreatic intraepithelial neoplasia: evidence of homozygous deletion in a noninvasive precursor lesion. Mod Pathol 2005;18:959–963.

22. Hingorani SR, Wang L, Multani AS, Combs C, Deramaudt TB, Hruban RH, Rustgi AK, Chang S, Tuveson DA: Trp53r172h and krasg12d cooperate to promote chromosomal instability and widely metastatic pancreatic ductal adenocarcinoma in mice. Cancer Cell 2005;7:469–483.

23. Baas IO, Mulder JW, Offerhaus GJ, Vogelstein B, Hamilton SR: An evaluation of six antibodies for immunohistochemistry of mutant p53 gene product in archival colorectal neoplasms. J Pathol 1994; 172:5–12.

24. Hahn SA, Hoque AT, Moskaluk CA, da Costa LT, Schutte M, Rozenblum E, Seymour AB, Weinstein CL, Yeo CJ, Hruban RH, Kern SE: Homozygous deletion map at 18q21.1 in pancreatic cancer. Cancer Res 1996;56:490–494.

25. Massague J, Blain SW, Lo RS: TGFbeta signaling in growth control, cancer, and heritable disorders. Cell 2000;103:295–309.

26. Kim BG, Li C, Qiao W, Mamura M, Kasprzak B, Anver M, Wolfraim L, Hong S, Mushinski E, Potter M, Kim SJ, Fu XY, Deng C, Letterio JJ: Smad4 signalling in T cells is required for suppression of gastrointestinal cancer. Nature 2006;441: 1015–1019.

27. Wilentz RE, Iacobuzio-Donahue CA, Argani P, McCarthy DM, Parsons JL, Yeo CJ, Kern SE, Hruban RH: Loss of expression of dpc4 in pancreatic intraepithelial neoplasia: evidence that dpc4 inactivation occurs late in neoplastic progression. Cancer Res 2000;60:2002–2006.

28. Vogelstein B, Kinzler KW: Cancer genes and the pathways they control. Nat Med 2004;10: 789–799.

29. D'Andrea AD, Grompe M: The fanconi anaemia/brca pathway. Nat Rev Cancer 2003;3:23–34.

30. Couch FJ, Johnson MR, Rabe KG, Brune K, de Andrade M, Goggins M, Rothenmund H, Gallinger S, Klein A, Petersen GM, Hruban RH: The prevalence of brca2 mutations in familial pancreatic cancer. Cancer Epidemiol Biomarkers Prev 2007; 16:342–346.

31. van der Heijden MS, Brody JR, Gallmeier E, Cunningham SC, Dezentje DA, Shen D, Hruban RH, Kern SE: Functional defects in the fanconi anemia pathway in pancreatic cancer cells. Am J Pathol 2004;165:651–657.

32. Luttges J, Galehdari H, Brocker V, Schwarte-Waldhoff I, Henne-Bruns D, Kloppel G, Schmiegel W, Hahn SA: Allelic loss is often the first hit in the biallelic inactivation of the p53 and dpc4 genes during pancreatic carcinogenesis. Am J Pathol 2001;158:1677–1683.

33. Yamano M, Fujii H, Takagaki T, Kadowaki N, Watanabe H, Shirai T: Genetic progression and divergence in pancreatic carcinoma. Am J Pathol 2000;156:2123–2133.

34. Kuroki T, Tajima Y, Kanematsu T: Role of hypermethylation on carcinogenesis in the pancreas. Surg Today 2004;34:981–986.

35. Baylin SB, Herman JG: DNA hypermethylation in tumorigenesis: epigenetics joins genetics. Trends Genet 2000;16:168–174.

36. Sato N, Fukushima N, Hruban RH, Goggins M: Cpg island methylation profile of pancreatic intraepithelial neoplasia. Mod Pathol 2008;21:238–244.

37. Peng DF, Kanai Y, Sawada M, Ushijima S, Hiraoka N, Kitazawa S, Hirohashi S: DNA methylation of multiple tumor-related genes in association with overexpression of DNA methyltransferase 1 (dnmt1) during multistage carcinogenesis of the pancreas. Carcinogenesis 2006;27:1160–1168.

38. Goggins M: Identifying molecular markers for the early detection of pancreatic neoplasia. Semin Oncol 2007;34:303–310.

39. Tanaka M, Komatsu N, Terakawa N, Yanagimoto Y, Oka M, Sasada T, Mine T, Gouhara S, Shichijo S, Okuda S, Itoh K: Increased levels of IgG antibodies against peptides of the prostate stem cell antigen in the plasma of pancreatic cancer patients. Oncol Rep 2007;18:161–166.

40. Foss CA, Fox JJ, Feldmann G, Maitra A, Iacobuzio-Donahue C, Kern SE, Hruban R, Pomper MG: Radiolabeled anti-claudin 4 and anti-prostate stem cell antigen: initial imaging in experimental models of pancreatic cancer. Mol Imaging 2007;6: 131–139.

41. Argani P, Iacobuzio-Donahue C, Ryu B, Rosty C, Goggins M, Wilentz RE, Murugesan SR, Leach SD, Jaffee E, Yeo CJ, Cameron JL, Kern SE, Hruban RH: Mesothelin is overexpressed in the vast majority of ductal adenocarcinomas of the pancreas: identification of a new pancreatic cancer marker by serial analysis of gene expression (sage). Clin Cancer Res 2001;7:3862–3868.

42. Li M, Bharadwaj U, Zhang R, Zhang S, Mu H, Fisher WE, Brunicardi FC, Chen C, Yao Q: Mesothelin is a malignant factor and therapeutic vaccine target for pancreatic cancer. Mol Cancer Ther 2008;7: 286–296.

43. Hassan R, Ebel W, Routhier EL, Patel R, Kline JB, Zhang J, Chao Q, Jacob S, Turchin H, Gibbs L, Phillips MD, Mudali S, Iacobuzio-Donahue C, Jaffee EM, Moreno M, Pastan I, Sass PM, Nicolaides NC, Grasso L: Preclinical evaluation of morab-009, a chimeric antibody targeting tumor-associated mesothelin. Cancer Immun 2007;7:20.

44. Segara D, Biankin AV, Kench JG, Langusch CC, Dawson AC, Skalicky DA, Gotley DC, Coleman MJ, Sutherland RL, Henshall SM: Expression of hoxb2, a retinoic acid signaling target in pancreatic cancer and pancreatic intraepithelial neoplasia. Clin Cancer Res 2005;11:3587–3596.

45. Klein WM, Hruban RH, Klein-Szanto AJ, Wilentz RE: Direct correlation between proliferative activity and dysplasia in pancreatic intraepithelial neoplasia (panin): additional evidence for a recently proposed model of progression. Mod Pathol 2002;15: 441–447.

46. Biankin AV, Kench JG, Morey AL, Lee CS, Biankin SA, Head DR, Hugh TB, Henshall SM, Sutherland RL: Overexpression of p21(waf1/cip1) is an early event in the development of pancreatic intraepithelial neoplasia. Cancer Res 2001;61:8830–8837.

47. Sarkar FH, Adsule S, Li Y, Padhye S: Back to the future: Cox-2 inhibitors for chemoprevention and cancer therapy. Mini Rev Med Chem 2007; 7:599–608.

48. Larsson SC, Giovannucci E, Bergkvist L, Wolk A: Aspirin and nonsteroidal anti-inflammatory drug use and risk of pancreatic cancer: a meta-analysis. Cancer Epidemiol Biomarkers Prev 2006;15:2561–2564.

49. Shiomi T, Okada Y: Mt1-mmp and mmp-7 in invasion and metastasis of human cancers. Cancer Metastasis Rev 2003;22:145–152.

50. Crawford HC, Scoggins CR, Washington MK, Matrisian LM, Leach SD: Matrix metalloproteinase-7 is expressed by pancreatic cancer precursors

51. and regulates acinar-to-ductal metaplasia in exocrine pancreas. J Clin Invest 2002;109:1437–1444.

51. Harvey SR, Hurd TC, Markus G, Martinick MI, Penetrante RM, Tan D, Venkataraman P, DeSouza N, Sait SN, Driscoll DL, Gibbs JF: Evaluation of urinary plasminogen activator, its receptor, matrix metalloproteinase-9, and von willebrand factor in pancreatic cancer. Clin Cancer Res 2003;9:4935–4943.

52. Varjosalo M, Taipale J: Hedgehog: functions and mechanisms. Genes Dev 2008;22:2454–2472.

53. Li C, Heidt DG, Dalerba P, Burant CF, Zhang L, Adsay V, Wicha M, Clarke MF, Simeone DM: Identification of pancreatic cancer stem cells. Cancer Res 2007;67:1030–1037.

54. Feldmann G, Fendrich V, McGovern K, Bedja D, Bisht S, Alvarez H, Koorstra JB, Habbe N, Karikari C, Mullendore M, Gabrielson KL, Sharma R, Matsui W, Maitra A: An orally bioavailable small-molecule inhibitor of hedgehog signaling inhibits tumor initiation and metastasis in pancreatic cancer. Mol Cancer Ther 2008;7:2725–2735.

55. Feldmann G, Dhara S, Fendrich V, Bedja D, Beaty R, Mullendore M, Karikari C, Alvarez H, Iacobuzio-Donahue C, Jimeno A, Gabrielson KL, Matsui W, Maitra A: Blockade of hedgehog signaling inhibits pancreatic cancer invasion and metastases: a new paradigm for combination therapy in solid cancers. Cancer Res 2007;67:2187–2196.

56. Thayer SP, di Magliano MP, Heiser PW, Nielsen CM, Roberts DJ, Lauwers GY, Qi YP, Gysin S, Fernandez-del Castillo C, Yajnik V, Antoniu B, McMahon M, Warshaw AL, Hebrok M: Hedgehog is an early and late mediator of pancreatic cancer tumorigenesis. Nature 2003;425:851–856.

57. Prasad NB, Biankin AV, Fukushima N, Maitra A, Dhara S, Elkahloun AG, Hruban RH, Goggins M, Leach SD: Gene expression profiles in pancreatic intraepithelial neoplasia reflect the effects of hedgehog signaling on pancreatic ductal epithelial cells. Cancer Res 2005;65:1619–1626.

58. Pasca di Magliano M, Biankin AV, Heiser PW, Cano DA, Gutierrez PJ, Deramaudt T, Segara D, Dawson AC, Kench JG, Henshall SM, Sutherland RL, Dlugosz A, Rustgi AK, Hebrok M: Common activation of canonical wnt signaling in pancreatic adenocarcinoma. PLoS ONE 2007;2:e1155.

59. Al-Aynati MM, Radulovich N, Riddell RH, Tsao MS: Epithelial-cadherin and beta-catenin expression changes in pancreatic intraepithelial neoplasia. Clin Cancer Res 2004;10:1235–1240.

60. Doucas H, Garcea G, Neal CP, Manson MM, Berry DP: Changes in the wnt signalling pathway in gastrointestinal cancers and their prognostic significance. Eur J Cancer 2005;41:365–379.

61. Hruban RH, Adsay NV, Albores-Saavedra J, Anver MR, Biankin AV, Boivin GP, Furth EE, Furukawa T,

Klein A, Klimstra DS, Kloppel G, Lauwers GY, Longnecker DS, Luttges J, Maitra A, Offerhaus GJ, Perez-Gallego L, Redston M, Tuveson DA: Pathology of genetically engineered mouse models of pancreatic exocrine cancer: consensus report and recommendations. Cancer Res 2006;66:95–106.

62. Feldmann G, Habbe N, Dhara S, Bisht S, Alvarez H, Fendrich V, Beaty R, Mullendore M, Karikari C, Bardeesy N, Oullette MM, Yu W, Maitra A: Hedgehog inhibition prolongs survival in a genetically engineered mouse model of pancreatic cancer. Gut 2008.

63. Faca VM, Song KS, Wang H, Zhang Q, Krasnoselsky AL, Newcomb LF, Plentz RR, Gurumurthy S, Redston MS, Pitteri SJ, Pereira-Faca SR, Ireton RC, Katayama H, Glukhova V, Phanstiel D, Brenner DE, Anderson MA, Misek D, Scholler N, Urban ND, Barnett MJ, Edelstein C, Goodman GE, Thornquist MD, McIntosh MW, DePinho RA, Bardeesy N, Hanash SM: A mouse to human search for plasma proteome changes associated with pancreatic tumor development. PLoS Med 2008;5:e123.

64. Funahashi H, Satake M, Dawson D, Huynh NA, Reber HA, Hines OJ, Eibl G: Delayed progression of pancreatic intraepithelial neoplasia in a conditional kras(g12d) mouse model by a selective cyclooxygenase-2 inhibitor. Cancer Res 2007;67:7068–7071.

65. Brune K, Abe T, Canto M, O'Malley L, Klein AP, Maitra A, Volkan Adsay N, Fishman EK, Cameron JL, Yeo CJ, Kern SE, Goggins M, Hruban RH: Multifocal neoplastic precursor lesions associated with lobular atrophy of the pancreas in patients having a strong family history of pancreatic cancer. Am J Surg Pathol 2006;30:1067–1076.

66. Canto MI, Goggins M, Hruban RH, Petersen GM, Giardiello FM, Yeo C, Fishman EK, Brune K, Axilbund J, Griffin C, Ali S, Richman J, Jagannath S, Kantsevoy SV, Kalloo AN: Screening for early pancreatic neoplasia in high-risk individuals: a prospective controlled study. Clin Gastroenterol Hepatol 2006;4:766–781; quiz 665.

67. Terhune PG, Phifer DM, Tosteson TD, Longnecker DS: K-ras mutation in focal proliferative lesions of human pancreas. Cancer Epidemiol Biomarkers Prev 1998;7:515–521.

68. Chari ST, Yadav D, Smyrk TC, DiMagno EP, Miller LJ, Raimondo M, Clain JE, Norton IA, Pearson RK, Petersen BT, Wiersema MJ, Farnell MB, Sarr MG: Study of recurrence after surgical resection of intraductal papillary mucinous neoplasm of the pancreas. Gastroenterology 2002;123:1500–1507.

69. Salvia R, Fernandez-del Castillo C, Bassi C, Thayer SP, Falconi M, Mantovani W, Pederzoli P, Warshaw AL: Main-duct intraductal papillary mucinous neoplasms of the pancreas: clinical predictors of malignancy and long-term survival following resection. Ann Surg 2004;239:678–685; discussion 685–677.

70. Silas AM, Morrin MM, Raptopoulos V, Keogan MT: Intraductal papillary mucinous tumors of the pancreas. AJR Am J Roentgenol 2001;176:179–185.

71. Maitra A, Fukushima N, Takaori K, Hruban RH: Precursors to invasive pancreatic cancer. Adv Anat Pathol 2005;12:81–91.

72. Terris B, Ponsot P, Paye F, Hammel P, Sauvanet A, Molas G, Bernades P, Belghiti J, Ruszniewski P, Flejou JF: Intraductal papillary mucinous tumors of the pancreas confined to secondary ducts show less aggressive pathologic features as compared with those involving the main pancreatic duct. Am J Surg Pathol 2000;24:1372–1377.

73. Farrell JJ, Brugge WR: Intraductal papillary mucinous tumor of the pancreas. Gastrointest Endosc 2002;55:701–714.

74. Tanaka M: Intraductal papillary mucinous neoplasm of the pancreas: iagnosis and treatment. Pancreas 2004;28:282–288.

75. Ban S, Naitoh Y, Mino-Kenudson M, Sakurai T, Kuroda M, Koyama I, Lauwers GY, Shimizu M: Intraductal papillary mucinous neoplasm (ipmn) of the pancreas. Its histopathologic difference between 2 major types. Am J Surg Pathol 2006;30: 1561–1569.

76. Adsay NV, Merati K, Andea A, Sarkar F, Hruban RH, Wilentz RE, Goggins M, Iocobuzio-Donahue C, Longnecker DS, Klimstra DS: The dichotomy in the preinvasive neoplasia to invasive carcinoma sequence in the pancreas: differential expression of muc1 and muc2 supports the existence of two separate pathways of carcinogenesis. Mod Pathol 2002;15:1087–1095.

77. Seidel G, Zahurak M, Iacobuzio-Donahue C, Sohn TA, Adsay NV, Yeo CJ, Lillemoe KD, Cameron JL, Hruban RH, Wilentz RE: Almost all infiltrating colloid carcinomas of the pancreas andxx periampullary region arise from in situ papillary neoplasms: a study of 39 cases. Am J Surg Pathol 2002;26:56–63.

78. Adsay NV, Pierson C, Sarkar F, Abrams J, Weaver D, Conlon KC, Brennan MF, Klimstra DS: Colloid (mucinous noncystic) carcinoma of the pancreas. Am J Surg Pathol 2001;25:26–42.

79. Biankin AV, Biankin SA, Kench JG, Morey AL, Lee CS, Head DR, Eckstein RP, Hugh TB, Henshall SM, Sutherland RL: Aberrant p16(ink4a) and dpc4/ smad4 expression in intraductal papillary mucinous tumours of the pancreas is associated with invasive ductal adenocarcinoma. Gut 2002;50:861–868.

80. Sasaki S, Yamamoto H, Kaneto H, Ozeki I, Adachi Y, Takagi H, Matsumoto T, Itoh H, Nagakawa T, Miyakawa H, Muraoka S, Fujinaga A, Suga T, Satoh M, Itoh F, Endo T, Imai K: Differential roles of alterations of p53, p16, and Smad4 expression in

the progression of intraductal papillary-mucinous tumors of the pancreas. Oncol Rep 2003;10:21–25.

81. Schonleben F, Qiu W, Ciau NT, Ho DJ, Li X, Allendorf JD, Remotti HE, Su GH: Pik3ca mutations in intraductal papillary mucinous neoplasm/carcinoma of the pancreas. Clin Cancer Res 2006;12:3851–3855.

82. Sato N, Fukushima N, Maitra A, Iacobuzio-Donahue CA, van Heek NT, Cameron JL, Yeo CJ, Hruban RH, Goggins M: Gene expression profiling identifies genes associated with invasive intraductal papillary mucinous neoplasms of the pancreas. Am J Pathol 2004;164:903–914.

83. Terris B, Blaveri E, Crnogorac-Jurcevic T, Jones M, Missiaglia E, Ruszniewski P, Sauvanet A, Lemoine NR: Characterization of gene expression profiles in intraductal papillary-mucinous tumors of the pancreas. Am J Pathol 2002;160:1745–1754.

84. Ohuchida K, Mizumoto K, Fujita H, Yamaguchi H, Konomi H, Nagai E, Yamaguchi K, Tsuneyoshi M, Tanaka M: Sonic hedgehog is an early developmental marker of intraductal papillary mucinous neoplasms: clinical implications of mrna levels in pancreatic juice. J Pathol 2006;210:42–48.

85. Nishikawa N, Kimura Y, Okita K, Zembutsu H, Furuhata T, Katsuramaki T, Kimura S, Asanuma H, Hirata K: Intraductal papillary mucinous neoplasms of the pancreas: an analysis of protein expression and clinical features. J Hepatobiliary Pancreat Surg 2006;13:327–335.

86. Cheung W, Darfler MM, Alvarez H, Hood BL, Conrads TP, Habbe N, Krizman DB, Mollenhauer J, Feldmann G, Maitra A: Application of a global proteomic approach to archival precursor lesions: deleted in malignant brain tumors 1 and tissue transglutaminase 2 are upregulated in pancreatic cancer precursors. Pancreatology 2008;8: 608–616.

87. Siveke JT, Einwachter H, Sipos B, Lubeseder-Martellato C, Kloppel G, Schmid RM: Concomitant pancreatic activation of kras(g12d) and tgfa results in cystic papillary neoplasms reminiscent of human ipmn. Cancer Cell 2007;12:266–279.

88. Hruban RH, Pitman MB, Klimstra DS: Tumors of the pancreas. Atlas of tumor pathology, 4th series, fascicle 6th edn. American Registry of Pathology and Armed Forces Institute of Pathology, Washington, DC, 2007.

89. Tanaka M, Chari S, Adsay V, Fernandez-del Castillo C, Falconi M, Shimizu M, Yamaguchi K, Yamao K, Matsuno S: International consensus guidelincs for management of intraductal papillary mucinous neoplasms and mucinous cystic neoplasms of the pancreas. Pancreatology 2006;6: 17–32.

90. Sahani DV, Saokar A, Hahn PF, Brugge WR, Fernandez-Del Castillo C: Pancreatic cysts 3 cm or smaller: how aggressive should treatment be? Radiology 2006;238:912–919.

91. Allen PJ, D'Angelica M, Gonen M, Jaques DP, Coit DG, Jarnagin WR, DeMatteo R, Fong Y, Blumgart LH, Brennan MF: A selective approach to the resection of cystic lesions of the pancreas: results from 539 consecutive patients. Ann Surg 2006;244:572–582.

92. Tada M, Kawabe T, Arizumi M, Togawa O, Matsubara S, Yamamoto N, Nakai Y, Sasahira N, Hirano K, Tsujino T, Tateishi K, Isayama H, Toda N, Yoshida H, Omata M: Pancreatic cancer in patients with pancreatic cystic lesions: a prospective study in 197 patients. Clin Gastroenterol Hepatol 2006;4:1265–1270.

93. Le Borgne J, de Calan L, Partensky C: Cystadenomas and cystadenocarcinomas of the pancreas: a multi-institutional retrospective study of 398 cases. French Surgical Association. Ann Surg 1999;230:152–161.

94. Zamboni G, Scarpa A, Bogina G, Iacono C, Bassi C, Talamini G, Sessa F, Capella C, Solcia E, Rickaert F, Mariuzzi GM, Kloppel G: Mucinous cystic tumors of the pancreas: clinicopathological features, prognosis, and relationship to other mucinous cystic tumors. Am J Surg Pathol 1999;23:410–422.

95. Albores-Saavedra J, Angeles-Angeles A, Nadji M, Henson DE, Alvarez L: Mucinous cystadenocarcinoma of the pancreas. Morphologic and immunocytochemical observations. Am J Surg Pathol 1987;11:11–20.

96. Fukushima N, Sato N, Prasad N, Leach SD, Hruban RH, Goggins M: Characterization of gene expression in mucinous cystic neoplasms of the pancreas using oligonucleotide microarrays. Oncogene 2004;23:9042–9051.

97. Lam MM, Swanson PE, Upton MP, Yeh MM: Ovarian-type stroma in hepatobiliary cystadenomas and pancreatic mucinous cystic neoplasms: an immunohistochemical study. Am J Clin Pathol 2008;129:211–218.

98. Mao J, Ligon KL, Rakhlin EY, Thayer SP, Bronson RT, Rowitch D, McMahon AP: A novel somatic mouse model to survey tumorigenic potential applied to the hedgehog pathway. Cancer Res 2006;66:10171–10178.

99. Izeradjene K, Combs C, Best M, Gopinathan A, Wagner A, Grady WM, Deng CX, Hruban RH, Adsay NV, Tuveson DA, Hingorani SR: Kras(g12d) and smad4/dpc4 haploinsufficiency cooperate to induce mucinous cystic neoplasms and invasive adenocarcinoma of the pancreas. Cancer Cell 2007;11:229–243.

6 Epigenetics and its Applications to a Revised Progression Model of Pancreatic Cancer

Gwen Lomberk · Raul Urrutia

| 1 | **Introduction** .... *144* |

| 2 | **Basic Concepts in Epigenetics** .... *144* |

3	**Evolving Paradigms in the Field of Transcription, Chromatin, and Epigenetics** *145*
3.1	The Universality of Promoters 145
3.2	The RNA Pol II Components and the General Transcription Factors 145
3.3	The Step-Wise Assembly of the RNA Pol II Complex Versus the Holoenzyme Complex 146
3.4	The Promoter-Bashing Paradigm, Cis-Regulatory Sequences, and Sequence-Specific Transcription Factors 146
3.5	The Coactivator-Corepressor Hypothesis 147
3.6	Chromatin Dynamics Forms the Basis of Epigenetics 148
3.6.1	The Histone Code and Subcode Hypotheses: Codifying Gene Activation and/or Silencing and Epigenetics 150
3.6.2	Nucleosome Remodeling Machines 150
3.6.3	Histone Chaperones 151
3.7	Nuclear Shape and Nuclear Domains 152

4	**Epigenetics: Developing a Novel and Comprehensive Genomic-Epigenomic Model for Pancreatic Cancer that Includes Chromatin Dynamics and Nuclear Shape** *154*
4.1	DNA Methylation 156
4.2	Histone Acetylation and Deacetylation 157
4.3	Histone H3-Methyl-K27 and Polycomb 158
4.4	Histone H3-Methyl-K9 and Heterochromatin Protein 1 159
4.5	Additional Non-Histone Chromatin Proteins as Epigenetic Targets 160
4.6	MicroRNAs and Pancreatic Cancer 160

| 5 | **Epigenetics, Chemoprevention and Chemotherapies** .... *161* |

| 6 | **Concluding Remarks** .... *163* |

J. P. Neoptolemos, R. Urrutia, J. L. Abbruzzese, M. W. Büchler (eds.), *Pancreatic Cancer*,
DOI 10.1007/978-0-387-77498-5_6, © Springer Science+Business Media, LLC 2010

Abstract: Defined as heritable changes in gene expression, which are not due to any alteration in the DNA sequence, epigenetic pathways are coming to the forefront of research in disease, and in particular, cancer. In fact, these pathways are altered far more prevalently in cancer than genetic alterations and most importantly, can be reversible, lending themselves as attractive therapeutic targets.

This chapter will cover the basic aspects of transcriptional gene regulation, epigenetics and chromatin dynamics and then discuss the intricacies of its application to pancreatic cancer biology and potential therapeutics. In addition, we propose a revised model for better understanding pancreatic cancer to expand the highly provocative and productive "mutation centric" progression model, as defined by Hruban and colleagues, into a new model that formally includes chromatin-induced and miRNA-induced epigenetic changes, as well as other alterations that could be caused by changes in nuclear shape. We are optimistic that this model may serve as a compass for further studies aimed at illuminating the field of pancreatic cancer biology, diagnosis, therapeutics, and chemoprevention, in a similar, fruitful manner as the original model.

1   Introduction

Elegant work, executed in particular during the last two decades, has revealed that the regulation of gene expression via chromatin modifications and remodeling underlies the phenomenon of epigenetics. An embryo, for instance, will be defined as human by the amount and sequence of DNA, which result from the fusion of the two parental gametes. However, as the embryo grows, cells will begin to differentiate from each other. The ultimate results of the differentiation process seen in a young adult clearly show that in spite of all cells within the same organism carrying the same DNA sequence, a neuron, for instance, is totally different than a pancreatic acinar cell. Meditating on this phenomenon can leave us breathless. If instead of thinking about these two cells as being part of a human, we imagine that they are independent unicellular organisms, we would never guess that they have the same genome. Therefore, when a cell phenotype is defined at the end of a differentiation process, one realizes that epigenetic mechanisms are responsible for making different cells by modulating the expression of the same genome in a different manner that is inheritable in each somatic cell division. Therefore, in the following paragraphs we will: (1) review the basic aspects of molecular mechanisms that are important for understanding gene regulation and epigenetics; (2) propose an updated model for better understanding pancreatic cancer, which will expand the extremely provocative and productive "mutation centric" model defined by Hruban et al. [1] into a new model that formally includes chromatin-induced and miRNA-induced epigenetic changes and other changes that could be caused by alterations in nuclear shape; and (3) briefly review drugs that may be important for the chemoprevention and/or treatment of pancreatic cancer.

2   Basic Concepts in Epigenetics

The study of epigenetics has been, for the authors of this chapter, an example of how applicable the epistemological concepts behind the Thomas Kuhn's seminal work, "The Structure of Scientific Revolutions," are to this science [2]. In this work, Kuhn proposes that science moves ahead not by the incessant generation of data but by work that changes preexistent paradigms. This is sometimes called by other philosophers as an epistemological fracture, meaning that the conceptual framework that was true yesterday has evolved into a new theoretical framework that better explains reality. Therefore, we will dissect the basis of epigenetics by discussing the paradigms that have dominated this science at different stages of its development until today. It would be desirable that the reader incorporates all these basic paradigms into a personal integrated picture of how chromatin and the transcriptional regulatory machinery work together in order to mediate epigenetic inheritance in somatic cells.

3   Evolving Paradigms in the Field of Transcription, Chromatin, and Epigenetics

3.1   The Universality of Promoters

This is the story of a remarkable journey since the work of Jacob and Monod [3] to the large amount of work that went into discovering the transcriptional mechanisms which regulate basal levels of expression before either activation or repression can occur (Basal Transcription). Prokaryotic cells have only one RNA polymerase that binds to the promoter of genes and, aided by a transcription factor (factor σ), initiates the synthesis of an RNA molecule (Transcription) (reviewed in [4]). A remarkable finding is that promoters from bacteria to human contain similar sequences (e.g., TATA box). This concept has supported the prediction that the regulation of gene expression throughout evolution has been mechanistically very similar. Today, most investigators accept that this level of similarity was remarkable in its time, but was far from the whole story. Hard-core evidence for the functional evolutionary-conservation thinkers has been further supported by the discovery that, at the atomic resolution, the tridimensional structure among RNA polymerases is strikingly high [5]. Thus, this theoretical framework paved the way for the search of eukaryotic molecules that mediate transcription.

3.2   The RNA Pol II Components and the General Transcription Factors

Work on understanding transcriptional regulation was highly stimulated by the discovery of an RNA polymerase from eukaryotic cells [6]. However, the complexity in jumping from bacteria to eukaryotes began to emerge, in particular, with the isolation of two additional RNA polymerases from higher organisms (reviewed in [7]). Today, we refer to these molecules as RNA polymerase I, RNA Polymerase II, and RNA polymerase III. This complexity became further evident upon attempts to reconstitute transcription from isolated RNA polymerase II complexes bound to the core promoter of genes involved in basal transcription [8,9]. Transcription initiation at RNA polymerase II promoters in eukaryotes, which is the focus of the current chapter due to its association with protein-encoding gene expression, involves the assembly of a megadalton, multiprotein complex, comprised of not only the polymerase itself, but a variety of associated factors, known as the General Transcription Factors (GTFs). These general transcription factors function to properly position RNA pol II on the promoter DNA, as well as to interact with transcriptional activators. The process of isolating and reconstituting transcription in vitro and derive the theoretical framework gained via these experiments took several decades, until we learned the details of the paradigm described in the following paragraph.

3.3 The Step-Wise Assembly of the RNA Pol II Complex Versus the Holoenzyme Complex

To focus on the process of transcriptional initiation, it is most logical to begin with a description of RNA polymerase II complex, the transcriptional enzyme complex, which includes the general transcription factors, responsible for making the protein-encoding RNA molecules. Two paradigms exist for how the occupancy of the promoter is initiated by the RNA pol II complex: individual general transcription factors and the enzyme may be assembled in situ on the promoter in a step-wise fashion or the entire machinery and its associated factors bind the promoter collectively as the polymerase II holoenzyme (reviewed in [10,11]). In eukaryotes, based on the step-wise assembly paradigm, the core promoter serves as a platform for the assembly of transcription preinitiation complex (PIC). The assembly of the PIC begins with TFIID binding to the TATA box, initiator, and/or downstream promoter element (DPE) found in most core promoters. The PIC was conceptualized primarily from in vitro reconstitution assays. These experiments led to the isolation of the GTFs that aid the RNA polymerase II by entering into the process of transcription in a step-wise manner. These proteins include, in order of association to the promoter, TFIID, TFIIB, TFIIA, TFIIF, TFIIE, and TFIIH (reviewed in [12]). As mentioned above, the initial step for PIC formation is the binding of the GTF, TFIID, which is the only GTF with site-specific DNA binding ability and in itself a complex containing the TATA-binding protein (TBP) and numerous TBP-associated factors, termed TAFIIs. Subsequently, TFIIB recognizes the TFIID-promoter complex and, along with TFIIA, stabilizes the nucleo-protein complex, which allows TFIIF to escort RNA pol II to the promoter. The interaction between TFIIB and RNA pol II is crucial for defining the proper start site of transcription [13,14]. Once RNA pol II is stably positioned, it is still unable to initiate RNA transcription until the recruitment of two additional GTFs, TFIIE and TFIIH. Transcriptional initiation requires two functions of the TFIIH, a helicase activity to open the double stranded DNA since the RNA polymerase will copy only a single strand of a gene, and a CDK kinase activity, which hyperphosphorylates the tail of the RNA polymerase II molecule to initiate transcription.

Two major discoveries performed during the last decade, the existence of the Mediator Complex [15], which is necessary for full function of the RNA polymerase II, as well as the possibility that the RNA pol II enzyme, GTFs, and Mediator could be pre-assembled to form the RNA Polymerase II holoenzyme (enzyme with all the parts) prior to the recruitment to promoter. This process forms the basis of the holoenzyme paradigm [11]. Fortunately, the knowledge derived from both, the step-wise assembly and the holoenzyme paradigm are both currently operational.

3.4 The Promoter-Bashing Paradigm, Cis-Regulatory Sequences, and Sequence-Specific Transcription Factors

While experiments aimed at understanding the mechanisms regulating basal transcription were actively underway, other investigators were searching for the basis of regulated transcription, namely transcriptional activation (gene induction) and/or transcriptional repression (gene silencing). Soon, investigators adopted concepts and tools to dissect this process, including fusing promoter regions to reporter genes and performing deletions and site-directed mutagenesis for teasing out potential sites that could bind sequence-specific transcriptional regulators, which provided fruitful information as the promoter-bashing paradigm. In addition, promoter footprinting and Electrophoretic Mobility Shift Assays (EMSAs) were utilized determining the binding of transcription factors to specific DNA sequences, called cis-regulatory sites [16]. These factors can act either as monomers, such as the pancreatic tumor suppressor and sequence-specific transcription factor, KLF11 [17], or as a complex, such as PTF1 [18], which recognizes the promoters of many acinar cell genes in a trimeric homeodomain complex including P48 and HEB. Some of this knowledge not only advanced the concept of transcription, but also generated useful tools for the Pancreatology field, since several tissue-enriched or developmental time-specific promoters (reviewed in [19]) are the key requirement for the creation of several animal models for pancreatitis and cancer.

3.5   The Coactivator-Corepressor Hypothesis

Studies designed to better decipher the way that sequence-specific transcription factors regulate gene expression led to the concept that these proteins behave as adaptors between the DNA and proteins that either induce or impede RNA pol II transcription. This concept was based upon the recognition this type of transcription factor were modular in structure, composed of a DNA binding domain and a transcriptional regulatory domain which influence the rate of mRNA synthesis (reviewed in [20–22]). Conceptually, proteins that promoted activation were called coactivators, while any corresponding repressor proteins were termed corepressors. Initially, some investigators searched for these factors among the hundreds of proteins that form the RNA Polymerase II holoenzyme. Indeed, the interaction of transcription factors with certain members of the holoenzyme was necessary for regulated transcription. However, at the same time, a new era in studying the role of chromatin proteins was being born and starting to dominate, at the mechanistic level, the field of gene expression and apoptosis, proliferation, senescence, stem cell biology, cell migration, oncogenesis, tumor suppression, DNA replication, DNA repair, ploidy, as well as other processes integrally associated with the development and maintenance of the pancreatic cancer phenotype. For instance, today, we know that histone deacetylases (HDACs) play significant regulatory roles in gene expression during cancer [23], in particular in silencing tumor suppressor genes, and inhibitors of these proteins are at different phases of clinical trials for the treatment of diverse malignancies [24]. HDACs are recruited into different protein corepressor complexes, which are recruited to promoters via the transcriptional regulatory domain of a distinct transcription factor bound to DNA (reviewed in [25]). As a result, this transcription factor effectively deacetylates histones, which serves as a signal for gene silencing (◉ Fig. 6-1). The reversal of this state is achieved through the function of histone acetylases enzymes (HATs), such as CREB binding protein (CBP)/P300 and P300/CBP-Associated Factor (PCAF) (reviewed in [26]). The deregulation of these types of enzymes can lead to the aberrant activation of oncogenes (◉ Fig. 6-2). Other non-histone chromatin proteins function either as coactivators or corepressors via distinct mechanisms, as mediators of histone methylation, ubiquitination, sumoylation, and other modifications, which inform the cell toward dynamically changing gene expression patterns according to the particular function being performed.

□ Fig. 6-1

Examples of epigenetic-mediated tumor suppressor gene silencing. This cartoon depicts a model for various roles of chromatin dynamics in tumor suppressor gene silencing, participating in the cancer phenotype. Several different mechanisms of epigenetic-mediated gene silencing can accomplish the same outcome of tumor suppressor gene silencing, including the HDAC system, polycomb proteins and HP1 proteins. For example, a sequence-specific transcription factor (ssTF) may recruit the Sin3a–HDAC complex to a target gene promoter. The recruitment of Sin3a–HDAC to the promoter facilitates the remodeling of surrounding chromatin with silencing marks, namely the deacetylation of histones. Removal of acetylation signals short-term repression of a target gene and in addition, primes the histone for receiving additional long-term silencing marks, such as methylation of K9 or K27 on histone H3, binding marks for HP1 and polycomb, respectively. The recruitment of HP1 to a gene promoter facilitates the further recruitment of the G9a methylase, which creates more methyl-K9 H3 silencing marks and thus, more HP1 binding sites. In addition, HP1 can recruit a DNA methyltransferase (Dnmt) to the promoter. In a similar manner for the polycomb group proteins, PRC1 recruitment results in the binding of the PRC2 complex, which contains the K27 H3 methylase EZH2. The PRC2 complex also is capable of recruiting the DNA methyltransferases.

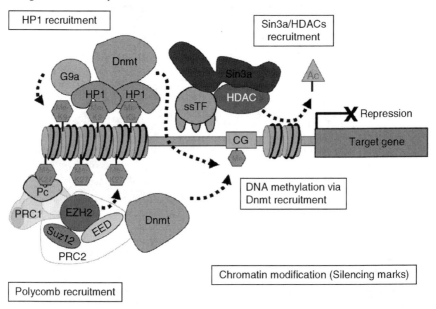

3.6 Chromatin Dynamics Forms the Basis of Epigenetics

Work on the role of histones in nuclear cell biology was very active in the 1970s with a detailed analysis of nucleosome composition and DNA packaging [27]. In terms of transcription, it was thought that histones and nucleosomes were rich solely in heterochromatin, which is transcriptionally silent, and relatively poor in euchromatin, which is transcriptionally active. Unfortunately, however, how these states could be interchanged, meaning that chromatin was more dynamic than previously speculated, remained poorly understood until the 1980s and received a boost at the turn of the century (reviewed in [28,29]). Research on transcriptional

☐ Fig. 6-2

Examples of epigenetic-mediated oncogene activation. This cartoon depicts a model for the role of chromatin dynamics in promoting the cancer phenotype through oncogene activation. In this model, a sequence-specific transcription factor (ssTF) triggers the recruitment of CBP/p300 (or PCAF) to a target gene promoter. The recruitment of CBP/p300 to the promoter also provides HAT activity, which facilitates the modification of surrounding histones to create "active" chromatin with acetylated histones. Addition of acetylated marks to histones signals activation of transcription through recruitment of other bromodomain-containing proteins, such as the SWI/SNF family of chromatin mechanochemical remodelers, which via the expenditure of ATP facilitate structural relaxation of chromatin and thus, access to transcriptional machinery. Additional players in the process of gene activation can include the histone chaperones, which through the exchange of histone variants, such as histone H3.3, provide activating signals. In addition, demethylation of DNA can trigger the activation of an oncogene promoter.

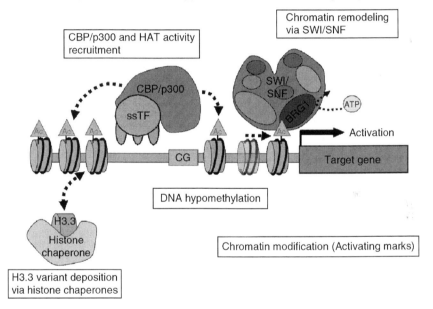

regulation and its relevance to biological and pathobiological processes grew significantly with the discovery that indeed, chromatin is dynamic, often switching from euchromatin to heterochromatin and vice versa. Chromatin dynamics is regulated by: (1) signaling events that form the basis of the histone code and subcodes; (2) mechanochemical enzymes that move nucleosomes from cis-regulatory sequences, an essential step in transcription; as well as c. histone chaperones, which remove histones from nucleosomes to either activate or silence gene expression. Noteworthy, it is chromatin dynamics which determines the epigenetic inheritance of either a phenotypic trait from the germ line (imprinting) or from one somatic cell to its daughter. Our DNA content is the same throughout the body, yet different types of cells with distinct characteristics and functions exist to create various organs and biological systems. We often do not consider it, but since the exact same DNA is in every cell, the distinctions in the type of cell it becomes lies within epigenetics, and in particular, chromatin dynamics. Following, we will describe these three areas of chromatin dynamics in further detail.

3.6.1 The Histone Code and Subcode Hypotheses: Codifying Gene Activation and/or Silencing and Epigenetics

Elegant work from many laboratories around the world found its conceptual integration in the development of the Histone Code hypothesis [30]. Before describing this theoretical framework for understanding transcription and epigenetics, one should remember that histones are small, basic proteins that are extremely conserved throughout evolution [31]. To illustrate how conserved histones are and better explain how the Histone Code hypothesis works, we will use histone H3 (H3) as an example, although the code considers all the histones and their genetic variants.

The first 24 amino acids of H3 are almost identical in most organisms, known as the histone H3 tail. Collectively, the histone "tails" have been defined from analysis of their crystal structure, as the regions of the histone sequences that extend from the nucleosomal disk [32]. The H3 tail contains several serine(S), threonine(T), and tyrosine(Y) residues, which can undergo phosphorylation, and other residues, such as lysine(K) and arginine(R), which can be extensively modified by methylation, acetylation, ubiquitination, and sumoylation [30]. In fact, the lysines in H3 even have the potential to be in different states of methylation, namely mono-, di-, and tri-methylated [33]. These histone modifications have come to be known as "marks" because in many cases, they are utilized as clues for epigenetics. For instance, the Polycomb complex, which keeps stem cells in their undifferentiated state, binds to trimethylated K27 of H3 in order to mediate heterochromatin formation on a target promoter and, as consequence of this event, gene silencing [34]. This is one of the mechanisms for epigenetic inheritance in human somatic cells where the K27 trimethyl mark must be removed in order to initiate the hierarchical cascade of gene expression that leads to a cell fate decision. Interestingly, as we will describe below, this epigenetic mechanism is often used for permanently silencing tumor suppressors without the need of gene mutation or deletion (◉ *Fig. 6-1*). Another protein is HP1, which binds to di- and tri-methylated K9 of H3 to perform a similar function in gene silencing. The Histone Code hypothesis predicts that the type, location, and combination of histone marks determine whether a gene would be expressed or silent under a particular set of circumstances. Recently, using HP1 as a model of a histone mark-binding protein, we have discovered that these non-histone proteins can also be modified by the same enzymes that are responsible of creating the Histone Code, appearing to act in the fine-tuning of the instructions given by the histone marks [35]. For instance, a required step for entering into cell senescence is the phosphorylation of HP1γ at residue S83 (S93 from alternative start site) [36], suggesting that this modification instructs HP1 to regulate the gene expression of key genes which will epigenetically influence the cell into senescence. Thus, the Histone Code and its subcodes have fueled a new era of great productivity and optimism in the field of transcription, chromatin dynamics, and epigenetics, in particular as it relates to cancer.

3.6.2 Nucleosome Remodeling Machines

Nucleosome remodeling machines, containing ATP-dependent mechanochemical activity (molecular motors), were discovered using biochemical methods and in vitro assays. Using these approaches, numerous laboratories have been able to isolate protein complexes that move nucleosomes along DNA thereby removing a repressive effect of histones on a particular cis-regulatory sequence. These nucleosome remodeling complexes include SWI/SNF, NuRD (nucleosome remodeling and deacetylation) and CHRAC (chromatin accessibility complex) (reviewed in [37]). Several of these molecular machines have been found to be conserved from organisms ranging from yeast to human. To demonstrate the basic mechanisms of these nucleosome remodelers, as an example, we will use the SWI/SNF complex, which is the human homolog to the *Drosophila* trithorax complex [38]. The function of complexes like SWI/SNF is essential for the expression of a myriad of genes via its recruitment to chromatin, hydrolysis of ATP and utilization of this energy to remodel nucleosomes (◉ *Fig. 6-2*). While *Drosophila* only possesses a single Swi2/Snf2 complex with ATPase activity, Brahma (Brm) [39], mammals have two homologues, BRM and BRG1 [40]. Although the amino acid sequences of these two are 75% identical with broad expression, these subunits are mutually exclusive, since a single SWI/SNF complex contains either BRM or BRG1. Thus, there are several subtypes of SWI/SNF complexes that can be divided based on the ATP-ase molecule that generates the mechano-chemical force for nucleosome movement. Interestingly, the genes encoding these subunits have been found to have mutations and/or loss of expression in some human tumor cell lines, as well as primary tumors. For instance, the *BRG1* gene has specific mutations identified in pancreatic, breast, lung and prostate cancer cell lines [41,42].

The trithorax complex recognizes methylated K4 of H3, actively participating in the epigenetics and chromatin dynamics of the cell. For instance, stem cells are characterized by having a subset of genes that have a dual mark, methylated at both, K4 and K27 of H3 (◉ *Fig. 6-3*). These gene promoters are known to be in a state called "poised," since they are repressed by polycomb in the stem cells, but after removal of the K27 mark, the remaining methylated K4 will signal for activation leading to the initiation of cell differentiation [43,44]. Therefore, although heterochromatin is repressive, nucleosome remodeling machines, by binding to specific histone marks, sometimes already present on a promoter along with the silencing mark, will convert it into active euchromatin. As we know, tumorigenesis exhibits the culmination of alterations in several genetic pathways. Therefore, as is the case with many of the global epigenetic effects discussed in this chapter, it would only take a single mutation to inactivate a large subset of SWI/SNF complexes (such as a BRG1 mutation) to perturb the regulation of numerous downstream genetic pathways and as a result, trigger robust growth-promoting effects (◉ *Fig. 6-2*).

3.6.3 Histone Chaperones

Histone chaperones constitute the later developments within the area of transcription [45]. The search for this type of proteins initiated from the understanding that there were many histones and histone variants that could occupy a nucleosome. For instance, histone H3 has four main isoforms in mammals [46]. Some of these variants act as activators, while others act as repressors when inside of a nucleosome [47]. For instance, deposition of histone variant H3.3 has been associated with transcriptionally active genes in plants, flies, and humans. In addition to the possibility of different histone variants occupying a nucleosome, these variants are also sub-strates of enzymes that create histone marks. Therefore, the combinatorial effect between the existence of the histone variants and their participation in the Histone Code, which is known as the histone "barcode" [47], creates the possibilities of regulating activation or repression significantly complex. An important contribution to the field was the discovery that some histone variants are rapidly exchanged from nucleosomes, leading to the finding that this nucleosome-histone exchange codifies for either gene activation or silencing. Therefore, histone chaperones cooperate with the Histone Code in instructing cells to regulate a particular program of gene expression (◉ *Fig. 6-2*). The exact role of histone chaperones in ATP-dependent

Dynamics of chromatin marks on promoters. The figure demonstrates three different promoter states of chromatin marks: active, "poised" and silenced (adapted from [44]). Nucleosomes encompassing the promoter region of a gene are shown. The numbers indicate the corresponding amino acid of the histone H3 tail. The orange circles represent the degree of methylation with multiple states possible for a given signal. For example, on active promoters, the chromatin marks are a signal of gene transcription, such as mono-, di- or tri-methylation of K4 of H3 and mono-methylation of H3-K9. Active promoters are also enriched in H3, H4, and H2A acetylation (not shown). On a "poised" promoter, a combination of active and repressive marks can leave genes ready for activation and forms a "bivalent domain." The promoter regions of this type are enriched in the repressive trimethyl-K27 H3 mark, whereas the region around the transcription start is also enriched in the active trimethyl-K4 H3 mark. Finally, a silenced promoter contains inactive chromatin marks. These nucleosomes are enriched in H3-K9 tri-methylation (and sometimes di-methylation, not shown) and H3-K27 di- and tri-methylation.

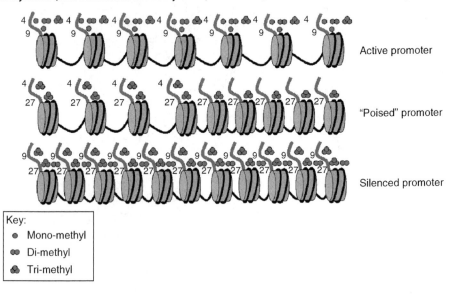

Active promoter

"Poised" promoter

Silenced promoter

Key:
- Mono-methyl
- Di-methyl
- Tri-methyl

remodeling and whether these chaperones serve to temporarily protect free histones or facilitate actual remodeling are all currently active areas of research.

3.7 Nuclear Shape and Nuclear Domains

The influence of nuclear shape in determining the tridimensional location of a particular gene within the nucleus in interphase is well-known (chromosome territory) [48]. In addition, the nucleus consists of distinct nuclear domains with various components, which suggests that various nuclear functions occur at precise locations within the nucleus (● *Fig. 6-4*). This knowledge supports the notion that changes in nuclear shape, by altering the nuclear position of the gene, can alter chromatin dynamics leading to aberrant gene expression. Clear support for this concept came from a naturally occurring mutation in the Lamin A gene [49]. Lamins are proteins that form intermediate filaments, which create a nuclear lamina covering the nucleus

■ Fig. 6-4

Chromosomal territories and nuclear domains. This cartoon of a mammalian nucleus illustrates the chromosomal territories and various nuclear bodies. Chromosomes occupy discrete territories in the nucleus. In addition, various functions within the nucleus occur in distinct locations, considered nuclear bodies or domains. Recent important and elegant work has demonstrated that alterations in nuclear shape will impact on these nuclear territories and domains, affecting gene expression in a manner resembles aging, polyploidy, and aneuploidy; all changes that are found in pancreatic cancer. Therefore, extending this area of research is of paramount importance for this field.

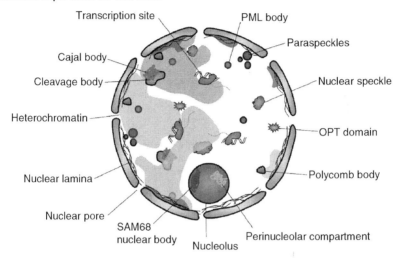

and extend toward the interior of this organelle to form a skeleton (reviewed in [50]). Thermodynamically speaking, the efficiency of a particular enzyme is better when in association to a surface rather than free floating in solution. Therefore, this lamin-based skeleton is necessary for all the processes that take place in the nucleus by helping to compartmentalize and concentrate specific molecular machineries into nuclear domains, which can be considered the nuclear equivalent of the cytoplasmic organelle, though they are not surrounded by membrane. Mutations in lamin A significantly change nuclear shape, generating a new pattern of gene expression, which is responsible of the phenotype of premature aging and cancer in the Hutchinson-Gilford progeria syndrome [49]. This has inspired our laboratory to predict that some of the gross nuclear changes observed early during the progression of histopathological lesions in pancreatic cancer are not a consequence of cancer; but rather these changes help in the development and/or maintenance of this malignant phenotype. Therefore, our laboratory has included nuclear shape as a candidate modifier of pancreatic cancer progression, since the transition of PanIN 1B to PanIN 2 requires changes in nuclear shape [51]. We hypothesize that these nuclear changes are responsible for extensively altering gene expression, independently of other mechanisms described, and thereby significantly contribute to the progression and maintenance of the pancreatic cancer phenotype. Since it has already been established that changes in DNA, such as mutation or deletion, are part of cancer progression and changes in chromatin are being increasingly recognized as well, we, here, integrate it with the addition layer of changes in nuclear structure to form what we call the "Triple Code Hypothesis" (◉ Fig. 6-5a).

4   Epigenetics: Developing a Novel and Comprehensive Genomic-Epigenomic Model for Pancreatic Cancer that Includes Chromatin Dynamics and Nuclear Shape

The revolution of somatic genetics in the field of cancer brought about by the model developed by Fearon and Vogelstein in colon [52], which later led to an adaptation to the pancreas by Hruban et al. [1], opened a fruitful era for pancreatic cancer research, spanning approximately two decades. The basic premise of somatic genetics in cancer is that if a gene, which is suspected to play a role related to cancer, is over-amplified, for instance, such as Myc in brain, it behaves as an oncogene, but if it is down-regulated, like p16 in pancreatic cancer, it behaves as a tumor suppressor. Due to this premise, in the pancreatic cancer field, the changes in expression of both oncogenes and tumor suppressors, according to the Hruban model, were originally believed to occur via mutation or deletion and later with the work of Goggins, by promoter methylation [53–55]. The validity of this model has been elegantly demonstrated using Genetically Engineered Models (GEM), primarily supported by NIH via the "Mouse Model Consortium" funded by NCI [56].

In addition to the recognition of the outstanding contribution this progression model of somatic genetics has had in advancing cancer research, we would like here to propose a new model that also takes into consideration the new theoretical framework of epigenetics, and in particular, changes that occur at the protein level in the absence of DNA changes, such as deletion, mutation, or even promoter methylation. For instance, upon reading through the Hruban model of pancreatic cancer, in which the underlying conceptual framework is genetic

⬛ Fig. 6-5

(a) The triple code hypothesis. This figure summarizes the integration of the well-known DNA-centric hypothesis for the establishment and maintenance of the cancer phenotype, which includes mutations and deletions, with changes in chromatin, signaled through the Histone Code, barcode and its subcodes, and alterations in nuclear structure to form what we call the "Triple Code Hypothesis." This "Triple Code Hypothesis" has formed the basis of the more comprehensive progression model for pancreatic cancer, proposed in *Fig. 6-5b*.

(b) Revised Comprehensive Progression Model for Pancreatic Cancer The model developed by Hruban and colleagues [1] was fundamental for expanding the work of many laboratories in the area of somatic genetics in pancreatic cancer to the point that today we understand the relationship between the morphological progression and mutations/deletion of important oncogenes and tumor suppressor pathways. However, the model cannot currently explain emerging knowledge on critical steps that occur between these mutations and even the potential cause of subsequent mutations and deletions. Most of these changes are epigenetic in nature with the underlying basic mechanisms of both, chromatin dynamics and nuclear shape. Thus, here, we propose a novel model for the progression of pancreatic cancer, which not only incorporates the elegant and extremely important data generated under the premise of the previous model but, in addition, formally includes chromatin-induced and miRNA-induced epigenetic changes, as well as other alterations caused by changes in nuclear shape. It is the hope that this model will serve as a compass to guide future experiments in these under-explored and yet crucial areas of knowledge. We believe that in the next 5 years, experiments aimed at addressing the contribution of these phenomena to pancreatic cancer progression and their potential translation to clinical applications will be among the most promising areas of our field.

⬛ Fig. 6-5 (continued)

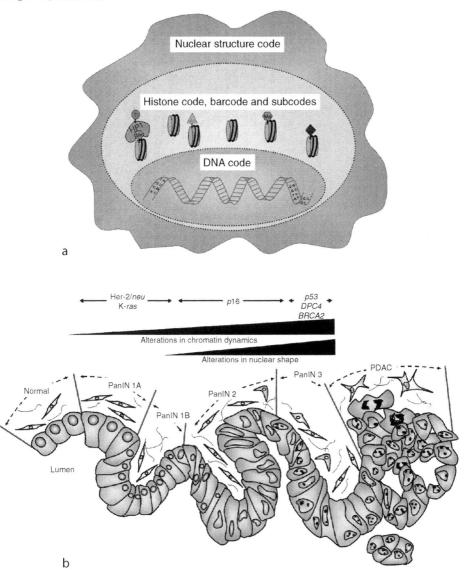

in nature, one can infer that pancreatic cancer progresses through multistep mechanisms with different lesions evolving via mutations in different genes. However, this model does not explain what protein-mediated epigenetic changes, which can take place between the occurrences of landmark mutations, are responsible for cancer progression, nor this model has proven that a later mutation is caused by an earlier one. Therefore, in the following paragraph, we will give examples of epigenetic changes that occur in time between mutations and can lead to tumor suppressor silencing, starting with DNA methylation and going through some modifiers of chromatin. These examples leave us with the scientific responsibilities of proposing an updated paradigm for the progression of pancreatic cancer which include two additional types of phenomena (besides genetics), namely changes in chromatin dynamics and nuclear shape (● *Fig. 6-5b*). Our intention in proposing this new paradigm is, for new investigators in this field, to dive into pancreatic cancer with a more in depth mechanistic approach than using only the tools of molecular pathology and a combination of a multitude of arrays for different purposes.

First, it is necessary to explain how changes in chromatin dynamics can silence tumor suppressor genes via mechanisms that are totally independent of either deletions or mutations of these genes. In fact, in the case of *p16*, which we will use as a prime example for pancreatic cancer in the following paragraphs, this mechanism leads to the final methylation of this gene, which should take the readers to consider that chromatin changes can occur before and lead to the inactivation of landmark mutations that were described in the original paradigm. Therefore, we will begin this journey with a brief description of this final read-out in epigenetics, DNA methylation, since, to date, it is the most commonly known epigenetic alteration, and continue temporally backwards in epigenetics toward changes in chromatin and their modifiers. In addition, we will briefly describe some recent studies in the epigenetics of microRNAs in pancreatic cancer, a neonate to the field within the past couple years.

4.1   DNA Methylation

As mentioned above, DNA methylation was the first type of epigenetic change to be studied as a mechanism for the inactivation of tumor suppressors [57]. DNA methylation occurs on dinucleotide CpGs, where cytosines that precede guanines. The process of DNA methylation entails the addition of a methyl group to the number 5 carbon of the cytosine pyrimidine ring, which ultimately silences gene expression. Noteworthy, DNA methylation normally has significant physiological significance, as with genomic imprinting to ensure monoallelic expression and hypermethylation of repetitive genomic sequences to prevent chromosomal instability, translocations, and gene disruption caused by the reactivation of transposable DNA sequences. However, during tumorigenesis, aberrant DNA methylation can assist the cancer phenotype.

In pancreatic cancer, DNA methylation has been known for a long time as a mechanism to inactivate tumor suppressor genes, such as well-known inactivation of the p16 promoter via methylation [58]. In addition, loss of methylation of a normally silenced promoter in pancreatic cells, such as the gene encoding the hematopoietic-specific guanine nucleotide exchange factor, *VAV1*, can lead to its misexpression [59]. Initial methodologies only provided insights at the single gene level, but fortunately, recent developments in methodologies have advanced enough to perform genome-wide scale gene methylation analysis. As an example, through the use of large-scale methylation analysis, KLF11, a tumor suppressor gene for pancreatic cancer and leukemia, was found to be methylated in these neoplastic diseases [60,61]. With validity to both methodologies, methylation analysis of a single gene is a specific candidate gene approach, while the genome-wide analysis possesses power in its unbiased approach. Several techniques utilized for methylation analysis include methylation-specific PCR, sequencing after bisulfite treatment, as well as mass spectrometry. However, we will now highlight some specific advances in methylation analysis of pancreatic cancer due to the significant power underlying these techniques.

Although individual genes were discovered to be methylated in advanced pancreatic cancer, as shown in the following two examples, current evidence supports the idea that aberrant methylation occurs very early during the histopathological progression of this neoplasia. Using a specific gene candidate approach, Rosty and colleagues demonstrated that PanIN lesions in patients with chronic pancreatitis show loss of *p16* expression [62], suggesting that this alteration may contribute to the predisposition of patients with chronic pancreatitis to develop pancreatic ductal adenocarcinoma. Interestingly, a study involving large-scale methylation analysis with subsequent confirmation via methylation-specific PCR, Sato and colleagues analyzed DNA samples from 65 PanIN lesions for methylation status of eight genes identified prior by a larger scale microarray approach as aberrantly hypermethy-lated in invasive pancreatic cancer [63]. Of the PanIN lesions examined in this study, methylation at any of these genes was identified in 68%. Even more importantly, the earliest lesions, which are the PanIN-1A, aberrant methylation was present in approximately 70%. Among the genes analyzed, methylation prevalence increased from PanIN-1 to PanIN-2 for *NPTX2*, and from PanIN-2 to PanIN-3 for *SARP2*, *Reprimo*, and *LHX1*. The most striking result from both of these studies is that aberrant CpG island hypermethylation begins in early stages of PanINs and its prevalance progressively increases during neoplastic progression.

Thus, evidence for methylation in tumor suppressor gene silencing continues to reconfirm its clear role in the progression of pancreatic cancer. Initially, some genes, such as *p16*, were believed to be methylated solely in the malignant pancreatic lesions. However, since the current evidence indicates that methylation also occurs earlier at the preneoplastic stage, pharmacological agents, which will be discussed in a subsequent section, that target methyla-tion may be useful not only for treatment but perhaps also for chemoprevention.

4.2   Histone Acetylation and Deacetylation

As mentioned previously, an important mechanism underlying the epigenetic regulation of gene expression is the acetylation and deacetylation of lysine residues within histone tails [64]. For acetylation, this process occurs via HATs, such as CBP, P300, and PCAF, to result in gene expression activation, whereas deacetylation is mediated by two different families of HDACs, resulting in gene silencing. Together, these enzymes provide a fine-tuned mechanism, which upon alteration, has the possibility to cause the activation of oncogenic pathways (◉ *Fig. 6-2*) and the silencing of tumor suppressors (◉ *Fig. 6-1*). However, differently from other epige-netic regulators, such as the polycomb complexes and HP1, which are discussed below, HATs and HDACs mediate short-term responses, a fact that should be taken into consideration when thinking about these molecules as potential therapeutic targets in cancer [64,65].

As discussed, transcriptional regulation is mediated by the DNA binding properties of sequence-specific transcription factors and the recruitment of trans-activators or repressors to ultimately cause epigenetic effects that alter chromatin structure. Studies have demonstrated that HDAC activity is increased in various tumors compared with normal tissue, and this increase in HDAC activity has been associated with transcriptional repression of tumor suppressor genes that cause growth inhibition and apoptosis [66]. In a study performed by Blasco and colleagues, the differential gene expression in a pancreatic cancer cell line upon induction of apoptosis was analyzed using cDNA arrays [67]. Among the genes differentially expressed, one that was studied for further validation was histone deacetylase 1 (HDAC1). Inhibition of HDAC activity led to an increase in the level of apoptosis, in parental cells and doxorubicin-resistant cells. Thus, this study suggested that HDAC1 could be a possible target to develop modulators in cancer chemotherapy that would increase or restore apoptosis. In another study performed by Ouaïssi et al., approximately 80% of pancreatic adenocarcinoma samples examined showed a significant increase of HDAC7 RNA and protein levels [68]. Interestingly, in contrast to the pancreatic adenocarcinoma samples, HDAC7 RNA levels were reduced in samples from chronic pancreatitis, serous cystadenoma, and intraductal papillary mucinous tumor of the pancreas (IMPN), suggesting that increased expression of HDAC7 can discriminate pancreatic adenocarcinoma from other pancreatic types of tumors. In addition, it has been shown that HDAC1 mediates transcriptional repression of the TGFβRII promoter in pancreatic ductal adenocarcinoma cells via recruitment to a specific Sp1 site [69]. Our laboratory has demonstrated that this Sp1 site can be occupied by TGFβ-inducible members of the KLF family, including KLF14 [70] and the pancreatic tumor suppressor, KLF11 [71]. Thus, it is clear that HDACs play an important role in the maintenance of the proper balance of chromatin marks on a given promoter, and if this balance is altered, such as HDAC expression in pancreatic cancer, the expected global effect on promoters is daunting. Potential therapeutic agents for targeting HDACs are discussed in a subsequent section.

4.3 Histone H3-Methyl-K27 and Polycomb

Polycomb proteins silence gene expression by specifically methylating histone H3, on K27 [64,72–74]. At the simple core of this pathway, polycomb group (PcG) proteins act via the stepwise recruitment of PRC2, containing the histone H3 K27 methylase activity, to chromatin. Subsequently, the trimethyl-K27-H3 mark deposited by PRC2 recruits the PRC1 complex, thereby completing the gene silencing complex formation. The enzymatic activity of the PCR2 complex involves the K27-H3 histone methylase, EZH2, but requires a complex with Suz12 and EED to function. The PCR1 complex contains the oncogene BMI1, as well as HPC1-3, HPH1-3, SCMH1, and the methyl-K27-H3-binding proteins, Cbx 2, 4, 6, 7, and 8. However, which of the Cbx proteins is active at different loci under different circumstances is not known.

The role of polycomb proteins in pancreatic cancer is an emerging area of research. For instance, new polycomb proteins have been discovered in pancreatic cancer cells [75]. More importantly, studies have demonstrated that loss of trimethylation at lysine 27 of histone H3, which is achieved by EZH2, is a predictor of poor outcome in pancreatic cancers [76]. In fact, together with tumor size and lymph node status, the level of trimethyl-K27-H3 was found to have a strong and independent prognostic influence in pancreatic cancer. In another recent study, nuclear accumulation of EZH2 was identified as a hallmark of poorly differentiated pancreatic adenocarcinoma and this nuclear overexpression of EZH2 contributes to pancreatic cancer cell proliferation, suggesting EZH2 as a potential therapeutic target for the treatment of pancreatic cancer [77]. Thus, although these initial studies inspire much more to learn about the composition and function of polycomb complexes in pancreatic cancer, the association of this pathway with poor survival of patients affected by this disease makes this area of research one of paramount importance.

Mechanistically, one of the outcomes of aberrant polycomb regulation is the silencing of the *p16* gene, which could occur prior to DNA methylation, via altered direct recruitment of members of this family to the *p16* promoter sequence [78]. Upon recent studies in human cells, EZH2 and DNA methyltransferases (DNMTs) were found to physically and functionally interact, evidenced by the PRC2 subunits, EZH2 and EED, co-immunoprecipitating with all three human DNMTs and the co-dependency of certain target gene silencing requiring both EZH2 and DNMTs [79]. Therefore, the presence of polycomb proteins on the *p16* promoter can recruit DNA methylases which then further inactivate the expression of *p16* via DNA methylation (⊙ Fig. 6-1). However, whether histone H3-K27 methylation and recruitment of DNMT leads to DNA methylation, which then ultimately leads to permanent mutation/deletion of the gene or all mechanisms of *p16* inactivation are independent remains to be discovered.

4.4   Histone H3-Methyl-K9 and Heterochromatin Protein 1

As described above, HP1 binds methylated K9 of histone H3, causing transcriptional repression [64,80]. This occurs through the N-terminal chromodomain of HP1, while the highly related C-terminal chromoshadow domain allows for dimerization of these HP1 molecules and serves as a docking site for various factors involved in a wide array of functions, from transcription to nuclear architecture. To mediate gene silencing via the formation of heterochromatin, HP1 isoforms must interact with two different H3-K9 histone methylases, G9a (EuHMTase-2) and Suv39h1 [64,80]. These methylases work in concert with HP1 in a circular manner to form silenced chromatin. When either of the methylases adds methyl groups to K9, this, in turn, forms an HP1 docking site on chromatin. Since HP1 also recruits the methylases, this cycle repeats, and the HP1-methylase pair can spread the formation of silenced chromatin to adjacent nucleosomes, causing long-term silencing of entire genes (⊙ Fig. 6-1).

Information regarding the function of HP1 proteins in both normal and tumor pancreatic cells is still emerging. However, HP1 proteins have altered expression in many different types of cancers, including breast, brain, ovarian, colon, and papillary thyroid cancers as well as leukemias [81–88]. Thus far, decreased expression of one or more HP1 isoforms has been associated with the cancer phenotype progression or invasiveness. Noteworthy, with the three human isoforms having over 80% similarity between them, the factors that influence these differences remain unknown. Unfortunately, in spite of the identification of numerous HP1 binding partners, distinct signaling cascades that mediate the interaction with these proteins in order to ultimately "switch on" or "switch off" gene silencing remain largely unknown. Although the discovery of the previously mentioned HP1-mediated subcode [35] certainly contributed to this understanding, it remains essential to carefully define these pathways to map useful networks of membrane-to-chromatin signaling cascades for better understanding of the regulation of activation, repression, as well as other cellular processes. The molecular mechanisms that operate as subcodes within the histone code trigger nuclear instructions imparted by K9-H3 methylation, which are subsequently translated as silencing, and thus, potentially participating in the silencing of tumor suppressor genes.

One specific example of how the methyl-K9 H3-HP1 type of chromatin dynamics can impact on the field of pancreatic cancer is the regulation of MUC1 expression. In pancreatic tumors, the MUC1 protein has been detected in >90% of samples examined via immunohistochemistry [89,90], as well as in the pancreatic juice of pancreatic adenocarcinoma patients by comprehensive proteomic analysis [91], and in the majority of pancreatic cancer cell lines [92]. The sialylated form of MUC1 is overexpressed in invading and metastatic pancreatic cancer cells, but absent in normal pancreas, cases of chronic pancreatitis, and pancreatic ductal hyperplasia [93], lending this molecule to be an interesting target for immunotherapeutic strategies [94]. Strikingly, studies have recently demonstrated that a mechanism responsible for changes in the expression of MUC1, which can in turn make proposed vaccines less than optimal, is regulated by DNA methylation and histone H3 lysine 9 (H3-K9) modification, which is bound by HP1, on the *MUC1* promoter [95]. Similar to polycomb, it is known that HP1 can recruit DNA methyl-transferases [96–98], which can lead to the silencing of this important molecule for pancreatic cancer (⊕ *Fig. 6-1*). MUC1-negative cancer cell lines correlated with high DNA methylation and H3 methyl-K9 levels, while MUC1-positive cell lines had low levels of these epigenetic marks, defining MUC1 as a new member of the group of genes controlled epigenetically. Therefore, chromatin dynamic-driven epigenetic changes have the potential to extend research beyond the minimal mutation paradigm to include other pathways that are also important for other key biological behaviors in pancreatic cancer.

4.5 Additional Non-Histone Chromatin Proteins as Epigenetic Targets

Our laboratory has done substantial work on the role of Sin3a–HDAC system in pancreatic cancer suppression [99]. Through this work, we have discovered that pancreatic cells express three different Sin3 proteins that are recruited by tumor suppressors, such as the Myc antagonist, Mad1, and KLF11, and these tumor suppressor proteins require binding to the Sin3a–HDAC complex to perform their function (⊕ *Fig. 6-1*). Thus, this system is both active and important for antagonizing pancreatic carcinogenesis. Although many other gene-silencing complexes exist in mammalian cells and have been shown to participate in several cancer-associated functions in other organs, studies on these proteins in the pancreas remain underrepresented and in most cases, absent. Some of these proteins include corepressors, such as N-CoR, SMART, the Mi-2/NuRD complex, TGIF, Groucho, CtBP, c-Ski, SnoN, among numerous others. Thus, the future anticipates studies of these complexes in pancreas, which may reveal a significant contribution to the initiation, maintenance, or spreading of pancreatic cancer or to cancer-associated function such as stem cell maintenance, DNA repair, metastasis, and therapeutic response.

4.6 MicroRNAs and Pancreatic Cancer

As a result of the discovery and increasing study of microRNAs (miRNAs), significantly more researchers are analyzing the miRNA signatures in pancreatic cancer. MiRNAs are endogenous non-coding RNA molecules ranging from 19–25 nucleotides in length that have been found to play important roles in the regulation of genes in animals and plants via a process involving their pairing to the mRNAs of protein-coding genes to direct their posttranscriptional repression [100]. In fact, miRNAs are currently predicted to control the activity of approximately 30% of all protein-coding genes in mammals [101]. During a recent global profiling study, several miRNAs were identified as aberrantly expressed in pancreatic cancer or desmoplasia [102]. Interestingly, some of these have been previously reported as differentially-expressed miRNAs in other human cancers, including miR-155, miR-21, miR-221, and miR-222, in addition to some novel ones not previously reported, such as miR-376a and miR-301. Typically, the most aberrantly expressed miRNAs were found to be downregulated in the tumor tissue.

In another study, several miRNAs, including miR-205, -18a, -31, -93, -221, and -224, were demonstrated to be over-expressed in primary neoplastic ductal cells and pancreatic cancer cell lines, representing promising biomarkers for pancreatic cancer [103]. Furthermore, 26 miRNAs were identified as the most significantly misregulated in pancreatic cancer and the analysis of only 2 miRNAs, miR-217 and -196a, allowed discrimination between normal and neoplastic tissues, further supporting the potential use of miRNAs for the diagnosis of pancreatic cancer.

Bloomston and colleagues also performed a global analysis to compare miRNA profiles of normal pancreas, chronic pancreatitis and pancreatic adenocarcinoma [104]. In 90% of the tested samples, 21 over-expressed and 4 down-regulated miRNAs were capable of differentiating pancreatic cancer from benign pancreatic tissues via cross validation. Additionally, 15 miRNAs demonstrated increased expression and 8 showed decreased expression, which could distinguish pancreatic cancer from chronic pancreatitis with 93% accuracy. Noteworthy, a subgroup of 6 miRNAs was able to discriminate node-positive disease between long-term survivors and patients who would succumb to the disease within 24 months. Poor survival of pancreatic cancer, with a median survival of 14.3 months versus 26.5 months, could be predicted with 95% confidence through high expression of miR-196a-2.

In summary, we propose a new paradigm for the better understanding and promoting further research in pancreatic cancer, which besides taking into consideration only mutations and deletions, as well as poorly-understood promoter methylation, now includes both chromatin dynamics and nuclear shape (⊙ Fig. 6-5a,b). As we write this review, it is noteworthy to underscore that although more work on chromatin dynamics is needed to understand pancreatic cancer development and phenotype, little has been done about the role of nuclear shape in this disease. Therefore, we are optimistic that this model will further fuel a new era of experiments that expand the scope of our field from a DNA-centric paradigm to a holistic and more inclusive model which takes into consideration protein-mediated epigenetics and the biology of the nucleus as an altered organelle in the progression of pancreatic tumors (⊙ Fig. 6-5a,b).

5   Epigenetics, Chemoprevention and Chemotherapies

The study of epigenetics also impacts the field of therapeutics. For instance, when the Hruban paradigm of pancreatic cancer was at its zenith of fame, many investigators were misled to think that fixing those mutations would be the step to take in order to replace other types of therapies. Unfortunately, this type of gene therapy research has almost died, as investigators have realized that replacement of a gene in a living human is not an easy undertaking and that in many instances it can even as dangerous as to cause death. The underlying problem of this type of gene therapy is that the replacement of a desired gene has to occur in somatic cells which carry deletions or mutations, which by their own nature are irreversible. Therefore, the gene therapy approach fueled a large amount of investigation, but unfortunately left us with nothing more than a proof of principle.

In stark contrast with genetic alterations, epigenetic changes have been proven to be reversible. For instance, methylation can be reversed through the use of 5-Aza-2′-Deoxycytidine or DNA methyltransferase inhibitors. Two types of DNMT inhibitors exist, namely, nucleoside and nonnucleoside (small molecule) inhibitors [105,106]. These types of pharmacologic DNMT inhibitors are currently being tested in phase I–III clinical trials. More importantly, the US Food and Drug Administration (FDA) has recently approved the prototypical DNMT inhibitor, 5-azacytidine (i.e., Vidaza; Pharmion Corp., Boulder, Colorado, USA) for the treatment of myelodysplastic syndrome [107].

Currently, among the most promising epigenetic treatments for cancer are the potential therapeutic agents that target histone deacetylation HDAC inhibitors (HDACIs) [108–112]. Intuitively, the proposed mechanisms of action for HDACs attempt to harness their ability to reactivate transcription of multiple genes found to be silenced in human tumors. However, the pleiotropic antitumor effects with selectivity for cancer cells, along with its potential to be beneficial for other diseases, elicit the possibility that they also act in other biological processes, though currently these other mechanisms remain poorly understood. In addition to being well-tolerated, several HDACIs show promising antitumor activity with more than 50 naturally occurring or synthetic HDACIs currently developed. Hydroxamic acid compounds, trichostatin A (TSA), and suberoylanilide hydroxamic acid (SAHA), are among the best known of these agents. In the same token, however, other equally promising, although less known, drugs can be classified into wider groups such as short-chain fatty acids (e.g., valproic acid), epoxides (e.g., trapoxin), cyclic peptides (e.g., apicidin), benzamides (e.g., CI-994, Nacetyldinaline), and hybrid compounds (e.g., SK-7068). Recent studies have shown that certain HDACIs can induce death of cultured pancreatic cells [113]. Additionally, conventional chemotherapeutic drugs, such as gemcitibine, in combination of some of these agents, can achieve a synergistic inhibition of pancreatic adenocarcinoma cell growth [114]. As a result of these promising studies, new agents that belong to this family of drugs, such as FR235222, have been discovered, which potentially could be used as therapeutic tools for this cancer [115]. Thus, the potential of HDACIs as potential agents to fight pancreatic cancer has been the central focus without yet the knowledge of the cellular, biochemical, and molecular work dealing with the characterization of histone deacetylases in pancreatic cancer. Noteworthy, HDACIs are in advanced phases of clinical trials, and therefore, may soon become part of the therapeutic regimen for oncologists treating this disease.

In addition, although not yet tested in the pancreas, the first generation of inhibitors is actively under development to target one of the HP1-associated methylases, G9a. Using G9a as the target enzyme, a recent study isolated seven compounds from a chemical library comprised of 125,000 preselected molecules in recombinant nonpancreatic cells [116]. One of these inhibitors, BIX-01294 (a diazepin-quinazolin-amine derivative) demonstrated selective inhibition of G9a, as well as the generation of dimethyl-H3-K9 in vitro. In cells incubated with BIX-01294, overall H3 dimethyl-K9 levels were significantly lower and in mouse embryonic stem cells and fibroblasts treated with this inhibitor, reversible reduction of promoter-proximal H3 dimethyl-K9 was shown at several G9a target genes via chromatin immunoprecipitation. The testing of this agent in pancreatic cancer remains to be done, however these results suggest BIX-01294 as a promising HMTase inhibitor that can modulate dimethyl-H3-K9 marks in mammalian chromatin.

Along the same lines, significant efforts are being made to identify small molecules that target and modulate the function of polycomb members. However, similar to the inhibitors of G9a methylases, these efforts are still at very early stages. Recently, 3-deazaneplanocin A (DZNep), a S-adenosylhomocysteine hydrolase inhibitor, demonstrated efficient induction of apoptotic cell death in cancer cells, while not affecting normal cells, by effectively depleting PRC2 levels (decreased EZH2, SUZ12, and EED) and thus, inhibiting histone H3 K27 methylation [117]. This discovery could provide a robust template upon which modification could assist the development of new direct therapies based upon the inhibition of these proteins. Thus far, however, the most common way to manipulate this pathway is indirect, despite how promising drugs that directly target polycomb proteins may be for the treatment of cancer. As an example, members of the polycomb complex, namely Bmi1 and EZH2, have been demonstrated to be downstream targets of Sonic hedgehog (Shh) [118], Notch [119], as well as estrogen and Wnt [120] signaling, providing a strong connection between epigenetic modulators (PcG) and developmental-signaling pathways (Shh, Notch, Wnt). Finally, inhibitors of cancer stem cell populations, such as cyclopamine, a hedgehog signaling inhibitor, 6-bromoindirubin-30-oxime (BIO), an inhibitor of GSK3, exisulind, along with other inhibitors of β-catenin signaling, and the tyrosine-kinase inhibitor, STI571/Gleevec (imatinib mesylate; Novartis Pharmaceuticals Corporation, East Hanover, New Jersey, USA), may provide potential therapies for polycomb-regulated targets [121]. It is our prediction that intense efforts will be made for the development of compounds that target this pathway and impact cancer-associated processes, taking into consideration the pivotal role of polycomb complexes in modulating the phenotype of both stem and cancer cells.

This type of approach leads to the re-expression of genes that have been silenced during tumor initiation and progression. Therefore, the reversibility of epigenetic changes bring hope again that one day we will have a collection of small drugs to reprogram lesions either before they become malignant (chemoprevention) or to reduced their burden at the malignant stage (chemotherapy). Certainly, the combination of several of these drugs will allow us to decrease individual doses, thereby reducing their potential toxic effect, while maintaining or even increasing their beneficial actions, thus providing an increased therapeutic index.

Lastly, we would like to point out that the knowledge on how nuclear shape alters cancer is still at its infancy. Without this knowledge, it is difficult to design drugs that can reverse such alterations. Similarly, as new roles for miRNAs in cancer continue emerging, the future for their use in the treatment of patients remains to be seen. However, taking into consideration the speed of how both of these lines of investigation are beginning to materialize, we are optimistic that the next decade may provide new therapeutic targets and small drugs to use this knowledge for developing novel therapeutic approaches.

6   Concluding Remarks

Increasing studies on chromatin dynamics are unveiling the existence of robust machineries that can mediate epigenetic changes in pancreatic cells. Unfortunately, however, a large portion of our research continues to focus only on somatic genetics, which certainly does not represent the full story for the mechanism of gene inactivation in pancreatic cancer. This important fact has led to one of the most important contributions of this article, the design of a more comprehensive model that can widely include the emerging data in the field of chromatin dynamics and nuclear shape. Guided by this model, we hope, the knowledge gathered on this disease can be more accurately mapped to a progression paradigm that will no doubt impact on many areas of pancreatic cancer research and practice. The era of epigenetics has emerged strongly, with well-justified and energetic beginnings, which will continue into a frontier area for pancreatic cancer research. The reversibility of the epigenetic changes, in itself, makes the journey worthwhile; however further insights into the mechanisms behind pancreatic cancer make the journey indisputable.

Key Research Points

- The field of epigenetics has evolved from the fusion of studies on RNA polymerase II transcription and chromatin. The current theoretical framework in this field has been distilled from different paradigms, which have evolved during almost half a century with some replacement of each other.
- Pancreatic cells are excellent models for developing knowledge of three types of transcriptional events, namely basal transcription, activated transcription (e.g., growth factor-inducible), and tissue-specific gene expression (e.g., secretory granule enzymes).
- Studies on chromatin dynamics, including miRNAs as well as nuclear structure and shape have recently begun in pancreatic cells. The emerging data from these studies are benefiting not only this field, but extending the knowledge of the biology of other cells in the body. In addition, current evidence links these phenomena to development, homeostasis control and diseases. Therefore, this area may constitute one of the most promising in basic and translational pancreatic cell research.

Future Scientific Directions

- Epigenetic mechanisms that are involved in stem cell biology, organ morphogenesis, and pancreatic cancer development constitute a new and very promising frontier. In particular, the discovery of how signaling and chromatin, together, determine cell fate during development and regeneration, as well as how epigenetics contributes to the cancer phenotype, are of paramount importance biologically and pathobiologically.
- Cell-specific mechanisms for regulating gene expression are well advanced only in acinar cells. Therefore, more studies are necessary to understand the biology of ductal cells. In addition, epigenetic mechanisms are known to take part in the processes of pattern formation, such as branching morphogenesis, which is better understood in *Drosophila melanogaster* where chromatin-mediated effects play a significant role in this process. Therefore, studies on chromatin may aid in better understanding the formation of the pancreatic duct and its branching, which is of significant biomedical interest.
- Animal models for studying the genetic mechanisms necessary for the progression of pancreatic cancer have been a major contribution to the field of pancreatic cancer. Unfortunately, models for studying epigenetic effects in pancreatic cells must follow, if we want to understand the role of epigenetics in the pancreas at the whole organism level.

Clinical Implications

- We are optimistic that the new "holo-genetic model for pancreatic cancer" described in this article may help to guide future research in pancreatic cancer in a similarly productive manner to the guidance provided by the previous genetic model for pancreatic cancer.
- It would be important to map key epigenetic changes that occur in the sequence of PanIN lesions along with the known mutations, so as to develop a better understanding of their potential mechanistic interrelationship. Therefore, we may develop new markers with good

predictive value for whether an earlier PanIN has the potential to transform into another more malignant lesion.

- The most relevant characteristic of epigenetics, which makes it extremely attractive for therapeutic purposes, is its reversibility. Due to the alarming difficulty of gene replacement, it is likely that gene therapy for pancreatic cancer will remain, at least for awhile, a hard-to-reach ideal. Therefore, due to its reversibility, epigenetics may provide attainable, useful tools for chemoprevention and chemotherapy.

- In general, nuclear proteins and miRNAs, which are shed by tumors into the bloodstream and are specific to detect pancreatic cancer, may be another prolific area of investigation with a great impact on diagnostics.

Acknowledgments

Work in the author's laboratory (R.U.) is supported by funding from the National Institutes of Health DK 52913 and Mayo Clinic Pancreatic SPORE (P50 CA102701).

References

1. Hruban RH, Goggins M, Parsons J, Kern SE: Progression model for pancreatic cancer. Clin Cancer Res 2000;6:2969–2972.

2. Kuhn TS: The Structure of Scientific Revolutions. Chicago: University of Chicago Press, 1996.

3. Jacob F, Monod J: Genetic regulatory mechanisms in the synthesis of proteins. J Mol Biol 1961;3:318–356.

4. McClure WR: Mechanism and control of transcription initiation in prokaryotes. Ann Rev Biochem 1985;54:171–204.

5. Ebright RH: RNA polymerase: structural similarities between bacterial rna polymerase and eukaryotic RNA polymerase II. J Mol Biol 2000;304:687–698.

6. Roeder RG, Rutter WJ: Multiple forms of DNA-dependent RNA polymerase in eukaryotic organisms. Nature 1969;224:234–237.

7. Chambon P: Eukaryotic nuclear RNA polymerases. Ann Rev Biochem 1975;44:613–638.

8. Roeder RG: Eukaryotic nuclear RNA polymerases. In RNA Polymerase. Losick R, Chamberlin (eds.). M Cold Spring Harbor, NY: Cold Spring Harbor Laboratory, 1976, pp. 285–329.

9. Weil PA, Luse DS, Segall J, Roeder RG: Selective and accurate initiation of transcription at the ad2 major late promotor in a soluble system dependent on purified rna polymerase II and DNA. Cell 1979;18:469–484.

10. Hori R, Carey M: The role of activators in assembly of RNA polymerase II transcription complexes. Curr Opin Genet Dev 1994;4:236–244.

11. Koleske AJ, Young RA: The RNA polymerase II holoenzyme and its implications for gene regulation. Trends Biochem Sci 1995;20:113–116.

12. Orphanides G, Lagrange T, Reinberg D: The general transcription factors of RNA polymerase II. Genes Dev 1996;10:2657–2683.

13. Li Y, Flanagan PM, Tschochner H, Kornberg RD: RNA polymerase II initiation factor interactions and transcription start site selection. Science 1994;263:805–807.

14. Pinto I, Ware DE, Hampsey M: The yeast SUA7 gene encodes a homolog of human transcription factor TFIIB and is required for normal start site selection in vivo. Cell 1992;68:977–988.

15. Myers LC, Kornberg RD: Mediator of transcriptional regulation. Ann Rev Biochem 2000;69:729–749.

16. Istrail S, Davidson EH: Logic functions of the genomic cis-regulatory code. In Proceedings of the National Academy of Sciences of the United States of America, vol. 102, 2005, pp. 4954–4959.

17. Cook T, Gebelein B, Mesa K, Mladek A, Urrutia R: Molecular cloning and characterization of tieg2 reveals a new subfamily of transforming growth factor-beta -inducible sp1-like zinc finger-encoding genes involved in the regulation of cell growth. J Biol Chem 1998;273:25929–25936.

18. Rose SD, Swift GH, Peyton MJ, Hammer RE, MacDonald RJ: The role of PTF1-P48 in pancreatic Acinar gene expression. J Biol Chem 2001;276:44018–44026.

19. Jan J: Gene regulatory factors in pancreatic development. Dev Dyn 2004;229:176–200.

20. Jones N: Structure and function of transcription factors. Semin Cancer Biol 1990;1:5–17.

21. Mitchell PJ, Tjian R: Transcriptional regulation in mammalian cells by sequence-specific DNA binding proteins. Science 1989;245:371–378.

22. Kadonaga JT: Regulation of RNA polymerase II transcription by sequence-specific DNA binding factors. Cell 2004;116:247–257.

23. Glozak MA, Seto E: Histone deacetylases and cancer. Oncogene 2007;26:5420–5432.

24. Lee MJ, Kim YS, Kummar S, Giaccone G, Trepel JB: Histone deacetylase inhibitors in cancer therapy. Curr Opin Oncol 2008;20:639–649.

25. Pazin MJ, Kadonaga JT: What's up and down with histone deacetylation and transcription? Cell 1997;89:325–328.

26. Sterner DE, Berger SL: Acetylation of histones and transcription-related factors. Microbiol Mol Biol Rev 2000;64:435–459.

27. Kornberg RD: Chromatin structure: a repeating unit of histones and DNA. Science 1974;184:868–871.

28. Kornberg RD, Lorch Y: Twenty-five years of the nucleosome, fundamental particle of the eukaryote chromosome. Cell 1999;98:285–294.

29. Li B, Carey M, Workman JL: The role of chromatin during transcription. Cell 2007;128:707–719.

30. Strahl BD, Allis CD: The language of covalent histone modifications. Nature 2000;403:41–45.

31. Rizzo PJ: Basic chromosomal proteins in lower eukaryotes: relevance to the evolution and function of histones. J Mol Evol 1976;8:79–94.

32. Luger K, Richmond TJ: The histone tails of the nucleosome. Curr Opin Gen Dev 1998;8:140–146.

33. Kustatscher G, Ladurner AG: Modular paths to 'decoding' and 'wiping' histone lysine methylation. Curr Opin Chem Biol 2007;11:628–635.

34. Schuettengruber B, Chourrout D, Vervoort M, Leblanc B, Cavalli G: Genome regulation by polycomb and trithorax proteins. Cell 2007;128:735–745.

35. Lomberk G, Bensi D, Fernandez-Zapico ME, Urrutia R: Evidence for the existence of an HP1-mediated subcode within the histone code. Nat Cell Biol 2006;8:407–415.

36. Zhang R, Chen W, Adams PD: Molecular dissection of formation of senescence-associated heterochromatin foci. Mol Cell Biol 2007;27:2343–2358.

37. Lusser A, Kadonaga JT: Chromatin remodeling by ATP-dependent molecular machines. Bioessays 2003;25:1192–1200.

38. Kennison JA: The polycomb and trithorax group proteins of drosophila: trans-regulators of homeotic gene function. Ann Rev Gen 1995;29:289–303.

39. Elfring LK, Deuring R, McCallum CM, Peterson CL, Tamkun JW: Identification and characterization of Drosophila relatives of the yeast transcriptional activator SNF2/SWI. Mol Cell Biol 1994;14:2225–2234.

40. Chiba H, Muramatsu M, Nomoto A, Kato H: Two human homologues of Saccharomyces cerevisiae SWI2/SNF2 and Drosophila brahma are transcriptional coactivators cooperating with the estrogen receptor and the retinoic acid receptor. Nucleic Acids Res 1994;22:1815–1820.

41. Decristofaro MF: Characterization of SWI/SNF protein expression in human breast cancer cell lines and other malignancies. J Cell Physiol 2001;186:136–145.

42. Wong AK: BRG1, a component of the SWI-SNF complex, is mutated in multiple human tumor cell lines. Cancer Res 2000;60:6171–6177.

43. Azuara V, Perry P, Sauer S, Spivakov M, Jorgensen HF, John RM, Gouti M, Casanova M, Warnes G, Merkenschlager M, Fisher AG: Chromatin signatures of pluripotent cell lines. Nat Cell Biol 2006;8:532–538.

44. Bernstein BE, Mikkelsen TS, Xie X, Kamal M, Huebert DJ, Cuff J, Fry B, Meissner A, Wernig M, Plath K, Jaenisch R, Wagschal A, Feil R, Schreiber SL, Lander ES: A bivalent chromatin structure marks key developmental genes in embryonic stem cells. Cell 2006;125:315–326.

45. Park Y-J, Luger K: Histone chaperones in nucleosome eviction and histone exchange. Curr Opin Struct Biol 2008;18:282–289.

46. Loyola A, Almouzni G: Marking histone H3 variants: how, when and why? Trends Biochem Sci 2007;32:425–433.

47. Hake SB, Allis CD: Histone H3 variants and their potential role in indexing mammalian genomes: The 'H3 barcode hypothesis'. Proc Natl Acad Sci USA 2006;103:6428–6435.

48. Heard E, Bickmore W: The ins and outs of gene regulation and chromosome territory organisation. Curr Opin Cell Biol 2007;19:311–316.

49. Merideth MA, Gordon LB, Clauss S, Sachdev V, Smith ACM, Perry MB, Brewer CC, Zalewski C, Kim HJ, Solomon B, Brooks BP, Gerber LH, Turner ML, Domingo DL, Hart TC, Graf J, Reynolds JC, Gropman A, Yanovski JA, Gerhard-Herman M, Collins MDFS, Nabel EG, Cannon RO III, Gahl WA, Introne WJ: Phenotype and Course of Hutchinson-Gilford progeria syndrome. N Engl J Med 2008;358:592–604.

50. Gruenbaum Y, Wilson KL, Harel A, Goldberg M, Cohen M: Review: nuclear lamins – structural proteins with fundamental functions. J Struct Biol 2000;129:313–323.

51. Hruban RH, Adsay NV, Albores-Saavedra J, Compton C, Garrett ES, Goodman SN, Kern SE, Klimstra DS, Kloppel G, Longnecker DS, Luttges J, Offerhaus GJ: Pancreatic intraepithelial neoplasia: a new nomenclature and classification system for pancreatic duct lesions. Am J Surg Pathol 2001;25:579–586.

52. Fearon ER, Vogelstein B: A genetic model for colorectal tumorigenesis. Cell 1990;61:759–767.

53. Sato N, Maitra A, Fukushima N, van Heek NT, Matsubayashi H, Iacobuzio-Donahue CA, Rosty C, Goggins M: Frequent hypomethylation of multiple genes overexpressed in pancreatic ductal adenocarcinoma. Cancer Res 2003;63:4158–4166.

54. Ueki T, Toyota M, Skinner H, Walter KM, Yeo CJ, Issa J-PJ, Hruban RH, Goggins M: Identification and characterization of differentially methylated cpg islands in pancreatic carcinoma. Cancer Res 2001;61:8540–8546.

55. Ueki T, Toyota M, Sohn T, Yeo CJ, Issa J-PJ, Hruban RH, Goggins M: Hypermethylation of multiple genes in pancreatic adenocarcinoma. Cancer Res 2000;60:1835–1839.

56. Frese KK, Tuveson DA: Maximizing mouse cancer models. Nat Rev Cancer 2007;7:654–658.

57. Esteller M: Epigenetics in cancer. N Engl J Med 2008;358:1148–1159.

58. Singh M, Maitra A: Precursor lesions of pancreatic cancer: molecular pathology and clinical implications. Pancreatology 2007;7:9–19.

59. Fernandez-Zapico ME, Gonzalez-Paz NC, Weiss E, Savoy DN, Molina JR, Fonseca R, Smyrk TC, Chari ST, Urrutia R, Billadeau DD: Ectopic expression of VAV1 reveals an unexpected role in pancreatic cancer tumorigenesis. Cancer Cell 2005;7:39–49.

60. Fernandez-Zapico M, Molina J, Ahlquist D, Urrutia R: Functional characterization of KLF11, a novel TGFb-regulated tumor suppressor for pancreatic cancer. Pancreatology 2003;3:429–441.

61. Gebhard C, Schwarzfischer L, Pham T-H, Schilling E, Klug M, Andreesen R, Rehli M: Genome-wide profiling of CpG methylation identifies novel targets of Aberrant Hypermethylation in Myeloid Leukemia. Cancer Res 2006;66:6118–6128.

62. Rosty C, Geradts J, Sato N, Wilentz RE, Roberts H, Sohn T, Cameron JL, Yeo CJ, Hruban RH, Goggins M: p16 Inactivation in pancreatic intraepithelial neoplasias (PanINs) arising in patients with chronic pancreatitis. Am J Surg Pathol 2003;27:1495–1501.

63. Sato N, Fukushima N, Maitra A, Matsubayashi H, Yeo CJ, Cameron JL, Hruban RH, Goggins M: Discovery of novel targets for aberrant methylation in pancreatic carcinoma using high-throughput microarrays. Cancer Res 2003;63:3735–3742.

64. Allis C, Jenuwein T, Reinberg D, Capparros ML, (eds.): Epigenetics. Cold Spring Harbor, NY: Cold Spring Harbor Laboratory Press, 2007.

65. Privalsky M (ed.): Transcriptional corepressors: mediators of eukaryotic gene expression. New York: Springer, 2001.

66. Cress W, Seto E: Histone deacetylases, transcriptional control, and cancer. J Cell Physiol 2000;184:1–16.

67. Blasco F, Peñuelas S, Cascalló M, Hernández JL, Alemany C, Masa M, Calbó J, Soler M, Nicolás M, Pérez-Torras S, Gómez A, Tarrasón G, Noé V, Mazo A, Ciudad CJ, Piulats J: Expression profiles of a human pancreatic cancer cell line upon induction of apoptosis search for modulators in cancer therapy. Oncology 2004;67:277–290.

68. Ouaïssi M, Sielezneff I, Silvestre R, Sastre B, Bernard J-P, Lafontaine J, Payan M, Dahan L, Pirrò N, Seitz J, Mas E, Lombardo D, Ouaissi A: High histone deacetylase 7 (hdac7) expression is significantly associated with adenocarcinomas of the pancreas. Ann Surg Oncol 2008;15:2318–2328.

69. Zhao S, Venkatasubbarao K, Li S, Freeman JW: Requirement of a specific Sp1 site for histone deacetylase-mediated repression of transforming growth factor {beta} type II receptor expression in human pancreatic cancer cells. Cancer Res 2003;63:2624–2630.

70. Truty MJ, Lomberk G, Fernandez-Zapico ME, Urrutia R: Silencing of the TGFbeta receptor II by kruppel-like factor 14 underscores the importance of a negative feedback mechanism in TGF beta signaling. J Biol Chem 2008;284:6291–6300.

71. Lomberk G, Zhang J, Truty M, Urrutia R: A new molecular model for regulating the tgf[beta] receptor ii promoter in pancreatic cells. Pancreas 2008;36:222–223.

72. Breiling A, Sessa L, Orlando V, Kwang WJ: Biology of polycomb and trithorax group proteins. Int Rev Cytology 2007;258:83–136.

73. Ringrose L: Polycomb comes of age: genome-wide profiling of target sites. Curr Opin Cell Biol 2007;19:290–297.

74. Cao R, Wang L, Wang H, Xia L, Erdjument-Bromage H, Tempst P, Jones RS, Zhang Y: Role of histone H3 lysine 27 methylation in polycomb-group silencing. Science 2002;298:1039–1043.

75. Grzenda AL, Lomberk G, Urrutia R: Different EZH2 isoforms are expressed in pancreatic cells: evidence for a polycomb-mediated subcode within the context of the histone code. Pancreas 2007;35:404.

76. Wei Y, Xia W, Zhang Z, Liu J, Wang H, Adsay N, Albarracin C, Yu D, Abbruzzese J, Mills G, Bast R, Hortobagyi G, Hung M: Loss of trimethylation at lysine 27 of histone H3 is a predictor of poor outcome in breast, ovarian, and pancreatic cancers. Mol Carcinog 2008;47:701–706.

77. Ougolkov AV, Bilim VN, Billadeau DD: Regulation of pancreatic tumor cell proliferation and chemoresistance by the histone methyltransferase enhancer

of zeste homologue 2. Clin Cancer Res 2008;14:6790–6796.

78. Kotake Y, Cao R, Viatour P, Sage J, Zhang Y, Xiong Y: pRB family proteins are required for H3K27 trimethylation and polycomb repression complexes binding to and silencing p16INK4a tumor suppressor gene. Genes Dev 2007;21:49–54.

79. Vire E, Brenner C, Deplus R, Blanchon L, Fraga M, Didelot C, Morey L, Van Eynde A, Bernard D, Vanderwinden J-M, Bollen M, Esteller M, Di Croce L, de Launoit Y, Fuks F: The polycomb group protein EZH2 directly controls DNA methylation. Nature 2006;439:871–874.

80. Lomberk G, Wallrath L, Urrutia R: The heterochromatin protein 1 family. Genome Biol 2006;7:228.

81. Espada J, Ballestar E, Fraga MF, Villar-Garea A, Juarranz A, Stockert JC, Robertson KD, Fuks F, Esteller M: Human DNA methyltransferase 1 is required for maintenance of the histone H3 modification pattern. J Biol Chem 2004;279:37175–37184.

82. Pomeroy SL, Tamayo P, Gaasenbeek M, Sturla LM, Angelo M, McLaughlin ME, Kim JYH, Goumnerova LC, Black PM, Lau C, Allen JC, Zagzag D, Olson JM, Curran T, Wetmore C, Biegel JA, Poggio T, Mukherjee S, Rifkin R, Califano A, Stolovitzky G, Louis DN, Mesirov JP, Lander ES, Golub TR: Prediction of central nervous system embryonal tumour outcome based on gene expression. Nature 2002;415:436–442.

83. Kirschmann DA, Lininger RA, Gardner LMG, Seftor EA, Odero VA, Ainsztein AM, Earnshaw WC, Wallrath LL, Hendrix MJC: Down-regulation of HP1Hs {{alpha}} expression is associated with the metastatic phenotype in breast cancer. Cancer Res 2000;60: 3359–3363.

84. Ruginis T, Taglia L, Matusiak D, Lee B-S, Benya RV: Consequence of gastrin-releasing peptide receptor activation in a human colon cancer cell line: a proteomic approach. J Proteome Res 2006;5:1460–1468.

85. Popova EY, Claxton DF, Lukasova E, Bird PI, Grigoryev SA: Epigenetic heterochromatin markers distinguish terminally differentiated leukocytes from incompletely differentiated leukemia cells in human blood. Exp Hematol 2006;34:453–462.

86. Lukasova E, Koristek Z, Falk M, Kozubek S, Grigoryev S, Kozubek M, Ondrej V, Kroupova I: Methylation of histones in myeloid leukemias as a potential marker of granulocyte abnormalities. J Leukoc Biol 2005;77:100–111.

87. Maloney A, Clarke PA, Naaby-Hansen S, Stein R, Koopman J-O, Akpan A, Yang A, Zvelebil M, Cramer R, Stimson L, Aherne W, Banerji U, Judson I, Sharp S, Powers M, deBilly E, Salmons J, Walton M, Burlingame A, Waterfield M, Workman P: Gene and protein expression profiling of human ovarian cancer cells treated with the heat shock protein 90

inhibitor 17-allylamino-17-demethoxygeldanamycin. Cancer Res 2007;67:3239–3253.

88. Wasenius V-M, Hemmer S, Kettunen E, Knuutila S, Franssila K, Joensuu H: Hepatocyte growth factor receptor, matrix metalloproteinase-11, tissue inhibitor of metalloproteinase-1, and fibronectin are upregulated in papillary thyroid carcinoma: A cDNA and tissue microarray study. Clin Cancer Res 2003;9:68–75.

89. Plate JM, Shott S, Harris JE: Immunoregulation in pancreatic cancer patients. Cancer Immunol Immunother 1999;48:270–279.

90. Qu CF, Li Y, Song YJ, Rizvi SMA, Raja C, Zhang D, Samra J, Smith R, Perkins AC, Apostolidis C, Allen BJ: MUC1 expression in primary and metastatic pancreatic cancer cells for in vitro treatment by 213Bi-C595 radioimmunoconjugate. Br J Cancer 2004;91:2086–2093.

91. Gronborg M, Bunkenborg J, Kristiansen TZ, Jensen ON, Yeo CJ, Hruban RH, Maitra A, Goggins MG, Pandey A: Comprehensive proteomic analysis of human pancreatic juice. J Proteome Res 2004;3:1042–1055.

92. Hollingsworth MA, Strawhecker JM, Caffrey TC, Mack DR: Expression of MUC1, MUC2, MUC3 and MUC4 mucin mRNAs in human pancreatic and intestinal tumor cell lines. Int J Cancer 1994;57:198–203.

93. Masaki Y, Oka M, Ogura Y, Ueno T, Nishihara K, Tangoku A, Takahashi M, Yamamoto M, Irimura T: Sialylated MUC1 mucin expression in normal pancreas, benign pancreatic lesions, and pancreatic ductal adenocarcinoma. Hepatogastroenterology 1999;46:2240–2245.

94. Mukherjee P, Basu GD, Tinder TL, Subramani DB, Bradley JM, Arefayene M, Skaar T, De Petris G: Progression of pancreatic adenocarcinoma is significantly impeded with a combination of vaccine and COX-2 inhibition. J Immunol 2009;182:216–224.

95. Yamada N, Nishida Y, Tsutsumida H, Hamada T, Goto M, Higashi M, Nomoto M, Yonezawa S: MUC1 expression is regulated by DNA methylation and histone H3 lysine 9 modification in cancer cells. Cancer Res 2008;68:2708–2716.

96. Gazzar ME, Yoza BK, Chen X, Hu J, Hawkins GA, McCall CE: G9a and HP1 couple histone and DNA methylation to TNF{alpha} transcription silencing during endotoxin tolerance. J Biol Chem 2008;283:32198–32208.

97. Smallwood A, Estève P-O, Pradhan S, Carey M: Functional cooperation between HP1 and DNMT1 mediates gene silencing. Genes Dev 2007;21:1169–1178.

98. Moss TJ, Wallrath LL: Connections between epigenetic gene silencing and human disease. Mut Res 2007;618:163–174.

99. Lomberk G, Urrutia R: The family feud: turning off Sp1 by Sp1-like KLF proteins. Biochem J 2005;392:1–11.

100. Bartel DP: MicroRNAs: target recognition and regulatory functions. Cell 2009;136:215–233.

101. Filipowicz W, Bhattacharyya SN, Sonenberg N: Mechanisms of post-transcriptional regulation by microRNAs: are the answers in sight? Nat Rev Genet 2008;9:102–114.

102. Lee E, Gusev Y, Jiang J, Nuovo G, Lerner M, Frankel W, Morgan D, Postier R, Brackett D, Schmittgen T: Expression profiling identifies microRNA signature in pancreatic cancer. Int J Cancer 2007;120:1046–1054.

103. Szafranska AE, Davison TS, John J, Cannon T, Sipos B, Maghnouj A, Labourier E, Hahn SA: MicroRNA expression alterations are linked to tumorigenesis and non-neoplastic processes in pancreatic ductal adenocarcinoma. Oncogene 2007;26:4442–4452.

104. Bloomston M, Frankel WL, Petrocca F, Volinia S, Alder H, Hagan JP, Liu C-G, Bhatt D, Taccioli C, Croce CM: MicroRNA expression patterns to differentiate pancreatic adenocarcinoma from normal pancreas and chronic pancreatitis. JAMA 2007;297:1901–1908.

105. Griffiths EA, Gore SD: DNA methyltransferase and histone deacetylase inhibitors in the treatment of myelodysplastic syndromes. Semin Hematol 2008;45:23–30.

106. Mund C, Brueckner B, Lyko F: Reactivation of epigenetically silenced genes by DNA methyltransferase inhibitors: basic concepts and clinical applications. Epigenetics 2006;1:7–13.

107. Ghoshal K, Bai S: DNA methyltransferases as targets for cancer therapy. Drugs Today (Barc) 2007;43:395–422.

108. Berger SL: Histone modifications in transcriptional regulation. Curr Opin Gen Dev 2002;12:142–148.

109. Hildmann C, Riester D, Schwienhorst A: Histone deacetylases – an important class of cellular regulators with a variety of functions. Appl Microbiol Biotechnol 2007;75:487–497.

110. Bruserud O, Stapnes C, Ersvaer E, Gjertsen BT, Ryningen A: Histone deacetylase inhibitors in cancer treatment: a review of the clinical toxicity and the modulation of gene expression in cancer cell. Curr Pharm Biotechnol 2007;8:388–400.

111. Glaser KB, Staver MJ, Waring JF, Stender J, Ulrich RG, Davidsen SK: Gene expression profiling of multiple histone deacetylase (hdac) inhibitors: defining a common gene set produced by hdac inhibition in t24 and mda carcinoma cell lines. Mol Cancer Ther 2003;2:151–163.

112. Pan LN, Lu J, Huang B: HDAC inhibitors: a potential new category of anti-tumor agents. Cell Mol Immunol 2007;4:337–343.

113. Ouaissi M, Cabral S, Tavares J, da Silva AC, Daude FM, Mas E, Bernard J, Sastre B, Lombardo D, Ouaissi A: Histone deacetylase (HDAC) encoding gene expression in pancreatic cancer cell lines and cell sensitivity to HDAC inhibitors. Cancer Biol Ther 2008;7:523–531.

114. Donadelli M, Costanzo C, Beghelli S, Scupoli MT, Dandrea M, Bonora A, Piacentini P, Budillon A, Caraglia M, Scarpa A, Palmieri M: Synergistic inhibition of pancreatic adenocarcinoma cell growth by trichostatin A and gemcitabine. Biochim Biophys Acta 2007;1773:1095–1106.

115. Singh EK, Ravula S, Pan C-M, Pan P-S, Vasko RC, Lapera SA, Weerasinghe SVW, Pflum MKH, McAlpine SR: Synthesis and biological evaluation of histone deacetylase inhibitors that are based on FR235222: a cyclic tetrapeptide scaffold. Bioorg Med Chem Lett 2008;18:2549–2554.

116. Kubicek S, O'Sullivan RJ, August EM, Hickey ER, Zhang Q, Teodoro MiguelL, Rea S, Mechtler K, Kowalski JA, Homon CA, Kelly TA, Jenuwein T: Reversal of H3K9me2 by a small-molecule inhibitor for the G9a histone methyltransferase. Mol Cell 2007;25:473–481.

117. Tan J, Yang X, Zhuang L, Jiang X, Chen W, Lee P, Karuturi R, Tan P, Liu E, Yu Q: Pharmacologic disruption of Polycomb-repressive complex 2-mediated gene repression selectively induces apoptosis in cancer cells. Genes Dev 2007;21:1050–1063.

118. Liu S, Dontu G, Mantle ID, Patel S, Ahn N-S, Jackson KW, Suri P, Wicha MS: Hedgehog signaling and Bmi-1 regulate self-renewal of normal and malignant human mammary stem cells. Cancer Res 2006;66:6063–6071.

119. Ferres-Marco D, Gutierrez-Garcia I, Vallejo DM, Bolivar J, Gutierrez-Avino FJ,Dominguez M: Epigenetic silencers and notch collaborate to promote malignant tumours by Rb silencing. Nature 2006;439:430–436.

120. Shi B, Liang J, Yang X, Wang Y, Zhao Y, Wu H, Sun L, Zhang Y, Chen Y, Li R, Zhang Y, Hong M, Shang Y: Integration of Estrogen and Wnt signaling circuits by the polycomb group protein EZH2 in breast cancer cells. Mol Cell Biol 2007;27:5105–5119.

121. Lomberk G, Mathison AJ, Grzenda A, Urrutia R: The sunset of somatic genetics and the dawn of epigenetics: a new frontier in pancreatic cancer research. Curr Opin Gastroenterol 2008;24:597–602.

7 Molecular Pathology of Pancreatic Endocrine Tumors

Gabriele Capurso · Stefano Festa · Matteo Piciucchi · Roberto Valente ·
Gianfranco Delle Fave

1	**Introduction**	**172**
2	**Inherited Pancreatic Endocrine Tumors**	**172**
2.1	Multiple Endocrine Neoplasia Type I (MEN-I)	173
2.2	Von Hippel-Lindau Disease (VHL)	175
2.3	Von Recklinghausen's Disease or Neurofibromatosis Type 1 (NF-1)	176
2.4	Tuberous Sclerosis Complex (TSC)	176
3	**Genetic Instability in Sporadic Pancreatic Endocrine Tumors**	**177**
3.1	Genome Wide Studies in Sporadic PETs	177
3.2	Prognostic Relevance	178
3.3	Final Considerations	185
4	**Genetic Alterations of Oncogenes and Tumor Suppressor Genes, and Expression of Growth Factors and Their Receptors**	**185**
4.1	Oncogenes	185
4.2	Tumor Suppressor Genes	186
4.3	Growth Factors and Their Receptors (Receptor Tyrosine Kinases)	187
4.4	The (PI3K)/Protein Kinase B/AKT/mTOR Pathway	188
5	**Microarray Studies**	**188**

J. P. Neoptolemos, R. Urrutia, J. L. Abbruzzese, M. W. Büchler (eds.), *Pancreatic Cancer*,
DOI 10.1007/978-0-387-77498-5_7, © Springer Science+Business Media, LLC 2010

Abstract: The molecular biology of Pancreatic Endocrine Tumors (PETs) carcinogenesis is poorly understood and is generally different from that of exocrine pancreatic neoplasms. PETs represent a rare group of neoplasms with heterogenous clinico-pathological features. They are generally sporadic but can also arise within very rare hereditary syndromes, such as Multiple Endocrine Neoplasia type I (MEN-I), von Hippel-Lindau disease (VHL), Neurofibromatosis type 1 (NF1) and Tuberous Sclerosis Complex (TSC). In these syndromes although a specific genotype/phenotype association with PETs has been described, exact mechanisms leading to tumors development are still debated. Some clinical and biological features of PETs associated with hereditary syndromes are similar in sporadic cases. Allelic imbalances (i.e., gain or loss of DNA sequences) have been explored by means of different techniques in different subtypes of sporadic PETs. Overall, main genomic changes involve gain of 17q, 7q, 20q, 9p, 7p, 9q and loss of 11q, 6q, 11p, 3p, 1p, 10q, 1q, that identify the region of putative candidate Oncogenes or Tumor Suppressor Genes (TSGs) respectively. For some of them a possible relevant prognostic role has been described. "Classical" oncogenes involved in exocrine neoplasms (k-Ras, c-Jun, c-Fos) are of limited relevance in PETs; on the contrary overexpression of Src-like kinases and cyclin DI oncogene (CCNDI) have been described. As for TSGs, p53, DPC4/Smad and Rb are not implicated in PETs tumorigenesis, while for p16^{INK4a}, TIMP-3, RASSF1A and hMLH1 more data are available, with data suggesting a role for methylation as silencing mechanism. Different molecular pathways, and the role of tyrosine kinase receptors have also been investigated in PETs (EGF, c-KIT) with interesting findings especially for VEGF and m-TOR, which encourage clinical development. Microarray analysis of expression profiles has recently been employed to investigate PETs, with a number of different strategies, even if these studies suffer from a number of limitations, mainly related with the poor repeatability and the poor concordance between different studies. However, apart from methodological limits, molecular biology studies are needed to better know this group of neoplasms, aiming at identifying novel markers and targets for therapy also highlighting relations with clinical outcome.

1   Introduction

The molecular biology of pancreatic endocrine tumors (PETs) is poorly understood, and overall oncogenes and tumor suppressor genes (TSGs) more frequently involved in exocrine neoplasms, and particularly in pancreatic cancer, are not relevant. PETs are generally sporadic, as their carcinogenesis is based on somatic mutations [1]. However oncosuppressors responsible for PETs can be involved by germline mutations [2]. This process may be spontaneous, without a previous family history, or more frequently inherited, as a part of well described syndromes. The present paragraph will review in depth existing evidences for the molecular pathogenesis of PETs, with a summary of data from studies of familial syndromes, genetic instability, as well as those examining the role of oncogenes, TSGs, and an insight into more recent microarray studies. A brief overview of the expression of growth factors and their receptors, as possible therapeutic targets will also be presented.

2   Inherited Pancreatic Endocrine Tumors

The following hereditary syndromes have been associated with PETs: Multiple Endocrine Neoplasia type I (MEN-I), von Hippel-Lindau disease (VHL), von Recklinghausen's disease

(Neurofibromatosis 1 or NF1) and tuberous sclerosis complex (TSC) [2,3]. The latter three are phakomatoses, rare neurocutaneous syndromes characterized by uncontrolled growth of ectodermal tissues from which endocrine tumors arise.

PETs occurring in these hereditary forms are primarily NF tumors or insulinomas, with different incidence, and don't differ from those detected as sporadic [3] (◑ *Table 7-1*).

2.1   Multiple Endocrine Neoplasia Type I (MEN-I)

The most frequent inherited syndrome causing PETs is MEN-I, a rare autosomal dominant disorder (incidence 1:20,000–40,000) clinically defined by the presence of two or more of the following neoplasms: gastroenteropancreatic neuroendocrine tumors, parathyroid gland adenomas, pituitary adenomas, with other neoplastic lesions (i.e., thyroid adenomas, multiple lipomas, bronchial or thymic carcinoids) occurring occasionally [4]. About 10% of PETs occur as a part of MEN-I.

MEN-I syndrome is the result of an inactivating mutation of the Menin gene, an onco-suppressor located on chromosome 11q13 [4].

This gene, consisting in 10 exons, encodes for a 68 KDa nuclear protein of 610 aminoacids, named Menin. Menin functions include binding and inactivation of many nuclear transcription factors (especially JunD but also SMAD3, mSin3a and trithorax family histone methyltransferase complex), upregulation of cell cycle inhibitors expression ($p27^{KIPI}$ and $p18^{Ink4c}$), influence on DNA repair process, all of which result in inhibition of cellular proliferation [5–8].

The spectrum of possible mutations is greatly various. In the last decade, more than 1,300 germline variants (the half of which with pathological effect) have been identified, and 10–12% of them occur without a positive family history. Some 23% are nonsense mutations, 9% splicing-site mutations, 41% frameshift deletions or insertions, 6% in-frame deletions or insertions, 20% missense mutations and 1% whole or partial gene deletions [4].

Even though any genotype/phenotype association with PETs have been described, the exact mechanism leading to the neoplasia is still debated and the role of Menin on cell cycle negative control and DNA stability is somehow controversial.

Gene mapping in MEN-I patients have shown loss of heterozygosis (LOH) in half of the cases, confirming the oncosuppressor function of Menin and the tumorigenesis Knudson's two-hit hypotesis. LOH of the Menin gene and other somatic mutations on wild-type allele behave as a second hit after a first hit germline, inherited mutation. LOH on Menin allele, as described in sporadic PETs, can also involve other terminal region of 11q, suggesting implications of additional genes in neoplastic development and progression [9,10].

PET patients with pathological Menin gene mutation don't differ from sporadic forms in terms of clinical features (age of onset, hormone and/or neoplasia related symptoms), but only 10% develop metastases, especially in the case of tumors larger than 3–5 cm (irrespectively to its histotype) [1,3].

In up to 80–90% of cases, endocrine pancreatic involvement consists in endocrine islet cell hyperplasia, without somatic LOH on Menin, and microadenomatosis (multiple indolent tumors <5 mm). These latter kind of lesions are characterized by trabecular structure and distinctive stroma, and, in spite of being asymptomatic and without metastases, in about 50% of the cases LOH of Menin gene is detectable [11–13].

In a variable percentage of MEN-I patients (20–60%), microadenomatosis is associated to one or multiple pancreatic "macro-tumors," which are larger than 5 mm but less than 3–5 cm.

Table 7-1

Described syndromes associated with inherited Pancreatic Endocrine Tumors, including clinical features and molecular defects

Syndrome	Gene	Gene function main molecular consequences	Major clinicals features	Patients with PET (%)	PETs Sub-type	Metastatic PET (%)
Multiple Endocrine Neoplasia type I	Menin (11q13)	Oncosuppressor Deregulation of JunD, SMAD3 p27^{KIPI} p18^{Ink4c}	2 or more between: (a) GEP-NET (b) Parathyroid adenomas (c) Pituitary adenoma	20–60%	80% NF 15% insulinomas 3% glucagonomas 1% gastrinomas and vipomas	<10%
von Hippel-Lindau disease	VHL (3p25–26)	Oncosuppressor Overexpression of HIF and VEGF	1 or 2 between: (a) Retinal or cerebellar hemangioblastomas (b) Renal cell carcinoma (c) Pheochromocytoma	5–17%	80–100% NF	<10%
Von Recklinghausen's disease	NF1 (17q11.2)	Oncosuppressor Deregulation of Ras pathway mTOR	(a) Café-au-lait skin spots (b) Neurofibromas of any type and localization	Rare	insulinomas and somatostinomas	–
Tuberous Sclerosis Complex	TSC 1 (9q34) TSC2 (16p13.3)	Oncosuppressor Deregulation of mTOR pathway	(a) Skin alterations (b) Renal angiomyiolipomas (c) Multiple and diffuse hamartomas, (d) Neurological alteration	Very rare	mainly NF	–

These neoplasms are NF PETs in about 80% of cases, 15–20% insulinomas, 3% glucagonomas and rarely VIPomas or gastrinomas [1–3].

These tumors are often clinically silent and just 10% of cases lead to metastases, but they are often associated with other symptomatic more aggressive gastrointestinal neuroendocrine tumors, especially duodenal gastrinomas and somatostatinomas [3,14,15].

In fact, although 20–60% of MEN-I patients have Zollinger-Ellison Syndrome (20–40% associated with gastric carcinoid type II), gastrinomas arise far more frequently in the duodenum as single or multiple small tumors (not unfrequently undetectable) rather than as PETs [3,16,17].

2.2   Von Hippel-Lindau Disease (VHL)

PETs also occur in a significant percentage of individuals affected by Von Hippel-Lindau disease (VHL). It is a very rare (1:30,000–1:50,000) autosomal dominant phakomatosis with a variable phenotype characterized by the presence of at least one of these major manifestations: single retinal or cerebellar hemangioblastoma (HB), renal cell carcinoma (RCC) or pheochromocytoma and other more rare multiorgan lesions such as pancreatic cysts or PETs, renal cysts, endo-lymphatic sac tumors, epididymal papillary cystoadenomas, paragangliomas, polycythaemia and other rare tumors [18].

The gene responsible for this disease is VHL gene, an oncosuppressor of 3 exons located on 3p25–26 that by alternative splicing can encode for 2 proteins (pVHL), respectively of 213 and 160 aminoacids [18].

The two VHL products accomplish to similar activities in the cytoplasm; in particular they make an ubiquitin complex with cullin-2, Rbx1 and elongins B named VBC, that in case of normoxia binds and inactivates hypoxia-inducible factor (HIF) [14].

Inactiving mutation of VHL gene causes an over-expression of HIF, especially of vascular endothelial growth factor which lines to tumorigenesis [15].

Until now, more than 300 germline mutations have been found, 60% of which are truncating or missense mutations while 40% are deletions. These mutations are associated with different phenotypical expressions: only patients with missense mutations develop pheochromocytoma (VHL type 2) associated (2b) or not (2a) to RCC, whereas patients affected by other mutations will develop the remaining related disease manifestations (VHL type 1) [15,18].

Disease penetrance grows by age (90% at 65 years), as germline mutations have to be followed by another somatic event in the wild-type allele.

As far as PETs, LOH in the VHL allele or, less frequently, methylation or neomutation are frequent findings [15,19]. Indeed, pancreatic involvement by multiple indolent cysts is typical of VHL (50–75%), but PETs are also frequent (5–17%) [20].

Strict associations between specific mutations and phenotypic expression of PET have been reported, but tumor cells show a typical LOH in chromosome 3p which is not limited to the VHL gene, but also involves other adjacent genes (such as Not papillary Renal Carcinoma-1) possibly implicated with tumorigenesis and progression [20].

Biological and clinical features of VHL-associated PETs are similar to sporadic forms: they are typically non-functioning and asymptomatic, generally expressing somatostatin receptors and in 30–50% of cases are multifocal in the pancreas [3,20,21].

However, PETs arising in VHL disease are usually small (<2–3 cm) and without liver metastases in about 80–90%, with a consequent better prognosis compared to sporadic ones. This difference is most likely due to earlier detection (at a mean of 35 vs. 58years) thanks to investigations due to other malignancies' symptoms [2,3,21].

2.3   Von Recklinghausen's Disease or Neurofibromatosis Type 1 (NF-1)

Occurence of gastroenteropancreatic NETs in NF-1 is less frequent than in MEN-I and VHL disease, and in particular the rate of pNET is very low [22].

NF-1 is an autosomal dominant phakomatoses (1:3,000–1:4,000) with high penetrance, defined by multiple café-au-lait skin spots, neurofibromas of any type and localization (10% malignant), and characterized by predisposition to various other malignancies development (3–30%) such as gliomas, myeloid leukemia and pheochromocytoma [23].

NF-1 arises from mutation of the NF-1 gene, a large oncosuppressor of 50 exons located on the 17q11.2 chromosome. Its product, called neurofibromin, is a GTPase acting as a negative regulator of mitonegic Ras pathway, especially of the mTOR signaling [24].

Many NF-1 gene mutations have been identified, of which up to 50% arising "de novo"; however all the significant genotype/phenotype association have been demonstrated [23].

Rate of associated PETs is undeterminable [3,25–27]. They arise from germline NF1 mutation and deletion; insulinomas and somatostatinomas are similar to sporadic forms as in the tumor cells there is low expression of NF-1. The risk of PETs development is often increased in this disease, probably because of mTOR pathway upregulation; however more cases are needed to study the genotype/phenotype relation.

2.4   Tuberous Sclerosis Complex (TSC)

The rarest inherited disease associated with gastroenteropancreatic NETs is TSC. This phakomatosis (1:10,000) is a hereditary multiorgan disease transmitted by autosomal dominant inheritance. TSC has a 100% penetrance and a highly variable expression; clinical manifestations are typical skin alterations, renal angiomyiolipomas, multiple and diffuse hamartomas, mental retardation, neurological alterations. PETs are occasionally associated [28].

Two genes are responsible for this disease: TSC1 (9q34) and TSC2 (16p13.3), that respectively encode for hamartin and tuberin. These two proteins make a dimer that multimodulates cell growth, interacting with phosphoinositide 3-kinase pathway-mTOR activity and insulin receptor signaling.

Several genotype/phenotype associations have been described and related to many different mutations (50% occurring de novo); somatic tumor cells show a secondary mutation or a large deletion, up to a complete LOH on the two alleles often involving large chromosomal region.

The described cases of PETs associated with this disease are mainly non functional, and few cases of insulinoma and somatostinoma, with a behavior similar to sporadic forms [5]. In particular, one case of PET described in literature, a non functional tumor identified in a child, exhibited a TSC2 gene LOH; this confirms its oncosuppressor role, such as in other TSC related neoplasm [29,30].

3 Genetic Instability in Sporadic Pancreatic Endocrine Tumors

Genetic instability represents the necessary condition for tumor development, through the clonal expansion of cancerous cells that have acquired a selective advantage. Among the different events (point mutations, chromosomal rearrangements, gene amplifications, microsatellite sequences alterations and epigenetic changes) occurring during the multistep process of somatic cells transformation, alterations in DNA copy number are the commonest events.

Allelic imbalances, that result from incorrect mitotic division and consequent abnormal chromosomal separation, may be revealed by a variety of methods including karyotyping, comparative genomic hybridization (CGH), microsatellite analysis or, more recently, single nucleotide polymorphisms (SNPs) allelotyping.

Conventional CGH is a molecular cytogenetic genome-wide technique for the analysis of copy number changes in DNA of tumor cells. Through this method, differentially labeled test DNA and normal reference DNA are hybridized simultaneously to normal chromosome spreads and the hybridization is detected with two different fluorochromes. Regions of gain or loss of DNA sequences, such as deletions, duplications, or amplifications, are seen as changes in the ratio of the intensities of the two fluorochromes along the target chromosomes. In brief, the regions frequently identified with decreased copy number are likely to harbor tumor suppressor genes (TSGs), whereas regions with increased copy number may contain dominant oncogenes.

Furthermore, allelotyping, that is the systematic analysis of the allelic losses in single chromosomes thus exploring Loss of Heterozigosity (LOH), is another strategy to determine the most probable locus of a TSG: it can be based on polymorphic microsatellite DNA or on SNPs, assaying the frequency and extent of lost regions on all chromosomal arms. SNPs allelotyping is more sensitive than microsatellite analysis and is also useful to detect DNA copy number.

3.1 Genome Wide Studies in Sporadic PETs

During the last decade several studies with different approaches have addressed to look for specific genomic defects in sporadic PETs [31–42]. As shown in ⊚ *Table 7-2*, CGH has been largely used to explore genetic aberrations. Most of the available data, refer to small, heterogeneous tumor series, and essentially regard well differentiated endocrine tumors/carcinomas. In addition, several different tumor classifications have been used by investigators in their studies during time making difficult a possible analysis of PETs subtypes. In this paragraph, data are presented separating Non-Functioning (NF) from Functioning PETs (F-PETs), and among these, further taking account of benign insulinomas, malignant insulinoma and gastrinomas to possibly identify specific genomic patterns.

In the nine published studies [31,32,35–38,40–42] of CGH/genomic wide-allelotyping, 101 Non-functioning pancreatic endocrine tumors have been studied (⊚ *Tables 7-3* and ⊚ *7-4*). The most frequent findings were losses of 11q (38,6%), 6q (37,6%), 11p (33,7%), 3p (26,7%), 1p (27,7%), 10q (25,7%) while the most frequent gains involved 17q (41%), 7q (35,9%), 12q (34,6%), 14q (34,6%), 4p (32%), 20q (30,7%).

As for the 31 gastrinomas investigated in seven studies, loss of 3p (19%) and gain of 9p (29%) represented the most common chromosomal aberrations [31,32,34–37,40].

In benign insulinomas (116 overall tumor samples in seven studies) most frequent losses were found on 11q (19%), Xq (18%), 1p (17%) while most frequent gains regarded 9q (41%), 7p

◘ Table 7-2

Main genome-wide studies of pancreatic endocrine tumors series

Method of study	N° PETs	PETs Subtypes	Reference
CGH	12	10 NF, 2 F	[31]
CGH	44	9 NF, 35 F	[32]
CGH	25	25 F	[33]
CGH	8	8 F	[34]
CGH	38	10 F, 28 F	[35]
CGH	45	14 NF, 31 F	[36]
CGH	9	3 NF,6 F	[37]
CGH	20	20 NF	[38]
CGH	62	62 F	[39]
Genome-wide Allelotyping	28	7 NF, 21 F	[40]
Genome-wide Allelotyping	32	32 NF	[41]
SNPs Allelotyping	15	13 NF, 2 F	[42]

CGH Comparative Genomic Hybridization, *SNPs* Single Nucleotide Polymorphisms
NF Non-Functioning, *F* Functioning

(20%), 7q e 5q (both 19%). Malignant insulinomas (30 tumor samples), defined by the presence of loco-regional advanced or metastatic disease, harbored more genomic alterations than benign counterpart [32, 33, 35–37, 39, 40]. In particular, most frequent losses were found on 6q (70%), Y (43%), 2q (33%), 3q (30%), 6p (30%), 10q, 11p, 11q and Xq (all 23%), while main gains involved 17q (57%), 17p (53%), 12q (53%). 14q (50%), 7q (47%), 20q and 9q (43%).

The identification of gains and losses on chromosomal regions helps to highlight loci potentially containing putative oncogenes and TSGs. ◉ *Tables 7-5* and ◉ *7-6* summarize main losses and gains, together with candidate TSGs and Oncogenes, the associated disorders for which a pathogenetic link has been already described and, finally, the prognostic significance of the particular genetic change.

On the whole, NF-PETs seem to present more genomic aberrations, then malignant insulinomas, with benign insulinomas and gastrinomas presenting the lowest amount of changes. This tendency is consistent with the finding by Speel and colleagues that PETs larger than 2 cm exhibited significantly more aberrations than lesions smaller than 2 cm given that NF-PETs are often larger than 2 cm at diagnosis [32].

All these observations strongly suggest that PETs subtypes may evolve along different molecular pathways: deciphering their specific signatures would help to implement PETs classification system, with obvious implications for a better understanding of this complex nosological entity.

3.2 Prognostic Relevance

Accumulated evidences showing that PETs from patients with advanced disease harbored significantly higher numbers of genetic aberrations than tumors from patients with localized disease suggest that malignant progression of PETs progression is driven by the progressive

□ Table 7-3

Frequence of chromosomal Losses (%) in pancreatic endocrine tumor subtypes

	n°	1p	1q	2p	2q	3p	3q	4p	4q	6p	6q	8p	8q	10p	10q	11p	11q	13q	15q	16p	16q	21p	21q	22p	22q	Xp	Xq	Y
	%																											
NF	101	26	24	21	23	27	25	2,9	9,9	24	37,6	19	20	24,8	25,7	34	38,6	12	19	13,9	16,8	12	19,8	11	20	5	5	5
B Ins	116	17	15	0	5	0	3	8	9	0	3	4	7	0	0	15	19	5	0	1	1	0	0	0	4	13	18	7
M Ins	30	27	20	10	33	20	30	13	10	30	70	3,3	10	6,6	23	23	23	17	3,3	6,6	10	0	13,3	0	10	13	23	43
Gas	31	3	10	0	0	19	10	0	0	0	0	0	3	0	3	3	13	3	3	3	3	0	0	0	0	0	0	0

NF non-functioning, *B* or *M Ins* benign or malignant Insulinoma, *Gas* Gastrinoma

☐ Table 7-4

Frequence of chromosomal Gains (%) in pancreatic endocrine tumor subtypes

	n°	% 2q	3q	4p	4q	5p	5q	6q	7p	7q	8p	8q	9p	9q	11q	12p	12q	13p	13q	14p	14q	15q	16p	16q	17p	17q	18p	18q	19p	19q	20p	20q	Xp	Xq	Y
NF	101	0	32	26	28	28	3	28	36	6	10	19	27	3	24	34	12	22	17	34	3	0	0	29	41	22	28	15	17	26	31	1,2	5	0	0
B Ins	107	0	1	2	1	13	19	5	20	19	1	1	6	41	3	3	4	0	1	3	8	11	0	0	3	5	3	2	10	10	5	12	5	1	2
M Ins	30	0	3	10	20	23	37	0	37	47	0	0	13	43	6	17	53	0	13	3	50	23	17	6	53	57	3	3	8	8	20	43	27	20	10
Gas	17	12	0	0	0	6	6	0	6	12	12	6	29	12	6	12	12	0	0	12	12	12	6	0	12	12	0	0	0	0	0	6	0	0	0

NF non-functioning, *B* or *M Ins* benign or malignant Insulinoma, *Gas* Gastrinoma

Table 7-5

Main losses in sporadic endocrine tumor of the pancreas

	% Loss						Prognostic relevance
Location	NF	B Ins	M Ins	Gas	Putative TSGs	Associated disorder	
11q	38,6	19	23	13	MEN-1	MEN-1 syndrome	
					PLCB3		
					SDHD	Intestinal Carcinoids, raganglioma, Pheochromocitoma	
					TSG11	Non small cell lung cancer	
					HHPT	Hereditary hyperparathyroid-jaw tumor syndrome	
					BRCC2	Breast Cancer	
					ZW10		
6q	37,6	3	70	0	AIM 1	Melanoma	Associated with liver metastasis [32,43]
					CCNC		
					PTPRK		
					LOT-1	Transient neonatal Diabetes mellitus	
					CX43	Oculodentodigital dysplasia, Hypoplastic left heart syndrome, Atrioventricular septal defect	
11p	33,7	15	23	3	WT1	Wilms tumor type 1, Denys-Drash syndrome, WAGR syndrome, Frasier syndrome, isolated diffuse Mesangial sclerosis	
3p	26,7	0	20	19,4	VHL	Von Hippel Lindau syndrome, Renal cell carcinoma	Associated with liver metastasis [32,44]
					hMLH1	Colorectal cancer, HNPCC	
					RAR-β		
					B-Catenin	Digestive endocrine tumors	
					RASSF1A	Lung cancer	
1p	27,7	17	26,6	3	p73	None	Associated with liver metastasis [45]
					p18/INK4		
					RUNX3		

◻ Table 7-5 **(continued)**

	% Loss						
Location	NF	B Ins	M Ins	Gas	Putative TSGs	Associated disorder	Prognostic relevance
10q	25,7	0	23	3	MGMT	Endometrial k, follicular thyroid k, meningioma	
					PTEN		
1q	24	15	20	10	HHPT2	Hereditary hyperparathyroid-jaw tumor syndrome	Associated with metastases and aggressive growth [46–49]
						Several cancer cell lines	
					MDA7/IL-24		

TSGs Tumor suppressor genes, *NF* non-functioning, *B or M Ins* benign or malignant Insulinoma, *Gas* Gastrinoma

accumulation of multiple genetic changes [32,36,39,50], as is also known to occur in other types of human carcinomas [46].

Another interesting issue is the possible relationship between molecular genetic defects (number and type of genomic changes) and tumor progression or malignancy in PETs.

Several LOH studies [45,47–49], using microsatellite markers, demonstrated that LOH at *chromosome 1*, and in particular of its long arm, is a common event among PETs subtypes (12/27 gastrinomas, 35/40 insulinomas, 10/29 different PET subtypes) and was significantly associated with the presence of hepatic metastases regardless of tumor type. Moreover, Chen and colleagues (2003) found in their series of gastrinomas that allelic loss at 1q31–32 as well as 1q21–23, significantly correlated with tumor aggressive growth and postoperative development of liver metastases [48]. Likewise, Yang and colleagues (2005) reported high frequency of LOH at 1q 21.3–23.2 and 1q31.3, significantly associated with malignancy of insulinomas suggesting in these two regions the presence of putative tumor suppressor genes important for aggressive growth of this tumors [49]. Although these two studies narrowed region of potential candidate genes, to date actual genes involved remain undefined (◉ *Table 7-5*).

As for *chromosome 3*, LOH was demonstrated to be a common event (frequency ranged from 33 to 83%) in PETs regardless of tumor subtypes and its frequency was significantly higher in malignant than in benign neoplasms, on the whole finding a correlation with clinically metastatic disease in several studies [44,51–53]. As common deleted region were different (3p14.2–21; 3p25.3-p23; 3q27-qter, all outside of the VHL locus) in the same studies, different putative tumor suppressor genes other than VHL on chromosome 3 may play a role in the latest steps of tumorigenesis of sporadic PETs.

Only one LOH study reported by Barghorn and colleagues (2001) described allelic loss at *chromosome 6* in 62.2% of cases in a heterogeneous cohort of PETs, the majority of which were insulinomas and NF PETs (with common deleted regions mapped at 6q22.1 and 6q23-q24), and it was significantly more common in tumors larger than 2 cm in diameter than below this threshold as well as in malignant than in benign tumors [43]. Previously, Speel and colleagues (1999), had reported an overall loss at 6q in 39% of PETs (with a common deleted region at 6q21–22) and in all of six insulinomas, again indicating a locus harboring a potential TSG involved in tumor development [32]. To further support this hypothesis, combined data from

⬛ Table 7-6

Main gains in sporadic endocrine tumor of the pancreas

Location	NF	B Ins	M Ins	Gas	Putative oncogenes	Associated disorder	Prognostic relevance
17q	41	5	57	12	Neu/ERB2	Breast cancer	Associated with malignant behavior in tumors <2 cm [35]
7q	35,9	19	47	12	HGF C-MET	Gastric cancer, Hepatocellular carcinoma	
20q	30,7	12	43	6	STK15/BTAK	Breast cancer, Ovarian and Digestive carcinomas	
9p	19,2	6	13	29	JAK2	Acute myelogenous leukemia, Myeloproliferative disorder	
					Oncogene ovc	Ovarian carcinoma	
					RAGA		
7p	28	20	37	6	EGFR/ERBB1	Bladder, Breast, Epidermoid carcinoma, Glioblastoma	
9q	26,9	41	43	12	VAV2	Breast cancer, Head & Neck squamous carcinoma	
					CDK9		
					cABL	Chronic Myeloid leukemia, Insulinoma rat cell lines	
					NOTCH-1	SCLC, T-cell acute lymphoblastic leukemia	
					LMX1B		

NF non-functioning, B or M Ins benign or malignant Insulinoma, Gas Gastrinoma

above mentioned genome wide studies show that 6q loss occurs in 70% of malignant insulinomas and in 37,6% of NF-PETs, as shown in ○ *Table 7-2.*

Chromosome 17. In a study of 20 mixed functioning and non-functioning pancreatic endocrine tumors Beghelli and colleagues (1998) found allelic losses on 17p13 in ~24% of the chromosomal loci analyzed with a higher frequency of allelic losses significantly associated with a high proliferation index and malignancy of the tumors [54]. Moreover the absence of p53 gene mutations in nearly all these tumors suggests the existence of another tumor suppressor gene in the same chromosomal area. However, according to genomic wide studies, loss of 17p is a rare event (<10%) and probably does not play a central role in the majority of endocrine tumors development. On the opposite, gain of 17q is a frequent event, especially in malignant insulinomas (>50%). The oncogene Her-2/Neu, frequently overexpressed in breast and esophageal cancer where identify more aggressive phenotype, is located on chromosome 17q21. Her-2/Neu gene amplifications were identified in 40% of 11 gastrinomas [55], the majority of which were locally advanced or metastatic, while in another study by Goebel (2002) the same gene was amplified in 14% of 43 gastrinomas and this time higher mRNA levels in tumor cells were correlated with liver metastases [56].

LOH on *chromosome 22q* was detected in 14 of 15 insulinomas (93%) by Wild and colleagues (2001). The shortest region of overlap implicated a deletion at 22q12.1-q12.2 where hSNF5/INI1 gene is located but no alteration was identified by single strand conformational polymorphism analysis, direct DNA sequencing, or RNA expression analysis [57]. The same group (Wild 2002), described LOH on chromosome 22q in 22 of 23 PETs (including Non-Functioning tumors, gastrinomas and Vipomas) showing a LOH rate of 85% at locus 22q12.1, with LOH strongly correlated with the presence or the development of distant metastases [58]. Moreover, LOH on 22q12.3 was significantly associated with distant metastases, an area where two putative candidate gene are located, that is, synapsin3 (SYN3) and tissue inhibitor of metalloproteinase-3 (TIMP-3). Also in this instance, Genome-wide studies tend to underestimate genetic changes: in particular, loss of 22q was found in ~20% of NF-PETs and in less than 10% of other PET subtypes.

Sex Chromosomes. According to combined data from genome-wide studies reported, Xq loss mainly occurs in insulinomas (~20% of cases) and one CGH-study also noted an association between Xq loss metastatic disease, raising the hypothesis that X chromosome changes plays a role in defining the more aggressive nature of endocrine lesions [32].

Aberration of X chromosome have been described mainly in gastric carcinoids and PETs, and in malignant compared with benign endocrine tumors. Pizzi et al. (2002) comparing PETs and endocrine tumors of the ileum and appendix, noted that LOH on chromosome X was evident in 60% of malignant gastric and pancreatic tumors but in only 4.5% of benign tumors. Similarly, none of the benign midgut tumors exhibited X chromosome LOH, whereas 15% of malignant tumors contained this aberration [59]. On the whole, an association between X chromosome LOH and malignancy clearly has been found. In LOH analysis, allelic losses on X chromosome were revealed in 50% of Type III gastric carcinoids, but not in Type I tumors. Again, tumors that exhibited LOH were associated with metastasis [60]. Also in a series of sixteen female patients with gastrinomas reported by Chen et al. 56% presented X chromosome LOH, was significantly associated with aggressive postoperative tumor growth and with increased primary tumor size [61]. Missiaglia and colleagues (2002), in their microsatellite and FISH analysis extended to chromosome Y, described that PETs from females had loss of chromosome X in 40% of cases whereas PETs from males showed loss of chromosome Y in 36% of case but never had loss of the X chromosome [62]. A significant association of sex chromosome loss with metastases, local invasion Ki-67 > 5% was also described. Sex chromosome loss was found to be an independent variable associated with a shorter survival period and an increased risk of death of approximately four fold.

Recently, in a comparative LOH analysis on X chromosome by Azzoni et al. (2006) higher rate of allelic loss were found in poorly differentiated endocrine carcinomas than in well differentiated endocrine carcinomas with two chromosomal regions, Xq25 and Xq26 showing LOH with a relatively high frequency [63]. Candidate tumor suppressor genes mapping at Xq25 are ODZ1, encoding Tenascin, a glycoprotein of the extracellular matrix involved in morphogenetic movements, tissue repair and tumor spreading and SH2D1A, whose mutation was described in X-linked lymphoproliferative disease and in non-Hodgkin Lymphomas [64]; while potential tumor suppressor genes for Xq26 are MEF, a transcription factor capable to suppress the transcription of the genes encoding for the matrix metalloproteinases, MMP-2 and MMP-9, and interleukin-8 as demonstrated in cell lines of human non small cell lung carcinoma [65]; and GPC-3, a heparan sulfate proteoglycan linked to the cell membrane, involved in the progression of several types of malignant tumors, including mesotheliomas, ovarian, and lung carcinomas [66].

3.3   Final Considerations

The limited resolution of the conventional CGH method, its low reliability (emerged from the observation that some regions – 1p32- pter, 16p, 19, and 22 – showed gains in negative control experiments) and its feature to be a laborious method remain the principal limits. On the other hand, LOH analysis, depending on number and type of microsatellite markers used, often offer contradictory results. For this reason, caution is needed in interpreting their results, awaiting further studies to confirm available data.

Array-CGH technology can improve the resolution of conventional CGH on metaphase chromosomes from 5 to 10 Mb to ≤1 Mb on arrayed DNA. In a series of 27 insulinomas Jonkers and colleagues (2006) performed a genome-wide array-based CGH analysis detecting in >50% of cases loss of chromosomes 11q and 22q and gains of chromosome 9q with the first two alterations only partially identified before by conventional CGH (11q loss and 22q loss were found in ~20% and ~10% of benign and malignant insulinomas, respectively) [67].

The chromosomal regions of interest included 11q24.1 (56%), 22q13.1 (67%), 22q13.31 (56%), and 9q32 (63%). Comparing their alteration frequencies in tumors with benign, uncertain, and malignant behavior according the most recent WHO classification, the authors suggest that gain of 9q32 and loss of 22q13.1 are early genetic events in insulinomas, occurring independently of the other alterations. Finally, in this study further evidence was found for the accumulation of chromosomal alterations which run parallel with increasing malignant potential.

4   Genetic Alterations of Oncogenes and Tumor Suppressor Genes, and Expression of Growth Factors and Their Receptors

4.1   Oncogenes

The role of k-Ras has been investigated by a number of authors, with findings suggesting limited relevance if any, thus differentiating pancreatic endocrine neoplasms from the exocrine counterpart. *K-ras* mutations were found in a risible proportion of cases [50,54,55,68–72], without any significant clinical association. Not surprisingly, the BRAF gene, one of the human isoforms of RAF, which is activated by ras, does not seem to have a role in tumorigenesis of PETs [73]. However, a possible role for the ras signaling pathway in PETs may depend on inactivation of the TSG RASSF1 (see below).

Similarly, there is limited evidence for a role of either *c-Jun* or *c-Fos* [71,74]. On the other hand *c-Myc* is over-expressed in most studies either at the RNA or protein level [50,68,75,76]. The proto-oncogene *Bcl-2*, which acts as an antiapoptotic factor, has been detected in up to 45% of examined PET samples [75], however, there are no data examining the overall balance of the pro/antiapoptotic machinery in PETs.

Src is a family of proto-oncogenic non-receptor tyrosine kinase including nine members. *Src-like kinases* act downstream of growth factor receptors and integrins transmitting messages that are crucial for several aspects of cell growth and metabolism, as for example cell cycle regulation, cell adhesion and motility. Overexpression of *Lck*, a member of *Src* family, has been recently demonstrated in metastatic progressive PETs in a microarray study [74]. The expression and activity of *Src* have been also described in PET cell lines and tissues, and inhibition of *Src* activity has been shown to interfere with adhesion, spreading and migration of cells [77].

As far as cell cycle, although animals with constitutive activation of CDK4 develop PETs [78], mutations have not been found in insulinomas [79]. A more relevant role for the cyclin DI oncogene (CCNDI) is suggested by findings of its overexpression, and relation with disease stage [80,81].

The Wnt signaling pathway is relevant for a number of neoplasms, and β-catenin activation is frequently detected in such cancers. However, no mutations of the β-catenin gene have been detected in a study including 108 PETs, and nuclear accumulation of the β-catenin protein seems a rare and late event [82].

In a further study, 52% of PETs showed abnormal β-catenin staining, which was related with loss of normal E-cadherin staining and more aggressive behavior [83].

4.2   Tumor Suppressor Genes

The role of MEN-I and VHL mutations, either in genetic or sporadic forms has been summarized in the previous paragraphs.

The role of the *p53* TSG has been investigated in a wide number of studies. A rationale for such investigations comes from studies of mice with *p53* mutations, and PET development. However, most studies found no mutations of *p53* and/or no over-expression of the mutated protein in human PETs [50,54,55,68,69,72,73,84–87]. These data suggest that findings of LOH at 17q13 may be related with other unknown TSGs.

Similarly, although LOH at 18q is fairly frequent in PETs, the DPC4/Smad gene has not been found to be mutated in the majority of published papers [50,68,88], and the Retinoblastoma TSG (Rb) is also not implicated [89].

On the other hand, the p16^{INK4a} TSG, which encodes for an inhibitor of CDK4, seems relevant for at least a portion of PETs. Particularly, inactivation of *p16*, either by mutations or by methylation is common in gastrinomas, but less frequent in NF PETs and insulinomas [55,68,90,91].

The expression of the putative tumor suppressor gene tissue inhibitor of metalloproteinase-3 (TIMP-3) has been found to be altered by either promoter hypermethylation or homozygous deletion. The predominant TIMP-3 in some 44% of examined PETs, with as significant relation with the metastatic process [92].

The Ras-association domain family 1A (RASSF1A) is a TSG, interacting with ras. It is inactivated in a variety of solid tumors, usually by epigenetic silencing of the promoter or by loss at 3p21.3. RASSF1A induces cell cycle arrest through inhibition of cyclin D1 accumulation. RASSF1A hypermethylation was detected in 10 out of 12 (83%) endocrine tumors [93], and in a further publication RASSF1A silencing by methylation and 3p21.3 deletion was associated with tumors from foregut only, and with malignant behavior [94].

Loss of expression of the p27 protein has instead been paradoxically related with well-differentiated PETs, with most indolent features, while its expression was associated with metastatic disease [95].

The aberrant promoter methylation of the mismatch repair gene, hMLH1, is associated with microsatellite instability (MSI). Hypermethylation of the hMLH1 promoter has been found in 23% of PETs. Some 50% of hMLH1-methylated PETs were found to be microsatellite unstable, and MSI was restricted to PETs with hMLH1 hypermethylation. Tumors with MSI-positive had a better survival compared with MSI-negative [96].

4.3   Growth Factors and Their Receptors (Receptor Tyrosine Kinases)

The expression of growth factors, and their receptors, generally tyrosine kinases, is an interesting issue, and offers the opportunity for targeted therapy. Angiogenesis has been studied in depth in transgenic mouse model (Rip1-Tag2) in which mice develop PETs [97]. Although PETs are highly vascular, some studies have suggested that they express VEGF, which correlates with a more aggressive tumor [98], while others detailed how PETs present a wide range of microvascular density (MVD) according to the malignant potential, with malignant tumors showing lower MVD and VEGF expression than benign ones [99].

The surface of PET cells presents several other growth factor receptors, including receptor tyrosine kinases such as the epidermal growth factor receptor (EGFR), the stem cell factor (SCF) receptor c-KIT and the platelet derived growth factor receptors (PDGFR) [100–103].

The EGFR (ErbB-1) is a member of a receptor tyrosine kinase family also including HER2/Neu (ErbB-2), HER-3 (ErbB-3) and HER-4 (ErbB-4), whose activation after interaction with their ligands leads to a number of downstream cascade molecular events involving cell proliferation and transformation. Although, the expression of the EGFR and its phosphorylation seems more relevant in carcinoids than PETs, phosphorylated-EGFR expression was found to be an unfavorable prognostic marker only in PETs [104]. As far as other members of the Erb family, the expression and amplification of HER-2/Neu were explored in patients with gastrinoma, with relevant data presented above [55,56].

c-KIT (CD117) is a type III tyrosine kinase receptor which, once activated by its ligand, stem cell factor (SCF), induces dimerization and autophosphorylation of the receptor at specific tyrosine regions, which acts as docking sites for other intracitosolic proteins important for intracellular signal transduction. Abnormal expression of c-KIT and/or SCF has been described in a variety of solid tumors, and activating mutations of c-KIT are a typical feature of gastrointestinal stromal tumors (GIST). Several studies have investigated the expression of c-KIT, together with other receptor tyrosine kinases in gastroenteropancreatic endocrine tumors, by immunohistochemistry [102,105]. The results are inconsistent and, as hypothesized for other cancer types, inter-studies disagreement may be explained by different antibodies employed or different immunohistochemistry protocols.

4.4 The (PI3K)/Protein Kinase B/AKT/mTOR Pathway

The mammalian target of rapamycin (mTOR) is a serine-threonine kinase involved in the mechanisms of regulation of cell growth and death trough apoptosis. It plays a critical role in transducing a number of different proliferative signals mediated through the phosphatidylinositol 3 kinase (PI$_3$K)/protein kinase B (AKT) pathway, principally by activating downstream protein kinases that are required for both ribosomal biosynthesis and translation of key mRNAs of proteins required for cell cycle progression.

The signaling pathways upstream of mTOR include several tumor suppressors, such as PTEN, NF1, the kinase LKB1, and oncogenes such as Ras and Raf. mTOR also mediates signaling downstream of a number of growth factors such as IGF-1 and VEGF (⊚ *Fig. 7-1*). These signaling pathways converge on the tuberous sclerosis complex (TSC1/TSC2), which inhibits the mTOR activator Rheb, a small GTPase. In turn, activation of the mTOR pathway enhances the activity of HIF1α and of VEGF itself [106,107].

Tumors exhibiting constitutively activated PI$_3$K/AKT/mTOR signaling due to mutations or loss of the above mentioned tumor suppressor genes (PTEN or TSC), or overexpression of upstream genes, are potentially susceptible to mTOR inhibitors, therefore making the investigation of this pathway particularly interesting for PETs.

5 Microarray Studies

Global expression profiling has been often employed in the past decade to better understand molecular changes occurring in a number of tumors. This approach has been proved useful to identify novel markers and targets for therapy, or to highlight relations with clinical outcome.

However, microarray studies suffer a number of limitations, mainly related with the poor repeatability, and the poor concordance between different studies [108].

Microarray analysis of expression profiles has recently been employed to investigate PETs, with a number of different strategies. These studies are summarized in ⊚ *Table 7-7* [74,109–114].

Overall the studies differ significantly in terms of different samples and design, different platforms and statistical/bioinformatics methods. Two of the studies [74,113] employed a wider platform. Two main different design subgroups can be identified: (1) comparison of PET samples versus purified pancreatic islets [74,109,110]. (2) comparison of metastatic versus non-metastatic PETs [112–114]. One other study compared expression profiles of pooled biopsy material of PETs with that obtained from other pancreatic pathologies and normal pancreata [111], making its comparison with the other studies of poor sense. However, some of these studies did not provide clinical or histopathologic data sufficient to determine the clinical behavior of the investigated patients, and only one of the studies also compared primary lesions versus liver metastases [74], with findings suggesting a striking similarity between matched primaries and metastases.

Fig. 7-1

Schematic representation of the PI₃K/AKT/mTOR pathway. A green color indicates overexpression or activation, red color indicates reduced expression or deactivating mutations. Overall the balance of such events suggests an important role for this signaling pathway in PETs. Notably, mutations of TSC1/TSC2 and PTEN may reduce the negative effect of hypoxia on the mTOR pathway.

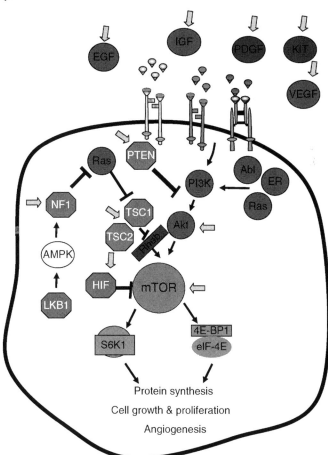

Overall, none of the studies could identify novel dysregulated genes associated with a certain clinical behavior or with prognosis or response to treatment. The overlap between the different gene lists is very poor, as previously reported for pancreatic adenocarcinoma [115]. However, some interesting candidates for further evaluation as prognostic factors or therapeutic factors may have been identified.

A single paper examined the expression of MicroRNAs in PETs [116]. MicroRNAs are small noncoding RNAs able to regulate gene expression by targeting specific mRNAs for degradation or translation inhibition. A role for microRNAs in tumor development and progression has been ascertained for many human cancers including pancreatic adenocarcinoma. Using a specific custom microarray, Roldo et al. explored the global microRNA

■ Table 7-7

Summary of gene expression profile studies of pancreatic endocrine tumors

Author [reference]	Samples	Comparison(s)	Platform	Upregulated genes	Downregulated genes	Relevant genes	Confirmation
Capurso [74]	13 NF PETs (8 primary, 5 metastasis), 3 cell lines (BON CM QGP), 4 purified islets	1. PETs versus islets	Affymetrix U133A + B	668	323	LCK, BIN1, BST2, SERPINA10	IHC qRT-PCR
		2. Primary versus Metastases		–	–		
Maitra [109]	8 NF PETs, 3 purified islets	PETs versus islets	Affymetrix U133A	66	119	IGFBP3, fibronectin, MIC2, p21	IHC
Dilley [110]	8 PETs samples from 6 MEN-I patients (2 insulinomas, 2 NF, 1 vipoma, 1 gastrinoma), 4 purified islets	PETs versus islets	Affymetrix U95AV2	45	148	IER3, IAPP, SST, PHLDA2	qRT-PCR
Bloomston [111]	Pooled biopsies from 9 PETs, normal pancreas, PDAC, CP	PETs versus normal pancreas	Affymetrix U133A	Ns	Ns	ANG2, NPDC1, ELOVL4, CALCR	IHC RT-PCR
Duerr [112]	24 PETs (9 insulinomas, 4 NF, 3 gastrinoma, 1 glucagonoma, 1 ACTHoma, 1 PTHRPoma), 6 GI Carcinoids	1. 12 WDETs versus 7 WDECs	Affymetrix U133A	71	41	FEV, NR4A2, ADCY2, GADD45β	qRT-PCR
		2. PETs versus carcinoids		228	157		
Hansel [113]	12 primary PETs	7 metastatic versus 5 non-metastatic	Affymetrix U133A + B	65	57	IGFB3, MET	IHC
Couvelard [114]	24 well-differentiated PETs (20 NF)	12 WDETs versus 12 WDECs	Sanger centre custom 10 k	72	51	CD-34, MDR1, E-selectin, MKK4	IHC

TSGs Tumor suppressor genes, *WDET* well-differentiated endocrine tumor, *WDEC* well-differentiated endocrine carcinoma, *NF* non-functioning

expression of 40 PETs (12 insulinomas, 28) compared to normal pancreas, and showed that a common pattern of microRNA distinguishes PET from normal pancreas. Specific microRNAs were identified, such as miR-204, primarily expressed in insulinomas and miR-21 which was strongly associated with both high Ki67 and liver metastases.

Key Research Points

- The molecular pathology of Pancreatic Endocrine Tumors is poorly understood, apart from these associated with inherited disorders such as MEN-I and VHL.
- CGH studies suggest a plausible role for a number of TSGs, which is partially confirmed by specific studies. The role of epigenetics changes, especially of methylation deserves more attention.
- Most oncogenes associated with pancreatic ductal adenocarcinoma have no role in PET carcinogenesis.
- A number of alterations of tyrosine kinase receptors (VEGFR), and molecular pathways (mTOR) expression and activity have been described.
- Data of microarray studies suffer of the poor heterogeneity of the samples and have not described a specific relation between expression profiles and prognosis or response to therapy.

Future Scientific Directions

- Future studies should always classify PET samples according to clinical and pathological standards, including WHO and TNM classification. Moreover, the tumor behavior (stable or progressive) is an issue in such an "indolent" tumor type.
- CGH array studies may help identifying putative oncogenes or TSGs.
- Microarray studies conducted in wide series of well-investigated PETs with a relation with clinical behavior and follow-up are needed.
- More in vitro models (animal models and cell lines) are sorely needed to better understand the process of tumor growth and progression, and possibly the role of novel therapies with targeted agents.
- The relation between PET cells and the surrounding stroma has not been investigated and may be important, similarly to pancreatic adenocarcinoma.

Clinical Implications

- Clinicians dealing with PETs should keep in mind the possibility of inherited disorders, as the diagnostic and therapeutic strategy is different from that of sporadic cases.
- Molecular alterations may somehow predict the clinical course, and possibly suggest the use of certain novel targeted therapies, such as VEGF and mTOR inhibitors.
- In this view, referral of patients to Centers with more experience in clinical and molecular aspects of neuroendocrine tumors should be recommended.

References

1. Metz DC, Jensen RT: Gastrointestinal neuroendocrine tumours: pancreatic endocrine tumours. Gastroenterology 2008;135(5):1469–1492.

2. Duerr EM, Chung DC: Molecular genetics of neuroendocrine tumours. Best Pract Res Clin Endocrinol Metab 2007;21(1):1–14.

3. Anlauf M, Garbrecht N, Bauersfeld J, Schmitt A, Henopp T, Komminoth P, Heitz PU, Perren A, Klöppel G: Hereditary neuroendocrine tumours of the gastroenteropancreatic system. Virchows Arch 2007;451(Suppl 1):S29–S38.

4. Lemos MC, Thakker RV: Multiple Endocrine Neoplasia Type 1 (MEN1): Analysis of 1336 Mutations Reported in the First Decade Following Identification of the Gene. Hum Mut 2008;29(1):22–32.

5. Milne TA, Hughes CM, Lloyd R, Yang Z, Rozenblatt-Rosen O, Dou Y, et al.: Menin and MLL cooperatively regulate expression of cyclin-dependent kinase inhibitors. Proc Natl Acad Sci USA 2005;102 (3):749–754.

6. Karnik SK, Hughes CM, Gu X, Rozenblatt-Rosen O, McLean GW, Xiong Y, Meyerson M, Kim SK: Menin regulates pancreatic islet growth by promoting histone methylation and expression of genes encoding p27Kip1 and p18INK4c Proc Natl Acad Sci USA 2005;102(41):14659–14664.

7. Bai F, Pei XH, Nishikawa T, Smith MD, Xiong Y: p18Ink4c, but not p27Kip1, collaborates with Men1 to suppress neuroendocrine organ tumours. Mol Cell Biol 2007;27(4):1495–1504.

8. Hughes CM, Rozenblatt-Rosen O, Milne TA, Copeland TD, Levine SS, Lee JC, et al.: Menin associates with a trithorax family histone methyltransferase complex and with the hoxc8 locus. Mol Cell 2004;13(4):587–597.

9. Bazzi W, Renon M, Vercherat C, Hamze Z, Lacheretz-Bernigaud A, Wang H, Blanc M, Roche C, Calender A, Chayvialle JA, Scoazec JY, Cordier-Bussat M: MEN1 Missense Mutations Impair Sensitization to Apoptosis Induced by Wild-Type Menin in Endocrine Pancreatic Tumour Cells. Gastroenterology 2008;135(5):1698–1709.

10. Anlauf M, Perren A, Henopp T, Rudolph T, Garbrecht N, Schmitt A, Raffel A, Gimm O, Weihe E, Knoefel WT, Dralle H, Heitz PU, Komminoth P, Klöppel G: Allelic deletion of the MEN1 gene in duodenal gastrin and somatostatin cell neoplasms and their precursor lesions. Gut 2007;56:637–644.

11. Machens A, Schaaf L, Karges W, Frank-Raue K, Bartsch DK, Rothmund M, Schneyer U, Goretzki P, Raue F, Dralle H: Age-related penetrance of endocrine tumours in multiple endocrine neoplasia type 1 (MEN1): a multicentre study of 258 gene carriers. Clin Endocrinol (Oxf) 2007;67(4):613–622.

12. Ballian N, Hu M, Liu SH, Brunicardi FC: Proliferation, hyperplasia, neogenesis, and neoplasia in the islets of Langerhans. Pancreas 2007;35(3):199–206.

13. Anlauf M, Perren A, Klöppel G: Endocrine precursor lesions and microadenomas of the duodenum and pancreas with and without MEN1: criteria, molecular concepts and clinical significance. Clin Endocrinol 2007;67:613–622.

14. Pereira T, Zheng X, Ruas JL, Tanimoto K, Poellinger L: Identification of residues critical for regulation of protein stability and the transactivation function of the hypoxia-inducible factor-1alpha by the von Hippel-Lindau tumour suppressor gene product. J Biol Chem 2003;278(9):6816–6823.

15. Woodward ER, Maher ER: Von Hippel-Lindau disease and endocrine tumour susceptibility. Endocr Relat Cancer 2006;13:415–425.

16. Berna MJ, Annibale B, Marignani M, Luong TV, Corleto V, Pace A, Ito T, Liewehr D, Venzon DJ, Delle Fave G, Bordi C, Jensen RT: A prospective study of gastric carcinoids and enterochromaffin-like cell changes in multiple endocrine neoplasia type 1 and Zollinger-Ellison syndrome: identification of risk factors. J Clin Endocrinol Metab 2008;93 (5):1582–1591.

17. Anlauf M, Garbrecht N, Henopp T, Schmitt A, Schlenger R, Raffel A, Krausch M, Gimm O, Eisenberger CF, Knoefel WT, Dralle H, Komminoth P, Heitz PU, Perren A, Klöppel G: Sporadic versus hereditary gastrinomas of the duodenum and pancreas: distinct clinico-pathological and epidemiological feature. World J Gastroenterol 2006;12(34): 5440–5446.

18. Corcos O, Couvelard A, Giraud S, Vullierme MP, Dermot O'Toole, Rebours V, Stievenart JL, Penfornis A, Niccoli-Sire P, Baudin E, Sauvanet A, Levy P, Ruszniewski P, Richard S, Hammel P: Endocrine pancreatic tumours in von Hippel-Lindau disease: clinical, histological, and genetic features. Pancreas 2008;37(1):85–93.

19. Lott ST, Chandler DS, Curley SA, Foster CJ, El-Naggar A, Frazier M, Strong LC, Lovel M, Killary AM: High frequency loss of Heterozygosity in von Hippel-Lindau (VHL)-associated and sporadic pancreatic islet cell tumours: evidence for a stepwise mechanism for malignant conversion in VHL tumourigenesis. Cancer Res 2002;62:1952–1955.

20. Mukhopadhyay B, Sahdev A, Monson JP, Besser GM, Reznek RH, Chew SL: Pancreatic lesions in von Hippel–Lindau disease. Clin Endocrinol 2002;57:603–608.

21. Chetty R, Kennedy M, Ezzat S, Asa SL: Pancreatic endocrine pathology in von Hippel-Lindau disease: an expanding spectrum of lesions. Endocr Pathol 2004;15:141–148.

22. Perren A, Wiesli P, Schmid S, Montani M, Schmitt A, Schmid C, Moch H, Komminoth P: Pancreatic endocrine tumours are a rare manifestation of the neurofibromatosis type 1 phenotype: molecular analysis of a malignant insulinoma in a NF-1 patient. Am J Surg Pathol 2006;30(8):1047–1051.

23. McClatchey AI: Neurofibromatosis. Annu Rev Pathol 2007;2:191–216.

24. Rosner M, Hanneder M, Siegel N, Valli A, Fuchs C, Hengstschläger M: The mTOR pathway and its role in human genetic diseases. Mutat Res 2008;659 (3):284–292.

25. Garbrecht N, Anlauf M, Schmitt A, Henopp T, Sipos B, Raffel A, Eisenberger CF, Knoefel WT, Pavel M, Fottner C, Musholt TJ, Rinke A, Arnold R, Berndt U, Plöckinger U, Wiedenmann B, Moch H, Heitz PU, Komminoth P, Perren A, Klöppel G: Somatostatin-producing neuroendocrine tumours of the duodenum and pancreas: incidence, types, biological behavior, association with inherited syndromes, and functional activity. Endocr Relat Cancer 2008;15(1):229–241.

26. Nesi G, Marcucci T, Rubio CA, Brandi ML, Tonelli F: Somatostatinoma: clinico-pathological features of three cases and literature reviewed. Gastroenterol Hepatol 2008;23(4):521–526.

27. Fujisawa T, Osuga T, Maeda M, Sakamoto N, Maeda T, Sakaguchi K, Onishi Y, Toyoda M, Maeda H, Miyamoto K, Kawaraya N, Kusumoto C, Nishigami T: Malignant endocrine tumour of the pancreas associated with von Recklinghausen's disease. J Gastroenterol 2002;37(1):59–67.

28. Curatolo P, Bombardieri R, Jozwiak S: Tuberous sclerosis. Lancet 2008;372(9639):657–668.

29. Rosner M, Hanneder M, Siegel N, Valli A, Hengstschläger M: The tuberous sclerosis gene products hamartin and tuberin are multifunctional proteins with a wide spectrum of interacting partners. Mutat Res 2008;658(3):234–246.

30. Francalanci P, Diomedi-Camassei F, Purificato C, Santorelli FM, Giannotti A, Dominici C, Inserra A, Boldrini R: Malignant pancreatic endocrine tumour in a child with tuberous sclerosis. Am J Surg Pathol 2003;27(10):1386–1389.

31. Terris B, Meddeb M, Marchio A, Danglot G, Fléjou JF, Belghiti J, Ruszniewski P, Bernheim A: Comparative genomic hybridization analysis of sporadic neuroendocrine tumours of the digestive system. Genes Chromosomes Cancer 1998;22 (1):50–56.

32. Speel EJ, Richter J, Moch H, Egenter C, Saremaslani P, Rütimann K, Zhao J, Barghorn A, Roth J, Heitz PU, Komminoth P: Genetic differences in endocrine pancreatic tumour subtypes detected by comparative genomic hybridization. Am J Pathol 1999;155 (6):1787–1794.

33. Stumpf E, Aalto Y, Höög A, Kjellman M, Otonkoski T, Knuutila S, Andersson LC: Chromosomal alterations in human pancreatic endocrine tumours. Genes Chromosomes Cancer 2000;29(1):83–87.

34. Yu F, Jensen RT, Lubensky IA, Mahlamaki EH, Zheng YL, Herr AM, Ferrin LJ: Survey of genetic alterations in gastrinomas. Cancer Res 2000;60 (19):5536–5542.

35. Speel EJ, Scheidweiler AF, Zhao J, Matter C, Saremaslani P, Roth J, Heitz PU, Komminoth P: Genetic evidence for early divergence of small functioning and nonfunctioning endocrine pancreatic tumours: gain of 9Q34 is an early event in insulinomas. Cancer Res 2001;61(13):5186–5192.

36. Zhao J, Moch H, Scheidweiler AF, Baer A, Schäffer AA, Speel EJ, Roth J, Heitz PU, Komminoth P: Genomic imbalances in the progression of endocrine pancreatic tumours. Genes Chromosomes Cancer 2001;32(4):364–372.

37. Tönnies H, Toliat MR, Ramel C, Pape UF, Neitzel H, Berger W, Wiedenmann B: Analysis of sporadic neuroendocrine tumours of the enteropancreatic system by comparative genomic hybridisation. Gut 2001;48(4):536–541.

38. Floridia G, Grilli G, Salvatore M, Pescucci C, Moore PS, Scarpa A, Taruscio D: Chromosomal alterations detected by comparative genomic hybridization in nonfunctioning endocrine pancreatic tumours. Cancer Genet Cytogenet 2005;156 (1):23–30.

39. Jonkers YM, Claessen SM, Perren A, Schmid S, Komminoth P, Verhofstad AA, Hofland LJ, de Krijger RR, Slootweg PJ, Ramaekers FC, Speel EJ: Chromosomal instability predicts metastatic disease in patients with insulinomas. Endocr Relat Cancer 2005;12(2):435–447.

40. Chung DC, Brown SB, Graeme-Cook F, Tillotson LG, Warshaw AL, Jensen RT, Arnold A: Localization of putative tumour suppressor loci by genome-wide allelotyping in human pancreatic endocrine tumours. Cancer Res 1998;58(16):3706–3711.

41. Rigaud G, Missiaglia E, Moore PS, Zamboni G, Falconi M, Talamini G, Pesci A, Baron A, Lissandrini D, Rindi G, Grigolato P, Pederzoli P, Scarpa A: High resolution allelotype of nonfunctional pancreatic endocrine tumours: identification of two molecular subgroups with clinical implications. Cancer Res 2001;61(1):285–292.

42. Nagano Y, Kim do H, Zhang L, White JA, Yao JC, Hamilton SR, Rashid A: Allelic alterations in pancreatic endocrine tumours identified by genome-wide single nucleotide polymorphism analysis. Endocr Relat Cancer 2007;14(2):483–492.

43. Barghorn A, Speel EJ, Farspour B, Saremaslani P, Schmid S, Perren A, Roth J, Heitz PU, Komminoth P: Putative tumour suppressor loci at 6q22 and 6q23-q24 are involved in the malignant progression of sporadic endocrine pancreatic tumours. Am J Pathol 2001;158(6):1903–1911.

44. Barghorn A, Komminoth P, Bachmann D, Rütimann K, Saremaslani P, Muletta-Feurer S, Perren A, Roth J, Heitz PU, Speel EJ: Deletion at 3p25.3-p23 is frequently encountered in endocrine pancreatic tumours and is associated with metastatic progression. J Pathol 2001;194(4):451–458.

45. Ebrahimi SA, Wang EH, Wu A, Schreck RR, Passaro E Jr., Sawicki MP: Deletion of chromosome 1 predicts prognosis in pancreatic endocrine tumours. Cancer Res 1999;59(2):311–315.

46. Vogelstein B, Kinzler KW: Cancer genes and the pathways they control. Nat Med 2004;10(8):789–799.

47. Guo SS, Wu AY, Sawicki MP: Deletion of chromosome 1, but not mutation of MEN-1, predicts prognosis in sporadic pancreatic endocrine tumours. World J Surg 2002;26(7):843–847.

48. Chen YJ, Vortmeyer A, Zhuang Z, Huang S, Jensen RT: Loss of heterozygosity of chromosome 1q in gastrinomas: occurrence and prognostic significance. Cancer Res 2003;63(4):817–823.

49. Yang YM, Liu TH, Chen YJ, Jiang WJ, Qian JM, Lu X, Gao J, Wu SF, Sang XT, Chen J: Chromosome 1q loss of heterozygosity frequently occurs in sporadic insulinomas and is associated with tumour malignancy. Int J Cancer 2005;117(2):234–240.

50. Pavelic K, Hrascan R, Kapitanovic S, Vranes Z, Cabrijan T, Spaventi S, Korsic M, Krizanac S, Li YQ, Stambrook P, Gluckman JL, Pavelic ZP: Molecular genetics of malignant insulinoma. Anticancer Res 1996;16(4A):1707–1717.

51. Chung DC, Smith AP, Louis DN, Graeme-Cook F, Warshaw AL, Arnold A: A novel pancreatic endocrine tumour suppressor gene locus on chromosome 3p with clinical prognostic implications. J Clin Invest 1997;100(2):404–410.

52. Nikiforova MN, Nikiforov YE, Biddinger P, Gnepp DR, Grosembacher LA, Wajchenberg BL, Fagin JA, Cohen RM: Frequent loss of heterozygosity at chromosome 3p14.2-3p21 in human pancreatic islet cell tumours. Clin Endocrinol (Oxf) 1999;51(1):27–33.

53. Guo SS, Arora C, Shimoide AT, Sawicki MP: Frequent deletion of chromosome 3 in malignant sporadic pancreatic endocrine tumours. Mol Cell Endocrinol 2002;190(1–2):109–114.

54. Beghelli S, Pelosi G, Zamboni G, Falconi M, Iacono C, Bordi C, Scarpa A: Pancreatic endocrine tumours: evidence for a tumour suppressor pathogenesis and for a tumour suppressor gene on chromosome 17p. J Pathol 1998;186(1):41–50.

55. Evers BM, Rady PL, Sandoval K, Arany I, Tyring SK, Sanchez RL, Nealon WH, Townsend CM Jr., Thompson JC: Gastrinomas demonstrate amplification of the HER-2/neu proto-oncogene. Ann Surg 1994;219(6):596–601; discussion 604–604.

56. Goebel SU, Iwamoto M, Raffeld M, Gibril F, Hou W, Serrano J, Jensen RT: Her-2/neu expression and gene amplification in gastrinomas: correlations with tumour biology, growth, and aggressiveness. Cancer Res 2002;62(13):3702–3710.

57. Wild A, Langer P, Ramaswamy A, Chaloupka B, Bartsch DK: A novel insulinoma tumour suppressor gene locus on chromosome 22q with potential prognostic implications. J Clin Endocrinol Metab 2001;86:5782–5787.

58. Wild A, Langer P, Celik I, Chaloupka B, Bartsch DK: Chromosome 22q in pancreatic endocrine tumours: identification of a homozygous deletion and potential prognostic associations of allelic deletions. Eur J Endocrinol 2002;147(4):507–513.

59. Pizzi S, D'Adda T, Azzoni C, Rindi G, Grigolato P, Pasquali C, Corleto VD, Delle Fave G, Bordi C: Malignancy-associated allelic losses on the X-chromosome in foregut but not in midgut endocrine tumours. J Pathol 2002;196(4):401–407.

60. D'Adda T, Candidus S, Denk H, Bordi C, Höfler H: Gastric neuroendocrine neoplasms: tumour clonality and malignancy-associate large X-chromosomal deletions. J Pathol 1999;189:394–401.

61. Chen YJ, Vortmeyer A, Zhuang Z, Gibril F, Jensen RT: X-chromosome loss of heterozygosity frequently occurs in gastrinomas and is correlated with aggressive tumour growth. Cancer 2004;100(7):1379–1387.

62. Missiaglia E, Moore PS, Williamson J, Lemoine NR, Falconi M, Zamboni G, Scarpa A: Sex chromosome anomalies in pancreatic endocrine tumours. Int J Cancer 2002;98(4):532–538.

63. Azzoni C, Bottarelli L, Pizzi S, D'Adda T, Rindi G, Bordi C: Xq25 and Xq26 identify the common minimal deletion region in malignant gastroenteropancreatic endocrine carcinomas. Virchows Arch 2006;448:119–126.

64. Brandau O, Schuster V, Weiss M, Hellebrand H, Fink FM, Kreczy A, Friedrich W, Strahm B, Niemeyer C, Belohradsky BH, Meindl A: Epstein–Barr virus-negative boys with non-Hodgkin lymphoma are mutated in the SH2D1A gene, as are patients with X-linked lymphoproliferative disease (XLP). Hum Mol Genet 1999;8:2407–2413.

65. Seki Y, Suico MA, Uto A, Hisatsune A, Shuto T, Isohama Y, Kai H: The ETS transcription factor MEF is a candidate tumour suppressor gene on the X chromosome. Cancer Res 2002 62:6579–6586.

66. Kim H, Xu GL, Borczuk AC, Busch S, Filmus J, Capurro M, Brody JS, Lange J, D'Armiento JM, Rothman PB, Powell CA: The heparan sulfate proteoglycan GPC3 is a potential lung tumour suppressor. Am J Respir Cell Mol Biol 2003;29:694–701.

67. Jonkers YM, Claessen SM, Feuth T, van Kessel AG, Ramaekers FC, Veltman JA, Speel EJ: Novel candidate tumour suppressor gene loci on chromosomes 11q23–24 and 22q13 involved in human insulinoma tumourigenesis. J Pathol 2006;210(4):450–458.

68. Moore PS, Orlandini S, Zamboni G, et al.: Pancreatic tumours: molecular pathways implicated in ductal cancer are involved in ampullary but in exocrine nonductal or endocrine tumourigenesis. Br J Cancer 2001;84:253–262.

69. Pellegata NS, Sessa F, Renault B, et al.: K-ras and p53 gene mutations in pancreatic cancer: ductal and nonductal tumours progress through different genetic lesions. Cancer Res 1994;54:1556–1560.

70. Yashiro T, Flton N, Hara H, et al.: Comparison of mutations of ras oncogene in human pancreatic exocrine and endoxrine tumours. Surgery 1993;114:758–764.

71. Hoffer H, Ruhri C, Putz B, et al.: Oncogene expression in endocrine pancreatic tumours. Virchows Arch B Cell Pathol Incl Mol Pathol 1998;55:355–361.

72. Sato T, Konishi K, Kimura H, et al.: Evaluation of PCNA, p53, K-ras and LOH in endocrine pancreas tumours. Hepatogastroenterology 2000;47:875–879.

73. Tannapfel A, Vomschloss S, Karhoff D, Markwarth A, Hengge UR, Wittekind C, Arnold R, Hörsch D: BRAF gene mutations are rare events in gastroenteropancreatic neuroendocrine tumours. Am J Clin Pathol 2005;123(2):256–260.

74. Capurso G, Lattimore S, Crnogorac-Jurcevic T, Panzuto F, Milione M, Bhakta V, Campanini N, Swift SM, Bordi C, Delle Fave G, Lemoine NR: Gene expression profiles of progressive pancreatic endocrine tumours and their liver metastases reveal potential novel markers and therapeutic targets. Endocr Relat Cancer 2006;13:541–558.

75. Wang DG, Johnston CF, Buchanan KD: Oncogene expression in gastroenteropancreatic neuroendocrine tumours: implications for pathogenesis. Cancer 1997;80:668–675.

76. Roncalli M, Springall DR, Varndell IM, et al.: Oncoprotein immunoreactivity in human endocrine tumours. J Pathol 1991;163:117–127.

77. Di Florio A, Capurso G, Milione M, Panzuto F, Geremia R, Delle Fave G, Sette C: Src family kinase activity regulates adhesion, spreading and migration of pancreatic endocrine tumour cells. Endocr Relat Cancer 2007;14(1):111–124.

78. Rane SG, Cosenza SC, Mettus RV, Reddy EP: Germ line transmission of the Cdk4(R24C) mutation facilitates tumourigenesis and escare from cellular senescence. Mol Cell Biol 2002;22:644–656.

79. Vax VV, Bibi R, Diaz-Cano S, et al.: Activating point mutations in cyclin-dependent kinase 4 are not seen in sporadic pituitary adenomas, insulinomas or Leydig cell tumours. J Endocrinol 2003;178:301–310.

80. Guo SS, Wu X, Shimoide AT, Wong J, Moatamed F, Sawicki MP: Frequent overexpression of cyclin D1 in sporadic pancreatic endocrine tumours. J Endocrinol 2003;179:73–79.

81. Chung DC, Brown SB, Graeme-Cook F, et al.: Overexpression of cyclin D1 in sporadic pancreatic endocrine tumours. J Clin Endocrinol Metab 2000;85:4373–4378.

82. Hervieu V, Lepinasse F, Gouysse G, et al.: J Clin Pathol 2006;59:1300–1304.

83. Chetty R, Serra S, Asa SL. Am J Surg Pathol 2008;32:413–419.

84. Wang DG, Johnston CF, Anderson N, et al.: Overexpression of the tumour suppressor p53 is not implicated in neuroendocrine tumour carcinogenesis. J Pathol 1995;175:397–401.

85. Yoshimoto K, Iwahana H, Fukuda A, et al.: Role of p53 mutations in endocrine tumourigenesis: mutation detection by polymerase chain reaction-single strand conformation polymorphism. Cancer Res 1992;52:5061–5064.

86. Lam KY, Lo CY: Role of p53 tumour suppressor gene in pancreatic endocrine tumours of Chinese patients. Am J Gastroenterol 1998;93:1232–1235.

87. Bartz C, Ziske C, Wiedenmann B, et al.: p53 tumour suppressor gene expression in pancreatic neuroendocrine tumour cells. Gut 1996;38:403–409.

88. Bartsch D, Hahn SA, Danichevski KD, et al.: Mutations of the DPC4/Smad4 gene in neuroendocrine pancreatic tumours. Oncogene 1999;18:2367–2371.

89. Chung DC, Smith AP, Louis DN, et al.: Analysis of the retinoblastoma tumour suppressor gene in pancreatic endocrine tumours. Clin Endocrinol (Oxf) 1997;47:423–428.

90. Bartsch D, Kersting M, Wild A: Low frequency of p16(INK4a) alterations in insulinomas. Digestion 2000;52:171–177.

91. Serrano J, Goebel SU, Peghini PL, et al.: Alterations in the p16 INK4a/CDKN2A tumour suppressor gene in gastrinomas. J Clin Endocrinol Metab 2000;85:4146–4156.

92. Wild A, Ramaswamy A, Langer P, Celik I, Fendrich V, Chaloupka B, Simon B, Bartsch DK: Frequent methylation-associated silencing of the tissue

inhibitor of metalloproteinase-3 gene in pancreatic endocrine tumours. J Clin Endocrinol Metab 2003;88(3):1367–1373.

93. Dammann R, Schagdarsurengin U, Liu L, Otto N, Gimm O, Dralle H, Boehm BO, Pfeifer GP, Hoang-Vu C: Frequent RASSF1A promoter hypermethylation and K-ras mutations in pancreatic carcinoma. Oncogene 2003;22(24):3806–3812.

94. Pizzi S, Azzoni C, Bottarelli L, Campanini N, D'Adda T, Pasquali C, Rossi G, Rindi G, Bordi C: RASSF1A promoter methylation and 3p21.3 loss of heterozygosity are features of foregut, but not midgut and hindgut, malignant endocrine tumours. J Pathol 2005;206(4):409–416.

95. Rahman A, Maitra A, Ashfaq R, Yeo CJ, Cameron JL, Hansel DE: Loss of p27 nuclear expression in a prognostically favorable subset of well-differentiated pancreatic endocrine neoplasms. Am J Clin Pathol 2003;120(5):685–690.

96. House MG, Herman JG, Guo MZ, Hooker CM, Schulick RD, Cameron JL, Hruban RH, Maitra A, Yeo CJ: Prognostic value of hMLH1 methylation and microsatellite instability in pancreatic endocrine neoplasms. Surgery 2003;134(6):902–908; discussion 909.

97. Parangi S, O'Reilly M, Christofori G, Holmgren L, Grosfeld J, Folkman J, et al.: Antiangiogenic therapy of transgenic mice impairs de novo tumour growth. Proc Natl Acad Sci (USA) 1996;93(5):2002–2007.

98. Zhang J, Jia Z, Li Q, Wang L, Rashid A, Zhu Z, et al.: Elevated expression of vascular endothelial growth factor correlates with increased angiogenesis and decreased progression-free survival among patients with low-grade neuroendocrine tumours. Cancer 2007;109(8):1478–1486.

99. Couvelard A, O'Toole D, Turley H, Leek R, Sauvanet A, Degott C, Ruszniewski P, Belghiti J, Harris AL, Gatter K: Microvascular density and hypoxia-inducible factor pathway in pancreatic endocrine tumours: negative correlation of microvascular density and VEGF expression with tumour progression. Br J Cancer 2005;92:94–101.

100. Wulbrand U, Wied M, Zofel P, Goke B, Arnold R, Fehmann H: Growth factor receptor expression in human gastroenteropancreatic neuroendocrine tumours. Eur J Clin Invest 1998;28(12):1038–1049.

101. Srivastava A, Alexander J, Lomakin I, Dayal Y: Immunohistochemical expression of transforming growth factor alpha and epidermal growth factor receptor in pancreatic endocrine tumours. Hum Pathol 2001;32(11):1184–1189.

102. Fjallskog ML, Lejonklou MH, Oberg KE, Eriksson BK, Janson ET: Expression of molecular targets for tyrosine kinase receptor antagonists in malignant endocrine pancreatic tumours. Clin Cancer Res 2003;9(4):1469–1473.

103. Welin S, Fjallskog ML, Saras J, Eriksson B, Janson ET. Expression of tyrosine kinase receptors in malignant midgut carcinoid tumours. Neuroendocrinology 2006;84(1):42–48.

104. Papouchado B, Erickson LA, Rohlinger AL, Hobday TJ, Erlichman C, Ames MM, et al.: Epidermal growth factor receptor and activated epidermal growth factor receptor expression in gastrointestinal carcinoids and pancreatic endocrine carcinomas. Mod Pathol 2005;18(10):1329–1335.

105. Koch CA, Gimm O, Vortmeyer AO, Al-Ali HK, Lamesch P, Ott R, et al.: Does the expression of c-kit (CD117) in neuroendocrine tumours represent a target for therapy? Ann NY Acad Sci 2006;1073:517–526.

106. Mita MM, Mita A, Rowinsky EK: The molecular target of rapamycin (mTOR) as a therapeutic target against cancer. Cancer Biol Ther 2003;4(Suppl 1):S169–S177.

107. Averous J, Proud CG: When translation meets transformation: the mTOR story. Oncogene 2006;25:6423–6435.

108. Tan PK, Downey TJ, Spitznagel EL Jr., Xu P, Fu D, Dimitrov DS, Lempicki RA, Raaka BM, Cam MC: Evaluation of gene expression measurements from commercial microarray platforms. Nucleic Acids Res 2003;31(19):5676–5684.

109. Maitra A, Hansel DE, Argani P, Ashfaq R, Rahman A, Naji A, Deng S, Geradts J, Hawthorne L, House MG: Global expression analysis of well-differentiated pancreatic endocrine neoplasms using oligonucleotide microarrays. Clin Cancer Res 2003;95:988–995.

110. Dilley WG, Kalyanaraman S, Verma S, Cobb JP, Laramie JM, Lairmore TC: Global gene expression in neuroendocrine tumours from patients with MEN-I syndrome. Mol Cancer 2005;4(1):9.

111. Bloomston M, Durkin A, Yang I, Rojiani M, Rosemurgy AS, Enkmann S, Yeatman TJ, Zervos EE: Identification of molecular markers specific for pancreatic neuroendocrine tumours by genetic profiling of core biopsies. Ann Surg Oncol 2004;11:413–419.

112. Duerr EM, Mizukami Y, Ng A, Xavier RJ, Kikuchi H, Deshpande V, Warshaw AL, Glickman J, Kulke MH, Chung DC: Defining molecular classifications and targets in gastroenteropancreatic neuroendocrine tumours through DNA microarray analysis. Endocr Relat Cancer 2008;15(1):243–256.

113. Hansel DE, Rahman A, House M, Ashfaq R, Berg K, Yeo CJ, Maitra A: Met proto-oncogene and insulin-like growth factor binding protein 3 overexpression correlates with metastatic ability in well-differentiated pancreatic endocrine neoplasms. Clin Cancer Res 2004;10:6152–6158.

114. Couvelard A, Hu J, Steers G, O'Toole D, Sauvanet A, Belghiti J, Bedossa P, Gatter K, Ruszniewski P, Pezzella F: Identification of potential therapeutic targets by gene-expression profiling in pancreatic endocrine tumours. Gastroenterology 2006;131 (5):1597–1610.

115. Grützmann R, Saeger HD, Lüttges J, Schackert HK, Kalthoff H, Klöppel G, Pilarsky C: Microarray-based gene expression profiling in pancreatic ductal carcinoma: status quo and perspectives. Int J Colorectal Dis 2004;19(5):401–413.

116. Roldo C, Missiaglia E, Hagan JP, Falconi M, Capelli P, Bersani S, Calin GA, Volinia S, Liu CG, Scarpa A, Croce CM: MicroRNA expression abnormalities in pancreatic endocrine and acinar tumours are associated with distinctive pathologic features and clinical behaviour. Clin Oncol 2006;24 (29):4677–4684.

8 Sporadic Pancreatic Endocrine Tumors

Volker Fendrich · Peter Langer · Detlef K. Bartsch

1	***Introduction***	***201***
1.1	Epidemiology	202
1.2	Molecular Genetics	202
1.3	Pathological Features	202
1.4	Natural History	203
2	***Insulinomas***	***204***
2.1	Clinical Symptoms	204
2.2	Differential Diagnosis	204
2.3	Diagnostic Procedures	205
2.3.1	Biochemical Testing	205
2.3.2	Imaging	205
2.4	Treatment	207
2.4.1	Benign Insulinoma	207
2.4.2	Malignant Insulinoma	209
2.5	Prognosis and Predictive Factors	211
3	***Gastrinomas (Zollinger-Ellison-Syndrome)***	***211***
3.1	Clinical Symptoms	211
3.2	Differential Diagnosis	212
3.3	Diagnostic Procedures	212
3.3.1	Biochemical Testing	212
3.3.2	Imaging	213
3.4	Treatment	214
3.4.1	Duodenal Gastrinomas	214
3.4.2	Pancreatic Gastrinomas	215
3.5	Prognosis and Predictive Factors	216
4	***Vipomas***	***216***
4.1	Clinical Symptoms	216
4.2	Localization	217
4.3	Treatment	217
4.4	Prognosis	217
5	***Glucagonomas***	***217***
5.1	Clinical Symptoms	217
5.2	Localization	218

J. P. Neoptolemos, R. Urrutia, J. L. Abbruzzese, M. W. Büchler (eds.), *Pancreatic Cancer*,
DOI 10.1007/978-0-387-77498-5_8, © Springer Science+Business Media, LLC 2010

5.3   Treatment 218
5.4   Prognosis 218

6   *Somatostatinomas* *219*
6.1   Clinical Symptoms 219
6.2   Localization 219
6.3   Treatment 219
6.4   Prognosis 219

7   *Non-Functioning Tumors* *220*
7.1   Clinical Symptoms 220
7.2   Differential Diagnosis 220
7.3   Diagnostic Procedures 220
7.3.1 Biochemical Testing 220
7.3.2 Imaging 220
7.4   Treatment 221
7.5   Prognosis and Predictive Factors 222

8   *Management of Metastases* *222*
8.1   Liver-directed Therapy 222
8.1.1 Liver Resection 222
8.1.2 Liver Transplantation 223
8.1.3 Radiofrequency Ablation 224
8.1.4 Embolization/Chemoembolization 224
8.1.5 Peptide-receptor Radionuclide Therapy 225
8.2   Biotherapy 227
8.2.1 Octreotide/Interferon 227
8.3   Chemotherapy 227

Abstract: Pancreatic endocrine tumors (PETs) are uncommon but fascinating tumors with an annual incidence of 1 per 100,000 people. PETs present as either functional tumors, causing specific hormonal syndromes like Zollinger-Ellison-Syndrome (ZES) or organic hyperinsulinism, or as non-functional pancreatic tumors (NFPTs). The natural history of PETs is highly variable. Small, benign neoplasms such as 90% of all insulinomas are readily curable by surgical resection. Most other functional and malignant NFPTs have a less favorable chance for cure. Patients with completely resected tumors generally have a good prognosis, and an aggressive surgical approach combined with conservative treatment options in patients with advanced disease often results in long-term survival.

1 Introduction

Pancreatic endocrine tumors (PETs) represent an important subset of pancreatic neoplasms (◐ *Table 8-1*). They account for 2–4% of all clinically detected pancreatic tumors. They consist of single or multiple benign or malignant neoplasms and are associated in 10–20% with multiple endocrine neoplasia type 1 (MEN1). PETs present as either functional

◘ Table 8-1

Neuroendocrine tumors of the pancreas

Tumor (Syndrome)	Incidence (%)	Presentation	Malignancy (%)
Insulinoma	70–80	Weakness, sweating, tremulousness, tachicardia, anxiety, fatigue, headache, dizziness, disorientation, seizures, and unconsciousness	<10
Gastrinoma	20–25	Intractable or recurrent peptic ulcer disease (hemorrhage, perforation), complications of peptic ulcer, diarrhea	50–60
VIPoma	4	Profuse watery diarrhea, hypotension, abdominal pain	80
Glucagonoma	4	Migratory, necrolytic skin rash, glossitis, stomatitis, angular cheilitis, diabetes, severe weight loss, diarrhea	80
Somatostatinoma	<5	weight loss, cholelithiasis, diarrhea, neurofibromatosis	50
Carcinoid	<1	Flushing, sweating, diarrhea, edema, wheezing	90
ACTHoma	<1	Cushing's syndrome	>90
GRFoma	<1	Acromegaly	30
PTH-like-oma	<1	Hypercalcemia, bone pain	>90
Neurotensinoma	<1	Hypotension, tachycardia, malabsorption	>80
Non-functional tumors	30–50	Obstructive jaundice, pancreatitis, epigastric pain, duodenal obstruction, weight loss, fatigue	60–90

tumors, causing specific hormonal syndromes, like Zollinger-Ellison-Syndrome or organic hyperinsulinism, or as non-functional PETs with symptoms similar to pancreatic adenocarcinoma. This chapter focuses on the management and surveillance of sporadic PETs.

1.1   Epidemiology

PETs are rare tumors. They occur in approximately 1 in 100, 000 people per year in Western countries [1]. The tumors show no significant gender predilection and occur at all ages. Overall, the sporadic form occurs 10–20 years earlier than inherited PETs (see following chapter).

1.2   Molecular Genetics

Whereas the molecular basis of familial PETs has been established, little is known about the oncogenesis and the molecular basis of the progression of sporadic tumors. In contrast to other human tumors, the activation of an oncogene is not a common event in PETs. Mutations in k-ras, p53, p16 myc, fos, jun, src and the Rb gene have not been implicated in the pathogenesis of sporadic PETs [2,3]. Recent cytogenetic and molecular studies have identified many chromosomal alterations in PETs. Comparative genomic hybridization studies demonstrate that chromosomal losses are more common than gains [4–10]. The most frequent gains were on chromosomes 7 and 20, whereas the most frequent losses were on chromosomes 2, 6q, 21q, and Y. According to these studies, the total number of genomic changes in the tumor tumor was associated with both tumor volume and disease stage. Thus large tumors with increased malignant potential harbor more genetic alterations than small and clinically benign neoplasms, suggesting a tumor suppressor pathway and genomic instability as important mechanisms associated with tumor progression. Losses of chromosome 1 and 11q as wells as gains on 9q appear to be early events in the development of PETs, since they are already present in small tumors. Prevalent chromosomal alterations common in metastases include gains of both chromosome 4 and 7 and losses of 21q, implying that these chromosome imbalances may contribute to tumor dissemination [9,11]. PETs belonging to the MEN-1 syndrome present deletions on chromosome 11q13. Studies on sporadic PETs have also detected relatively common losses at 11q13 or elsewhere on the short arm of chromosome 11 (70%), but specific *MEN1* gene mutations are present in only 20% of the PETs, suggesting involvement of another tumor-suppressor gene [12]. These findings indicate that another as yet unknown tumor suppressor gene might be involved. The von-Hippel-Lindau syndrome (VHL), which is less common than the MEN-1 syndrome also predisposes to the development of PETs. The gene associated with VHL is located on chromosome 3p25.2, but is not involved in the development of sporadic PETs [13].

1.3   Pathological Features

The gross appearance of sporadic PETs is generally that of a solitary, circumscribed, solid mass, showing a white–yellow or pink–brown color. The size varies from below 1 cm for duodenal gastrinomas or insulinomas to more than 5 cm for non-functioning PETs [1]. The characteristic histological appearance of PETs is a uniform cytology with scant mitoses.

■ Fig. 8-1
H&E staining with the typical trabecular pattern of a PET (here gastrinoma).

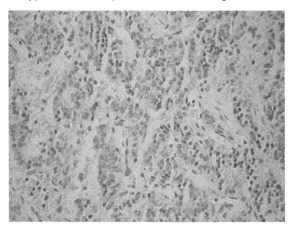

Cellular patterns can be either solid, acinar or trabecular. However, these different patterns exhibit no difference in biological behavior. The trabecular pattern is particularly characteristic (see ● *Fig. 8-1*). PETs can clearly be identified by using antibodies to markers common to all or most neuroendocrine cells: i.e., chromogranin A (CgA), pancreatic polypeptide (PP), synaptophysin, neuron-specific enolase [14]. CgA is a 49 kDa, monomeric, hydrophilic, acidic glucoprotein which is widely expressed in neuroendocrine cells and constitutes one of the most abundant components of secretory granules. CgA immunohistochemistry is the main step in the diagnosis of neuroendocrine tumors. It is released into the circulation and is a useful marker for PETs. Increased levels of CgA have been reported in 50–80% of all PETs, with the highest levels reported in non-functioning PETs [15]. In a recent study, combination of CgA with measurement of PP increased the sensitivity from 84 to 96% in non-functioning tumors and from 74 to 94% in functioning tumors [16].

PETs are categorized on the basis of their clinical manifestation into functioning and non-functioning tumors. Functioning tumors are associated with a clinical syndrome caused by inappropriate secretion or release of hormones. Within this group are insulinomas, gastrinomas, VIPomas, glucagonomas, somatostatinomas, and other extremely rare tumors (● *Table 8-1*). Non-functioning tumors are not associated with a distinct hormonal syndrome, but may still show elevated hormone levels in the blood or immunoreactivity in tissue sections, especially PP. They encompass 40–50% of all patients with PETs. Tumors with a majority of cells expressing and secreting pancreatic polypeptide are included in the group of non-functioning tumors. Many somatostatin-producing tumors are also clinically silent, because they do not cause a distinct hormonal syndrome [17].

1.4   Natural History

The natural history of PETs is highly variable (see below). Small, benign neoplasms such as 90% of all sporadic insulinomas are readily curable by surgical resection. Most other functional and malignant non-functional PETs have a less favorable prognosis. Approximately

50–80% of these neoplasms recur or metastasize, and up to one-third of patients already have metastases at initial presentation [18]. Historic controls with untreated liver metastases have a 5-year survival of only 20 to 30% [19].

2   Insulinomas

Insulinomas are the most frequent of all functioning PETs. The incidence was reported to be 2–4 patients per million population and year. Insulinomas have been diagnosed in all age groups with a highest incidence found at age 40–60 years. Females seem to be slightly more frequently affected [20]. The etiology and pathogenesis of insulinomas are unknown. No risk factors have been associated with these tumors. Virtually all insulinomas are located in the pancreas or are directly attached to it. Tumors are equally distributed within the gland. Approximately 90% of insulinomas are solitary; the remaining 10% are multiple and are associated with MEN1-syndrome [21]. Most insulinomas are small. Forty percent are less than 1 cm in diameter, 66% are less than 1.5 cm, and 90% are less than 2 cm. The most common sites of metastases are the peripancreatic lymph nodes with occasional hepatic metastases. Only 10% of the tumors are malignant at time of diagnosis.

2.1   Clinical Symptoms

Insulinomas are characterized by fasting hypoglycemia and neuroglycopenic symptoms, and occasionally sympathoadrenal autonomic symptoms [22]. The episodic nature of the hypoglycaemic attacks is due to the intermittent insulin secretion by the tumor. The severity of symptoms does not always predict malignancy or the size of the tumor. Most important symptoms of central nervous system dysfunction include diplopia, blurred vision, confusion, abnormal behavior and amnesia. Some patients might develop loss of consciousness and coma or even permanent brain damage. The release of catecholamines produces symptoms such as sweating, weakness, hunger, tremor, nausea, anxiety and palpitation. Whipple developed a symptom triad bearing his name to identify patients with insulinoma more accurately. These symptoms include signs and symptoms of hypoglycemia after fasting or exercise, blood glucose of less than 45 mg/dL when symptomatic, and symptoms relieved by intravenous or oral glucose. These symptoms usually occur when serum glucose is less than 40 mg/dL [23].

2.2   Differential Diagnosis

Insulinomas are an uncommon cause of hypoglycemia. The differential diagnosis of hypoglycemia includes reactive hypoglycemia, hormonal deficiencies, hepatic insufficiency, exogenous hyperinsulinism, medications and drugs. Occasionally, differentiating insulinoma from these other causes of hypoglycemia can be quite difficult [17]. The hypoglycemia of insulinoma is typically during a fasting state or after exercise which sets this diagnosis apart from the far more common postprandial or reactive hypoglycemia. Patients with multiple myeloma or systemic lupus erythematosus and hypoglycemia may have antiinsulin antibodies. These patients can be distinguished from patients with insulinoma by an anti-insulin antibody test. Neisidioblastosis is a rare disorder which may require intraoperative biopsy to differentiate it from insulinoma. This disorder is characterized by replacement of normal pancreatic islets with diffuse hyperplasia of the islets [24].

2.3 Diagnostic Procedures

2.3.1 Biochemical Testing

A fasting test that may last up to 72 h is regarded as the most sensitive test. Usually insulin, proinsulin, C-peptide and blood glucose are measured in 1–2 h intervals to demonstrate an inappropriately high secretion of insulin in relation to blood glucose. About 80% of insulinomas are diagnosed by this test, most of them in the first 24 h [25]. In most reports one-third of patients develop symptoms within 12 h, at least 80% within 24 h, 90% in 48 h, and 100% in 72 h [25,26]. Continuous C-peptide level demonstrate the endogenous secretion of insulin and exclude factitious hypoglycaemia by insulin injection. An example of a fasting test is given in ❯ Fig. 8-2.

2.3.2 Imaging

Imaging studies should be initiated after the biochemical diagnosis is established. Most endocrine surgeons would agree that imaging is only needed to exclude diffuse liver metastases by either computer tomography (CT) or magnetic resonance imaging (MRI). This is because there is evidence that intraoperative exploration of the pancreas as well as in the use of intraoperative US (IOUS) is the best method to localize insulinomas [25,27,28]. Today,

❑ Fig. 8-2

Example of a typical fasting test of a patient with an insulinoma.

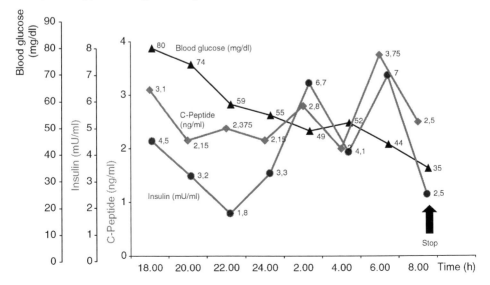

a variety of preoperative imaging modalities for the detection of insulinomas are available beside CT and MRI, such as ultrasound (US), somatostatin receptor scintigraphy (SRS), and various invasive methods, including endosonography (EUS), selective angiography (SA), selective portal venous sampling (PVS), and selective hepatic venous sampling after arterial stimulation (modified Imamura procedure). EUS is the most sensitive preoperative procedure. It was initially introduced in the 1980s and provides direct visualization of the pancreas and is able to detect tumors down to 0.3–0.5 cm in diameter (see ❯ *Fig. 8-3*). An early study by Rösch and colleagues in 1992 [29] identified endocrine tumors by EUS in the head of the pancreas in 95% of their patients and in the body and tail in 78 and 60%, respectively. One year later, Palazzo et al. [30] underlined its accuracy for localizing small PETs. 13 insulinomas below 15 mm in diameter were imaged by EUS, US and CT. Accuracy for these procedures was 79, 7 and 14%, respectively. Since then, more studies confirmed these results, showing that EUS is superior to CT, US, MRI, SA and SRS [25,31,32]. On the basis of these results, EUS is the method of choice if one wants to use preoperative imaging. It is mandatory before reoperation or if a laparoscopic approach is planned (see below). Transabdominal US offers a less invasive alternative, but is extremely operator dependent, its sensitivity ranges from 0 to 62% [33,34].

The majority of insulinomas are isodense on unenhanced CT and will not be seen without intravenous contrast enhancement, appearing then as hypervascular lesions [35]. Both arterial and portal venous phase images can identify intrapancreatic and hepatic lesions and should be performed as part of the imaging protocol for these tumors [36,37]. Fifty per cent of insulinomas measure <1 cm, so it is important to catch the vascular blush for the diagnosis. Dynamic or dual-face helical CT scans allows multiphase imaging and can achieve high sensitivities [38]. These sensitivities are directly related to the size of the tumor. For tumors

◘ Fig. 8-3

Endosonography shows a typical hypoechoic insulinoma (arrow) in the head of the pancreas.

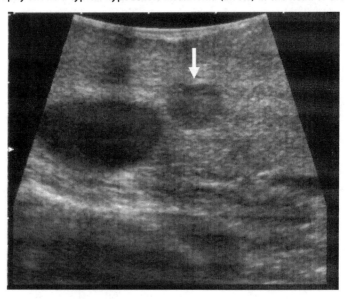

less than 1 cm, sensitivity is less than 10%. For tumors 3–4 cm, the sensitivity increases to 40%. A comparative study showed that T1-weighted MRI is equivalent to delayed dynamic CT. MRI is considered to be the most sensitive modality for detection of liver and bone metastases in patients with neuroendocrine tumors [39].

SRS was believed to be a promising method after the initial data were published. This has been thought because large numbers of somatostatin-receptors (SS-R) are found on most PETs. At least five different human SS-R subtypes have been cloned. Octreotide binds with high affinity to SS-R subtype 2 (sst2) and sst5. The efficacy of SRS in PETs is quite different [40]. The sensitivity of 111In-pentetreotide scintigraphy for the detection of gastrinomas, vasoactive intestinal polypeptide-secreting tumors, and glucagonomas as well as clinically non-functioning lesions is 75–100%. However, for insulinoma this is 50–60% owing to the low incidence of sst2 on insulinoma cells.

In the 1970s selective angiography (SA) selective portal venous sampling (PVS) were considered as a useful imaging procedures for the regionalization of insulinomas. Different series have shown high sensitivities. However, because of the invasive character that can be associated with serious complications, a decrease in its use has been noted [41,42]. In this context, a modification of the Imamura method is also worth mentioning. In this procedure, known as "arterial stimulation and venous sampling" (ASVS), calcium gluconate is injected into various gastroduodenal and splenic arteries [43]. After the injection, blood is obtained for insulin assay from the hepatic veins. Doppmann demonstrated high (88–100%) sensitivity rates [43] of this method, that is less painful, less difficult for the interventional radiologist to perform, and is associated with fewer complications than transhepatic catheterization of the pancreatic veins. Nowadays, PVS and ASVS is only indicated before reexploration for recurrent or persistent hyperinsulinism.

Preoperative diagnostic studies, however, are still beset by limitations in their ability to assess the site of an insulinoma. It has to be mentioned again, that intraoperative exploration of the pancreas by an experienced surgeon with combination of IOUS might be the best method to localize insulinomas. In a recent survey of 40 patients with insulinoma the tumor was correctly localized before operation in 65% by EUS, 37% by SA, 33% by CT and US, 15% by MRI and 0% by SRS. On the other hand, all tumors were identified using IOUS and bidigital palpation of the pancreas after extensive mobilization of the gland [25]. This is true in open surgery. In laparoscopic surgery, palpation is not possible. If a laparoscopic resection of the tumor is planned, preoperative localization, mainly by EUS, is crucial [44,45]. Furthermore, minimally invasive surgery for PETs should only be undertaken if laparoscopic ultrasound (LapUS) is available. LapUS helps the surgeon to determine the type and level of procedure, enucleation or resection, based on the relationship of the tumor to the main pancreatic duct or large blood vessels.

2.4 Treatment

2.4.1 Benign Insulinoma

Surgical cure rates in patients with the biochemical diagnosis of insulinoma range from 77 to 100% [27]. At surgical exploration, the abdomen is initially explored for evidence of metastatic disease. Then a meticulous surgical exploration should follow, i.e., an extended Kocher maneuver to be able to palpate the head, and mobilization of the distal pancreas and the spleen should follow to explore the body and tail of the gland to examine the distal pancreas carefully and completely. IOUS should then be used to confirm the presence of the insulinoma or to detect nonpalpable lesions and also to realize the relation of the tumor to the pancreatic duct. Identification of the pancreatic duct and determination of its proximity to the insulinoma can guide safe enucleation of the tumor. This approach can minimize the likelihood of a postoperative pancreatic fistula. Tumor enucleation, when feasible, is the technique of choice. If the tumor is located in the pancreatic tail, a distal spleen-preserving pancreatic resection might be the procedure of choice.

Postoperatively, blood sugar levels begin to rise in most patients within the first hour after of removal of an insulinoma (reactive hyperglycaemia). To preserve pancreatic function and reduce the risk of iatrogenic diabetes mellitus, patients in whom tumor localization is not successful at operation should not undergo blind resection [46]. They should be carefully evaluated to ascertain the diagnosis. These patients should be referred to an experienced endocrine surgeon for confirmation of the diagnosis and further treatment.

Recent advances in laparoscopic technique and instrumentation have enabled surgeons to approach complex procedures laparoscopically. This is also true for insulinomas [44,45,47].

The patient is placed in halflateral position with the left-side up for tumors located in the body or tail of the pancreas, or with the right-side up for tumors in the head of the gland, and in the reverse Trendelenburg position. Four 10–12 mm trocars are inserted in the abdominal wall: 3–4 cm above the umbilicus, in the xiphoid area, subcostal on the midaxillary line, and in the subcostal midclavicular line (see ◉ *Fig. 8-4*). The pancreas is exposed after opening the lesser sac after mobilizing its head. Laparoscopic ultrasound can be used to identify nonvisible tumors and determine the relationship of the lesion to surrounding veins and the

◘ Fig. 8-4

Laparoscopic operation for PETs. The patient is placed in a half-lateral decubitus position with the left side uppermost for tumors in the body/tail of the pancreas. The surgeon and assistant stand on the left of the patient, the cameraman and scrub nurse on the opposite side. Two monitors are used. Typical port sites for resection of lesions in the body/tail of the pancreas are shown.

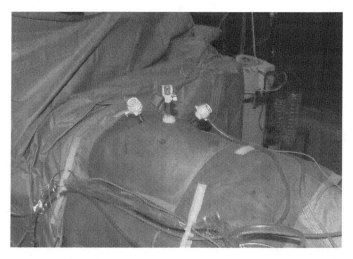

pancreatic duct. Laparoscopic ultrasound can be particularly helpful in identifying lesions in the tail that are often missed by endoscopic ultrasound. For superficial ventral tumors, laparoscopic enucleation is undertaken with electrocautery or laparoscopic coagulating shears (see ⊙ Fig. 8-5). Small pancreatic vessels can be clipped and cut. Tumors located deep in the body or tail of the pancreas and those in close proximity to the pancreatic duct require distal pancreatectomy. In cases where visualization and ultrasound fail, a hand port can be used to allow palpation of the gland. Tumors situated very distally near the splenic hilum are especially difficult to identify. It is worthwhile preserving the spleen during this procedure if it can be accomplished safely. The pancreatic tail and/or body should be meticulously dissected from the splenic vessels or these vessels may be resected together with the pancreas, leaving the spleen vascularized by the short gastric vessels [48]. Given the current data, laparoscopic enucleation or resection of benign insulinoma is feasible and safe, so that it might be become the future procedure of choice for imageable insulinomas (⊙ Table 8-2) [47,49–52].

For patients with benign insulinoma a follow-up is not necessary.

2.4.2   Malignant Insulinoma

To be considered malignant these tumors must show evidence of either local invasion into surrounding soft tissue or verification of lymph node or liver metastasis. Malignant insulinomas account for only about 5–10% of all insulinomas. Aggressive attempts for resection are indicated, since there is no effective medical treatment option to control hypoglycaemia. In addition, these tumors are much less malignant than their malignant ductal exocrine counterparts. Ten-year survival of 29% has been reported in malignant insulinomas [20]. Malignant

◘ Fig. 8-5
Laparoscopic enucleation of a insulinoma in the pancreatic tail.

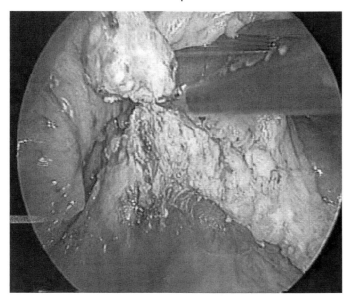

Table 8-2

Results of laparoscopic resection of PETs

Author	Year	Design of study	Patients (MEN1)	Tumor	Operative procedures	Conversion (n)	Duration of operation (h)	Time in hospital (days)	Complications
Assalia	2004	Meta analysis	93 (1)	81 Insulinomas 3 Gastrinomas	39 E	15/93	2,8 E	5 E	22/78 (28%)
Fernández-Cruz	2005	Single center	11 (20)	1 Vipoma 7 nfNEPTs 11 Insulinomas	39 DPR 7 E 3 DPR	1/11	3,7 DPR 3 E 3 DPR	6 DPR 5 E 10 DPR	14 fistula (18%, 12 E, 2 DPR) 3 E 1 DPR
Ayav	2005	Multicenter (9)	36	36 Insulinomas	19 E 12 DPR 5 sonstige	11/36	2,5 h	11	30%
Mabrut	2005	Multicenter (25)	127 (5)	25 Insulinoas 21 nfNEPT	NA	16/127	2 E 3,2 DPR	7	31%
Marburg	2008	Single center (unpublished)	10 (1)	9 Insulinoas 1 nfNEPT	5 E 5 DPR	4/10	3,3 h	11	20%

E Enucleation; *DPR* Distal pancreatic resection

insulinomas located in the body or tail of the pancreas are effectively treated by distal pancreatectomy with splenectomy and lymphadenectomy. For tumors located in the head of the gland, resection requires pancreaticoduodenectomy [53]. The management of metastases is described below.

2.5   Prognosis and Predictive Factors

No immunohistochemical markers are available which reliably predict a biological behavior of insulinoma. The percentage of malignant insulinomas is about 10. Insulinomas of <2 cm in diameters without signs of angioinvasion or metastases and <2% Ki67 positive cells are considered benign (see Chapter Molecular Pathology of Ampullary, Intra-Pancreatic Bile Duct and Duodenal Cancers).

3   Gastrinomas (Zollinger-Ellison-Syndrome)

Gastrinomas are functionally active endocrine tumors of the pancreas accounting for about 20% of PETs, second in frequency to insulinomas. Gastrinomas were first described in 1955 In 1955, when Zollinger and Ellison, of the Ohio State University Medical School, described two patients with islet cell tumors associated with atypical peptic ulceration of the jejunum [54]. Approximately 0.1% of patients with duodenal ulcers have evidence of Zollinger–Ellison syndrome. The reported incidence is between 0.5 and 4 per million of the population per year. Zollinger–Ellison syndrome is more common in males than in females, with a ratio of 3:2. The mean age at the onset of symptoms is 38 years, range 7–83 years in some series [55]. The etiology and pathogenesis of sporadic gastrinomas are unknown. Approximately 20% of gastrinomas are part of MEN-1 (see next chapter). No other risk factors are known. At the time of diagnosis 60–90% of tumors are malignant. The anatomical area harboring the vast majority of these tumors encomprise the head of the pancreas, the superior and descending portion of the duodenum and the relevant lymph nodes and has been termed the "gastrinoma triangle" (see ◉ Fig. 8-6), since it [56]. Up to 50% of sporadic gastrinomas are located in the duodenum [57]. More than 90% of the duodenal gastrinomas are located in the first and second part of the duodenum and are limited to the submucosa in 54% of patients. Pancreatic gastrinomas occur more frequently in the head of the pancreas.

3.1   Clinical Symptoms

In patients with ZES abdominal pain is the most frequent complaint either alone, or with diarrhea, followed by heartburn, nausea, or bleeding. The abdominal pain is primarily due to peptic ulcer disease or gastroesophageal reflux disease (GERD) and is indistinguishable in character from that seen in ordinary ulcer patients. The mean age of onset of symptoms is 41 years; however, there is an average 5.9-year delay in the diagnosis of ZES [55]. All of the symptoms early in the course of ZES are due to the gastric acid hypersecretion secondary to the ectopic secretion of gastrin by the tumor.

☐ Fig. 8-6

Gastrinoma triangle.

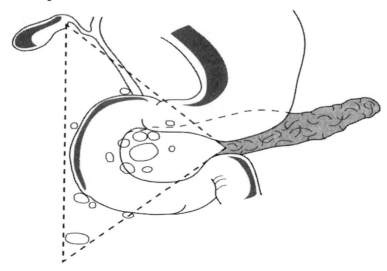

3.2 Differential Diagnosis

In the study of Roy et al. 164 of 168 (98%) patients with ZES were misdiagnosed before the diagnosis of ZES could be established [55]. The most common misdiagnoses were idiopathic peptic ulcer disease, chronic idiopathic diarrhea, GERD, Crohn's disease, and irritable bowel syndrome.

Hypergastrinemia can be caused by conditions other than ZES. Hypergastrinemia can be associated with increased gastric acid (e.g., retained gastric antrum, short bowel syndrome, gastric outlet obstruction) or with little or no gastric acid (e.g., pernicious anemia, chronic atrophic gastritis or vagotomy).

3.3 Diagnostic Procedures

3.3.1 Biochemical Testing

If the patient presents gastric pH below 4.0 and serum gastrin concentration above 1,000 pg/mL (normal <100 pg/mL) then the diagnosis of ZES is confirmed. Unfortunately, the majority (40–50%) of patients present serum gastrin concentrations between 100 and 500 pg/mL, and in these patients a secretin test should be performed. The secretin stimulation test can differentiate between patients with ZES and those with other causes of hypergastrinemia. Patients with pernicious anemia or chronic atrophic gastritis have a lost antral gastrin release, due to their achlorhydria. In contrast to ZES, these patients can be identified by gastric pH greater than 4. The patients receive 2 μg/kg of secretin intravenously. A rise in serum gastrin by more than 200 pg/mL is typically considered positive. This test has a sensitivity and specificity of >90% for detecting gastrinomas [58].

3.3.2 Imaging

Eighty to 90% of all gastrinomas are located in the so called gastrinoma triangle, which includes the duodenum, the pancreatic head, and the hepatoduodenal ligament [56] (see ⊙ *Fig. 8-6*). In more than 90% duodenal gastrinomas are situated in the first and second part of the duodenum [59]. The size of gastrinomas varies with the site of the tumors: pancreatic gastrinomas are often larger than 1 cm (see ⊙ *Fig. 8-7*), whereas gastrinomas of the duodenum are usually smaller [60]. For duodenal microgastrinomas, conventional imaging studies fail to localize the tumor in 80% of patients. In contrast, in patients with pancreatic gastrinomas these methods identify a gastrinoma in 50–72% of patients. In 1999, Norton and colleagues [61] presented their results of surgical resection in more than 150 patients with ZES. Sporadic gastrinomas were detected by US in 24%, by CT in 39%, by MRI in 46% and by selective angiography in 48%. In approximately one third of patients with sporadic gastrinomas, the results of conventional imaging studies were negative. EUS is also able to detect only pancreatic gastrinomas. Zimmer and colleagues found pancreatic gastrinomas by EUS in 79% [62]. Anderson et al. have been able to localize all 36 pancreatic gastrinomas investigated by EUS [31].

The European multicenter trial to evaluate the efficacy of somatostatin receptor scintigraphy (SRS) showed positive results in pancreatic gastrinomas in 73% [40]. Gibril et al. compared the sensitivity of SRS using [111In-DTPA-DPhe1] octreotide with that of other imaging methods in the localization of gastrinomas and their metastases in 80 patients [63]. Among patients with a possible primary tumor, US was positive in 9%, CT was positive in 31%, MRI was positive in 30%, angiography was positive in 28%, and SRS was positive in 58%. In 24 patients who had histologically proven metastatic liver disease, sensitivities for the detection of any metastatic liver lesions were 46% for US, 42% for CT, 71% for MRI, 62% for angiography, and 92% for SRS, respectively. The authors concluded that SRS is the single most sensitive method for imaging either the primary or the metastatic lesions in patients with the Zollinger-Ellison syndrome. Because of its sensitivity, simplicity, and cost-effectiveness, it should be the first imaging method used in these patients.

▢ Fig. 8-7

Enhanced computed tomographic scan demonstrates a large pancreatic gastrinoma (large arrow) with diffuse liver metastases (arrowheads).

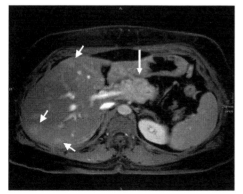 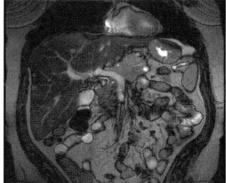

Portal venous sampling and the selective intra-arterial injection of secretin combined with venous sampling (Imamura technique), show a comparatively high sensitivity of 77 and 100%, respectively; however, they allow only a regionalization and not an exact localization of the gastrinoma [64].

The best method for localization is surgical exploration and IOUS. The sensitivities of palpation and IOUS are 91 and 95%, respectively. A study from the National Institutes of Health tested four different intraoperative procedures [60]. All 31 duodenal tumors were detected after longitudinal incision of the second part of the duodenum and a separate palpation of the posterior and anterior walls. The second best result was achieved by intraoperative endoscopy and transillumination of the duodenal wall (64%). Standard palpation without duodenotomy and IOUS, on the other hand, detected only 61 and 26% of gastrinomas, respectively. Recently, Norton and colleagues underlined the importance of duodenotomy in all patients with ZES [65].

3.4   Treatment

As with all PETs, the only chance for cure of gastrinoma is complete surgical resection, which is achieved in 26 to 100% of patients (see ❯ *Table 8-3*). A recent study compared 160 patients with ZES undergoing resection with 35 patients who had a similar stage of disease but did not undergo surgical exploration [72]. After a follow-up of 12 years, 41% of patients were cured with surgery and significantly more patients developed liver metastases with conservative treatment (29 vs. 5%; $P < 0.001$). Fifteen-year disease-related survival was 98% after surgery and 74% after medical treatment ($P < 0.001$). These results demonstrate that routine surgical exploration increases survival in patients with ZES by increasing disease-related survival and reducing the rate of advanced disease. Therefore, routine surgical exploration should be performed in all patients with sporadic gastrinomas without evidence of diffuse hepatic metastases, and who are fit for surgery.

3.4.1   Duodenal Gastrinomas

Duodenotomy (DUODX) should be routinely performed for all patients with ZES. Recently, Norton and colleagues underlined the importance of DUODX in patients with ZES [65]. They performed DUODX in 79 patients and no DUODX was performed in 64 patients. Gastrinoma was found in 98% with DUODX compared with 76% with no DUODX. They could show that the use of routine DUODX increases the short-term and long-term cure rate. Duodenal exploration is undertaken via longitudinal duodenotomy in the descending part of the duodenum. Small tumors can be identified by palpation. Duodenal tumors smaller than 5 mm can be enucleated with the overlying mucosa (see ❯ *Fig. 8-8*); larger tumors are excised with full thickness excision of the duodenal wall. After completion of this exploration the duodenotomy is cautiously sutured longitudinally.

Because of the high incidence of lymph node metastases associated with duodenal gastrinomas, prophylactic lymph node dissection should be done. In a recent study, the distribution of lymph node metastases found at the time of operation in 38 patients with sporadic duodenal gastrinomas were analyzed by mapping their location in relation to the duodenal primary [57]. Patients who had primary duodenal tumors located above the ampulla of Vater,

■ Table 8-3

Surgical cure rates for gastrinoma

Author (Reference)	n (total)	Sporadic	Cure-rate (%)	MEN1	Cure-rate (%)	Follow up (years)
Norton et al. [61]	151	123	34	28	0	10
Norton et al. [65][a]	79	79	52	0	–	8.8
Ellison et al. [66]	106	80	26	26	4	6
Zogakis et al. [57][a]	63	63	60	0	–	10
Thodiyil et al. [67]	13	10	80	3	66	7.5
Stadil et al. [68][b]	12	9	100	3	66	6
Bartsch et al. [69]	11	0	–	11	77	10.3
Tonelli et al. [70]	13	0	–	13	77	0.5
Melvin et al. [71]	19	0	–	19	5	12

[a]Only duodenal gastrinomas
[b]Only Pancreatectomies were performed
MEN1 Multiple endocrine neoplasia type 1

■ Fig. 8-8

Duodenal gastrinoma after duodenotomy.

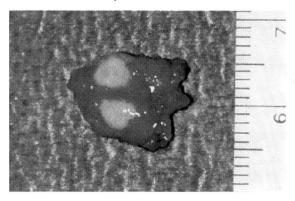

in general, harbored positive lymph nodes in the superior periduodenal area, celiac axis, or periportal area. Those with primary tumors in the third and fourth portions of the duodenum had positive lymph nodes located most commonly in the superior mesenteric artery or inferior periduodenal areas. Lymph nodes were found close to the primary tumor in most cases.

3.4.2   Pancreatic Gastrinomas

The role of operative exploration in patients with sporadic gastrinomas is relatively well defined. Most of these non-MEN1 gastrinomas are solitary, identifiable at laparotomy, and resectable with simple enucleation. Formal pancreatic resections are typically reserved for patients with local tumor invasion. In practice, this leads to distal pancreatic resection, splenectomy and peripancreatic lymph node dissection for gastrinomas in the pancreatic body or tail. Most of the pancreatic gastrinomas are located in the head of the gland or uncinate process. An enucleation with peripancreatic lymph node dissection is the procedure of choice in gastrinomas of the pancreatic head. For large pancreatic head gastrinomas a pylorus-preserving pancreaticoduodenectomy (PPPD) is justified.

After removal of a gastrinoma, serum gastrin should be measured before discharge of the patient and then at 3-month intervals for the first year. Hypergastrinemia indicated residual gastrinoma tissue. A normal gastrin level may indicate a surgical cure, but a positive secretin provocative test unmasks some patients who still harbor tumor tissue. In a study of Jaskowiak et al. 120 patients with ZES underwent gastrinoma resection, 78 patients had recurrent or persistent ZES after operation; of which 17 (15 with sporadic disease) patients with imageable disease underwent reoperation and 30% of these patients remained disease free [73]. Patients with persistent ZES after a failed primary operation should be send to tertiary referral centers [18].

3.5   Prognosis and Predictive Factors

Although most gastrinomas grow slowly, 60 to 90% are malignant at the time of initial diagnosis. Progression of a malignant gastrinoma has been the cause of death with 5-year survival rates in 20 to 38% for patients with metastatic gastrinoma. Studies have provided information on the biologic behavior of pancreatic and duodenal gastrinomas. It has been shown that both locations are equally malignant (40 to 70% metastases), and the postoperative disease-free intervals are similar [74,75]. However, duodenal tumors are smaller, less likely to metastasize to the liver, and have a better prognosis than pancreatic gastrinomas [75].

4   Vipomas

Vasointestinal peptide-secreting tumors, also called VIPomas, Verner–Morrison syndrome or WDHA (watery diarrhoea, hypokalaemia, and acidosis), account for fewer than 5% of islet cell tumors [76]. The two patients described by Verner and Morrison in1958 died from dehydration and renal failure in spite of attempted intravenous hydration. The VIP directly inhibits gastric acid secretion causing achlorhydria. Sporadic VIPomas are solitary tumors, arising from the VIP-secreting cells that are usually located in the region of the pancreatic tail and body [77]. More than 60% of these tumors are malignant and metastasize to lymph nodes, liver, and bone [77].

4.1   Clinical Symptoms

The Verner–Morrison syndrome is characterized by watery diarrhoea, hypokalaemia and achlorhydria or, more often, hypochlorhydria. The secretory diarrhoea ranges between 0.5 and 15 L/24 h and is usually the most prominent symptom at presentation. It results in severe loss of potassium and bicarbonate, which in turn lead to metabolic acidosis and dehydration [1]. Additional features include hypercalcaemia with normal parathyroid hormone levels, hyperglycaemia, and occasionally flushing of the face and the chest. The diagnosis of a VIPoma is confirmed by measurement of plasma VIP, and levels above 60 pmol/L are diagnostic.

4.2   Localization

Analogous to the other islet cell tumors, VIPomas can be localized by transabdominal ultrasonography, CT, MRI, endoscopic ultrasonography and 111In-pentetreotide scintigraphy [40]. The imaging is fairly easy in most symptomatic patients, since most tumors are >5 cm in size when symptomatic.

4.3   Treatment

Nearly all patients with functional islet cells tumors should have abdominal exploration with the intent of complete resection of tumor. The goals of operative exploration are not only complete resection, but also preparation for non-operative management, if a complete resection is not possible. Total surgical removal of the primary tumor may be curative in approximately 40% of patients with either benign VIPomas or non-metastatic malignant tumors [77]. In patients with metastatic VIPomas, cytoreductive debulking surgery may result in considerable palliation. All patients, regardless of disease stage should have cholecystectomy to facilitate later somatostatin analogue treatment, should this become necessary. The patients often require an intensive intravenous supplementation of fluid losses (often exceeding 10 L/day) and a careful correction of electrolyte and acid–base abnormalities. Somatostatin analogues reduce tumoral VIP secretion by more than 50% and inhibit intestinal water and electrolyte secretion. Via this mechanism, these drugs control the secretory diarrhoea in more than 50% of patients, and significant clinical improvement is attained in another 25% [78].

4.4   Prognosis

The 5-year survival rate is 60% for patients with metastases and over 90% for patients without distant metastases [78].

5   Glucagonomas

Glucagonomas arise from the glucagon-producing a-cells of the pancreas. Around 60% of patients already have liver metastases at the time of diagnosis [76].

5.1   Clinical Symptoms

Tumors that produce excessive glucagon cause a specific syndrome of diabetes mellitus, a skin rash (necrolytic migratory erythema), hypoaminoacidemia, and a tendency for deep venous thrombosis. Patients also often have stomatitis, glossitis and cheilosis associated with the skin rash (see ◉ Fig. 8-9). The syndrome is diagnosed by elevated plasma levelof glucagon. Levels greater than 1,000 pg/mL are diagnostic of the syndrome, while levels between 150 and 1,000 pg/mL

◘ Fig. 8-9
Necrolytic migratory erythema in a patient with a malignant glucagonoma.

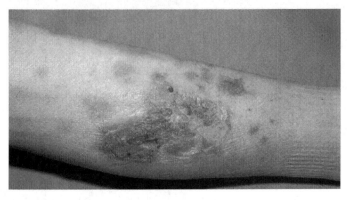

are suggestive. Once the syndrome is diagnosed, surgical resection of the tumor is indicated whenever possible. Preoperatively a management with somatostatin analogues and nutritional supplementation is indicated [79] to correct the nutritional deficiency and resolve the rash.

5.2   Localization

Analogous to VIPomas, glucagonomas can be localized by a broad spectrum of imaging modalities without difficulties [40] due the generally large tumor size (>5 cm).

5.3   Treatment

For localized glucagonoma the treatment of choice is an oncological pancreatic resection, either PPPD or distal pancreatectomy with splenectomy. However, total surgical removal may provide long-term cure only for patients with localized disease. In patients with more extensive disease, cytoreductive debulking surgery can effectively reduce symptoms even without necessarily normalizing plasma glucagon levels. Diabetic patients may require insulin therapy. Aspirin therapy has been used to prevent thrombosis. Single or repeated hepatic artery embolization of the metastases initially results in symptomatic relief in the majority (more than 80%) of patients, but in more than 50% of patients the symptoms will aggravate within 6 months. In both benign and malignant disease, octreotide is effective in controlling the rash, but it is less effective in the management of weight loss and diabetes mellitus and ineffective in reducing the incidence of venous thrombosis.

5.4   Prognosis

Approximately 60–70% of glucagonomas are already metastatic at the time of diagnosis. Even small glucagonomas are considered tumors of uncertain behavior; these tumors tend to grow slowly, and patients mostly survive for many years [79].

6   Somatostatinomas

Somatostatinomas are rare, mostly malignant, somatostatin-producing endocrine tumors with a prevalence estimated to be only one in 40 million people. Most somatostatinomas arise in the periampullary area of the pancreas or in the gastrointestinal tract.

6.1   Clinical Symptoms

Somatostatin generally inhibits different secretory processes, both endocrine and exocrine, as well as the motor function of the stomach and the gallbladder, over excretion by tumor tissue results in multisecretory insufficiency and gastrointestinal symptoms collectively termed, the somatostatinoma-syndrome. The classic triad of the syndrome is hyperglycemia, cholelithiasis and maldigestion [80]. The majority of the pancreatic tumors have been associated with a somatostatin syndrome, whereas this is very rare in duodenal somatostatinomas [81]. Thus, the clinical presentation of the duodenal somatostatinoma is not determined by hormonal excess, but by non-specific symptoms such as icterus, abdominal pain, weight loss or gastrointestinal bleeding.

6.2   Localization

Normally the tumor is detectable by abdominal ultrasonography, endosonography, computed tomography or MRI. Duodenal tumors were usually visualized during endoscopy.

6.3   Treatment

The optimal treatment of somatostatinomas has not been defined, as little long term follow-up information is available on the natural history of this rare neoplasm. Small tumors (<2 cm) arising in the duodenum may be adequately treated with local excision or wedge resection. In one study, four patients with proved duodenal somatostatinomas were treated by simple wedge resection [82]. In all of these patients, the tumors were <2 cm and confined to the bowel wall without evidence of liver metastases. These patients were followed-up for two years, with no clinical evidence of tumor recurrence. Large tumors (>2 cm) arising in the periampullary region of the duodenum or within the head of the pancreas should be managed by partial pancreatoduodenectomy. Large tumors arising in the body or tail of the pancreas should undergo distal pancreatectommy with splenectomy. Large somatostatinomas often have simultaneous liver metastases. Based on the limited information in the literature, resection of the primary tumor and the liver metastases can be associated with long term survival and appears justified in selected patients [82].

6.4   Prognosis

The number of patients undergoing successful complete resection ranges from 60 to 80%. In a review of the literature, there was no statistically significant difference in the rate of metastases and malignancy between pancreatic and extrapancreatic tumors. The overall 5-year survival rate ranges between 60 and 75% when metastases are present [83].

7   Non-Functioning Tumors

Clinically non-functioning pancreatic endocrine tumors (NFPETs) produce none, or insufficient quantities of peptides, or hormones, such as pancreatic polypeptide, that do not cause any hormonal symptoms [1]. Because of modern imaging modalities, they have been diagnosed more frequently and now represent at least 50% of PETs. At operation these tumors are generally larger than their functional counterparts and are located equally throughout the pancreas [84].

7.1   Clinical Symptoms

Patients usually present late owing to the lack of a clinical/ hormonal marker of the tumor's activity. Therefore, in contrast to functioning PETs, patients with NFPETs present with various nonspecific symptoms, sometimes jaundice, distant metastases, or invasion of surrounding structures [85]. Symptoms can include abdominal pain, weight loss, and pancreatitis. In some cases, liver metastases are the first symptom or finding.

7.2   Differential Diagnosis

Because an aggressive surgical approach is justified even in locally advanced or metastatic NFPETs, differentiation from the more aggressive pancreatic adenocarcinomas is extremely important (◐ *Table 8-4*).

7.3   Diagnostic Procedures

7.3.1   Biochemical Testing

Measurement of detectable serum or plasma levels of various hormones can establish the diagnosis of a non-functional endocrine tumor of the pancreas. Chromogranin A (CgA) is considered the best tumor marker currently available for the evaluation and follow-up of patients with non-functioning PETs, as these tumors do not reliably produce any other suitable marker. Plasma CgA is elevated in 60 to 100% of patients with NFPETs. Furthermore, up to 75% of non-functioning PETs are associated with increased serum levels of pancreatic polypeptide [85]. The combination of chromogranin A with measurement of PP increased the sensitivity from 84 to 96% in non-functioning tumors.

7.3.2   Imaging

Preoperatively US, CT or MRI scan are the procedures of choice and are usually effective, because these tumors are relatively large, usually more than 5 cm in diameter [86]. Also SRS

■ Table 8-4

Differences between pancreatic cancer and non-functioning endocrine tumors of the pancreas (NFPET)

	Pancreatic cancer	NFPET
Tumor size	<5 cm	>5 cm
CT-Scan	Hypodensity	Hyperdensity
	No calcifications	Calcifications possible
Chromogranin A in blood	Negative	Positive
Somatostatin-Receptor-Szintigraphy	Negative	Positive

can be performed to differentiate endocrine from nonendocrine pancreatic tumors. Since almost all exocrine pancreatic carcinomas are SRS-negative, a positive SRS is highly suggestive for neuroendocrine carcinoma. Therefore, the potential value of SRS is mainly the determination of the tumor type and its extent, rather than its correct localization. Recognition of NFPETs is imperative because of their good resectability and good long term survival compared to that of ductal pancreatic carcinoma.

7.4   Treatment

In patients with presumed sporadic NFPETs, complete surgical resection of the primary tumor is the treatment of choice if technically possible. The goals of surgery are to improve local disease control, and to increase quality and length of patient survival. Today, most authors advocate an aggressive surgical approach for the management of malignant NFPETs even in the presence of localized metastases [18,53]. The major goal is a potentially curative resection with no tumor tissue left behind. This may require partial pancreatoduodenectomy with resection and reconstruction of the superior mesenteric artery and/or the superior mesenteric-portal venous confluence as well as the synchronous resection of liver metastases (see ◉ Fig. 8-10). Using an aggressive approach potentially curative resections are possible in up to 62% and overall 5-year survival rates around 65% can be achieved [18,53,86]. Even debulking resections may have a place in this concept [87]. Removal of the primary tumor in nonmetastatic patients may significantly improve survival compared to that of patients who have not undergone successful primary tumor resection [88,89]. Solorzano et al. reported survival data for 163 patients with NFPETs [89]. As expected, patients with localized, non-metastatic disease at the time of diagnosis had a significantly superior median survival compared to those with metastatic disease (7.1 years compared to 2.2 years, P < 0.0001). Among those with localized disease, an additional survival advantage was demonstrated for patients who underwent complete resection of the primary tumor compared to those with locally advanced unresectable tumors (median survival of 7.1 years for patients with localized, resectable disease vs. 5.2 years for patients with locally advanced unresectable tumors).

Patients with NFPETs may be candidates for laparoscopic surgery if their lesions are <2 cm and without signs of malignancy. Unfortunately, most present with tumors over 5 cm in diameter, virtually all of which are malignant. Still, in selected patients for whom only palliative treatment is intended laparoscopic surgery remains a good option.

☑ Fig. 8-10

Large non-functioning PET (arrow) presenting with a liver metastases (asterix).

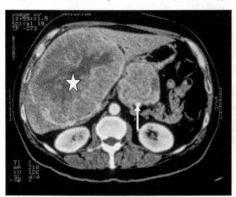 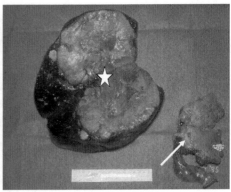

7.5   Prognosis and Predictive Factors

About 70% of all NFPETs are malignant. Overall 5- and 10-year survival rates of 65 and 49%, respectively, have been described (❯ *Table 8-5*) [18,53,84,86]. When comparing nonfunctioning with functioning pancreatic endocrine neoplasms, the non-functioning neoplasms seem to have a poorer prognosis.

8   Management of Metastases

The most important predictor of poor survival in patients with PETs is hepatic metastases [18,75,93]. In patients with liver metastases, different treatment modalities have been adopted. Overall, an aggressive approach is justified.

8.1   Liver-directed Therapy

8.1.1   Liver Resection

An increasing number of studies on surgical treatment of neuroendocrine liver metastases have been published [93–99]. Although none of these studies was a randomized clinical trial, and most of them pooled patients with PETs and patients with midgut carcinoid tumors, important conclusions can be drawn. In these studies, a total of 118 patients with hepatic metastases from PETs were treated, mostly by surgical resection. There was an average operative mortality of 3% and a 5-year survival rate of 64%. In a recent study by Touzios et al. [93] the median and 5-year survival was only 20 months or 25% for patients with non-surgically treated liver metastases versus 96 months or 72% for patients who underwent hepatic resection and/or radiofrequency ablation of their liver metastases. In a study by Norton and colleagues, 19 patients with liver metastases from gastrinomas underwent major hepatic surgery and 17 of them were able to have all identifiable gastrinoma resected. The 5-year survival rate was 85%. Five of the 17 completely resected patients remained disease free at a median follow-up of

8

■ Table 8-5

Surgical cure rates for non-functioning PETs

Author	Year	Patients (n)	Resection rate (%)	5-Year/ 10-Year-survival rate (%)
Kent et al. [90]	1981	25	60	60/44
Broughan et al. [91]	1986	21	57	63/55
Thompson et al. [92]	1988	27	51	58
Lo et al. [53]	1996	34	52	49
Solorzano et al. [89]	2001	163	38	43
Marburg (unpublished)	2008	50	85	72/56

5.5 years. Besides a lack of controlled clinical trials, patients with functional neuroendocrine tumors and liver metastases are often considered together with those with non-functional neuroendocrine tumors when evaluating the value of liver resection. Patients with advanced liver metastases from functional neuroendocrine tumors, in whom the symptoms are not well controlled medically, may benefit from cytoreductive surgery. Because the medical antitumor treatment of advanced liver metastases in patients with gastrinomas is generally unsatisfactory, our approach at present is to perform surgical resection in any patient in whom, based on imaging studies, all or at least 90% of the gross tumor can be removed [18].

8.1.2 Liver Transplantation

- Approximately, 120–130 cases of orthotopic liver transplantation (OLT) for PETs have been published, but follow-up after OLT is limited, and the individual series are rather small (largest single-center study, 19 cases) [100]. Indication for OLT is given, if the following criteria are fulfilled:
- patient <55 years
- metastases not resectable
- primary resected
- no extrahepatic disease
- good or moderate differentiation
- low Ki67-index (<10%)
- (tumor load <50% of liver volume)

Prior to OLT an extensive staging should be performed to exclude extrahepatic disease. Dopa-PET might be the best staging procedure as supplementary imaging modality to SRS, CT or MRI.

However, the limited data in the literature indicate that long-term cure by transplantation is rare. The largest single-centre analysis was recently published by Rosenau et al. reporting on 19 patients who received an OLT for metastatic NET [101]. The authors reported 1-, 5- and 10-year survival rates of 89, 80 and 50%, respectively. All deaths during long-term follow-up were tumor-associated. Recurrence was diagnosed in 12 patients between 2 weeks and 48 months after OLT. Survival in the five patients with a low Ki67 and regular E-cadherin staining was significantly better than in the 12 patients with a high Ki67 or aberrant E-cadherin expression (7-year survival 100 vs. 0% respectively; log rank $P < 0.007$). Olausson et al. reported on OLTs in nine patients [102]. Four patients developed recurrent tumors 9–36 months after OLT. The authors proposed a Ki67 cut-off of 10% as an appropriate criterion for the selection of patients. Le Treut et al. [103] carried out a retrospective multicentric study. There were 15 cases of metastatic carcinoid tumor and 16 cases of islet cell carcinoma. Hormone-related symptoms were present in 16 cases. The primary tumor was removed at the time of OLT in 11 cases. Of seven patients undergoing upper abdominal exenteration, only two survived longer than 4 months. Actuarial survival rates after OLT were 59% at 1 year, and 36% at 5 years. Survival rates were significantly higher for metastatic carcinoid tumors (69% at 5 years) than for PETs (8% at 4 years). Given the shortage of donor organs, OLT should be only considered in selected young patient with metastases limited to the liver and a previously resected primary PET who require relief from hormonal or tumor symptoms.

8.1.3 Radiofrequency Ablation

Radiofrequency ablation (RFA) is being used increasingly in patients with PETs with hepatic metastases, either alone or in combination with other treatments [104]. Percutaneous RFA may be more attractive because it avoids laparotomy and offers a minimally invasive procedure. On the other hand, intra-abdominal ultrasound performed during open surgery may be the most sensitive way of imaging the liver to identify liver metastases. Factors limiting its application include tumor size (usually used in tumors <3.5 cm) and number (usually used in cases with <5 lesions) [105]. Morbidity is low (<15%), although occasional cases of hemorrhage or abscess formation occur. Although there are yet no prospective trials proofing that RFA treatment of PET liver metastases is superior to other treatment options, the first reports are promising. Response rates from 80 to 95% are reported and responses have lasted up to 3 years [105].

8.1.4 Embolization/Chemoembolization

Liver metastasis derive their blood supply from hepatic artery branches, in contrast to native liver tissue, which derives the majority of its blood supply from the portal vein (see ❯ Fig. 8-11). Recent studies have shown that liver metastases show rapid growth in less than 50% of patients and up to 30% show no growth on follow-up evaluation [105]. Selective deprivation of blood supply to metastases for the palliative management of metastatic disease can be achieved by surgical ligation, but interventional radiologic approaches via intra-arterial catheterization of the iliac/brachial arteries without (hepatic artery embolization (HAE)) or with co-administration of chemotherapeutic agents (HACE) permits a similar result (see ❯ Fig. 8-12). Absolute contraindications to HAE/HACE are portal venous thrombosis, and liver failure, whereas relative contraindications are hepatic tumor loads greater than 50%, contrast allergy, extensive extrahepatic disease, and poor performance status. There are no randomized studies comparing embolization alone (HAE) with those with embolization combined with chemotherapeutic agents (HACE) such as 5-fluorouracil, cisplatin, mitomycin C, or streptozotocin [105]. The usual approach to HAE/HACE is sequential catheterization of peripheral radicals of the hepatic artery in one liver lobe followed by repeated administration of therapy on the other side about 6–8 weeks later [105]. In various studies 55–100% of

☐ Fig. 8-11

Diffuse liver metastases of a NFPET. Angiography (left) and chemoembolization of the right liver lobe (right).

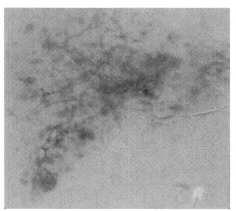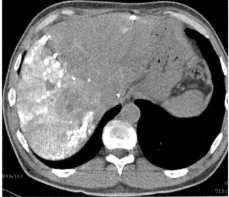

patients with malignant PETs treated by HAE/HACE have symptomatic improvement and 20–80% had an objective response with tumor reduction [106]. Overall mortality rate is less than 3%, but pain develops in nearly all patients, together with nausea and vomiting, and fever/ leukocytosis in 50%. In 5–15% of patients serious side effects can occur including hepatic failure, bleeding, gallbladder necrosis, hepatic abscess formation, and renal failure. At present there is no uniform agreement on when HAE/HACE should be used in patients with malignant PET [106]. In patients with functional PETs not responding to other therapies, or malignant PETs with diffuse hepatic metastases, this procedure may be considered and may be quite helpful in controlling symptoms.

8.1.5   Peptide-receptor Radionuclide Therapy

Somatostatin (SS) receptors are overexpressed in almost all PETs, despite insulinoma. SS receptors and internalize radiolabeled SS agonist analogues, facilitating the delivery of cytotoxic doses of localized radiation to the PET [107]. Three different radiolabeled SS analogues have been investigated in patients with malignant PETs including analogues labeled with 111In, 90Y, and 177Lu [107]. The effect of 111In-DPTA-octreotide was examined in 2 studies [107,108] including 52 patients with malignant progressive PETs and complete tumor regression was seen in 0%, partial regression was seen in 0–8%, and tumor stabilization was seen in 42–81%. [90YDOTA,Tyr3]-octreotide, [90Y-DOTA]lanreotide or [90YDOTA-, Tyr3]octreotate were examined in 7 studies involving more than 280 patients with malignant PETs and complete tumor responses occurred in 0–3%, partial responses in 6–37%, and stabilization in 44–88% [107,108]. One study reported results with 129 patients with malignant PETs treated with [177Lu- DOTA,Tyr3]octreotate and found a complete tumor response in 2%, a partial response in 32%, and stabilization in 34% [107,108]. In general, peptide-receptor radionuclide therapy has been safe. Around 30% of the patients develop acute side effects (nausea, pain, vomiting) that usually are mild and can be controlled with symptomatic therapy. More severe side effects include hematologic toxicity and renal toxicity [107]. Although no controlled studies have been conducted so far, to prove that peptide-receptor radionuclide therapy extends survival, it seems an attractive treatment option for diffuse metastasizing disease.

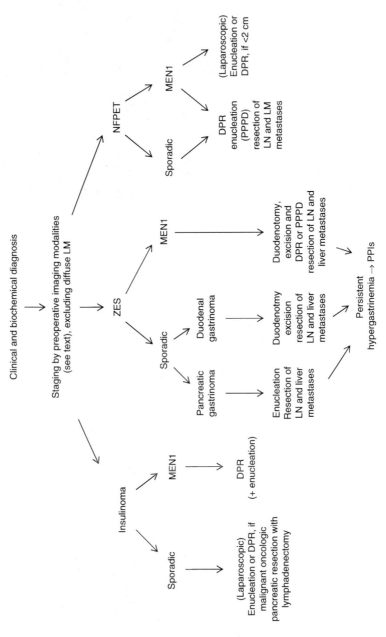

◘ Fig. 8-12

Algorithm of clinical management of PETs.

ZES = Zollinger-ellision-syndrome; NFPET = Non-functioning endocrine tumors of the pancreas; LM = Liver metastases; LN = Lymph node metastases; PPPD = Pylorus-preserving pankreaticoduodenectomy; PPI = Proton Pump Inhibitors

8.2   Biotherapy

8.2.1   Octreotide/Interferon

SS analogues frequently are used first because these agents are well tolerated and numerous studies suggest they have a tumoristatic effect, causing a decrease or cessation of growth in 30–80% of cases, without tumor regression in most cases [109] and with no studies that clearly have shown a prolonged survival. It is presumed that this tumoristatic effect will result in improved survival, but at present this remains unproven. The exact mechanism of SS analogue action in PETs is not completely resolved, however, they induce apoptosis and in various cells activate phosphatases, suppress release of growth factors, inhibit insulin-like growth factor-1 signaling, have immunomodulatory effects, and inhibit angiogenesis, respectively [110].

Interferon therapy also is used frequently for the treatment of metastatic disease but, as with octreotide, its major effect is tumor growth stabilization rather than inducing regression [109]. Similar to SS analogues it is hoped that this tumoristatic effect will result in improved survival, but at present this is also unproven [109]. The mechanism of interferon's antiproliferative effect in PETs is not completely known, however, it increases tumor expression of bcl-2, resulting in decreased cell proliferation and in other cells inhibits protein and hormone synthesis and angiogenesis and stimulates the immune system. Unfortunately, interferon therapy causes frequent side effects including flu-like symptoms (which may improve with prolonged therapy); fatigue; weight loss; leukopenia, which may persist and interfere with the acceptability of long-term treatment [109]. Because both interferon and octreotide therapy are tumoristatic by different mechanisms, combination therapy was believed to have promise. Nonrandomized studies were suggestive of additive effects, but a recent prospective study showed no additivity [111].

8.3   Chemotherapy

If biotherapy fails or the tumor is rapidly growing or poorly differentiated, chemotherapy frequently is used. Many different chemotherapeutic agents have been tried in the quest to find one regimen most effective against PETs. As with many of the trials involving therapies for these tumors, the data regarding chemotherapy can be difficult to interpret. Many of the series are small with pooled cohorts of both carcinoid tumors and PETs. In general the response rate of PETs is better than the rate for carcinoid tumors [17]. Chemotherapy becomes an option for PETs when the tumor symptoms are not treatable by other methods or the size of the tumor is rapidly growing in size. Single agent chemotherapy has proven to be inadequate treatment for malignant PETs with response rates around 20% and is not standard of care at this time [112]. Streptozocin in combination with other chemotherapeutic agents is currently the most effective regimen being widely used. Streptozocin plus 5-fluorouracil has proven to be superior to streptozocin alone with response rates of 63 and 36% respectively. When streptozocin plus doxorubicin is compared to streptozocin plus 5-fluorouracil the streptozocin and doxorubicin combination had superior response rates (69 vs. 45%) and improved median survival (2.2 vs.1.4 years) [113].

Key Practice Points

Insulinomas
- 90% are single, benign, small tumors of the pancreas.
- Don't rely on preoperative imaging procedures.
- (Laparoscopic) Enucleation is procedure of choice.
- Avoid occult distal pancreatic resection.
- Treat also metastatic insulinomas aggressively.

Gastrinomas
- Most gastrinomas are located in the 'gastrinoma triangle'.
- 50–60% of tumors are malignant at the time of diagnosis.
- Duodenotomy is an essential part of the operation.
- Biochemical evidence justifies operation.

VIPomas
- WDHA syndrome (watery diarrhoea, hypokalaemia, and acidosis).
- Treat tumor and metastases aggressively to reduce symptoms.

Glucagonomas
- Necrolytic migratory erythema and diabetes mellitus in more than 70% of patients.
- Cytoreductive debulking surgery can effectively reduce symptoms.

Somatostatinomas
- Pancreatic somatostatinomas usually present with somatostatinoma-syndrome.
- Duodenal somatostatinomas usually present with local effects of the tumor.

Non-Functioning Tumors
- Symptoms similar to pancreatic carcinoma.
- 60–90% malignancy rate.
- An aggressive surgical approach is justified even in patients with metastase.

Published Guidelines

- W.W. de Herder, D. O'Toole and G. Rindi et al., ENETS consensus guidelines for the diagnosis and treatment of neuroendocrine gastrointestinal tumors: part 2—midgut and hindgut tumors, *Neuroendocrinology* 87 (2008), pp. 1–63.
- U. Plockinger, G. Rindi and R. Arnold et al., Guidelines for the diagnosis and treatment of neuroendocrine gastrointestinal tumors A consensus statement on behalf of the European Neuroendocrine Tumour Society (ENETS), *Neuroendocrinology* 80 (2004), pp. 394–424.

Future Research Directions

- Genetic background of sporadic PETs has to be studied further.
- Randomized control trials are necessary to generate more evidence-based data for the treatment of PETs.
- Evaluation of reliable prognostic factors.

References

1. Öberg K, Eriksson B: Endocrine tumors of the pancreas. Best Pract Res Clin Gastroenterol 2005;19:753–781.

2. Rindi G, Candusso ME Solcia E: Molecular aspects of the endocrine tumours of the pancreas and the gastrointestinal tract. Ital J Gastroenterol Hepatol 1999;31(Suppl. 2):S135–S138.

3. Moore PS, Orlandini S, Zamboni G, Capelli P, Rigaud G, Falconi M, Bassi C, Lemoine NR, Scarpa A: Pancreatic tumours: molecular pathways implicated in ductal cancer are involved in ampullary but not in exocrine nonductal or endocrine tumorigenesis. Br J Cancer 2001;84:253–262.

4. Speel EJ, Richter J, Moch H, et al.: Genetic differences in endocrine pancreatic tumor subtypes detected by comparative genomic hybridization. Am J Pathol 1999;155:1787–1794.

5. Stumpf E, Aalto Y, Hoog A, Kjellman M, Otonkoski T, Knuutila S, et al.: Chromosomal alterations in human pancreatic endocrine tumors. Genes Chromosomes Cancer 2000;29:83–87.

6. Terris B, Meddeb M, Marchio A, Danglot G, Flejou JF, Belghiti J, et al.: Comparative genomic hybridization analysis of sporadic neuroendocrine tumors of the digestive system. Genes Chromosomes Cancer 1998;22:50–56.

7. Kytola S, Hoog A, Nord B, Cedermark B, Frisk T, Larsson C, et al.: Comparative genomic hybridization identifies loss of 18q22—qter as an early and specific event in tumorigenesis of midgut carcinoids. Am J Pathol 2001;158:1803–1808.

8. Tonnies H, Toliat MR, Ramel C, Pape UF, Neitzel H, Berger W, et al.: Analysis of sporadic neuroendocrine tumours of the enteropancreatic system by comparative genomic hybridisation. Gut 2001;48:536–541.

9. Zhao J, Moch H, Scheidweiler AF, et al.: Genomic imbalances in the progression of endocrine pancreatic tumors. Genes Chromosomes Cancer 2001;32:364–372.

10. Zikusoka MN, Kidd M, Eick G, Latich I, Modlin IM: The molecular genetics of gastroenteropancreatic neuroendocrine tumors. Cancer 2005;104:2292–2309.

11. Rigaud G, Missiaglia E, Moore PS, et al.: High resolution allelotype of nonfunctional pancreatic endocrine tumors: identification of two molecular subgroups with clinical implications. Cancer Res 2001;61:285–292.

12. Debelenko LV, Zhuang Z, Emmert-Buck MR, et al.: Allelic deletions on chromosome 11q13 in multiple endocrine neoplasia type 1-associated and sporadic gastrinomas and pancreatic endocrine tumors. Cancer Res 1997;57:2238–2243.

13. Chung DC, Smith AP, Louis DN, et al.: A novel pancreatic endocrine tumor suppressor gene locus on chromosome 3p with clinical prognostic implications. J Clin Invest 1997;100:404–410.

14. Heitz PU, Kasper M, Polak JM, Kloppel G: Pancreatic endocrine tumors. Hum Pathol 1982;13:263–271.

15. Bajetta E, Ferrari L, Martinetti A, et al.: Chromogranin A, neuron specific enolase, carcinoembryonic antigen, and hydroxyindole acetic acid evaluation in patients with neuroendocrine tumors. Cancer 1999;86:858–865.

16. Panzuto F, Severi C, Cannizzaro R, et al.: Utility of combined use of plasma levels of chromogranin A and pancreatic polypeptide in the diagnosis of gastrointestinal and pancreatic endocrine tumors. J Endocrinol Invest 2004;27:6–11.

17. Mansour JC, Chen H: Pancreatic endocrine tumors. J Surg Res 2004;120:139–161.

18. Fendrich V, Langer P, Celik I, Bartsch DK, Zielke A, Ramaswamy A, Rothmund M: An aggressive surgical approach leads to long-term survival in patients with pancreatic endocrine tumors. Ann Surg 2006;244:845–851; discussion 852–853.

19. Hochwald SN, Zee S, Conlon KC, Colleoni R, Louie O, Brennan MF, Klimstra DS: Prognostic factors in pancreatic endocrine neoplasms: an analysis of 136 cases with a proposal for low-grade and intermediate-grade groups. J Clin Oncol 2002;20:2633–2642.

20. Service FJ, McMahon MM, O'Brien PC, Ballard DJ: Functioning insulinoma-incidence, recurrence, and long-term survival of patients: a 60-year study. Mayo Clin Proc 1991;66:711–719.

21. Burns AR, Dackiw APB: Insulinoma. Curr treat Options Oncol 2003;4:309–317.

22. Service FJ: Hypoglycemic disorders. New Engl J Med 1995;332:1144–1152.

23. Whipple AO: Adenomas of the islet cells with hyperinsulinism. Ann Surg 1935;101:1299.

24. Kaczirek K, Niederle B: Nesidioblastosis: an old term and a new understanding. World J Surg 2004;28:1227–1230.

25. Fendrich V, Bartsch DK, Langer P, Zielke A, Rothmund M: Diagnosis and therapy in 40 patients with insulinoma. Dtsch Med Wochenschr 2004;129:941–946.

26. van Heerden JA, Edis AJ: Insulinoma: diagnosis and management. Surg Rounds 1980;42–51.

27. Rothmund M, Angelini L, Brunt M, et al.: Surgery for benign insulinoma: an international review. World J Surg 1990;14:393–398.

28. Van Heerden JA, Grant CS, Czako PF, Service FJ, Charboneau JW: Occult functioning insulinomas:

Which localizing studies are indicated? Surgery 1992;112:1010–1014.

29. Rösch T, Lightdale CJ, Botet JF, et al.: Localization of pancreatic endocrine tumors by endoscopic ultrasonography. N Eng J Med 1992;326:1721.

30. Palazzo L, Roseau G, Chaussade S, et al.: Pancreatic endocrine tumors: contribution of ultrasound endoscopy in the diagnosis of localization. Ann Chir 1993;47:419.

31. Anderson MA, Carpenter S, Thompson NW, et al.: Endoscopic ultrasound is highly accurate and directs management in patients with neuroendocrine tumors of the pancreas. Am J Gastroenterol 2000;95:2271.

32. Kann P, Bittinger F, Engelbach M, et al.: Endosonography of insulin-secreting and clinically nonfunctioning neuroendocrine tumors of the pancreas: criteria for benignancy and malignancy. Eur J Med Res 2001;6:385.

33. Bottger TC, Weber W, Beyer J, Junginger T: Value of tumor localization in patients with insulinomas. World J Surg 1990;14:07.

34. Hashimoto LA, Walsh RM: Preoperative localization of insulinomas is not necessary. Am Coll Surg 1999;189:368.

35. King CM, Reznek RH, Dacie JE, et al.: Imaging islet cell tumours. Clin Radiol 1994;49:295–303.

36. Power N, Reznek RH: Imaging pancreatic islet cell tumours. Imaging 2002;14:147–159.

37. Noone TC, Hosey J, Firat Z, Semelka RC: Imaging and localization of islet-cell tumours of the pancreas on CT and MRI. Best Pract Res Clin Endocrinol Metab 2005;19:195–211.

38. Van Hoe L, Gryspeerdt S, Marchal G, et al.: Helical CT for the preoperative localization of islet cell tumors of the pancreas: value of arterial and parenchymal phase images. ARJ Am J Roentgenol 1995;165:1437–1439.

39. Debray MP, Geoffroy O, Laissy JP, et al.: Imaging appearances of metastases from neuroendocrine tumours of the pancreas. Br J Radiol 2001;74: 1065–1070.

40. de Herder WW, Kwekkeboom DJ, Valkema R, Feelders RA, van Aken MO, Lamberts SW, van der Lely AJ, Krenning EP: Neuroendocrine tumors and somatostatin: imaging techniques. J Endocrinol Invest. 2005;28 (11 Suppl International):132–136.

41. Won JG, Tseng HS, Yang AH, Tang KT, Jap TS, Kwok CF, Lee CH, Lin HD: Intra-arterial calcium stimulation test for detection of insulinomas: detection rate, responses of pancreatic peptides, and its relationship to differentiation of tumor cells. Metabolism. 2003;52:1320–1329.

42. Hiramoto JS, Feldstein VA, LaBerge JM, Norton JA: Intraoperative ultrasound and preoperative localization detects all occult insulinomas. Arch Surg. 2001;136:1020–1025.

43. Doppmann JL, Miller DL, Chang R, et al.: Insulinomas: Localization with selective intraarterial injection of calcium. Radiology 1991;178:237.

44. Fernandez-Cruz L, Cesar-Borges G: Laparoscopic strategies for resection of insulinomas. J Gastrointest Surg 2006;10:752–760.

45. Fendrich V, Langer P: Minimally invasive surgery for pancreatic endocrine tumours. Br J Surg 2007;94: 1187–1188.

46. Hirshberg B, Libutti SK, Alexander HR, et al.: Blind distal pancreatectomy for occult insulinoma, an inadvisable procedure. J Am Coll Surg 2002;194: 761–764.

47. Langer P, Bartsch DK, Fendrich V, Kann PH, Rothmund M, Zielke A: Minimal-invasive operative treatment of organic hyperinsulinism. Dtsch Med Wochenschr 2005;130:508–513.

48. Carrere N, Abid S, Julio CH, Bloom E, Pradere B: Spleen-preserving distal pancreatectomy with excision of splenic artery and vein: a case-matched comparison with conventional distal pancreatectomy with splenectomy. World J Surg. 2007;31:375–382.

49. Assalia A, Gagner M: Laparoscopic pancreatic surgery for islet cell tumors of the pancreas. World J Surg 2004;28:1239–1247.

50. Ayav A, Bresler L, Brunaud L, Boissel P; SFCL (Societe Francaise de Chirurgie Laparoscopique); AFCE (Association Francophone de Chirurgie Endocrinienne): Laparoscopic approach for solitary insulinoma: a multicentre study. Langenbecks Arch Surg. 2005;390:134–140.

51. Fernandez-Cruz L, Martinez I, Cesar-Borges G, Astudillo E, Orduna D, Halperin I, Sesmilo G, Puig M: Laparoscopic surgery in patients with sporadic and multiple insulinomas associated with multiple endocrine neoplasia type 1. J Gastrointest Surg. 2005;9:381–388.

52. Mabrut JY, Fernandez-Cruz L, Azagra JS, Bassi C, Delvaux G, Weerts J, Fabre JM, Boulez J, Baulieux J, Peix JL, Gigot JF; Hepatobiliary and Pancreatic Section (HBPS) of the Royal Belgian Society of Surgery; Belgian Group for Endoscopic Surgery (BGES): Club Coelio. Laparoscopic pancreatic resection: results of a multicenter European study of 127 patients. Surgery 2005;137:597–605.

53. Lo CY, van Heerden JA, Thompson GB, Grant CS, Soreide JA, Harmsen WS: Islet cell carcinoma of the pancreas. World J Surg 1996;20:878.

54. Zollinger RM, Ellison EH: Primary peptic ulcerations of the jejunum associated with islet cell tumors of the pancreas. Ann Surg 1955;142:709–723.

55. Roy P, Venzon DJ, Shojamanesh H, et al.: Zollinger-Ellison syndrome: clinical presentation in 261 patients. Medicine 2000;79:379–411.

56. Stabile BE, Morrow DJ, Passaro E : The gastrinoma triangle: Operative implications. Am J Surg 1987; 209:550.

57. Zogakis TG, Gibril F, Libutti SK, et al.: Management and outcome of patients with sporadic gastrinoma arising in the duodenum. Ann Surg 2003; 238:42–48.

58. Jensen RT, Gardner JD: Gastrinoma. In: Go VLW, Di Magno EP, Gardner JD (eds.). The Pancreas: Biology, Pathobiology and Disease, 2nd ed. Raven Press, New York, 1993, pp. 931.

59. Hoffmann KM, Furukawa M, Jensen RT: Duodenal neuroendocrine tumors: Classification, functional syndromes, diagnosis and medical treatment. Best Pract Res Clin Gastroenterol 2005;19:675–697.

60. Sugg SL, Norton JA, Fraker DL, et al.: A prospective study of intraoperative methods to find and resect duodenal gastrinomas. Ann Surg 1993;218:138.

61. Norton JA, Fraker DL, Alexander HR, et al.: Surgery to cure the Zollinger-Ellison syndrome. N Engl J Med 1999;341:635.

62. Zimmer T, Scherübl H, Faiss S, et al.: Endoscopic ultrasonography of neuroendocrine tumors. Digestion 2000;62(Suppl1):45.

63. Gibril F, Reynolds JC, Doppmann JL, et al.: Somatostatin receptor scintigraphy: its sensitivity compared with that of other imaging methods in detecting primary and metastatic gastrinomas. A prospective study. Ann Intern Med 1996;125:26.

64. Imamura M, Takahashi K, Isobe Y, et al.: Curative resection of multiple gastrinomas aided by selective arterial secretin injection test and intraoperative secretin test. Ann Surg 1989;210:710.

65. Norton JA, Alexander HR, Fraker DL, et al.: Does the use of routine duodenotomy (DUODX) affect rate of cure, development of liver metastases, or survival in patients with Zollinger-Ellison syndrome? Ann Surg 2004;239:617.

66. Ellison EC, Sparks J, Verducci JS, Johnson JA, Muscarella P, Bloomston M, Melvin WS: 50-year appraisal of gastrinoma: recommendations for staging and treatment. J Am Coll Surg 2006;202: 897–905.

67. Thodiyil PA, El-Masry NS, Williamson RC: Achieving eugastrinaemia in Zollinger-Ellison syndrome: resection or enucleation? Dig Surg 2001;18:118–123.

68. Stadil F, Bardram L, Gustafsen J, Efsen F: Surgical treatment of the Zollinger-Ellison syndrome. World J Surg 1993;17:463–467.

69. Bartsch DK, Fendrich V, Langer P, Celik I, Kann PH, Rothmund M: Outcome of duodenopancreatic resections in patients with multiple endocrine neoplasia type 1. Ann Surg 2005 Dec; 242:757–764, discussion 764–766.

70. Tonelli F, Fratini G, Nesi G, et al.: Pancreatectomy in multiple endocrine neoplasia type 1-related gastrinomas and pancreatic endocrine neoplasias. Ann Surg 2006;244:61–70.

71. Melvin WS, Johnson JA, Sparks J, Innes JT, Ellison EC: Long-term prognosis of Zollinger-Ellison syndrome in multiple endocrine neoplasia. Surgery 1993;114:1183–1188.

72. Norton JA, Fraker DL, Alexander HR, Gibril F, Liewehr DJ, Venzon DJ, et al.: Surgery increases survival in patients with gastrinoma. Ann Surg 2006;244:410–419.

73. Jaskowiak NT, Fraker DL, Alexander HR, et al.: Is reoperation for gastrinoma excision indicated in Zollinger-Ellison syndrome? Surgery 1996;120: 1055–1063.

74. Weber HC, Venzon DJ, Fishbein VA, et al.: Determinants of metastatic rate and survival in patients with Zollinger-Ellison syndrome: a prospective long-term study. Gastroenterology 1995;108:1637–1649.

75. Yu F, Venzon DJ, Serrano J, et al.: Prospective study of the clinical course, prognostic factors, causes of death, and survival in patients with long-standing Zollinger-Ellison syndrome. J Clin Oncol 1999;17: 615–630.

76. de Herder WW, Lamberts SW: Clinical endocrinology and metabolism. Gut endocrine tumours. Best Pract Res Clin Endocrinol Metab. 2004;18:477–495.

77. Perry RR, Vinik AI: Clinical review 72: diagnosis and management of functioning islet cell tumors. J Clin Endocrinol Metab 1995;80:2273–2278.

78. Soga J, Yakuwa Y: Vipoma/diarrheogenic syndrome: a statistical evaluation of 241 reported cases. J Exp Clin Cancer Res 1998;17:389–400.

79. Chastain MA: The glucagonoma syndrome: a review of its features and discussion of new perspectives. Am J Med Sci 2001;321:306–320.

80. Krejs GJ, Orci L, Conlon JM, et al.: Somatostatinoma syndrome. N Engl J Med 1979;301:285.

81. Mao C, Shah A, Hanson D, Howard J: Von Recklinghausen's Disease associated with duodenal somatostatinoma: contrast of duodenal versus pancreatic somatostatinomas. J Surg Oncol 1995;59:67.

82. O'Brien TD, Chejfec G, Prinz RA: Clinical features of duodenal somatostatinomas. Surgery 1993;114:1144.

83. Soga J, Yakuwa Y: Somatostatinoma/inhibitory syndrome: a statistical evaluation of 173 reported cases as compared to other pancreatic endocrinomas. J Exp Clin Cancer Res 1999;18:13–22.

84. Grant CS: Surgical management of malignant islet cell tumors. World J Surg 1993;17:498–503.

85. Kouvaraki MA, Solorzano CC, Shapiro SE, Yao JC, Perrier ND, Lee JE, Evans DB: Surgical treatment of non-functioning pancreatic islet cell tumors. J Surg Oncol 2005;89:170–185.

86. Bartsch DK, Schilling T, Ramaswamy A, et al.: Management of non-functioning islet cell carcinomas. World J Surg 2000;24:1418.

87. Sarmiento JM, Farnell MB, Que FG, et al.: Pancreaticoduodenectomy for islet cell tumors of the head of the pancreas: long-term survival analysis. World J. Surg. 2002;26:1267–1271.

88. Evans DB, Skibber JM, Lee JE, et al.: Nonfunctioning islet cell carcinoma of the pancreas. Surgery 1993;114:1175–1182.

89. Solorzano CC, Lee JE, Pisters PWT, et al.: Nonfunctioning islet all carcinoma of the pancreas: survival results in a contemporary series of 163 patients. Surgery 2001;130:1078–1085.

90. Kent RB, van Heerden JA, Weiland LH, et al.: Nonfunctioning islet cell tumors. Ann Surg 1981;193: 185–190.

91. Broughan TA, Leslie JD, Soto JM, et al.: Pancreatic islet cell tumors. Surgery 1986;99:671–678.

92. Thompson GB, van Heerden JA, Grant CS, et al.: Islet cell carcinoma of the pancreas: a twenty-year experience. Surgery 1988;104:1011–1017.

93. Touzios JG, Kiely JM, Pitt SC, Rilling WS, Quebbeman EJ, Wilson SD, et al.: Neuroendocrine hepatic metastases: does aggressive management improve survival? Ann Surg 2005;241:776–785.

94. Dousset B, Saint-Marc O, Pitre J, et al.: Metastatic endocrine tumors: medical treatment, surgical resection, or liver transplantation. World J Surg 1996;20:908–914.

95. Que FG, Nagorny DM, Batts KP, et al.: Hepatic resection for metastatic neuroendocrine carcinomas. Am J Surg 1995;169:36–42.

96. Chen H, Hardacre JM, Uzar A, Cameron JL, Choti MA: Isolated liver metastases from neuroendocrine tumors: does resection prolong survival? J Am Coll Surg 1998;187:88–192.

97. Chamberlain RS, Canes D, Brown KT, et al.: Hepatic neuroendocrine metastases: does intervention alter outcomes? J Am Coll Surg 2000;190:432–435.

98. Nave H, Mossinger E, Feist H, et al.: Surgery as primary treatment in patients with liver metastases from carcinoid tumors: a retrospective, unicentric study over 13 years. Surgery 2001;129:170–175.

99. Sarmiento JM, Heywood G, Rubin J, et al.: Surgical treatment of neuroendocrine metastases to the liver: a plea for resection to increase survival. J Am Coll Surg 2003;197:29–37.

100. Pascher A, Klupp J, Neuhaus P: Transplantation in the management of metastatic endocrine tumours. Best Pract Res Clin Gastroenterol 2005;19:637–648.

101. Rosenau J, Bahr MJ, von Wasielewski R, et al.: Ki67, E-cadherin, and p53 as prognostic indicators of longterm outcome after liver transplantation for metastatic neuroendocrine tumours. Transplantation 2002;73:386–394.

102. Olausson M, Friman S, Cahlin C, et al.: Indications and results of liver transplantation in patients with neuroendocrine tumours. World J Surg 2002;26: 998–1004.

103. Le Treut YP, Delpero JR, Dousset B, et al.: Results of liver transplantation in the treatment of metastatic neuroendocrine tumors. A 31-case French multicentric report. Ann Surg 1997;225:355–364.

104. Hellman P, Ladjevardi S, Skogseid B et al.: Radiofrequency tissue ablation using cooled tip for liver metastases of endocrine tumors. World J Surg 2002;26:1052–1056.

105. O'Toole D, Ruszniewski P: Chemoembolization and other ablative therapies for liver metastases of gastrointestinal endocrine tumours. Best Pract Res Clin Gastroenterol 2005;19:585–594.

106. Toumpanakis C, Meyer T, Caplin ME : Cytotoxic treatment including embolization/chemoembolization for neuroendocrine tumours. Best Pract Res Clin Endocrinol Metab 2007;21:131–144.

107. Forrer F, Valkema R, Kwekkeboom DJ, et al.: Neuroendocrine tumors. Peptide receptor radionuclide therapy. Best Pract Res Clin Endocrinol Metab 2007;21:111–129.

108. Kwekkeboom DJ, Mueller-Brand J, Paganelli G, et al.: Overview of results of peptide receptor radionuclide therapy with 3 radiolabeled somatostatin analogs. J Nucl Med 2005;46(Suppl 1): 62S–66S.

109. Plockinger U, Wiedenmann B: Biotherapy. Best Pract Res Clin Endocrinol Metab 2007;21:145–162.

110. Guillermet-Guibert J, Lahlou H, Pyronnet S, et al.: Somatostatin receptors as tools for diagnosis and therapy: molecular aspects. Best Pract Res Clin Gastroenterol 2005;19:535–551.

111. Faiss S, Pape UF, Bohmig M, et al.: Prospective, randomized, multicenter trial on the antiproliferative effect of lanreotide, interferon alfa, and their combination for therapy of metastatic neuroendocrine gastroenteropancreatic tumors—the International Lanreotide and Interferon Alfa Study Group. J Clin Oncol 2003;21:2689–2696.

112. Moertel CG, Hanley JA, Johnson LA: Streptozocin alone compared with streptozocin plus fluorouracil in the treatment of advanced islet-cell carcinoma. N Engl J Med 1980;303:1189.

113. Moertel CG, Lefkopoulo M, Lipsitz S, Hahn RG, Klaassen D: Streptozocin-doxorubicin, streptozocin-fluorouracil or chlorozotocin in the treatment of advanced islet-cell carcinoma. N Engl J Med 1992;326:519.

9 Molecular Pathology of Ampullary, Intra-Pancreatic Bile Duct and Duodenal Cancers

Patrick Michl · Albrecht Neesse · Thomas M. Gress

1	*Introduction*	**235**
2	*Sporadic Periampullary Cancers*	**237**
2.1	Ampullary Cancer	237
2.1.1	Epidemiology	237
2.1.2	Prognosis	237
2.1.3	Morphological Appearance	238
2.1.4	Histological Classification	238
2.1.5	Correlation Between Molecular Markers and Histological Morphology	238
2.1.6	Genetic Alterations	240
2.1.7	Cytogenetic Alterations	240
2.1.8	Prognostic Markers	241
2.1.9	Ampullary Adenomas as Precursor Lesions	242
2.1.10	Molecular Markers Characterising the Adenoma-Carcinoma Sequence	242
2.2	Duodenal Cancer	243
2.2.1	Epidemiology	243
2.2.2	Prognosis	244
2.2.3	Morphological Appearance	244
2.2.4	Molecular Alterations	244
2.2.5	Precursor Lesions	245
2.3	Distal Bile Duct Cancer	245
2.3.1	Epidemiology	245
2.3.2	Prognosis	246
2.3.3	Molecular Alterations	246
3	*Periampullary Cancers in Familial Cancer Syndromes*	**247**
3.1	Ampullary and Duodenal Cancers in Familial Adenomatous Polyposis (FAP)	247
3.1.1	Epidemiology	247
3.1.2	Prognosis	247
3.1.3	Molecular Alterations	248
3.2	Ampullary and Duodenal Cancers in Hereditary Nonpolyposis Colorectal Cancer (HNPCC)	248

J. P. Neoptolemos, R. Urrutia, J. L. Abbruzzese, M. W. Büchler (eds.), *Pancreatic Cancer*,
DOI 10.1007/978-0-387-77498-5_9, © Springer Science+Business Media, LLC 2010

3.2.1 Epidemiology 248
3.2.2 Molecular Alterations 248

4   Outlook **248**

Abstract: Periampullary cancers include carcinomas of the pancreatic head, ampullary cancers at the papilla of Vater, duodenal cancers and distal bile duct cancers. Due to their anatomical location close to the orifice of the biliary tract into the duodenum, they often present with similar symptoms. Likewise, curative treatment approaches such as Whipple procedure or its variants, are applied similarly for most periampullary cancers. However, striking differences in survival are consistently being observed between the different periampullary tumor types, and histological classification is sometimes difficult due to overlapping histopathological phenotypes. During recent years, increasing effort has been made to elucidate the molecular alterations underlying the observed histopathological and prognostic differences among periampullary tumors. This chapter concentrates on the molecular pathology of the three non-pancreatic carcinoma types located in the periampullary region: Ampullary, duodenal and distal bile duct cancer. Immunohistochemically, ampullary carcinomas are subclassified into an intestinal-type and a pancreaticobiliary-type. Intestinal-type ampullary cancers closely resemble duodenal cancers and both are molecularly related to other bowel cancers such as colorectal cancer. In contrast, distal bile duct carcinomas and ampullary carcinomas of the pancreatico-biliary type are more related to ductal pancreatic cancer. However, the prognosis varies considerably, with survival rates being greatest for ampullary and duodenal cancers and least for pancreatic cancer. Periampullary cancers may be associated with familial cancer syndromes such as familial adenomatous polyposis (FAP) or hereditary non-polypous colon cancer (HNPCC). In these cases, the underlying molecular alterations have been elucidated. In contrast, data on the molecular patterns characterizing sporadic periampullary non-pancreatic cancers are still fragmentary and further studies are required to better understand their genetic, transcriptional and epigenetic characteristics.

1   Introduction

Obstructive jaundice is one of the cardinal symptoms of pancreatic ductal adenocarcinomas located in the head of the pancreas. Most frequently, this is caused by obstruction of the distal common bile duct close to the ampulla of Vater. The ampulla of Vater represents the common channel formed by the distal bile duct and the main pancreatic duct in the duodenal wall, which empties through the papilla [1].

Pancreatic cancer is the most prevalent, but by far not the only cause of malignant distal bile duct obstruction. All cancers located close to the ampulla of Vater, known as periampullary cancers, may lead to distal bile duct obstruction. By definition, periampullary cancers encompass four different types of tumors arising from different anatomic locations within 2 cm of the major papilla of Vater [2]: (1) Adenocarcinoma of the head of the pancreas, (2) ampullary cancer, (3) duodenal cancer, and (4) intrapancreatic distal bile duct cancer. A graphic overview of the different anatomic locations is depicted in ❯ *Fig. 9-1*, the frequency of the different tumor types among resected periampullary cancers is listed in ❯ *Table 9-1*. In addition to these four periampullary adenocarcinomas, very rare tumor entities exist which may also be found in the periampullary regions, such as duodenal carcinoids, mixed acinar-endocrine tumors, lymphomas, gastrointestinal stromal tumors (GIST), and hamartomas in patients with Peutz-Jeghers syndrome. This chapter will focus on the periampullary adenocarcinomas, the rare non-carcinomatous malignancies will be discussed elsewhere.

Determining the exact origin of adenocarcinomas arising in the periampullary region is sometimes difficult due to overlapping histopathological characteristics. However, the

◘ Fig. 9-1

Schematic overview on the different locations of periampullary cancers: (1) Ampullary carcinoma, intestinal-type; (2) Ampullary carcinoma, pancreaticobiliary-type; (3) Duodenal cancer; (4) Distal bile duct cancer; (5) Pancreatic ductal adenocarcinoma. Modified from [13].

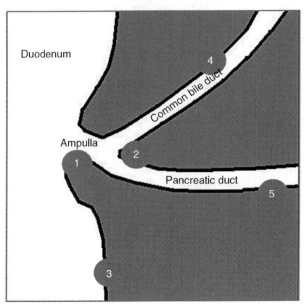

◘ Table 9-1

Proportion of the different tumor types among resected periampullary cancers [73]

Cancer type	Proportion of resected cancers
Ampullary carcinoma	15–25%
Duodenal carcinoma	10%
Distal bile duct carcinoma	10%
Pancreatic carcinoma	50–70%

prognosis of the four cancers varies considerably, with survival rates being greatest for duodenal and ampullary cancers, intermediate for distal biliary cancers and least for pancreatic cancer [2]. Radical resection involves a Whipple procedure or its variants similarly for all four cancer entities. However, even after radical resection, marked discrepancies in survival among periampullary cancers remain [2].

Several explanations exist for these striking differences in survival [1]: Small tumors arising directly from the ampulla or the periampullary duodenum may cause obstructive jaundice as an early symptom, whereas biliary obstruction caused by pancreatic cancers is usually a sign for advanced disease. However, there are also differences in both macroscopic and microscopic growth patterns between the tumor types. For example, ampullary and duodenal cancers show less vascular and perineural invasion compared to pancreatic cancer and distal bile duct cancer which are both characterized by a highly invasive growth pattern [1,3].

During recent years, research has started to focus on differences between the cancer entities in their molecular and genetic growth characteristics. Preliminary data so far indicate that each tumor type drives a distinct molecular program underlying its macroscopic and microscopic phenotype. However, some molecular alterations seem to be shared among several tumor types suggesting that some periampullary tumor types might be genetically closer related than others.

This article aims to summarize the data available in the literature on the molecular pathology of non-pancreatic periampullary cancers. In the future, increasing knowledge of the highly complex molecular alterations defining the different growth characteristics of the tumors will hopefully lead to improvements in diagnosis and tumor-type specific therapy.

2   Sporadic Periampullary Cancers

2.1   Ampullary Cancer

The papilla of Vater lies at the end of the intramural portion of the common bile duct and is located on the postermedial wall of the second part of the duodenum. The ampulla is the common pancreatico-biliary channel below the junction of the two ducts within the papilla (depicted schematically in ◉ Fig. 9-1) [4]. Therefore, the papilla encompasses the border between two completely different types of mucosa, the intestinal duodenal mucosa and the mucosa of the pancreatico-biliary channel [5]. Due to this close regional anatomy, the periampullary region is being exposed to three different juices, i.e., pancreatic, bile and duodenal juice, making it to an hot spot for malignant tumors of the small intestine [5].

2.1.1   Epidemiology

As compared to pancreatic ductal carcinoma, ampullary carcinomas are uncommon accounting for approximately 6–8% of the periampullary tumors [1,5,6], with age-standardized incidence rates of 3.8/1,000,000 in males and 2.7/1,000,000 in females [7]. Incidental ampullary cancers have been observed in 0.2% of all routine autopsies [2]. Although most ampullary carcinomas develop sporadically, several genetic disorders are known to predispose to this cancer type. Patients with familial adenomatous polyposis (FAP) frequently develop adenomas or carcinomas in the periampullary region. Therefore, these patients have to undergo frequent surveillance upper GI endoscopies to detect ampullary and duodenal adenomas [8]. In addition, neurofibromatosis type I seems to be associated with a higher incidence of both carcinomas and neuroendocrine tumors of the ampullary region [9].

2.1.2   Prognosis

The prognosis of ampullary carcinomas significantly exceeds the prognosis of pancreatic adenocarcinomas. Moreover, it exceeds also the prognosis of the other periampullary cancers, distal bile duct carcinoma and duodenal cancer. In a recent series from Büchler et al. mean survival time after curative resection was 60.9 months for ampullary cancer as compared to 42.9 or 45.4 months for distal bile duct or duodenal carcinomas, respectively [10]. A Korean series by Woo et al. further supported these data, observing 5-year survival rates of 68% in ampullary cancer versus 54% in distal cholangiocarcinomas [11]. Apart from these data from single cancer centers, nation-wide survival rates, however, may be considerably lower: A recent national population-based study from the US found a markedly lower 5-year survival rate after resection for ampullary cancer of 37%, indicating a bias towards better survival rates in single-center studies [12].

2.1.3   Morphological Appearance

Ampullary cancers can be morphologically classified as polypoid or ulcerating. Ulcerating carcinomas are usually diagnosed at more advanced stages with a higher likelihood of lymphatic or hematogenous spread, which is associated with a poor prognosis [5].

2.1.4   Histological Classification

Due to a broad histomorphologic spectrum of ampullary carcinomas, a reproducible histological classification is difficult [13]. Kimura et al. proposed two main histological types of ampullary carcinomas, an intestinal type and a pancreatico-biliary type [14]. In addition, several rare histological types such as mucinous, neuroendocrine or signet-ring cell carcinomas have been described [5].

Ampullary carcinomas showing intestinal differentiation are characterized by the presence of goblets cells and frequently have adenomatous components within the tumor [1,6]. In contrast, carcinomas of the pancreaticobiliary type more closely resemble carcinomas of the pancreas or extrahepatic bile ducts [5].

Conflicting data have been reported on the frequency of these two histological types [15]. In two case series published by Kimura [14] and Fischer [5], the pancreaticobiliary type predominated over the intestinal type. However, two other published cohorts show a higher frequency of intestinal-type cancers [16,17]. These discrepancies reflect the difficulties in classifying the subtypes of ampullary cancer by histological measures alone.

2.1.5   Correlation Between Molecular Markers and Histological Morphology

To allow a more reliable differentiation between the two subtypes of ampullary cancers, immunohistochemical analysis of selected mucins (MUC) has been applied. Two major mucin families can be distinguished: secreted mucins (MUC2, 5A, 5B, 6) and membrane-bound mucins (MUC1, 3, 4, 12, 17). Furthermore, certain cytokeratins (CKs) and the intestine-specific transcription factor CDX2 have been used for differentiation. Similar to intestinal epithelium, intestinal-type adenocarcinomas are characterized by positivity for CK20, CDX2 and secreted MUC2 (◉ *Fig. 9-2*) whereas CK7 and CK17 are absent. In contrast, pancreaticobiliary-type carcinomas display immunoreactivity for CK7, CK17 and membrane-bound MUC1 (◉ *Fig. 9-2*), but lack MUC2 and frequently also CK20 [5,18]. Recently, Paulsen et al. found two other mucins, MUC7 and MUC8, as expressed in normal duodenal mucosa, but absent in the ampulla of Vater and pancreaticobiliary-type cells. The authors speculate that

◘ Fig. 9-2

Immunohistochemical characterization of intestinal-type versus pancreaticobiliary-type ampullary carcinomas: Intestinal-type carcinomas are positive for mucin-2 (MUC2) and cytokeratin-20 (CK20) (left column), whereas pancreaticobiliary-type carcinomas are positive for mucin-1 (MUC1) and cytokeratin-7 (CK7) (right column), as detected immunohistochemically by specific antibodies. The intestinal-type ampullary cancer histologically resembles duodenal carcinomas, the hepatobiliary-type is similar to distal bile-duct carcinomas. Courtesy of Prof. G. Klöppel, Dept. of Pathology, University of Kiel, Germany.

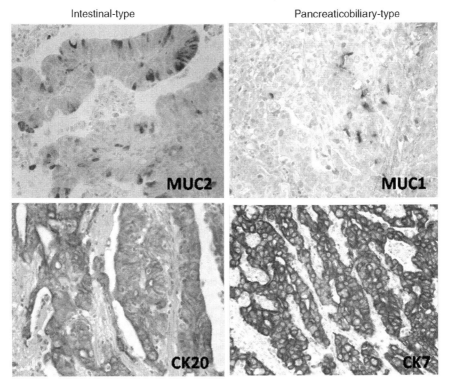

both mucins could serve as useful molecular markers to further facilitate the classification of ampullary cancers [19]. Vice versa, Zhou et al. showed that pancreaticobiliary-type cancers are positive for MUC5A, one of the secreted mucins, whereas intestinal-type carcinomas express carcinoembryonic antigen (CEA). The positivity of intestinal-type ampullary cancers for CEA further supports its relationship with other adenocarcinomas of the small and large intestine.

Interestingly, alterations in mismatch repair proteins such as loss of MLH1 or MSH2 or microsatellite instability, were observed only in intestinal-type carcinomas [15]. In addition, Perrone et al. described COX2 expression as another marker to distinguish between intestinal- and pancreaticobiliary-type tumors: COX2 was significantly overexpressed in intestinal-type versus pancreaticobiliary carcinomas [20]. These data add further evidence to the hypothesis that intestinal-type ampullary carcinomas and colorectal cancer are indeed pathogenetically closely related.

In analogy to survival rates of colon and pancreatic cancers, several studies observed a better prognosis of patients with intestinal-type ampullary cancer as compared to patients with pancreaticobiliary-type cancer [5,14,15].

Thus, immunohistological analysis allows a more precise classification with prognostic relevance into the two categories «intestinal» and «pancreaticobiliary» in cases which have remained unspecified after routine histomorphological examination [13].

2.1.6   Genetic Alterations

During recent years, increasing effort has been made to elucidate the molecular alterations underlying the observed histopathological and prognostic differences among periampullary tumors. Unfortunately, the different subtypes of ampullary carcinomas have not been specified in most studies.

Overall, carcinomas of the ampulla of Vater appear to share some molecular analogies with both colorectal and pancreatic cancers. However, the frequency of these alterations varies considerably between ampullary, colorectal and pancreatic cancers. For example, K-ras mutations are detected in all three cancers. In ductal pancreatic carcinomas, however, the frequency of K-ras mutations is markedly higher (up to 90%) as compared to both ampullary and colorectal carcinomas (ranging from 13 to 50%) [1,21,22]. Likewise, the overall frequency and the patterns of K-ras mutations in ampullary carcinomas resemble those of colorectal cancers. For example, codon 13 mutations occur rarely in pancreatic cancer, but account for up to 20% of the ampullary carcinomas, similar to colorectal cancers [1]. These findings underscore differences existing at the molecular level between pancreatic and ampullary cancer which may at least in part account for the lower aggressiveness of the latter [1].

In contrast, mutations in tumor suppressor genes such as p53 and DPC4/SMAD4 are found in both pancreatic and ampullary cancers with a similar frequency [23]: The tumor suppressor p53 is mutated in 14% of carcinoma-associated adenomas, 32% of early-stage and 53% of advanced ampullary carcinomas, suggesting that p53 mutations represent a late event in ampullary carcinogenesis and indicate the transition to high-grade, invasive cancers, similarly as described in both colon and pancreatic cancers [1]. Interestingly, the p53 status seems to influence the macroscopic growth pattern in ampullary cancers. Ulcerating carcinomas are more often associated with overexpression of p53 protein than polypoid carcinomas (67% vs. 32%) [24].

A growth factor receptor, the transforming growth factor $-\beta$-receptor-II (TGF-βR-II) is found to be mutated in 78% of ampullary cancers [25]. Mutated TGF-βR-II blocks the growth-inhibitory action of TGF-β, thereby promoting tumor progression. Mutations in TGF-βR-II might at least in part explain the invasive phenotype of advanced ampullary cancers which become resistant to the growth-inhibitory functions of TGF-β, but remain still sensitive to its proinvasive effects acting via alternative pathways.

2.1.7   Cytogenetic Alterations

On a chromosomal level, allelic loss of chromosome 17p and 18q has been detected in 55 and 36% of the ampullary cancer cases, respectively. Both LOHs were associated with poor prognosis in univariate analysis. 17p LOH which contains the p53 locus, served also as independent negative predictor of survival in multivariate analysis [26]. Furthermore, ampullary carcinomas with a complete loss of p53 function (one mutated p53 allele and 17p LOH), showed faster disease progression [27]. In another smaller series, additional allelic loss of 11p or 11q was described [28].

2.1.8   Prognostic Markers

Several genes have been identified as putative prognostic or diagnostic marker for ampullary carcinomas, including intracellular oncogenic signaling and effector molecules, surface markers and matrix components (see also ⊙ Table 9-2):

Santini et al. recently investigated the expression of effectors of the apoptotic machinery, Bax, Bcl-2, and p53, in patients with radically resected ampullary cancer. They identified a positive staining for the pro-apoptotic bcl-2 family member Bax as an independent positive predictor of survival [29]. Vice versa, increased cyclin D expression significantly correlated with increased tumor cell proliferation and worse clinical outcome [30].

Defects in DNA mismatch repair systems have been reported for numerous cancers including colon cancer, but are relatively uncommon in pancreatic cancer. Microsatellite instability (MSI) indicating defects in DNA repair mechanisms has been reported in 20% of ampullary cancers and was associated with better survival as compared to MSI-negative cases in a series by Achille et al. [26,31].

In contrast, other molecular markers indicating a poor prognosis in colon cancer, such as COX2 expression or telomerase activity, could not be validated as prognostic predictors in ampullary cancer [32,33].

Several growth factors as well as their receptors have been examined for their expression and prognostic relevance: Chen et al. reported VEGF expression and increased microvessel density to be associated with poor survival, suggesting that targeting VEGF might be a promising therapeutic strategy in ampullary carcinomas [34].

☐ Table 9-2

Prognostic markers in ampullary carcinomas

Gene/Alteration	Function	Pos./negative association with prognosis	Reference
Bax	Pro-apoptotic	+	[29]
Cyclin D	Cell cycle	−	[74]
Microsatellite instability	DNA repair	+	[31]
VEGF	Angiogenesis	−	[34]
ENT1	Nucleosid transport	−	[36]
KL-6	Mucin	−	[37]
CD44 variant 6	Cell adhesion	−	[38]
E-cadherin	Cell-cell contact	+	[39]
Osteonectin	Extracellular matrix	−	[40]

Interestingly, the expression of the epidermal growth factor receptor (EGFR) which acts as an upstream activator of several oncogenic signaling cascades including the Ras/raf pathway, was lower in ampullary cancer as compared to pancreatic cancer [35]. These findings indicate that EGFR targeting by small molecule inhibitors or monoclonal antibodies as routinely performed in colon and pancreatic cancer, might not be a promising therapeutic approach in ampullary cancer.

In addition, several other surface markers and membrane-bound molecules have been examined for their potential as prognostic indicators:

Recently, Santini et al. reported a correlation between short survival and expression of the equilibrative nucleoside transporter 1 hENT1, which is clinically relevant due to its function as transporter of the chemotherapeutic drug gemcitabine into the cell [36].

Another group suggested that expression of the transmembrane KL-6 mucin, a member of the MUC1 protein family, was associated with poor survival [37].

A variant of the cell adhesion molecule CD44 was found to be highly expressed in ampullary carcinomas and correlated with poor prognosis in advanced ampullary cancers [38]. The cell adhesion molecule CD44 was found to be highly expressed in ampullary carcinomas and correlated with poor prognosis in advanced ampullary cancers. Disruption of the cell-cell adhesion complex E-cadherin/beta-catenin was shown to be significantly associated with shorter survival: Expressional loss of E-cadherin and loss of membranous beta-catenin staining was correlated with poor survival [39].

In addition to intracellular and membrane-bound molecules, secreted matrix components have also been evaluated for their prognostic significance: Osteonectin, a matrix component also known as SPARC, was also correlated with worse prognosis and increased invasiveness, indicating that extracellular matrix components play a role in tumor progression in ampullary carcinomas [40].

2.1.9 Ampullary Adenomas as Precursor Lesions

In histological sections of ampullary carcinomas, residual adenomatous areas are found in 30–91% of the cases [5]. Vice versa, in about 23% of biopsied tubular adenomas and in up to 60% of biopsied villous adenomas, invasive cancers are detected after complete histological work-up of the resected specimens [4]. These observations suggest that ampullary carcinomas arise from preneoplastic adenomas, and follow an adenoma-carcinoma sequence as established in the colorectum [5]. Like colon adenomas, the majority of ampullary adenomas show a tubular, villous or tubulo-villous growth pattern. In addition, increasing grades of dysplasia ranging from low- to high-grade dysplastic lesions occur in ampullary adenomas, indicating a stepwise progression to invasive cancer. Low-grade adenomas show little mucous depletion with differentiated cells such as Paneth cells or goblet cells still present. In high-grade dysplasia, the epithelial polarity disappears, and the mitotic activity ratio as well as the nuclear/cytoplasmic ratio is increased [4].

2.1.10 Molecular Markers Characterising the Adenoma-Carcinoma Sequence

Several reports investigated immunohistochemical markers accompanying the transition from ampullary adenomas to invasive cancers (see also ❯ Fig. 9-3). Park et al. showed that loss of

◘ Fig. 9-3

Schematic overview of the present knowledge on accumulating molecular alterations characterizing the transition from normal epithelium via adenomas to invasive ampullary carcinomas.

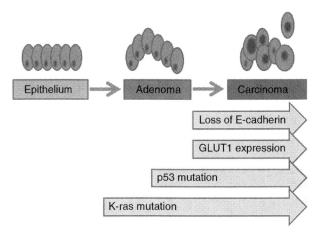

E-cadherin occurred rarely in adenomas, but was frequently found in invasive carcinomas [39]. Kim et al. examined the expression of the glucose transporter GLUT1, which is known to be increased in malignant tumors due to the higher metabolic needs of proliferating cell populations. GLUT1 was found to be over-expressed in 58% of the ampullary carcinomas, but only in 17% of the adenomas, suggesting that GLUT1 is associated with malignant transition and could serve as marker for malignancy [41].

The mutation patterns of K-ras and p53 have been extensively studied in ampullary adenomas versus carcinomas:

Takashima et al. evaluated p53 immunoreactivity indicating the presence of inactivating mutations in ampullary tumors. The authors report p53 positivity in 0% of pure adenomas, 36% of the adenomatous areas of carcinomas with adenomatous areas and 62% in the carcinomatous areas of carcinomas with adenomatous areas, and 56% in pure carcinoma [42]. These data suggest that p53 abnormality in ampullary tumors occurs during malignant transformation from adenoma to carcinomas and continues during tumor progression in invasive carcinomas.

K-ras mutations have been found in both adenomas and carcinomas of the ampulla. In particular, adenomas adjacent to a carcinoma harboring K-ras mutations showed the same mutation in over 95% of the cases. These data add to the growing body of evidence that K-ras mutations are an early event in ampullary carcinogenesis and are not suitable to distinguish adenomas from carcinomas [43].

2.2 Duodenal Cancer

2.2.1 Epidemiology

Like ampullary carcinomas of the intestinal-type, duodenal cancers arise from intestinal mucosa. However, the exact site of origin is not located in the ampulla, but in the adjacent duodenal wall (◉ *Fig. 9-1*).

In general, carcinomas of the small intestine represent a rare tumor entity with an incidence of approximately 1/100,000 [44]. Within the small bowel, the majority of carcinomas develop most frequently in the duodenum. Duodenal carcinomas account for approximately 0.5% of all malignancies in the gastrointestinal tract [45] and for 4–6% of all periampullary tumors [44] with a peak incidence in the seventh decade [46]. About 45% of duodenal carcinomas arise from the third and fourth parts of the duodenum. [47].

As for ampullary cancer, genetic predispositions include familial adenomatous polyposis (FAP) and hereditary nonpolyposis colorectal cancer (HNPCC). In addition, Crohn's disease and celiac disease are associated with increased risk for duodenal cancer [44].

2.2.2 Prognosis

In contrast to ampullary cancers, which usually present early with obstructive jaundice, the diagnosis of duodenal cancers is often hampered by non-specific and late symptoms such as weight loss, melena, bowel obstruction and biliary obstruction. Compared to ampullary cancer, clinical symptoms occur later in duodenal cancer due to the greater anatomical distance to the ampulla. The overall 5-year survival rate of non-ampullary duodenal adenocarcinomas ranges between 38 and 48%, according to two series published by Heniford et al. and Kelsey et al. [48,49]. If surgical resection as curative option is possible, 5-year survival increases up to 67% [50]. Interestingly, patients presenting with weight loss or obstructive symptoms had a markedly worse prognosis compared to patients presenting with melena, suggesting that patients with bowel obstruction and weight loss suffer from a more advanced disease at time of diagnosis.

2.2.3 Morphological Appearance

Duodenal cancers can be classified morphologically as polypoid, flat elevated and ulcerative-invasive. The polypoid phenotype is associated with superior prognosis compared to the flat-elevated and ulcerative cancers [2].

2.2.4 Molecular Alterations

Very few data exist on the molecular pathology of duodenal cancers. The available data in the literature suggest that the molecular profile of duodenal cancer resembles ampullary carcinomas, especially intestinal-type ampullary cancers.

Zhu et al. examined the expression levels of p53, c-neu, TGF-alpha, CEA, and mucin-1 in duodenal adenocarcinoma and ampullary adenocarcinoma by immunohistochemistry and found similar levels in both tumor entities [51].

Kim et al. compared genetic alterations in duodenal cancers to those found in distal bile duct and ampullary cancers [52]. They found microsatellite instability in approximately one third of the cases, indicating a relationship to intestinal-type ampullary cancers. Furthermore, they observed comparable levels of K-ras mutations (33%) and p53 mutations (45%) [52]. Based on the similarity of histological appearance and molecular alterations, Sarmiento et al. suggested to classify intestinal-type ampullary cancers as duodenal cancers [2]. A comparison

■ Table 9-3

Immunohistochemical and molecular characteristics of the non-pancreatic periampullary carcinomas

Cancer type	Typical Molecular markers	Genetic alterations
Ampullary carcinoma-intestinal subtype	CK20+, CDX2+, MUC2+, CEA+, COX2+, CK7−, CK17−	Microsatellite instability+, K-ras mutation 13–50%*, p53 mutation 11–53%*, TGFβR-II mutation 22–78%*, LOH 17p 55%*, LOH 18q 36%*
Duodenal carcinoma	CK7−, CK20+, CEA+	Microsatellite instability 33%, K-ras mutation 33%, p53 mutation 45%, TGFβR-II mutation 22%,
Ampullary carcinoma-hepatobiliary subtype	CK7+, CK17+, MUC1+, MUC5A+, MUC2−, CK20−, COX2−,	No microsatellite instability, K-ras mutation 13–50%*, p53 mutation 11–53%*, TGFβR-II mutation 22–78%*, LOH 17p 55%*, LOH 18q 36%*
Distal bile duct carcinoma	CK7+, MUC1+	p53 mutation 30%, K-ras mutation 17%, TGFβR-II mutation 0%,

*Analysis did not distinguish between intestinal- and hepatobiliary subtypes

of the typical immunohistochemical markers of duodenal cancer and intestinal-type ampullary cancer as compared to distal bile duct and hepatobiliary-type ampullary cancer is listed in ◗ *Table 9-3*. Further studies are warranted to better define the molecular profiles of duodenal and ampullary carcinomas in order to justify classification of both cancers as one entity.

2.2.5 Precursor Lesions

As for colon cancers and for ampullary carcinomas of the intestinal-type, duodenal carcinomas arise from adenomatous precursor lesions following the adenoma-carcinoma-sequence. Duodenal adenomas were seen in about 0.4% of all patients referred to diagnostic endoscopy [53]. The incidence of malignancy in duodenal adenomas reaches up to 50%, which is worse than the malignant propensity of villous adenomas in the colorectum that reaches approximately 30% [54]. Similar to colon cancer and intestinal-type ampullary cancers, several levels of dysplasia (low-grade and high-grade) as well as invasiveness (non-invasive adenoma vs. invasive adenocarcinoma) may be present within a single tumor after complete histological work-up of the surgical specimen. Generally, the likelihood for malignancy increases with size or ulcerative growth shape [54].

2.3 Distal Bile Duct Cancer

2.3.1 Epidemiology

As for the other periampullary cancers, distal bile duct carcinoma is a rare malignancy: Cholangiocellular carcinomas (CCCs) account for about 2% of all reported cancers, and can be classified in intrahepatic, perihilar and distal bile duct cancers. Distal cholangiocarcinomas, mostly arising from the bile duct located within the pancreatic head, account for approximately 27–40% of all cholangiocarcinomas [55,56]. They represent 5–14% of the periampullary carcinomas [57].

Risk factors for distal bile duct cancers include long-standing inflammatory processes such as primary sclerosing cholangitis (PSC), choledochus cysts and congenital anomalies, such as abnormal pancreaticobiliary junctions. These are defined as a common channel with a length of 8 mm or more. The abnormal pancreaticobiliary junction has been well recognized as risk factor for cholangiocellular carcinomas and gall bladder cancers in case series with Japanese patients. Recently, a cohort analysis from the United States confirmed in a Western population, that a common pancreaticobiliary channel of 8 mm or more was present in 44.8% of patients with biliary tract carcinomas compared to 6.2% of controls, suggesting that the length of the common channel with simultaneous exposure to pancreatic juice and bile acids posed a risk factor for biliary cancer [58].

2.3.2 Prognosis

The prognosis of distal extrahepatic cholangiocarcinomas is worse than ampullary and duodenal cancers. The 5-year survival after resection of distal bile duct cancer reaches only 27–54% versus 68% in ampullary cancer [11,59]. The median survival time in patients with distal cholangiocellular carcinoma ranges from 18 to 30 months [55,60]. Clinically and histologically, hepatic metastasis and lymph node involvement were more frequent in distal bile duct cancers compared to ampullary carcinomas [11]. Independent factors negatively influencing survival include distant metastasis, lymph node and/or venous invasion, histological grading and pancreatic infiltration [60].

2.3.3 Molecular Alterations

Similar to duodenal cancers, the data available on molecular alterations in distal bile duct cancers, is fragmentary, and has to be inferred from reports on the molecular pathogenesis of CCCs in general, not distinguishing between the intrahepatic, perihilar and distal/intrapancreatic locations. All CCCs arise from biliary epithelial cells undergoing a stepwise malignant transformation.

The tumor suppressor p53 is mutated in approximately 30% of cholangiocarcinomas, accompanied by its immunohistochemical overexpression. Cheng et al. described p53 overexpression as one of the most powerful negative predictors of survival in patients with distal cholangiocarcinoma [57].

Interestingly, two novel members of the p53 family, p63 and p73, were also found to be over-expressed in extrahepatic bile duct cancers, with p63 being significantly associated with distal location [61]. Since the effects of p63 and p73 and their different splice variants on tumor progression are still under debate, the functional relevance of these findings remains to be elucidated.

Recently, Ney et al. proposed a marker to distinguish distal bile duct and duodenal cancers from pancreatic cancers. They analysed the expression of Podocalyxin-like protein 1

(PODXL1), which plays a role as marker of precursor cells and poorly differentiated cells, in periampullary cancers. Interestingly, a high expression of PODXL1 in 44% of ductal pancreatic adenocarcinomas was found, whereas no or weak PODXL1 expression was detected in extrahepatic bile duct cancers and duodenal cancers [62].

3 Periampullary Cancers in Familial Cancer Syndromes

3.1 Ampullary and Duodenal Cancers in Familial Adenomatous Polyposis (FAP)

Familial adenomatous polyposis (FAP) is an autosomal dominant disorder caused by germline mutations in the adenomatous polyposis coli (APC) gene which is located on the long arm of chromosome 5 (5q21) [63].

In addition to colorectal neoplasias, the periampullary region is the second important hotspot for the development of ampullary or duodenal adenomas or carcinomas in patients with FAP.

3.1.1 Epidemiology

As shown for the sporadic tumors, ampullary and duodenal carcinomas in FAP patients arise from adenomas following the adenoma-carcinoma-sequence. This underscores the importance of detecting duodenal and ampullary adenomas as premalignant conditions in this patient group. High-resolution endoscopy and random biopsies revealed high rates of duodenal and ampullary adenomas in more than 70% of the patients, among them microadenomas in macroscopically normal appearing mucosa [63]. Frequently, numerous lesions can be found, most commonly in the second and third parts of the duodenum [64]. Interestingly, most duodenal adenomas distant from the ampullary region show microscopically a tubular structure with mild dysplasia, whereas adenomas in the periampullary region more frequently develop high-grade dysplasia and show a villous growth pattern [63]. Spigelman proposed a staging system for the severity of duodenal adenomatosis, with number, size, histology and dysplasia of the biopsied duodenal polyps as discriminating parameters. Stage I indicates mild duodenal polyposis, whereas stage IV indicates severe disease.

According to a prospective multi-national surveillance study of FAP patients by Bülow et al. the cumulative incidence rate of cancer detected by surveillance endoscopy in the duodenal region was 4.5% at age 57 years. The risk was significantly higher in patients with Spigelman stage IV at their first endoscopy than in those with stages 0-III. This underscores the need for regular surveillance upper GI endoscopy in FAP patients.

3.1.2 Prognosis

Due to the prophylactic colectomy prior to the development of colorectal cancer, periampullary tumors, in particular ampullary and duodenal cancers, nowadays account for 5–10% of deaths in FAP patients [1]. The cumulative 5-year survival for FAP-associated duodenal cancer was 44%, similar to sporadic duodenal cancers [65].

3.1.3   Molecular Alterations

On a molecular level, APC-inactivating mutations in FAP result in a stabilization and nuclear translocation of beta-catenin which leads to increased proliferation and oncogenic transformation. APC-inactivating mutations could be confirmed in the majority of duodenal adenomas in FAP patients [66].

Interestingly, somatic mutations within the APC gene are also quite common in sporadic ampullary carcinomas, ranging from 17% [67] up to 47% [68] in two independent series. This underlines once more the close relationship of at least a significant portion of ampullary cancers and colon cancers. The latter are well known to frequently harbor APC mutations. In contrast, pancreatic cancers, rarely carry APC mutations. Moreover, LOH at 5q21 where the APC gene is located, occurs in up to 70% of sporadic ampullary cancers, similarly to colon and gastric cancers. In pancreatic cancers, however, LOH 5q is uncommon [69].

3.2   Ampullary and Duodenal Cancers in Hereditary Nonpolyposis Colorectal Cancer (HNPCC)

Hereditary nonpolyposis colorectal cancer (HNPCC) represents the most common form of hereditary colorectal cancer, which is also associated with frequent development of extracolonic malignancies such as small bowel tumors including periampullary cancers.

3.2.1   Epidemiology

In HNPCC patients, the lifetime risk for small bowel cancers ranges from 1 to 4%, which is >100 times the risk in the general population. Most of the tumors occurred in the proximal small bowel, with equal distribution between the duodenum and the jejunum. Moreover, cancers of the small bowel may be the first and only cancer manifestation in HNPCC patients [70].

3.2.2   Molecular Alterations

HNPCC is an autosomal dominant trait with incomplete penetrance. HNPCC patients carry germ line mutations in the DNA mismatch repair genes, which include MLH1, MSH2, PMS2, and MSH6. About 90% of the identified germline mutations in the mismatch repair genes are found in two genes, MLH1 and MSH2 [71].

Interestingly, Park et al. observed a different mutation pattern in HNPCC patients with or without small bowel involvement and MSH2 mutations. Patients with HNPCC-associated small bowel cancers had fewer mutations in the MutL homolog interaction domain of MSH2 as compared to the control HNPCC group without small bowel cancers. However, an increased frequency of mutations in codons 626 to 733 was detected, a domain that has not previously been associated with a known function [71].

4   Outlook

Our current knowledge on the molecular pathology of the periampullary cancers, in particular non-pancreatic carcinomas, remains fragmentary. Given the overlapping histological appearance, conventional histopathological work-up may fail to identify the exact cellular origin of a particular periampullary tumor. Due to the different underlying tumor biology and the resulting prognostic differences, a more precise analysis of the molecular profiles of periampullary cancers is essential. Although the use of immunohistochemical marker proteins somewhat improved our ability to differentiate between the tumors, more systematic approaches are needed in order to reliably classify the cancer types, to make individual prognostic estimates and to individually tailor therapies.

DNA microarray technology represents a promising approach to screen for molecular differences in a high-throughput manner. By analyzing the expression of hundreds or thousands of genes simultaneously, an expression pattern rather than the expression levels of individual genes can be exploited to discriminate between tumor types. Expression profiling has already been applied to identify novel markers and expression patterns of ampullary carcinomas compared to normal duodenal tissues [72]. In the group of the authors of this chapter, experiments are in progress to establish gene expression profiles, which allow to discriminate between ampullary adenocarcinomas and pancreatic ductal adenocarcinomas. Preliminary results suggest that it is indeed feasible to discriminate between these tumor types with high accuracy by using expression profiles derived from tumor samples and even from low-volume fine needle aspirates. If these results can be corroborated, DNA expression profiles will be applied to obtain a molecular profile-based tissue diagnosis and, hopefully, information on the tumor biology, allowing to tailor targeted therapies for each individual.

Key Research Points

- Periampullary cancers include carcinomas of the pancreatic head, ampullary cancers, duodenal cancers and distal bile duct cancers.
- Due to overlapping histopathological phenotypes and close anatomical locations, accurate morphological and histological classification is sometimes difficult.
- Ampullary carcinomas are subclassified into an intestinal-type and a pancreaticobiliary-type.
- Intestinal-type ampullary cancers closely resemble duodenal cancers and both are molecularly related to other bowel cancers such as colorectal cancer. Distal bile duct carcinomas and ampullary carcinomas of the pancreatico-biliary type, however, are more related to ductal pancreatic cancer.

Future Scientific Directions

- Efforts should be made to further elucidate the molecular pathology underlying the observed histopathological and prognostic differences among the periampullary tumors, in particular the non-pancreatic adenocarcinomas.
- DNA microarray technology represents a promising approach to screen for molecular differences in a high-throughput manner.
- Detailed information on the tumor biology on a genome-wide expression level will offer the possibility to apply individually targeted therapies.

Clinical Implications

- The prognosis of periampullary cancers varies considerably, with survival rates being greatest for ampullary and duodenal cancers, intermediate for distal bile duct cancer and least for pancreatic cancer.
- Due to the differences in tumor behavior and survival, accurate classification of the periampullary cancers is crucial for an adequate prognostic estimate and an individualized therapeutic decision. Due to the lack of unambiguous molecular markers, accurate classification remains difficult and may not be possible in certain cases. It is thus of utmost importance to identify novel molecular signatures or sets of molecular markers that will assist both the pathologists and the clinicians in classifying periampullary tumors.
- Familial cancer syndromes such as familial adenomatous polyposis (FAP) or hereditary non-polypous colon cancer (HNPCC) show a high incidence of periampullary cancers. Patients with these genetic predispositions should therefore undergo a close surveillance program using upper gastrointestinal endoscopy.

Acknowledgment

We are indebted to Prof. G. Klöppel, Institute of Pathology, University of Kiel, Germany, for providing the immunohistochemical pictures of ampullary carcinomas.

References

1. Esposito I, Friess H, Buchler MW: Carcinogenesis of cancer of the papilla and ampulla: pathophysiological facts and molecular biological mechanisms. Langenbecks Arch Surg 2001;386(3):163–171.
2. Sarmiento JM, Nagomey DM, Sarr MG, Farnell MB: Periampullary cancers: are there differences? Surg Clin North Am 2001;81(3):543–555.
3. Yamaguchi K, Enjoji M, Tsuneyoshi M: Pancreato-duodenal carcinoma: a clinicopathologic study of 304 patients and immunohistochemical observation for CEA and CA19–9. J Surg Oncol 1991; 47(3):148–154.
4. Wittekind C, Tannapfel A: Adenoma of the papilla and ampulla – premalignant lesions? Langenbecks Arch Surg 2001;386(3):172–175.
5. Fischer HP, Zhou H: Pathogenesis of carcinoma of the papilla of Vater. J Hepatobiliary Pancreat Surg 2004;11(5):301–309.
6. Howe JR, Klimstra DS, Moccia RD, Conlon KC, Brennan MF: Factors predictive of survival in ampullary carcinoma. Ann Surg 1998;228(1):87–94.
7. Benhamiche AM, Jouve JL, Manfredi S, Prost P, Isambert N, Faivre J: Cancer of the ampulla of Vater: results of a 20-year population-based study. Eur J Gastroenterol Hepatol 2000;12(1):75–79.
8. Iwama T, Tomita H, Kawachi Y, Yoshinaga K, Kume S, Maruyama H, Mishima Y: Indications for local excision of ampullary lesions associated with familial adenomatous polyposis. J Am Coll Surg 1994;179(4):462–464.
9. Costi R, Caruana P, Sarli L, Violi V, Roncoroni L, Bordi C: Ampullary adenocarcinoma in neurofibromatosis type 1. Case report and literature review. Mod Pathol 2001;14(11):1169–1174.
10. Berberat PO, Kunzli BM, Gulbinas A, Ramanauskas T, Kleeff J, Muller MW, Wagner M, Friess H, Buchler MW: An audit of outcomes of a series of periampullary carcinomas. Eur J Surg Oncol 2009; 35(2):187–191.
11. Woo SM, Ryu JK, Lee SH, Yoo JW, Park JK, Kim YT, Jang JY, Kim SW, Kang GH, Yoon YB: Recurrence and prognostic factors of ampullary carcinoma after radical resection: comparison with distal extrahepatic cholangiocarcinoma. Ann Surg Oncol 2007;14(11):3195–3201.
12. O'Connell JB, Maggard MA, Manunga J, Jr., Tomlinson JS, Reber HA, Ko CY, Hines OJ: Survival after resection of ampullary carcinoma: a national population-based study. Ann Surg Oncol 2008; 15(7):1820–1827.

13. Zhou H, Schaefer N, Wolff M, Fischer HP: Carcinoma of the ampulla of Vater: comparative histologic/immunohistochemical classification and follow-up. Am J Surg Pathol 2004;28(7):875–882.

14. Kimura W, Futakawa N, Zhao B: Neoplastic diseases of the papilla of Vater. J Hepatobiliary Pancreat Surg 2004;11(4):223–231.

15. Sessa F, Furlan D, Zampatti C, Carnevali I, Franzi F, Capella C: Prognostic factors for ampullary adenocarcinomas: tumor stage, tumor histology, tumor location, immunohistochemistry and microsatellite instability. Virchows Arch 2007;451(3):649–657.

16. Matsubayashi H, Watanabe H, Yamaguchi T, Ajioka Y, Nishikura K, Kijima H, Saito T: Differences in mucus and K-ras mutation in relation to phenotypes of tumors of the papilla of vater. Cancer 1999;86(4):596–607.

17. McCarthy DM, Hruban RH, Argani P, Howe JR, Conlon KC, Brennan MF, Zahurak M, Wilentz RE, Cameron JL, Yeo CJ, Kern SE, Klimstra DS: Role of the DPC4 tumor suppressor gene in adenocarcinoma of the ampulla of Vater: analysis of 140 cases. Mod Pathol 2003;16(3):272–278.

18. Chu PG, Schwarz RE, Lau SK, Yen Y, Weiss LM: Immunohistochemical staining in the diagnosis of pancreatobiliary and ampulla of Vater adenocarcinoma: application of CDX2, CK17, MUC1, and MUC2. Am J Surg Pathol 2005;29(3):359–367.

19. Paulsen FP, Varoga D, Paulsen AR, Corfield A, Tsokos M: Prognostic value of mucins in the classification of ampullary carcinomas. Hum Pathol 2006;37(2):160–167.

20. Perrone G, Santini D, Zagami M, Vincenzi B, Verzi A, Morini S, Borzomati D, Coppola R, Antinori A, Magistrelli P, Tonini G, Rabitti C: COX-2 expression of ampullary carcinoma: correlation with different histotypes and clinicopathological parameters. Virchows Arch 2006;449(3):334–340.

21. Howe JR, Klimstra DS, Moccia RD, Conlon KC, Brennan MF: Factors predictive of survival in ampullary carcinoma. Ann Surg 1998;228(1):87–94.

22. Chung CH, Wilentz RE, Polak MM, Ramsoekh TB, Noorduyn LA, Gouma DJ, Huibregtse K, Offerhaus GJ, Slebos RJ: Clinical significance of K-ras oncogene activation in ampullary neoplasms. J Clin Pathol 1996;49(6):460–464.

23. Moore PS, Orlandini S, Zamboni G, Capelli P, Rigaud G, Falconi M, Bassi C, Lemoine NR, Scarpa A: Pancreatic tumours: molecular pathways implicated in ductal cancer are involved in ampullary but not in exocrine nonductal or endocrine tumorigenesis. Br J Cancer 2001;84(2):253–262.

24. Younes M, Riley S, Genta RM, Mosharaf M, Mody DR: p53 protein accumulation in tumors of the ampulla of Vater. Cancer 1995;76(7):1150–1154.

25. Imai Y, Tsurutani N, Oda H, Inoue T, Ishikawa T: Genetic instability and mutation of the TGF-beta-receptor-II gene in ampullary carcinomas. Int J Cancer 1998;76(3):407–411.

26. Iacono C, Verlato G, Zamboni G, Scarpa A, Montresor E, Capelli P, Bortolasi L, Serio G: Adenocarcinoma of the ampulla of Vater: T-stage, chromosome 17p allelic loss, and extended pancreaticoduodenectomy are relevant prognostic factors. J Gastrointest Surg 2007;11(5):578–588.

27. Scarpa A, Di PC, Talamini G, Falconi M, Lemoine NR, Iacono C, Achille A, Baron A, Zamboni G: Cancer of the ampulla of Vater: chromosome 17p allelic loss is associated with poor prognosis. Gut 2000;46(6):842–848.

28. Moore PS, Missiaglia E, Beghelli S, Bragantini E, Mina MM, Zamboni G, Falconi M, Scarpa A: Allelotype of ampulla of Vater cancer: highly frequent involvement of chromosome 11. J Cancer Res Clin Oncol 2004;130(6):339–345.

29. Santini D, Tonini G, Vecchio FM, Borzomati D, Vincenzi B, Valeri S, Antinori A, Castri F, Coppola R, Magistrelli P, Nuzzo G, Picciocchi A: Prognostic value of Bax, Bcl-2, p53, and TUNEL staining in patients with radically resected ampullary carcinoma. J Clin Pathol 2005;58(2):159–165.

30. Yamazaki K, Hanami K, Nagao T, Asoh A, Sugano I, Ishida Y: Increased cyclin D1 expression in cancer of the ampulla of Vater: relevance to nuclear beta catenin accumulation and K-ras gene mutation. Mol Pathol 2003;56(6):336–341.

31. Achille A, Biasi MO, Zamboni G, Bogina G, Iacono C, Talamini G, Capella G, Scarpa A: Cancers of the papilla of vater: mutator phenotype is associated with good prognosis. Clin Cancer Res 1997;3(10):1841–1847.

32. Kim HJ, Sohn TS, Lee KT, Lee JK, Paik SW, Rhee JC: Expression of cyclooxygenase-2 and its correlation with clinicopathologic factors of ampulla of vater cancer. J Korean Med Sci 2003;18(2):218–224.

33. Balcom JH, Keck T, Warshaw AL, Antoniu B, Graeme-Cook F, Fernandez-del CC: Telomerase activity in periampullary tumors correlates with aggressive malignancy. Ann Surg 2001;234(3):344–350.

34. Chen L, Tao SF, Zheng YX: Prognostic significance of vascular endothelial growth factor expression and microvessel density in carcinoma of ampulla of Vater. Hepatogastroenterology 2006;53(67):45–50.

35. Smeenk HG, Erdmann J, van DH, van MR, Hop WC, Jeekel J, van Eijck CH: Long-term survival after radical resection for pancreatic head and ampullary cancer: a potential role for the EGF-R. Dig Surg 2007;24(1):38–45.

36. Santini D, Perrone G, Vincenzi B, Lai R, Cass C, Alloni R, Rabitti C, Antinori A, Vecchio F, Morini S,

Magistrelli P, Coppola R, et al.: Human equilibrative nucleoside transporter 1 (hENT1) protein is associated with short survival in resected ampullary cancer. Ann Oncol 2008;19(4):724–728.

37. Tang W, Inagaki Y, Kokudo N, Guo Q, Seyama Y, Nakata M, Imamura H, Sano K, Sugawara Y, Makuuchi M: KL-6 mucin expression in carcinoma of the ampulla of Vater: association with cancer progression. World J Gastroenterol 2005;11(35): 5450–5454.

38. Yokoyama Y, Hiyama E, Murakami Y, Matsuura Y, Yokoyama T: Lack of CD44 variant 6 expression in advanced extrahepatic bile duct/ampullary carcinoma. Cancer 1999;86(9):1691–1699.

39. Park S, Kim SW, Lee BL, Jung EJ, Kim WH: Expression of E-cadherin and beta-catenin in the adenoma-carcinoma sequence of ampulla of Vater cancer. Hepatogastroenterology 2006;53(67):28–32.

40. Bloomston M, Ellison EC, Muscarella P, Al-Saif O, Martin EW, Melvin WS, Frankel WL: Stromal osteonectin overexpression is associated with poor outcome in patients with ampullary cancer. Ann Surg Oncol 2007;14(1):211–217.

41. Kim SJ, Lee HW, Kim DC, Rha SH, Hong SH, Jeong JS: Significance of GLUT1 expression in adenocarcinoma and adenoma of the ampulla of Vater. Pathol Int 2008;58(4):233–238.

42. Takashima M, Ueki T, Nagai E, Yao T, Yamaguchi K, Tanaka M, Tsuneyoshi M: Carcinoma of the ampulla of Vater associated with or without adenoma: a clinicopathologic analysis of 198 cases with reference to p53 and Ki-67 immunohistochemical expressions. Mod Pathol 2000;13(12):1300–1307.

43. Howe JR, Klimstra DS, Cordon-Cardo C, Paty PB, Park PY, Brennan MF: K-ras mutation in adenomas and carcinomas of the ampulla of vater. Clin Cancer Res 1997;3(1):129–133.

44. Berkhout M, Nagtegaal ID, Cornelissen SJ, Dekkers MM, van de Molengraft FJ, Peters WH, Nagengast FM, van Krieken JH, Jeuken JW: Chromosomal and methylation alterations in sporadic and familial adenomatous polyposis-related duodenal carcinomas. Mod Pathol 2007;20(12):1253–1262.

45. Hurtuk MG, Devata S, Brown KM, Oshima K, Aranha GV, Pickleman J, Shoup M: Should all patients with duodenal adenocarcinoma be considered for aggressive surgical resection? Am J Surg 2007;193(3):319–324.

46. Hung FC, Kuo CM, Chuah SK, Kuo CH, Chen YS, Lu SN, Chang Chien CS: Clinical analysis of primary duodenal adenocarcinoma: an 11-year experience. J Gastroenterol Hepatol 2007;22(5):724–728.

47. Tocchi A, Mazzoni G, Puma F, Miccini M, Cassini D, Bettelli E, Tagliacozzo S: Adenocarcinoma of the third and fourth portions of the duodenum: results of surgical treatment. Arch Surg 2003;138(1):80–85.

48. Heniford BT, Iannitti DA, Evans P, Gagner M, Henderson JM: Primary nonampullary/periampullary adenocarcinoma of the duodenum. Am Surg 1998;64(12):1165–1169.

49. Kelsey CR, Nelson JW, Willett CG, Chino JP, Clough RW, Bendell JC, Tyler DS, Hurwitz HI, Morse MA, Clary BM, Pappas TN, Czito BG: Duodenal adenocarcinoma: patterns of failure after resection and the role of chemoradiotherapy. Int J Radiat Oncol Biol Phys 2007;69(5):1436–1441.

50. Sohn TA, Yeo CJ, Cameron JL, Lillemoe KD, Talamini MA, Hruban RH, Sauter PK, Coleman J, Ord SE, Grochow LB, Abrams RA, Pitt HA: Should pancreaticoduodenectomy be performed in octogenarians? J Gastrointest Surg 1998;2(3): 207–216.

51. Zhu L, Kim K, Domenico DR, Appert HE, Howard JM: Adenocarcinoma of duodenum and ampulla of Vater: clinicopathology study and expression of p53, c-neu, TGF-alpha, CEA, and EMA. J Surg Oncol 1996;61(2):100–105.

52. Kim SG, Chan AO, Wu TT, Issa JP, Hamilton SR, Rashid A: Epigenetic and genetic alterations in duodenal carcinomas are distinct from biliary and ampullary carcinomas. Gastroenterology 2003; 124(5):1300–1310.

53. Jepsen JM, Persson M, Jakobsen NO, Christiansen T, Skoubo-Kristensen E, Funch-Jensen P, Kruse A, Thommesen P: Prospective study of prevalence and endoscopic and histopathologic characteristics of duodenal polyps in patients submitted to upper endoscopy. Scand J Gastroenterol 1994;29(6): 483–487.

54. Cavallini M, Cavaniglia D, Felicioni F, Vitale V, Pilozzi E, Ziparo V: Large periampullary villous tumor of the duodenum. J Hepatobiliary Pancreat Surg 2007;14(5):526–528.

55. DeOliveira ML, Cunningham SC, Cameron JL, Kamangar F, Winter JM, Lillemoe KD, Choti MA, Yeo CJ, Schulick RD: Cholangiocarcinoma: thirty-one-year experience with 564 patients at a single institution. Ann Surg 2007;245(5):755–762.

56. Nakeeb A, Pitt HA, Sohn TA, Coleman J, Abrams RA, Piantadosi S, Hruban RH, Lillemoe KD, Yeo CJ, Cameron JL: Cholangiocarcinoma. A spectrum of intrahepatic, perihilar, and distal tumors. Ann Surg 1996;224(4):463–473.

57. Cheng Q, Luo X, Zhang B, Jiang X, Yi B, Wu M: Distal bile duct carcinoma: prognostic factors after curative surgery. A series of 112 cases. Ann Surg Oncol 2007;14(3):1212–1219.

58. Roukounakis N, Manolakopoulos S, Tzourmakliotis D, Bethanis S, McCarty TM, Cuhn J: Biliary tract malignancy and abnormal pancreaticobiliary junction in a Western population. J Gastroenterol Hepatol 2007;22(11):1949–1952.

59. Murakami Y, Uemura K, Hayashidani Y, Sudo T, Hashimoto Y, Ohge H, Sueda T: Prognostic significance of lymph node metastasis and surgical margin status for distal cholangiocarcinoma. J Surg Oncol 2007;95(3):207–212.

60. Ebata T, Nagino M, Nishio H, Igami T, Yokoyama Y, Nimura Y: Pancreatic and duodenal invasion in distal bile duct cancer: paradox in the tumor classification of the American Joint Committee on Cancer. World J Surg 2007;31(10):2008–2015.

61. Hong SM, Cho H, Moskaluk CA, Yu E, Zaika AI: p63 and p73 expression in extrahepatic bile duct carcinoma and their clinical significance. J Mol Histol 2007;38(3):167–175.

62. Ney JT, Zhou H, Sipos B, Buttner R, Chen X, Kloppel G, Gutgemann I: Podocalyxin-like protein 1 expression is useful to differentiate pancreatic ductal adenocarcinomas from adenocarcinomas of the biliary and gastrointestinal tracts. Hum Pathol 2007;38(2):359–364.

63. Kadmon M, Tandara A, Herfarth C: Duodenal adenomatosis in familial adenomatous polyposis coli. A review of the literature and results from the Heidelberg Polyposis Register. Int J Colorectal Dis 2001;16(2):63–75.

64. Kashiwagi H, Spigelman AD, Debinski HS, Talbot IC, Phillips RK: Surveillance of ampullary adenomas in familial adenomatous polyposis. Lancet 1994;344 (8936):1582.

65. Bulow S, Bjork J, Christensen IJ, Fausa O, Jarvinen H, Moesgaard F, Vasen HF: Duodenal adenomatosis in familial adenomatous polyposis. Gut 2004; 53(3):381–386.

66. Toyooka M, Konishi M, Kikuchi-Yanoshita R, Iwama T, Miyaki M: Somatic mutations of the adenomatous polyposis coli gene in gastroduodenal tumors from patients with familial adenomatous polyposis. Cancer Res 1995;55(14):3165–3170.

67. Achille A, Scupoli MT, Magalini AR, Zamboni G, Romanelli MG, Orlandini S, Biasi MO, Lemoine NR, Accolla RS, Scarpa A: APC gene mutations and allelic losses in sporadic ampullary tumours: evidence of genetic difference from tumours associated with familial adenomatous polyposis. Int J Cancer 1996;68(3):305–312.

68. Imai Y, Oda H, Tsurutani N, Nakatsuru Y, Inoue T, Ishikawa T: Frequent somatic mutations of the APC and p53 genes in sporadic ampullary carcinomas. Jpn J Cancer Res 1997;88(9):846–854.

69. Achille A, Baron A, Zamboni G, Di PC, Orlandini S, Scarpa A: Chromosome 5 allelic losses are early events in tumours of the papilla of Vater and occur at sites similar to those of gastric cancer. Br J Cancer 1998;78(12):1653–1660.

70. Aarnio M, Sankila R, Pukkala E, Salovaara R, Aaltonen LA, de la CA, Peltomaki P, Mecklin JP, Jarvinen HJ: Cancer risk in mutation carriers of DNA-mismatch-repair genes. Int J Cancer 1999; 81(2):214–218.

71. Park JG, Kim DW, Hong CW, Nam BH, Shin YK, Hong SH, Kim IJ, Lim SB, Aronson M, Bisgaard ML, Brown GJ, Burn J, et al.: Germ line mutations of mismatch repair genes in hereditary nonpolyposis colorectal cancer patients with small bowel cancer: International Society for Gastrointestinal Hereditary Tumours Collaborative Study. Clin Cancer Res 2006;12(11 Pt 1):3389–3393.

72. Van Heek NT, Maitra A, Koopmann J, Fedarko N, Jain A, Rahman A, Iacobuzio-Donahue CA, Adsay V, Ashfaq R, Yeo CJ, Cameron JL, Offerhaus JA, et al.: Gene expression profiling identifies markers of ampullary adenocarcinoma. Cancer Biol Ther 2004;3(7):651–656.

73. Yeo CJ, Cameron JL, Sohn TA, Lillemoe KD, Pitt HA, Talamini MA, Hruban RH, Ord SE, Sauter PK, Coleman J, Zahurak ML, Grochow LB, et al.: Six hundred fifty consecutive pancreaticoduodenectomies in the 1990s: pathology, complications, and outcomes. Ann Surg 1997;226(3):248–257.

74. Yamazaki K, Hanami K, Nagao T, Asoh A, Sugano I, Ishida Y: Increased cyclin D1 expression in cancer of the ampulla of Vater: relevance to nuclear beta catenin accumulation and K-ras gene mutation. Mol Pathol 2003;56(6):336–341.

10 Miscellaneous Non-Pancreatic Non-Endocrine Tumors

John D. Abad · Keith D. Lillemoe

1	*Epidemiology*	*257*
2	*Pathology*	*257*
2.1	Ampullary Neoplasms	257
2.1.1	Benign Ampullary Tumors	258
2.1.2	Malignant Ampullary Tumors	259
2.2	Distal Common Bile Duct Neoplasms	261
2.2.1	Benign Distal Bile Duct Tumors	261
2.2.2	Malignant Distal Bile Duct Tumors	262
2.3	Duodenal Neoplasms	263
2.3.1	Benign Duodenal Tumors	263
2.3.2	Malignant Duodenal Tumors	264
2.4	Rare Periampullary Tumors	264
2.4.1	Mesenchymal Neoplasms	264
2.4.2	Lymphomas, Metastatic Tumors and Pseudotumors	265
3	*Clinical Presentation*	*265*
4	*Diagnostic Evaluation*	*266*
4.1	Laboratory Data	266
4.2	Imaging Studies	266
4.2.1	Ultrasonography	266
4.2.2	Computed Tomography	267
4.2.3	Magnetic Resonance Cholangiopancreatography	268
4.2.4	Endoscopy/Endoscopic Ultrasound	268
4.2.5	Endoscopic Retrograde Cholangiopancreatography	270
4.2.6	Percutaneous Transhepatic Cholangiography	271
4.3	Preoperative Staging	272
5	*Surgical Management*	*273*
5.1	Endoscopic Resection	273
5.2	Local Excision	273
5.3	Pancreaticoduodenectomy	275

J. P. Neoptolemos, R. Urrutia, J. L. Abbruzzese, M. W. Büchler (eds.), *Pancreatic Cancer*,
DOI 10.1007/978-0-387-77498-5_10, © Springer Science+Business Media, LLC 2010

5.4   Segmental Resection 276
5.5   Palliative Procedures 276

6   *Adjuvant and Neoadjuvant Therapy* *276*

7   *Survival* *277*

Abstract: Non-endocrine, non-pancreatic periampullary tumors are generally classified as arising from the ampulla of Vater, distal common bile duct or duodenum. The most common clinical finding on presentation is obstructive jaundice. These lesions may occur spontaneously or as part of a hereditary syndrome (familial adenomatous polyposis, Gardner's syndrome, inflammatory bowel disease). The most effective diagnostic strategies for determining extent of disease and resectability of periampullary tumors include dual-phase computed tomography and endoscopic ultrasound. Small, benign periampullary lesions may be amenable to endoscopic resection. For benign lesions <3 cm that are unable to be completely removed endoscopically, transduodenal local resection should be considered. Appropriate surgical candidates with larger lesions >3 cm or suspicion of invasive carcinoma should undergo a pancreaticoduodenectomy. Five-year survival for duodenal, ampullary, and distal common bile duct carcinomas are 51–59, 37–39 and 23–27%, respectively. For each of these tumors, both lymph node status and negative margins are significant predictors of outcome. At this point, neoadjuvant and adjuvant therapies have not clearly demonstrated a survival benefit for non-pancreatic periampullary cancers. The future success in treating these cancers likely rests in the development of novel biological and targeted therapies in the setting of well designed multi-institutional clinical trials. This chapter will focus on benign and malignant non-pancreatic and non-neuroendocrine periampullary tumors and will include the pathology, clinical presentation, diagnostic work-up, and management strategies to approach these neoplasms.

1 Epidemiology

The majority of periampullary tumors are malignant, with pancreatic adenocarcinoma being the most common followed by cancers of the ampulla of Vater, distal common bile duct, and duodenum, respectively. Periampullary adenocarcinoma has a yearly incidence in the United States of approximately 30,000 cases which has remained stable over the last few decades [1]. Pancreatic adenocarcinoma likely accounts for up to 90% of these cases, although without surgical resection and pathologic analysis, the actual specific organ of origin can be difficult to determine. The relative frequency of malignant periampullary neoplasms in resected specimens is shown in ⊙ *Table 10-1* [2]. The percentage of non-pancreatic malignancies is higher in surgical resection series since such tumors have a higher rate of resection compared to primary pancreatic cancers.

2 Pathology

2.1 Ampullary Neoplasms

Tumors of the ampulla can be either benign or malignant. In most series, the majority of ampullary neoplasms are malignant. Compared with other neoplasms of the gastrointestinal tract, the incidence of ampullary neoplasms is low. Autopsy studies demonstrate an incidence of approximately 0.04–0.12% [3–5]. Overall, ampullary carcinomas represent only 0.2% of gastrointestinal cancers [6].

2.1.1 Benign Ampullary Tumors

Benign adenomas are the most commonly diagnosed ampullary neoplasm. The incidence of sporadic adenomas appears to be increasing and is likely the direct result of increased detection due to the increased utilization of upper endoscopy. Ampullary adenomas are classified by their microscopic findings as either intestinal-type or biliary type. Intestinal-type may occur either as sporadic tumors or in patients with familial adenomatous polyposis (FAP). Sporadic ampullary adenomas usually occur during the sixth decade of life and are an average diameter of 2 cm [7,8] (◐ Fig. 10-1). There appears to be a slight increase in incidence in women over men.

Tumors of the ampulla can also occur in association with hereditary disorders such as familial adenomatous polyposis (FAP). Ampullary adenomas are present in 50–85% of FAP patients; however, the cumulative life-time risk is near 100% [9,10]. The ratio of male to female appears to be equal in cases associated with familial polyposis syndromes. The median

◐ Table 10-1

Relative frequency periampullary neoplasms in resected specimens

Location	Percentage (%)
Head of pancreas	56
Ampulla of Vater	21
Distal common bile duct	17
Duodenum	3

◐ Fig. 10-1

Endoscopic appearance of benign villous adenoma.

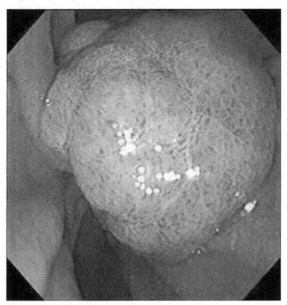

age at presentation for familial adenomas is earlier than the sporadic cases with a median age of 30–40 years. The diagnosis of periampullary adenomas associated with FAP usually occurs well after the diagnosis of colonic polyps typically at a mean follow up of 17 years after colectomy [4]. At presentation, these lesions can often be multiple and involve both the ampulla and duodenal mucosal surface simultaneously.

Similar to the well defined transformation of colonic adenomas into adenocarcinoma, ampullary adenomas have the potential for malignant degeneration. The likelihood of malignancy is related to the size and type of adenoma. Adenocarcinoma is present in approximately 20% of tubular adenomas and 60% of villous adenomas [11]. FAP patients represent a 100–200 fold increase in the life-time risk of ampullary adenocarcinoma [12]. However, in a multicenter study of 1,262 patients with FAP, only 4% developed periampullary carcinoma [13]. Regardless, close screening and follow-up is extremely important in this population.

2.1.2 Malignant Ampullary Tumors

Ampullary carcinoma is classified as four types based on macroscopic features: intra-ampullary (24%), periampullary duodenal (6%), mixed exophytic (31%) and mixed ulcerated (39%) (❯ *Fig. 10-2*). Overall, intra-ampullary cancers have a better prognosis than other sub-types as these tumors usually present smaller lesions with less angiolymphatic invasion, fewer lymph node metastases, and less direct invasion of the pancreas.

Adenocarcinomas of the ampulla are further divided into intestinal-type (50%) and pancreaticobiliary type (20%) based on histologic features. The most prevalent type of ampullary adenocarcinomas are intestinal-type which resemble primary adenocarcinomas of the colon pathologically with simple or cribriform glands lined by atypical cells with features

◻ Fig. 10-2

Surgical specimen demonstrating an ulcerated ampullary carcinoma. The papilla is replaced by an exophytic papillary and ulcerated tumor. (Reprinted from Mino and Lauwers, [14].)

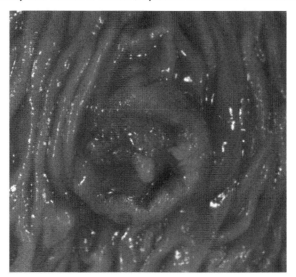

of intraluminal necrosis and inflammation (❯ *Fig. 10-3*). Pancreaticobiliary-type resembles primary pancreatic and biliary adenocarcinomas. These tumors are composed of simple glands lined with low columnar cells with features of atypical nuclei and surrounding desmoplastic stroma (❯ *Fig. 10-4*). Compared to the intestinal type, the pancreaticobiliary type more often demonstrates perineural invasion, but angiolymphatic invasion is less common. In instances where both microscopic features of intestinal and pancreaticobiliary are present, these tumors are classified as intestinal, unless there is a predominant pancreaticobiliary phenotype. A recent series from the University of California San Francisco of

❑ Fig. 10-3
Adenocarcinoma, intestinal type. The tumor is composed of complexed glands lined by atypical cells. Note the typical luminal inflammation. (Reprinted from Mino and Lauwers, [14].)

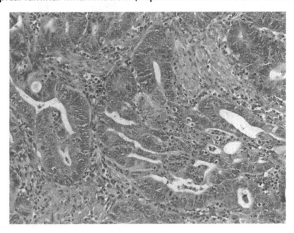

❑ Fig. 10-4
Adenocarcinoma, pancreatobiliary type. The tumor is composed of simple malignant glands lined by low columnar cells. Note the markedly atypical nuclei and the surrounding desmoplasia. (Reprinted from Mino and Lauwers, [14].)

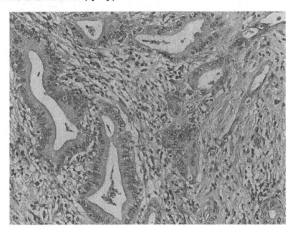

118 patients with ampullary adenocarcinomas noted patients with pancreaticobiliary type presented with jaundice more frequently and had significantly worse survival compared to those with intestinal type [15].

There are several unusual sub-types of ampullary cancers including papillary, mucinous and signet-ring carcinomas. Papillary carcinomas are uncommon and are reported in 6% of ampullary carcinomas. They are classified as either invasive or noninvasive. Invasive papillary carcinomas appear as complex branching papillary structures with fibrovascular cores and/or micro papillary structures without fibrovascular cores. These are lined by either intestinal or pancreatobiliary-type cells. In contrast, noninvasive papillary carcinomas are exophytic tumors arising in the intra-ampullary mucosa and lined by pancreatobiliary-type epithelium. The neoplasms are similar to noninvasive papillary carcinomas of the extrahepatic bile ducts and noninvasive intraductal papillary mucinous neoplasms of the pancreas.

Mucinous or colloid carcinomas represent only 4–7% of ampullary carcinomas. These neoplasms demonstrate two particular morphologies both with greater than 50% containing extracellular mucin. These carcinomas are composed of columnar epithelium with nuclear atypia or contain clusters of neoplastic cells.

Signet-ring cell carcinomas of the ampulla are extremely rare. These neoplasms contain cells with nuclei forced to the periphery by intracytoplasmic mucin. In order to diagnose these tumors, greater than 50% of the tumors must contain signet-ring cells with a diffuse growth pattern, and a primary from another site must be excluded.

2.2   Distal Common Bile Duct Neoplasms

The common bile duct (CBD) is divided into four parts: (1) supraduodenal, (2) retroduodenal, (3) intrapancreatic, and (4) intraduodenal. The periampullary distal CBD is considered to include the intrapancreatic and intraduodenal segments. Tumors of epithelial, non-epithelial, and mesenchymal origin can arise from the distal CBD.

2.2.1   Benign Distal Bile Duct Tumors

Adenomas are extremely rare lesions of the distal common bile duct and are less common than carcinomas. These lesions are usually small, often single and may appear as pedunculated or sessile polyps and are histologically classified similarly to adenomas of the colon: tubular, tubulovillous, and villous. Reports of distal common bile duct adenomas have been reported in familial adenomatous polyposis and Gardner's syndrome [16].

Cystadenomas are mucinous cystic tumors that can arise from various structures in the upper gastrointestinal tract, most commonly, the liver, pancreas, and extrahepatic bile ducts. These tumors occur in the biliary tree of middle-aged females and may grow as large as 20 cm. Malignant transformation is rare, although dysplasia is seen in 13% of these tumors [17]. Complete local excision for symptomatic lesions is necessary due to a high rate of recurrence if incompletely resected.

Biliary papillomatosis is a rare phenomenon of multicentric complex papillary neoplasms which involve the extra and intrahepatic biliary systems, gallbladder and may extend into the pancreatic ducts. It affects both males and females equally during the sixth decade of life. Surgical resection is difficult and recurrence is common. The treatment of choice is total hepatectomy and liver transplantation.

Granular cell tumors are neoplasms of the extrahepatic biliary system usually involving the common bile duct. These tumors typically occur in young women (median age 34 years). Patients typically present with jaundice and abdominal pain. Granular cell tumors are occasionally multicentric with lesions in the gallbladder, skin, omentum, esophagus, and stomach. Within the common bile duct, these lesions appear as small (<2 cm), firm, submucosal nodules that invade the lumen. These tumors are not malignant, however may invade into periductal tissue and adjacent pancreas. Diagnosis usually occurs by ultrasound with subsequent MRCP/ERCP. These lesions are clinically similar to malignant distal common bile duct tumors and often require operative resection to make the diagnosis.

2.2.2 Malignant Distal Bile Duct Tumors

The incidence of extrahepatic biliary malignancy in the United States is low, approximately 0.54 cases per 100,000, and approximately 2,000 new cases of distal bile duct cancers per year [18]. Although the etiology is unknown, there are several well documented risk factors. Patients with ulcerative colitis and sclerosing cholangitis have a relative risk of 30% in developing bile duct carcinoma and typically present at an earlier age (median age 42 years) [19,20]. Several reports from Japan have demonstrated that an abnormal choledochopancreatic junction predisposes to common bile duct, as well as, gallbladder carcinoma. An abnormally long common channel involving the pancreatic and bile duct results in reflux of pancreatic juice into the common bile duct and induces metaplastic changes. These changes may lead to dysplastic changes which further progress to carcinoma in situ and invasive cancer. This phenomenon is also believed to contribute to the increased risk of cholangiocarcinoma in patients with congenital biliary cystic disease (i.e., choledochal cysts, Caroli's disease). Hepatolithiasis and biliary parasitic infestation (*Clonorchis sinensis* or *Opisthorchis viverrini*), both prevalent in parts of Asia, also have well documented increased risks for cholangiocarcinoma.

Using the classification of cholangiocarcinoma proposed by Nakeeb and colleagues, these lesions are divided into intrahepatic, perihilar, and distal subgroups [21]. The majority of cholangiocarcinomas arise in the perihilar region. The distal common bile duct is the site of origin of 20–30% of all cholangiocarcinomas and represents approximately 5–10% of all periampullary tumors [18,21–23]. The majority of these tumors occur in older males (median age 68 years) with the incidence similar between blacks and whites.

Adenocarcinoma is the primary histologic subtype in the distal common bile duct malignancies. The three macroscopic classifications of cholangiocarcinoma are sclerosing, nodular, and papillary. Sclerosing lesions are the most common and appear as thickening of the bile duct with diffuse infiltration of adjacent tissues. Nodular tumors are irregular nodules that invade into the lumen of the bile duct. Nodular-sclerosing lesions, as implied, have characteristics of both. Papillary subtype represents only 10% of cholangiocarcinomas and is more common in the distal bile duct than the hepatic bifurcation [24]. These tumors are soft polypoid lesions with limited transmural involvement that expands the duct with an intraductal growth pattern. These lesions often have little or no invasive component and generally have a more favorable prognosis compared with the sclerosing subtype [25,26]. These tumors spread longitudinally along the duct wall beneath the epithelial lining. As a result, preoperative imaging and intraoperative examination may not appreciate the extent of submucosal spread, highlighting the importance of intraoperative frozen section to determine adequate margins for resection (*Table 10-2*).

◘ Table 10-2
Tumor Classification Table

Miscellaneous Non-Pancreatic Non-Neuroendocrine Tumors Periampullary Tumor Classification
1. Ampullary Neoplasms
A. Benign adenomas
B. Adenocarcinomas (intestinal-type, pancreaticobiliary-type)
C. Papillary carcinoma (invasive, noninvasive)
D. Mucinous or colloid carcinomas
E. Signet-ring carcinomas
2. Distal Common Bile Duct Neoplasms
A. Benign adenomas
B. Cystadenomas
C. Biliary papillomatosis
D. Granular cell tumors
E. Cholangiocarcinoma (sclerosing, nodular, papillary)
3. Duodenal Neoplasms
A. Benign adenomas (tubular, villous, Brunner gland)
B. Lipomas
C. Hamartomas
D. Hemangiomas
E. Primary duodenal adenocarcinomas
4. Mesenchymal Neoplasms
A. Leiomyomas, lipomas
B. Neurogenic tumors (neurofibromas, ganglioneuromas)
C. Vascular tumors (hemangiomas, lymphangiomas)
D. Granular cell tumors
E. Schwann cell tumors
F. Gastrointestinal stromal tumors (GIST)
5. Lymphomas (B-cell lymphomas)
6. Metastatic tumors (renal cell carcinoma, melanoma, breast cancer, squamous cell carcinoma, endometrioid adenocarcinoma, osteosarcoma)
7. Psuedotumors (myoepithelial hamartoma, Brunner gland hyperplasia)

2.3   Duodenal Neoplasms

2.3.1   Benign Duodenal Tumors

Small bowel tumors are rare and represent only 1–1.5% of all gastrointestinal neoplasms. Depending on the series, the proportion of benign small bowel tumors ranges from 14 to 52% [27]. Familial syndromes, such as Gardner's syndrome and familial adenomatous polyposis are often associated with duodenal adenomas. Adenomas are comprised of three types: (1) tubular, (2) villous, and (3) Brunner gland. Tubular adenomas are usually pedunculated and generally have low risk for invasive carcinoma. Villous adenomas have a higher malignant potential, especially when greater than 2 cm. Brunner gland adenomas originate from hyperplastic exocrine glands in the proximal duodenum and carry no malignant risk.

Lipomas are rare tumors of the duodenum and are usually identified as incidental findings on CT as circumscribed tumors of fat density in the bowel wall. If symptomatic, they present as bleeding or obstruction. If small (<2 cm) and asymptomatic, they do not require resection. However, symptomatic, large or increasing size on serial CT requires endoscopic or segmental resection to rule out the possibility of liposarcoma.

Hamartomas are lesions seen almost exclusively in Peutz-Jeghers syndrome, an autosomal dominant condition characterized by multiple GI hamartomas throughout the bowel with mucocutaneous pigmentation. Rarely, these tumors cause obstruction or bleeding. Malignant transformation is rare, but requires that these patients have close surveillance. Surgical intervention should be considered for symptomatic lesions or concern for the development of malignancy.

Hemangiomas are rare congenital lesions that present as acute or chronic bleeding during midlife. They are usually single and have no malignant potential. If these tumors are symptomatic, treatment consists of endoscopic or segmental resection. Additional treatment modalities including endoscopic sclerotherapy or angiographic embolization have also been described.

2.3.2   Malignant Duodenal Tumors

The incidence of small bowel cancer in the United States is approximately 5,300 cases per year with 1,100 deaths per year as a result [28]. The majority of small bowel adenocarcinomas arise in the duodenum and up to half of primary duodenal adenocarcinomas occur in the periampullary region [29]. The incidence is higher in older patients and males more than females. Most cancers of the duodenum are sporadic. Familial adenomatous polyposis is the most prominent genetic predisposing factor with a relative risk of over 300 times that of the normal population. Hereditary nonpolyposis colorectal cancer, celiac sprue and Crohn's disease are also associated with duodenal cancer.

Most of these tumors are solitary, sessile lesions, which often appear in association with adenomas. They are usually moderately well differentiated. These lesions are similar to the malignant transformation of adenocarcinomas found in the colon with similar pathologic features.

2.4   Rare Periampullary Tumors

2.4.1   Mesenchymal Neoplasms

Benign and malignant periampullary mesenchymal tumors are extremely uncommon. The most common benign neoplasms are leiomyomas or lipomas. Other more rare benign lesions consist of neurogenic tumors (neurofibromas, ganglioneuroma), vascular tumors (hemangiomas, lymphangioma), or granular cell tumors of Schwann cell origin. Neurogenic tumors involving the ampulla may arise in patients with neurofibromatosis.

Malignant mesenchymal tumors mostly consist of gastrointestinal stromal tumors (GISTs). Periampullary stromal tumors compose about 3–5% of all GI stromal tumors. The sub-proliferation in the majority of gastrointestinal stromal tumors is thought to be driven by gain-of-function mutations of the *KIT* gene, which encodes a type of tyrosine kinase receptor. Activating mutations of *KIT* can be found in most periampullary stromal tumors. These tumors can occur at any age and usually present with gastrointestinal bleeding associated with a growth of a large size with central necrosis. Complete surgical excision is the treatment of choice. Because lymph node metastasis are rare, local resection can be employed selectively. Larger tumors, however, may require pancreaticoduodenectomy.

2.4.2 Lymphomas, Metastatic Tumors and Pseudotumors

Other rare periampullary tumors include lymphomas and metastatic tumors. Most reports of lymphoma involving the ampulla of Vater involve high-grade B-cell lymphoma and marginal zone B-cell lymphoma. Metastatic disease involving the periampullary region is often from direct extension from an adjacent locally advanced tumor. Hematogenous spread from a primary neoplasm is extremely rare, but most commonly reported with renal cell carcinoma. Other malignant tumors reported to metastasize to the periampullary region include melanoma, breast cancer, squamous cell carcinoma of the larynx, endometrioid adenocarcinoma, and osteosarcoma. Pseudotumors are recognized as 23% of tumors identified in the ampullary region [30]. They include myoepithelial hamartoma and Brunner gland hyperplasia, which collectively are more common than adenomas. It can be challenging to discern pseudotumors from neoplastic lesions, and often result to unnecessary surgery.

3 Clinical Presentation

Benign periampullary and duodenal adenomas are often asymptomatic and discovered incidentally or during surveillance for familial syndromes. Common symptoms depend on location and size of the tumors and can include jaundice, bleeding, and obstruction such as are seen with malignant periampullary tumors.

Generally, periampullary and pancreatic carcinomas are difficult to diagnose in their early stages. Symptoms tend to be nonspecific and often the diagnosis is not made until patients develop jaundice. Compared to pancreatic primaries however, tumors of the Ampulla of vater, distal common bile duct, and periampullary duodenum present at an earlier stage with jaundice. The mean diameter in one series of 149 patients diagnosed with ampullary cancer (2.7 cm) was significantly smaller, compared to pancreatic head cancer (3.5 cm) [31]. This generally translates to higher resectability rates than pancreatic cancers. Usually jaundice is progressive and relentless and may be associated with significant pruritus. Occasionally however, ampullary carcinomas may present with intermittent jaundice due to the "ball valve" effect of a polypoid tumor or necrosis during the growth phase leading to extrahepatic biliary obstruction. The development of jaundice is more commonly associated with a periampullary carcinoma (70%) than a benign tumor (20–30%) [32–36].

Periampullary neoplasms may also present with abdominal pain, anorexia, nausea, weight loss, and gastrointestinal bleeding. Partial biliary or pancreatic duct obstruction may result in complaints of abdominal pain prior to the development of jaundice. This pain is usually dull, moderate intensity, located in either the epigastrium or right upper quadrant, possibly radiating to the back, and aggravated by eating. Vomiting secondary to duodenal obstruction is usually a late manifestation of periampullary cancers in general, but may occur earlier in bulky duodenal cancers. Ampullary or duodenal cancers may present with chronic or intermittent gastrointestinal bleeding. An episode of acute pancreatitis of unclear etiology should raise suspicion for an underlying periampullary neoplasm and initiate a thorough evaluation once the acute episode has resolved. In a report by Rattner et al., acute pancreatitis was the presenting symptom in 25% of patients diagnosed with ampullary neoplasms [37].

Duodenal adenocarcinomas not immediately adjacent to the ampulla of Vater may present with vague complaints of abdominal pain, weight loss, symptoms of bowel obstruction or bleeding. These lesions tend to represent more advanced disease than periampullary adeno- carcinomas, which are often diagnosed earlier when presenting with jaundice.

Past medical and family history may be extremely significant in evaluating a patient for a possible periampullary neoplasm. Patients with Gardner's syndrome and familial poly- posis may carry a 200-fold increased risk for ampullary and duodenal carcinomas [12]. These patients will often have multiple polyps involving a significant portion of the duodenal mucosa.

Aside from jaundice, physical examination findings are commonly absent in patients with periampullary tumors. Hepatomegaly may be present and usually reflects hepatic congestion from biliary obstruction, not necessarily the presence of metastatic disease. Ascites, however, may represent advanced disease. A palpable gallbladder may be present in approximately 25% of patients. Occult fecal blood may be seen in those with bleeding periampullary cancers as well.

4 Diagnostic Evaluation

4.1 Laboratory Data

Nearly all patients with periampullary cancers present with abnormal liver function tests which includes increased plasma bilirubin and alkaline phosphatase, characteristic of extrahepatic obstruction. Transaminase levels may also be increased, but usually not as significantly as alkaline phosphatase levels. In cases of longstanding extrahepatic obstruction, the prothrombin time may be prolonged. Anemia may be present with any periampullary cancers arising from the ampulla or duodenum secondary to gastrointestinal bleeding. Tumor markers, CEA and CA19–9 are generally not valuable as they are not specific for malignancy and may be elevated in benign causes of extrahepatic obstruction.

4.2 Imaging Studies

Early diagnosis of periampullary cancers is dependent on prompt evaluation of the jaundiced patient. Current imaging modalities provide detailed information regarding the level and etiology of biliary obstruction. Once these lesions are identified, a focused surgical approach gives these patients the best chance for long-term survival.

4.2.1 Ultrasonography

Transabdominal ultrasound (US) is often used in the initial evaluation of patients presenting with abdominal pain or obstructive jaundice, as it documents the presence of biliary obstruction with a dilated biliary tree and can define the level of biliary obstruction thereby narrowing the differential diagnosis. Other important findings that can be visualized with US include gallstones, ascites, and liver metastases. A major limitation of US is the frequent inability to identify a periampullary tumor and the 15–20% rate of technically inadequate studies, which can result from patient body habitus, the presence of intervening bowel gas, or technical limitations of the operator. Conversely, the lack of radiation exposure and its relatively low cost are some of the advantages offered by US.

4.2.2   Computed Tomography

Despite the advantages of US, the high accuracy and reproducibility of computed tomography (CT) and its widespread availability, make it the most useful, and often the most cost-effective test in the evaluation of a patient with a suspected periampullary malignancy [38]. CT can detect the presence of a periampullary mass of at least 2 cm in size and also provides important information about the level of biliary obstruction with respect to the pancreatic parenchyma, if no mass is seen (❍ *Fig. 10-5*). Pancreatic duct dilatation may also be seen. The optimal technique for evaluation of the periampullary region involves administration of both intravenous and oral contrast and obtaining 1- to 3-mm slices within a single breathhold during both the arterial and portal venous phase of intravenous contrast enhancement [39,40]. Scans obtained during the rapid intravenous injection of an iodinated contrast agent result in an increase in the pancreatic parenchymal attenuation, as well as excellent contrast enhancement of the major peripancreatic blood vessels. This technique not only results in clear delineation of the tumor, but may also demonstrate involvement of adjacent major visceral vessels, such as the portal/superior mesenteric vein complex or superior mesenteric or hepatic arteries, suggesting unresectability. CT also has nearly 100% sensitivity for the detection of liver metastases at least 1.5 cm in size [41]. It can also demonstrate ascites and often evidence of peritoneal metastases. The value of CT lies in the virtual absence of technically unsatisfactory

❍ Fig. 10-5

Computed tomography scan of a patient with obstructive jaundice due to ampullary carcinoma: (a) Scan demonstrated a 3-cm ampullary mass (black arrow) and (b) scan at higher level demonstrating bile duct dilation within pancreatic parenchyma indicating distal duct obstruction (white arrow).

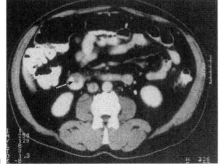
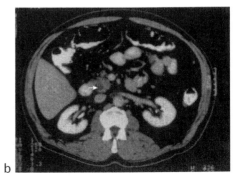

a   b

examinations and in its high accuracy in both the detection and staging of periampullary carcinoma. The positive predictive value associated with CT-determination of unresectability is greater than 90% [39]. Magnetic resonance imaging (MRI) is equivalent to, but not superior to CT, for either detection or staging of periampullary tumors and has a higher cost [42]. However, it does offer the advantages of avoiding exposure to radiation or ionic contrast, and so is a more suitable test for patients with contrast allergies or renal insufficiency.

4.2.3   Magnetic Resonance Cholangiopancreatography

Magnetic resonance cholangiopancreatography (MRCP) is emerging as a non-invasive method to determine the most likely etiology of a pancreaticobiliary abnormality. It is most helpful in evaluating abnormalities of the proximal bile ducts and liver. In periampullary lesions, the thick slab MR images will delineate the biliary and pancreatic ductal anatomy with detail that is similar to the more invasive techniques of endoscopic retrograde cholangiopancreatography (ERCP). The other MR sequences will define the presence or absence of a mass, the level of the obstruction and the location of any given abnormality relative to the regional vessels.

The pattern on cholangiopancreatography can be characteristic for ampullary bile duct and pancreatic carcinomas. Cancers of the ampulla or duodenum will obstruct both the pancreatic and bile duct at the ampulla whereas pancreatic cancer will show the classic "double duct" sign. Distal bile duct cancers show a characteristic "apple core" appearance, with a normal appearing pancreatic duct.

4.2.4   Endoscopy/Endoscopic Ultrasound

Simple upper endoscopy can define the extent, size, and gross appearance of a periampullary lesion suspected of being malignant and allows for simultaneous performance of an endoscopic biopsy and cytologic brushings. The endoscopic appearance of an ampullary lesion, however, is often similar for benign and malignant tumors. Furthermore, endoscopic biopsies with periampullary malignancies may be inaccurate in 15–25% of patients, yielding false negative results, largely due to sampling error. (15,47,48) The demonstration of malignancy on biopsy specimens is definitive and will in most cases indicate the need for pancreaticoduodenectomy. However, a diagnosis of a benign adenoma does not rule out the presence of an adenocarcinoma elsewhere in the adenoma. Finally, an important consideration is that ampullary adenomas are considered a pre-malignant condition since they tend to progress to carcinoma [43]. Therefore, regardless of whether the biopsy shows a malignant or benign histology, complete resection (either operative or endoscopic) is warranted.

Endoscopic ultrasonography (EUS) is a relatively new diagnostic modality, which combines and modifies the techniques of gastrointestinal endoscopy and US. This combination decreases the distance between the ultrasonic source and the organ of interest, thereby markedly improving the resolution and imaging of the surrounding structures. Real-time EUS enables one to evaluate and integrate, on the same examination, mucosal, vascular, ductal, and parenchymal abnormalities. It allows detection of periampullary tumors, evaluation of their size and depth of invasion, as well as assessment of regional lymph nodes. EUS appears to be superior to CT and MRI for the detection of small pancreatic tumors (<2 cm)

[44]. However, the sensitivity of EUS decreases in the setting of chronic pancreatitis [39]. EUS is able to demonstrate depth of invasion (T stage) of mucosal based ampullary and duodenal tumors with an overall accuracy of 74% and increasing accuracy with higher T stages [45] (◐ *Fig. 10-6*). This feature is of importance in detecting noninvasive benign periampullary neoplasms from malignant tumors with invasion through the bowel wall. Although results are not conclusive, several reports have also indicated that EUS has greater sensitivity and accuracy in detecting vascular invasion than CT [44,46].

The value of defining a benign versus a malignant periampullary mucosal based tumor is the opportunity to provide local excision for benign lesion as opposed to pancreaticoduodenectomy needed for malignant tumors. However, since frozen section analysis of resected specimens can fail to detect malignancy in 14% of patients [47], the surgeon always risks the possibility of a final diagnosis of cancer following local excision. The use of EUS provides another method of selecting patients for local resection. EUS cannot differentiate a T1 carcinoma (limited to the mucosa) from an adenoma, however T3 and T4 tumors are easily differentiated from an adenoma or early carcinoma by EUS. In a series reported by Mukai and colleagues, EUS accurately defined wall-depth penetration in 78% of ampullary carcinomas [48]. Under-estimating the depth of the tumor penetration seldom occurs, while overestimation is more common and is often due to edema of the submucosa from associated pancreatitis, which occurs in up to one-third of T1 lesions [49]. Finally, EUS can determine the presence or absence of enlarged regional lymph nodes. Reported accuracies of EUS-assessment of lymph node status have ranged from 63 to 84%, which is at least equivalent to CT [39,44,45,50]. Furthermore, EUS offers the ability to perform fine-needle aspiration (FNA) of both the lesion and suspicious regional lymph nodes.

◨ Fig. 10-6

Endoscopic ultrasonography scan of ampullary tumor, represented by the hypoechoic area on the right. An endoprosthesis (small black arrows) can be seen running through the center of the tumor. The tumor infiltrates beyond the muscularis propria (open arrows) into the pancreas.

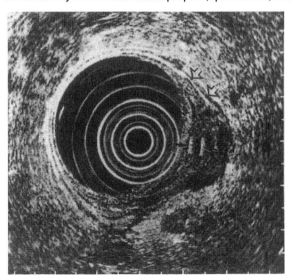

Limitations of EUS include its need for skill in both operating and interpreting, its invasive nature, and its limited view, which does not allow evaluation for distant sites of metastases. The combination of CT and EUS is better than either alone in detecting resectability in patients with periampullary cancers. The strategy of obtaining a CT for all patients with suspected periampullary malignancies, followed by EUS in those patients in whom CT does not clearly demonstrate unresectability has been shown to be the most cost-effective strategy for preoperative staging of and determination of resectability in these tumors [46,50].

4.2.5 Endoscopic Retrograde Cholangiopancreatography

With advances in cross sectional imaging and the introduction of endoscopic ultrasound and MRCP, the role of endoscopic retrograde cholangiopancreatography (ERCP) in the diagnosis of periampullary lesions has become limited (❱ *Fig. 10-7*). The most common current indication for ERCP in patients with periampullary tumors is for placement of a temporary

☐ Fig. 10-7

(a) Endoscopic retrograde cholangiopancreatography (ERCP) showing ampullary carcinoma obstructing the distal common bile duct, (b) ERCP with distal common bile duct carcinoma. Note the normal appearance of the main pancreatic duct, indicating a bile duct origin for the tumor, and (c) ERCP of a pancreatic carcinoma, with partial obstruction of both the main pancreatic duct and the common bile duct ("double-duct" sign).

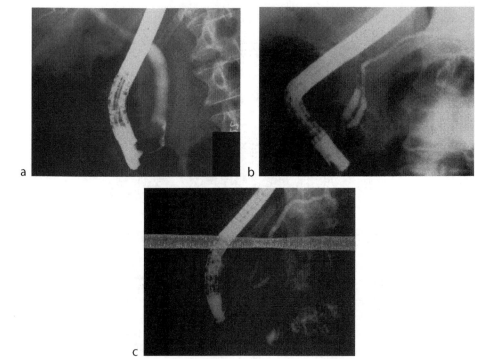

a

b

c

stent in the common bile duct to relieve biliary obstruction preoperatively or as palliation (◉ *Fig. 10-8*). Although stent placement will lead to colonization of the biliary tree and a higher perioperative infection rate in resected patients, it is appropriate in a number of clinical circumstances: (1) patients who present with symptoms of cholangitis requiring immediate intervention to treat the biliary infection, (2) patients presenting with intractable pruritus that can be relieved during the period of preoperative evaluation, and (3) patients with hyperbilirubinemia associated with renal insufficiency, which will correct with relief of the biliary obstruction. Under these circumstances, at least 2–3 weeks should be allowed prior to definitive resection to allow the metabolic derangements to normalize and to ensure the absence of active infection after instrumentation. Endoscopic stenting can provide relief of jaundice in patients in whom delay in surgery may be necessary to allow referral to a high volume institution or for planned neoadjuvant therapy.

4.2.6   Percutaneous Transhepatic Cholangiography

As with ERCP, percutaneous transhepatic cholangiography (PTC) for diagnosis of a periampullary malignancy is seldom indicated due to noninvasive options. It does remain a therapeutic option in some patients, particularly when the endoscopic route is unsuccessful

◘ Fig. 10-8

Endoscopic photo of biliary stent placed through an obstructing ampullary carcinoma.

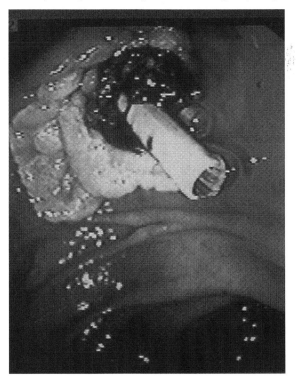

due to complete obstruction of the ampulla by tumor or the ampulla is not accessible due to a prior surgical procedure such as gastric bypass. PTC is often technically easier with a dilated biliary tree and is useful in defining the proximal biliary system, which is critical in the decision making process concerning biliary reconstruction. Percutaneously placed catheters can be helpful during operative management for either resection or palliation, especially in re-operative cases or in the early postoperative period to allow biliary decompression in order to protect the biliary anastomosis. In most patients, however, PTC offers little advantage over ERCP, has a greater morbidity, and should be considered only if ERCP is technically not possible.

4.3   Preoperative Staging

Although the presentation of non-pancreatic periampullary cancer with jaundice early in the course may lead to a higher rate of resectability, preoperative staging remains important. The modalities currently considered most useful in staging patients with periampullary neoplasms are dual phase CT, EUS and diagnostic laparoscopy. The dynamic spiral CT scan is currently the most valuable of these studies, playing a role in both diagnosis and staging of periampullary neoplasms. Its primary advantages are the lower cost and non-invasive nature of the technique. Computed tomography can detect liver metastases (>1.0 cm) or larger peritoneal implants. Obstruction and/or encasement of the major visceral arteries and veins in the region can be defined by loss of the perivascular fat planes and encroachment on the vessel lumen or the development of venous collaterals in the area.

EUS has high accuracy for evaluating T stage and defining malignancy by demonstrating invasion. The technique can also be used to perform an FNA for histologic evaluation of suspicious lymph nodes. However, EUS cannot be used as the sole modality for staging. Given its inability to adequately rule out peritoneal or hepatic metastases, it should be combined with CT or laparoscopy for complete staging.

One of the limitations of CT is its poor sensitivity for detecting lesions in the liver, omentum, or peritoneal surface that are less than 1 cm in size. In an attempt to identify such metastases in a minimally invasive manner, laparoscopy has been suggested as a method for further staging. In the past, advocates of laparoscopy have reported that more than 40% of patients with pancreatic cancer previously staged by CT were found to have small metastases at laparoscopy [51]. Nevertheless, with the introduction of dual phase imaging, CT has become more effective at picking up suspicious small volume metastases. Although reaching different conclusions about whether laparoscopy should be utilized, more recent reports have shown that staging laparoscopy subsequent to CT staging, even when combined with laparoscopic ultrasound, has the potential to identify only an additional 10–14% of patients with unresectable disease [52,53]. This yield is even lower for patients with ampullary and duodenal tumors leading many surgeon to avoid this step in patients with these tumors [53].

The decision to stage patients with periampullary neoplasms via laparoscopy is largely dependent on the treatment algorithms of the surgeon. Those surgeons favoring surgical palliation as opposed to nonoperative palliation of unresectable tumors consider laparoscopy unnecessary. Whereas those surgeons who feel endoscopic palliation is adequate for most patients suggest that laparoscopy can save a substantial number of patients from the morbidity of a non-curative laparotomy. Those centers currently investigating neoadjuvant chemotherapeutic and radiation protocols also feel that laparoscopy is important in order to document the absence of liver or peritoneal metastases.

The goal of preoperative staging is to determine which tumors are potentially resectable and have not already metastasized to distant sites or directly invaded the major peripancreatic vessels. Improvements in preoperative imaging and the addition of EUS to our clinical armamentarium has allowed for better selection of patients for operation with fewer patients being found to be unresectable at the time of operation, thereby minimizing unnecessary morbidity. Nonoperative techniques for the management of obstructive jaundice secondary to a periampullary tumor have also improved and can provide adequate palliation for most patients with unresectable neoplasms. Although the response is less durable than surgical palliation, nonoperative palliation is often the most appropriate therapy for patients with a short life expectancy. These improvements in nonoperative management have made appropriate preoperative staging more important. In the past, laparotomy was required in all patients to establish the diagnosis and, thereafter, resection or operative palliation was performed. However, as noted earlier, preoperative staging is less important in patients with non-pancreatic periampullary neoplasms because of the much higher rate of resectability in this group.

5   Surgical Management

5.1   Endoscopic Resection

Benign periampullary tumors and small, ampullary tubular adenomas with very low malignant potential may be endoscopically resected. Small, pedunculated adenomas of the distal common bile duct can also be successfully treated and excised endoscopically. For tubular duodenal and Brunner gland adenomas, endoscopic excision is the most suitable option. With villous duodenal adenomas, transduodenal local excision should be considered depending on the size of the lesion. Endoscopic resection of a villous adenoma may be performed only if the entire lesion can be safely removed (◉ *Fig. 10-9*). Close followup with repeat endoscopy is indicated in such cases, as recurrence rates can be seen in 10–25% of cases. Finally it is reasonable to consider endoscopic resection as a palliative option with patients that cannot tolerate general anesthesia to perform even a local excision for periampullary cancers.

Complications following endoscopic resection of ampullary tumors includes pancreatitis (5–15%), bleeding (4–15%), perforation (<2%), and cholangitis (<2%). Mortality, however, remains very uncommon.

5.2   Local Excision

Local resection of an ampullary tumor with reimplantation of the pancreatic and common bile ducts was first described by Halsted in 1899. Initially, this procedure was associated with high operative mortality and low long-term survival; however, with improvements in technique and preoperative staging, transduodenal ampullary resection has regained popularity. Local resection of the ampulla of Vater has been suggested for benign ampullary tumors or low grade ampullary carcinomas. Histologic confirmation of malignancy or large size or

⬛ Fig. 10-9

(a) Endoscopic appearance of a benign periampullary adenoma, (b and c). Endoscopic cautery excision of lesion, and (d) Final appearance after complete endoscopic excision.

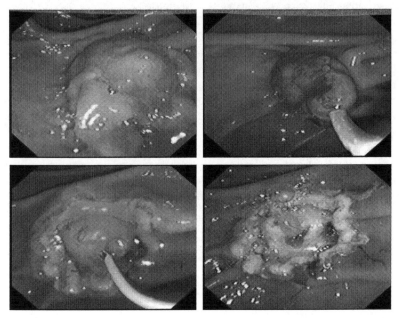

extensive extension into the common bile duct or pancreatic duct can preclude local excision. Furthermore, the false negative rate of endoscopic biopsy (up to 25%) or even intraoperative frozen section (up to 14%) requires that complete histologic diagnosis of the entire resected specimen be completed. If invasive cancer is found in permanent sections, return to the OR for pancreaticoduodenectomy is necessary.

The operation begins with an exploration of the abdomen through a right subcostal or upper midline incision to rule out metastatic disease. An extended Kocher maneuver is performed to mobilize the duodenum. A longitudinal duodenotomy is made over the junction of the second and third portions of the duodenum. Stay sutures are placed to expose the ampullary lesion, and the common bile duct is cannulated through the center of the mass. If the common bile duct cannot be directly entered, passage of a biliary Fogarty catheter from above via cannulation through the cystic duct following cholecystectomy is advisable. Next, a resection margin of 0.5–1.0 cm of normal tissue is created by scoring the mucosal surface with electrocautery (⬗ *Fig. 10-10*). The lesion is excised by dissecting lateral to medial in the submucosal plane. In this approach, the common bile duct located at 11 o'clock, is transected prior to the pancreatic duct and located at 5 o'clock. The specimen is sent to pathology for frozen-section analysis. If a negative margin is not accomplished or an invasive component is identified, then a pancreaticoduodenectomy should be performed. In a series of 39 patients undergoing ampullectomy at Duke University Medical Center, the negative predictive values of frozen-section analysis was 94% [35]. If the lesion is benign and negative margins are achieved, then the common channel between the common bile duct and pancreatic duct is reconstructed by dividing the intervening septum with scissors. Next, the circumferential

☐ Fig. 10-10

The ampulla is exposed via a longitudinal duodenotomy, and the common bile duct is cannulated. (Reprinted from Clary et al., [54].)

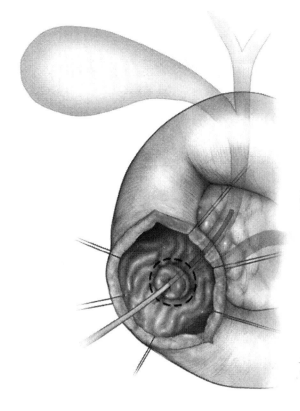

anastomosis between the duodenal mucosa to the common channel is performed with 5–0 Vicryl interrupted sutures. Lastly, the duodenum is closed transversely in two layers.

Recurrence rates after local excision in patients with sporadic adenomas are 0–26% [34–36,54,56]. Significantly increased rates of recurrences are seen in patients with polyposis syndromes and approximately 25% of all recurrences are invasive carcinomas [36]. This highlights the importance of surveillance endoscopy following ampullectomy. Most series demonstrated complication rates of 20–25% which included delayed gastric emptying, duodenal leak, pancreatitis, cholangitis, and common bile duct stricture.

5.3   Pancreaticoduodenectomy

Since its introduction by Whipple et al. in 1935, pancreaticoduodenectomy has been the most effective treatment for periampullary carcinomas [57]. Either classic or pylorus-preserving pancreaticodenectomy is appropriate for most periampullary cancers, with the exception of patients with extensive duodenal polyposis associated with FAP. In such cases all duodenal mucosa should be removed, and therefore the total duodenectomy approach of the classic resection is appropriate. A prospective randomized study by Yeo and colleagues, showed no advantage to an extended retroperitoneal lymphadenectomy when performing a pancreatico-duodenectomy for periampullary adenocarcinomas including ampullary and distal common bile duct primaries [58].

Perioperative morbidity and mortality rates have continued to improve over the past decade with mortality rates of 5% or less and morbidity rates of 30–40% expected in patients treated at high volume centers [59–61]. One of the complications of pancreaticoduodenect-omy that is often increased is the rate of pancreatic anastomotic leak due to the often soft texture of the pancreas usually seen with non-pancreatic tumors. On the other hand, since local vascular invasion by periampullary non-pancreatic tumors is uncommon, the procedures are often technically easier.

To date, no study has directly compared local ampullary resection with pancreaticoduo-denectomy for small ampullary cancers. There are several series with subsets of patients with T1 lesions that local resection was performed, usually in high-risk patients that were poor candidates for the more radical resection [34,37,62,63]. Although these subsets are not prospectively randomized, patients that underwent pancreaticoduodenectomy for T1 tumors generally experienced both higher disease-free and overall survival rates [6,33,34,64,66]. As a result, local excision is only acceptable for patients with small ampullary cancers that are unable to tolerate a pancreaticoduodenectomy.

5.4 Segmental Resection

Surgery options for duodenal adenocarcinomas include segmental resection and pancreatico-duodenectomy. For lesions involving the proximal first and second portions of the duodenum, the treatment of choice is a Whipple procedure. Patients with more distal tumors involving the third and fourth portions of the duodenum, an en bloc segmental resection of the distal duodenum and proximal jejunum with lymphadenectomy is appropriate. Previous studies have demonstrated that pancreaticoduodenectomy has an improved disease free interval and overall survival compared to segmental resections. This difference is most likely due to the earlier detection of periampullary duodenal adenocarcinomas than more distal tumors.

5.5 Palliative Procedures

In patients with unresectable or metastatic disease found at exploration, palliative operative gastric or biliary bypass should be strongly considered and performed especially if patient is symptomatic. For those with recurrent disease or known metastatic disease prior to explora-tion, palliative biliary stents and duodenal wall stents placed endoscopically may be the most appropriate local therapy to relieve symptoms and avoid delaying any additional systemic therapies being considered. In patients with bulky bleeding tumors, gastrojejunostomy (potentially performed laparoscopically) and radiation therapy can usually control symptoms.

6 Adjuvant and Neoadjuvant Therapy

The use of adjuvant and neoadjuvant therapies for non-pancreatic periampullary cancers has been reported. Due to the relatively fewer numbers of these lesions, series which include these reports remain low powered and non-randomized. The use of neoadjuvant strategies for treatment of periampullary malignancies is becoming more popular. These approaches are mostly observed with pancreatic adenocarcinoma and very little published data exists at this point regarding non-pancreatic periampullary primaries. The theoretical advantages include the delivery of a systemic therapy to well-oxygenated tissues, and the potential for down-staging unresectable and borderline resectable lesions. In a series from Duke University, neoadjuvant chemoradiation did not increase the mortality or morbidity of pancreaticoduo-denectomy for periampullary cancers, and interestingly yielded fewer pancreatic leaks and leak-associated morbidity and mortality compared to those not receiving neoadjuvant therapy [67]. Critics of neoadjuvant protocols for potentially resectable periampullary cancers point to selection biases based on favorable biology in those that proceed on to resection following chemoradiation treatment.

The role of adjuvant therapy in ampullary cancer has been assessed in numerous small studies. In a series from Stanford, 12 patients with resected ampullary cancers having lymph node metastases, positive margins, tumor size >2 cm, poorly differentiated, or neurovascular invasion were given adjuvant chemoradiation resulting in an 89% actuarial 1-year survival [68]. In another series from Johns Hopkins, 17 of 106 patients with a resected ampullary cancer received adjuvant therapies without any survival benefit [32]. In the European Organization for Research and Treatment of Cancer (EORTC) Trial 40891, there was no benefit of adjuvant chemoradiation over observation for non-pancreatic periampullary malignancies [69]. Due to these results, many oncologists consider only chemotherapy with regimens similar to those used for colon cancer rather than the more aggressive chemoradiation protocols.

Adjuvant therapies for cholangiocarcinoma are also not well defined. A Japanese rando-mized, multi-institutional trial of 139 patients with bile duct cancer showed no difference in 5-year survival for patients receiving adjuvant chemotherapy [70]. In contrast there is some data to support its use from a recent retrospective study. From 1994 to 2003 at Johns Hopkins, 34 patients with distal bile duct adenocarcinomas were treated with pancreaticoduodenect-omy with subsequent adjuvant chemoradiation and compared with historical controls from the same institution. For both lymph node positive and negative patients, overall survival was improved in patients that received surgery plus adjuvant chemoradiation [71]. Although a prospective, randomized trial would be necessary to determine if there exists a role for current adjuvant chemoradiation in this population, the rarity of distal bile duct cancer would make such a trial difficult.

Due to the relative rare incidence of primary duodenal adenocarcinomas, current data regarding its utility has not been able to identify a role for adjuvant therapy. The group at Johns Hopkins recently published a small retrospective series of 14 patients with stage III/IV periampul-lary adenocarcinoma of the duodenum that were treated with pancreaticoduodenectomy and adjuvant chemoradiotherapy. Comparing their results with historic controls, there was no difference in overall 5-year survival between surgery plus adjuvant chemoradiation vs. surgery alone [72]. Despite the lack of data to justify adjuvant therapies for primary duodenal adenocarcinoma at this time, most medical oncologists would recommend its use for advanced stage disease.

7   Survival

Overall the survival following surgical resection for non-pancreatic periampullary cancers are substantially better than periampullary pancreatic cancer (◉ *Fig. 10-11*). In the series from

☐ Fig. 10-11

The tumor-specific actual 5-year survival curves for the cohort of 242 patients treated by pancreaticoduodenectomy for periampullary adenocarcinoma. (Reprinted from [73].)

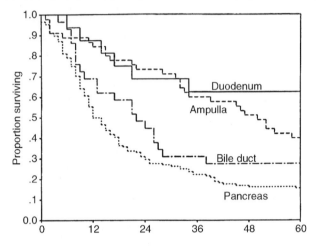

Johns Hopkins, duodenal and ampullary cancers demonstrate the 5-year survival rates of 51–59 and 37–39%, respectively [2,73]. In the same series, distal cholangiocarcinomas and pancreatic cancers have the lowest 5-year survival rates, 23–27 and 15–17%, respectively. In the Memorial Sloan-Kettering experience, ampullary carcinomas had the highest overall survival rates (median 43.6 months) and resectability (82.1%) for periampullary tumors [66]. Beger et al. reviewed 171 consecutive ampullary cancer treated by local or radical resection. The 5-year survival rates by stage in that series were 84% (stage I), 70% (stage II), and 27% (stage III) and 0% (stage IV) [34]. Poor prognostic indicators for recurrence after resection of ampullary adenocarcinoma are advanced T stage, lymph node involvement, positive margins, neural invasion and poor differentiation [32,33,64,66]. The two most important factors commonly found among different series are T stage and nodal status, where the rate of lymph node involvement is a reflection of the T stage progression. For T1/2 and T3/4 tumors the percent of lymph node positivity is approximately 20 and 50%, respectively [34]. However, as previously stated, there is no advantage to an extended retro-peritoneal lymphadenectomy when performing a pancreaticoduodenectomy for any periam-pullary adenocarcinoma [58].

With complete resection of distal cholangiocarcinoma, 5-year survivals range from 14 to 40% [18,22,23,74]. Resection rates are generally between 40 and 85%. In the series from DeOliveira et al., reviewing 564 patients with bile duct cancer undergoing surgery, overall 5-year survival for all patients and those after R0 resection were 18 and 30%, respectively. For 239 patients with distal cholangiocarcinoma in that series, the overall 5-year survival for all patients and those after R0 resection were 23 and 27%, respectively. The significant predictors of survival for patients with distal cholangiocarcinoma included negative margins, lymph node involve-ment, size >2 cm, and degree of differentiation [75]. The Memorial experience from Fong et al. demonstrated a resection rate of 43.3% for lower bile duct cancers and a 5-year survival

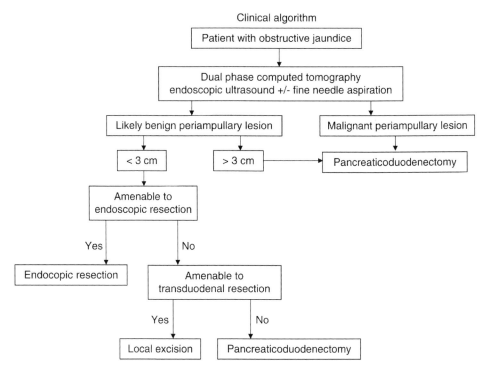

Clinical algorithm

Note: If Invasive carcinoma discovered on endoscopic or local resection, proceed with pancreaticoduodenectomy

of 27% [18]. In this series, the 5-year survival rate for radically resected node negative distal cholangiocarcinomas was 54%. Predictors of favorable outcomes in this population were negative lymph nodes and resectability. The Japanese have compiled their extensive experience of distal cholangiocarcinomas into a national registry demonstrating a similar 5-year survival of 26% [76].

The most significant predictors of long-term survival for primary duodenal carcinoma include margin negative resection and lymph node involvement. For node-negative patients, overall 5-year survival following resection varies from 38 to 83%. For node-positive patients, the 5-year survival drops to 15–56%. In a recent series from the Mayo Clinic of 101 consecutive patients undergoing surgery for adenocarcinoma of the duodenum, lymph node involvement, stage III or greater, positive margin, and weight loss each carried a significantly negative impact on survival [77]. In the same series, the tumor grade, size and location within the duodenum had no impact on survival (5-year survival, 54%). In the Memorial series, the survival benefit between node-positive (5-year survival, 56%) and node-negative (5-year survival, 83%) tumors demonstrated in patients with ≥15 nodes sampled did not carry a similar positive prognostic impact on survival when <15 lymph nodes were sampled [78]. The Hopkins group published their retrospective experience of 55 patients surgically treated primary adenocarcinoma of the duodenum [79]. Similar to other series, the 5-year survival was 53%. In this series, negative margins, pancreaticoduodenectomy, and tumors involving the first and second portions of the duodenum were favorable predictors of long-term survival. Nodal status, tumor diameter and grade did not influence survival in this study.

Key Practice Points

- Non-pancreatic periampullary malignancies originate from the distal common bile duct, ampulla of Vater, and duodenum.
- Clinical findings of biliary obstruction require cross sectional imaging and evaluation of the biliary system to exclude periampullary malignancies.
- Patients with familial syndromes (FAP, Gardner's syndrome, inflammatory bowel disease) must undergo close surveillance for periampullary cancers.
- Preoperative staging with CT and endoscopic ultrasound are the most cost effective diagnostic strategies for determining resectability.
- In general, due to the higher rate of resectability of non-pancreatic periampullary neoplasms, pre-operative staging and laparoscopic exploration are less important than pancreatic primary tumors.
- Small, benign periampullary lesions may undergo endoscopic resection.
- Transduodenal resection should be considered for small (<3 cm) ampullary tumors or low grade ampullary malignancies in patients unable to tolerate a pancreaticoduodenectomy.
- For large periampullary lesions (>3 cm) and invasive periampullary malignancies, pancreaticoduodenectomy remains the standard treatment.
- Adjuvant and neoadjuvant treatments for non-pancreatic periampullary tumors have been investigated; however, no clear survival benefit has been identified.
- Actual 5-year survival rates following surgical resection for non-pancreatic periampullary cancers as 51% for duodenal cancer, 37% for ampullary cancer, and 23% for distal common bile duct cancer.
- Poor prognostic indicators for ampullary adenocarcinoma include advanced T stage, lymph node involvement, positive margins, neural invasion and poor differentiation.
- Significant predictors of survival for distal cholangiocarcinoma include negative margins, lymph node involvement, size >2 cm, and degree of differentiation.
- Significant predictors of survival for duodenal carcinoma include margin negative resection and lymph node involvement.

Future Research Directions

- Translational investigations to better understand the molecular biology of periampullary tumors to improve early detection and targeted therapies.
- Technologic advances to improve local endoscopic diagnosis, staging, and management.
- Multi-institutional clinical trials to investigate adjuvant and neoadjuvant therapies for resectable periampullary cancers.

References

1. Riall TS, et al.: Pancreaticoduodenectomy with or without distal gastrectomy and extended retroperitoneal lymphadenectomy for periampullary adenocarcinoma – part 3: update on 5-year survival. J Gastrointest Surg 2005;9(9):1191–1204.

2. Riall TS, et al.: Resected periampullary adenocarcinoma: 5-year survivors and their 6- to 10-year follow-up. Surgery 2006;140(5):764–772.

3. Stolte M, Pscherer C: Adenoma-carcinoma sequence in the papilla of Vater. Scand J Gastroenterol 1996;31(4):376–382.

4. Galandiuk S, et al.: Villous tumors of the duodenum. Ann Surg 1988;207(3):234–239.

5. Rosenberg J, et al.: Benign villous adenomas of the ampulla of Vater. Cancer 1986;58(7):1563–1568.

6. Roder JD, et al.: Number of lymph node metastases is significantly associated with survival in patients with radically resected carcinoma of the ampulla of Vater. Br J Surg 1995;82(12):1693–1696.

7. Blackman E, Nash SV: Diagnosis of duodenal and ampullary epithelial neoplasms by endoscopic biopsy: a clinicopathologic and immunohistochemical study. Hum Pathol 1985;16(9):901–910.

8. Yamaguchi K, Enjoji M: Carcinoma of the ampulla of Vater. A clinicopathologic study and pathologic staging of 109 cases of carcinoma and 5 cases of adenoma. Cancer 1987;59(3):506–515.

9. Noda Y, et al.: Histologic follow-up of ampullary adenomas in patients with familial adenomatosis coli. Cancer 1992;70(7):1847–1856.

10. Bjork J, et al.: Periampullary adenomas and adenocarcinomas in familial adenomatous polyposis: cumulative risks and APC gene mutations. Gastroenterology 2001;121(5):1127–1135.

11. Wittekind C, Tannapfel A: Adenoma of the papilla and ampulla – premalignant lesions? Langenbecks Arch Surg 2001;386(3):172–175.

12. Iwama T, et al.: Indications for local excision of ampullary lesions associated with familial adenomatous polyposis. J Am Coll Surg 1994;179(4):462–464.

13. Spigelman AD, et al.: Evidence for adenoma-carcinoma sequence in the duodenum of patients with familial adenomatous polyposis. The Leeds Castle Polyposis Group (Upper Gastrointestinal Committee). J Clin Pathol 1994;47(8):709–710.

14. Mino M, Lauwers GY: Pathology of periampullary tumors. In: Von Hoff DD, Evans DB, Hruban RH, (eds.): Pancreatic Cancer. Jones and Bartlett, 2005: 686–702.

15. Carter JT, et al.: Tumors of the ampulla of Vater: histopathologic classification and predictors of survival. J Am Coll Surg 2008;207(2):210–218.

16. Komorowski RA, et al.: Assessment of ampulla of Vater pathology. An endoscopic approach. Am J Surg Pathol 1991;15(12):1188–1196.

17. Devaney K, Goodman ZD, Ishak KG: Hepatobiliary cystadenoma and cystadenocarcinoma. A light microscopic and immunohistochemical study of 70 patients. Am J Surg Pathol 1994;18(11): 1078–1091.

18. Fong Y, et al.: Outcome of treatment for distal bile duct cancer. Br J Surg 1996;83(12):1712–1715.

19. Mir-Madjlessi SH, Farmer RG, Sivak MV Jr: Bile duct carcinoma in patients with ulcerative colitis. Relationship to sclerosing cholangitis: report of six cases and review of the literature. Dig Dis Sci 1987;32(2):145–154.

20. Bergquist A, et al.: Hepatic and extrahepatic malignancies in primary sclerosing cholangitis. J Hepatol 2002;36(3):321–327.

21. Nakeeb A, et al.: Cholangiocarcinoma. A spectrum of intrahepatic, perihilar, and distal tumors. Ann Surg 1996;224(4):463–473.

22. Wade TP, et al.: Experience with distal bile duct cancers in U.S. Veterans Affairs hospitals: 1987–1991. J Surg Oncol 1997;64(3):242–245.

23. Yeo CJ, et al.: Six hundred fifty consecutive pancreaticoduodenectomies in the 1990s: pathology, complications, and outcomes. Ann Surg 1997;226(3):248–257.

24. Weinbren K, Mutum SS: Pathological aspects of cholangiocarcinoma. J Pathol 1983;139(2):217–238.

25. Pitt HA, et al.: Malignancies of the biliary tree. Curr Probl Surg 1995;32(1):1–90.

26. Jarnagin WR, et al.: Papillary phenotype confers improved survival after resection of hilar cholangiocarcinoma. Ann Surg 2005;241(5):703–712.

27. Howe JR, et al.: The American College of Surgeons Commission on Cancer and the American Cancer Society. Adenocarcinoma of the small bowel: review of the National Cancer Data Base, 1985–1995. Cancer 1999;86(12):2693–2706.

28. Jemal A, et al.: Cancer statistics, 2003. CA Cancer J Clin 2003;53(1):5–26.

29. Joesting DR, et al.: Improving survival in adenocarcinoma of the duodenum. Am J Surg 1981;141(2):228–231.

30. Leese T, et al.: Tumours and pseudotumours of the region of the ampulla of Vater: an endoscopic, clinical and pathological study. Gut 1986;27(10):1186–1192.

31. Yamaguchi K, Enjoji M: Tsuneyoshi, Pancreatoduodenal carcinoma: a clinicopathologic study of 304 patients and immunohistochemical observation for CEA and CA19-9. J Surg Oncol 1991;47(3):148–154.

32. Talamini MA, et al.: Adenocarcinoma of the ampulla of Vater. A 28-year experience. Ann Surg 1997;225 (5):590–599.

33. Klempnauer J, et al.: Carcinoma of the ampulla of Vater: determinants of long-term survival in 94 resected patients. HPB Surg 1998;11(1):1–11.

34. Beger HG, et al.: Tumor of the ampulla of Vater: experience with local or radical resection in 171 consecutively treated patients. Arch Surg 1999;134 (5):526–532.

35. Clary BM, et al.: Local ampullary resection with careful intraoperative frozen section evaluation for presumed benign ampullary neoplasms. Surgery 2000;127(6):628–633.

36. Farnell MB, et al.: Villous tumors of the duodenum: reappraisal of local vs. extended resection. J Gastrointest Surg 2000;4(1):13–21, discussion 22–23.

37. Rattner DW, et al.: Defining the criteria for local resection of ampullary neoplasms. Arch Surg 1996; 131(4):366–371.

38. Balthazar EJ, Chako AC: Computed tomography of pancreatic masses. Am J Gastroenterol 1990;85 (4):343–349.

39. Walsh RM, Connelly M, Baker M: Imaging for the diagnosis and staging of periampullary carcinomas. Surg Endosc 2003;17(10):1514–1520.

40. Wyatt SH, Fishman EK: Spiral CT of the pancreas. Semin Ultrasound CT MR 1994;15(2):122–132.

41. Legmann P, et al.: Pancreatic tumors: comparison of dual-phase helical CT and endoscopic sonography. AJR Am J Roentgenol 1998;170(5):1315–1322.

42. Steiner E, et al.: Imaging of pancreatic neoplasms: comparison of MR and CT. AJR Am J Roentgenol 1989;152(3):487–491.

43. Ross WA, Bismar MM: Evaluation and management of periampullary tumors. Curr Gastroenterol Rep 2004;6(5):362–370.

44. Rivadeneira DE, et al.: Comparison of linear array endoscopic ultrasound and helical computed tomography for the staging of periampullary malignancies. Ann Surg Oncol 2003;10(8):890–897.

45. Kubo H, et al.: Pre-operative staging of ampullary tumours by endoscopic ultrasound. Br J Radiol 1999;72(857):443–447.

46. Tierney WM, et al.: The accuracy of EUS and helical CT in the assessment of vascular invasion by peripapillary malignancy. Gastrointest Endosc 2001;53 (2):182–188.

47. Sharp KW, Brandes JL: Local resection of tumors of the ampulla of Vater. Am Surg 1990;56 (4):214–217.

48. Mukai H, et al.: Evaluation of endoscopic ultrasonography in the pre-operative staging of carcinoma of the ampulla of Vater and common bile duct. Gastrointest Endosc 1992;38(6):676–683.

49. Souquet JC, et al.: Endosonography-guided treatment of esophageal carcinoma. Endoscopy 1992;24 (Suppl. 1):324–328.

50. Soriano A, et al.: Preoperative staging and tumor resectability assessment of pancreatic cancer: prospective study comparing endoscopic ultrasonography, helical computed tomography, magnetic resonance imaging, and angiography. Am J Gastroenterol 2004;99(3):492–501.

51. Warshaw AL, Tepper JE, Shipley WU: Laparoscopy in the staging and planning of therapy for pancreatic cancer. Am J Surg 1986;151(1):76–80.

52. Friess H, et al.: The role of diagnostic laparoscopy in pancreatic and periampullary malignancies. J Am Coll Surg 1998;186(6):675–682.

53. Brooks AD, et al.: The value of laparoscopy in the management of ampullary, duodenal, and distal bile duct tumors. J Gastrointest Surg 2002;6(2):139–145.

54. Clary BM, Pappas TN, Tyler DS. Transduodenal local resection for periampullary neoplasms. In: Evans DB, Abbruzzese JL, Pisters PW, (eds.): Pancreatic Cancer: M.D. Anderson Solid Tumor Oncology Series. New York: Springer-Verlag; 2007: 181–191.

55. Posner S, et al.: Safety and long-term efficacy of transduodenal excision for tumors of the ampulla of Vater. Surgery 2000;128(4):694–701.

56. Cahen DL, et al.: Local resection or pancreaticoduodenectomy for villous adenoma of the ampulla of Vater diagnosed before operation. Br J Surg 1997;84 (7):948–951.

57. Whipple AO, Parsons WB, Mullins CR: Treatment of Carcinoma of the Ampulla of Vater. Ann Surg 1935;102(4):763–779.

58. Yeo CJ, et al.: Pancreaticoduodenectomy with or without distal gastrectomy and extended retroperitoneal lymphadenectomy for periampullary adenocarcinoma, part 2: randomized controlled trial evaluating survival, morbidity, and mortality. Ann Surg 2002;236(3):355–366.

59. Wray CJ, et al.: Surgery for pancreatic cancer: recent controversies and current practice. Gastroenterology 2005;128(6):1626–1641.

60. Schmidt CM, et al.: Pancreaticoduodenectomy: a 20-year experience in 516 patients. Arch Surg 2004;139(7):718–725.

61. Stephens J, et al.: Surgical morbidity, mortality, and long-term survival in patients with peripancreatic cancer following pancreaticoduodenectomy. Am J Surg 1997;174(6):600–603.

62. Klein P, et al.: Is local excision of pT1-ampullary carcinomas justified?. Eur J Surg Oncol 1996;22 (4):366–371.

63. Branum GD, Pappas TN, Meyers WC: The management of tumors of the ampulla of Vater by local resection. Ann Surg 1996;224(5):621–627.

64. Su CH, et al.: Factors affecting morbidity, mortality and survival after pancreaticoduodenectomy for carcinoma of the ampulla of Vater. Hepatogastroenterology 1999;46(27):1973–1979.

65. Roberts RH, et al.: Pancreaticoduodenectomy of ampullary carcinoma. Am Surg 1999;65(11):1043–1048.

66. Howe JR, et al.: Factors predictive of survival in ampullary carcinoma. Ann Surg 1998;228(1):87–94.

67. Cheng TY, et al.: Effect of neoadjuvant chemoradiation on operative mortality and morbidity for pancreaticoduodenectomy. Ann Surg Oncol 2006;13(1):66–74.

68. Mehta VK, et al.: Adjuvant chemoradiotherapy for "unfavorable" carcinoma of the ampulla of Vater: preliminary report. Arch Surg 2001;136(1):65–69.

69. Smeenk HG, et al.: Long-term survival and metastatic pattern of pancreatic and periampullary cancer after adjuvant chemoradiation or observation: long-term results of EORTC trial 40891. Ann Surg 2007;246(5):734–740.

70. Takada T, et al.: Is postoperative adjuvant chemotherapy useful for gallbladder carcinoma? A phase III multicenter prospective randomized controlled trial in patients with resected pancreaticobiliary carcinoma. Cancer 2002;95(8):1685–1695.

71. Hughes MA, et al.: Adjuvant concurrent chemoradiation for adenocarcinoma of the distal common bile duct. Int J Radiat Oncol Biol Phys 2007;68(1):178–182.

72. Swartz MJ, et al.: Adjuvant concurrent chemoradiation for node-positive adenocarcinoma of the duodenum. Arch Surg 2007;142(3):285–288.

73. Yeo CJ, etal.: Periampullary adenocarcinoma. Analysis of 5-year survivors. Ann Surg 1998;227(6):821–831.

74. Nagorney DM, et al.: Outcomes after curative resections of cholangiocarcinoma. Arch Surg 1993;128(8):871–877.

75. DeOliveira ML, et al.: Cholangiocarcinoma: thirty-one-year experience with 564 patients at a single institution. Ann Surg 2007;245(5):755–762.

76. Nagakawa T, et al.: Biliary tract cancer treatment: results from the Biliary Tract Cancer Statistics Registry in Japan. J Hepatobiliary Pancreat Surg 2002;9(5):569–575.

77. Bakaeen FG, et al.: What prognostic factors are important in duodenal adenocarcinoma? Arch Surg 2000;135(6):635–641.

78. Sarela AI, et al.: Adenocarcinoma of the duodenum: importance of accurate lymph node staging and similarity in outcome to gastric cancer. Ann Surg Oncol 2004;11(4):380–386.

79. Sohn TA, et al.: Adenocarcinoma of the duodenum: factors influencing long-term survival. J Gastrointest Surg 1998;2(1):79–87.

11 Molecular Relationships Between Chronic Pancreatitis and Cancer

Craig D. Logsdon · Baoan Ji · Rosa F. Hwang

1	*Introduction*	*287*
2	*Defining CP and PDAC*	*287*
3	*Observed Relationships Between CP and PDAC*	*288*
3.1	CP and PDAC Share Histopathological Features	288
3.2	CP is a Risk Factor for PDAC	288
3.3	Both CP and PDAC Possess Preneoplastic Lesions	290
3.4	CP and PDAC Share Genetic Alterations	291
3.5	CP and PDAC Have Similar Patterns of Gene Expression	292
3.6	CP and PDAC Mouse Models	294
3.6.1	Genetic Model of Hereditary CP	294
3.6.2	Mouse Models Involving Inflammatory Mediators	294
3.6.3	Mouse Models Involving K-Ras Mutations	294
4	*Pancreatic Stellate Cells Link Pancreatitis and Pancreatic Carcinoma*	*295*
4.1	Identification of Pancreatic Stellate Cells in CP	296
4.2	PSCs are Present in PDAC and Interact with Cancer Cells	297
4.3	Pancreatic Cancer Cells Influence PSCs	298
4.4	PSCs Influence Pancreatic Cancer Cells	299
4.5	PSCs Contribute to Chemo- and Radiation- Resistance	300
4.6	Summary of PSC and Cancer Cell Communication	301
5	*Speculations on the Associations Between CP and PDAC*	*301*
5.1	Inflammation as the Link Between CP and PDAC	301
5.2	K-Ras Activity may be a Common Cause of Inflammation in CP and PDAC	301
5.3	Modeling the Relationship Between CP and PDAC	302
6	*Clinical Implications*	*304*
6.1	Targeting Stroma as a Therapy for Pancreatic Cancer	304
6.2	Modulation of Tumor-associated Stroma to Overcome Resistance to Chemotherapy and Radiation	305

J. P. Neoptolemos, R. Urrutia, J. L. Abbruzzese, M. W. Büchler (eds.), *Pancreatic Cancer*,
DOI 10.1007/978-0-387-77498-5_11, © Springer Science+Business Media, LLC 2010

6.3   Targeting Stroma as a Chemoprevention Strategy 305

7   *Future Scientific Directions* *306*
7.1   Further Characterization/development of Mouse Models 306
7.2   Further Characterization of PSCs 306
7.3   Influence of PSC on Immune Responses 306

Abstract: Chronic pancreatitis (CP) and pancreatic ductal adenocarcinoma (PDAC) have long been known to be related diseases of the exocrine pancreas, however much of the existing literature is focused on identifying the differences between these two diseases. Thus, the exact nature of the relationship between CP and PDAC is unclear. CP is a major risk factor for PDAC, but the mechanisms of the increased risk have not been well characterized. PDAC is always associated with areas of histological CP, but whether CP is a cause, a precursor or a consequence of PDAC is unknown. Recently, novel mouse models of PDAC and CP have been developed that are providing new insights into these relationships. Moreover, the most obvious connection between CP and PDAC is the common characteristic of a prominent desmoplastic stroma. It is now understood that this stroma is the product of pancreatic stellate cells. New information about the function and regulation of these cells provides new insights into the relationships between these diseases. Clearly there is much to learn by considering the similarities between CP and PDAC, rather than continuing to focus on differences.

1 Introduction

The relationship between chronic pancreatitis (CP) and pancreatic ductal adenocarcinoma (PDAC) remains an enigma. Many different observations indicate the existence of an important relationship between these two diseases, but whether CP is a consequence, a precursor, or an independently associated pathology to PDAC remains controversial. Whatever the causal relationship, these two diseases share the presence of a complex stroma which is nearly but not completely identical. This stroma is produced by a specialized cell called the pancreatic stellate cell (PSC) and has profound influence clinically as well as biologically in both diseases. In this review we will provide background on the epidemiological and molecular evidence for a relationship between CP and PDAC and will provide a model for the potential causal connection between these diseases. We will also focus on shared aspects of the fibrotic microenvironment by describing what is known concerning the contributions of the PSCs to both diseases. Finally, we will address future directions for research and the clinical implications of the relationship between these diseases.

2 Defining CP and PDAC

Before discussing the relationships between CP and PDAC it is necessary to clearly define these terms. Tumors within the pancreas may appear in a variety of forms including endocrine tumors, acinar cell carcinoma, solid pseudopapillary tumors, lymphoplasmacytic sclerosing pancreatitis, and primary pancreatic lymphoma [1]. Furthermore, a number of histological variants of pancreatic cancer have been described such as adenosqamous carcinoma, medullary carcinoma, hepatoid carcinoma, and undifferentiated carcinoma [2]. However, nearly 90% of malignant pancreatic cancers are defined histologically as pancreatic ductal adenocarcinoma (PDAC). Therefore, for this review PDAC will be the focus. Fortunately, much is known concerning the histology, clinical course, genetics and molecular characteristics of PDAC and the readers are referred to several excellent reviews [3–6].

Despite all of the excellent information that has been gathered characterizing PDAC, the cell of origin of this disease remains controversial. The proposed cellular origins for PDAC include virtually all cell types in adult pancreas: ductal cells [7], acinar cells [8,9], islet cells [10], and centroacinar cells [11]. In addition, some have suggested that the cell of origin for PDAC is not an adult pancreatic cell but rather an undifferentiated progenitor cell [3,12,13]. It may also be possible that more than one type of cell is capable of developing into PDAC. In the current review we will not try to specifically deal with this issue. However, the cell of origin of PDAC determines whether the relationship between CP and PDAC is direct (acinar for both) or indirect (acinar for CP, other for PDAC). Therefore, we will mention the implications of different cells of origin.

CP is a chronic inflammatory condition of the pancreas that leads to irreversible deterioration of the structure and function of the organ. Clinical CP has been difficult to classify, as it occurs in many forms related to different etiologies. Currently diagnosis depends on independent analysis of imaging, histology and pancreatic function tests [14]. For most of the clinical manifestations of the disease, such as recurrent abdominal pain and pancreatic insufficiency, the extent of damage must be considerable. Histologically, CP is primarily defined by loss of normal parenchyma, presence of inflammatory cells, and extensive fibrosis [15] (❯ *Fig. 11-1c,d*). These histological manifestations can vary greatly in extent and may occur without overt clinical symptoms. Thus, it is not well defined when focal histological fibrosis becomes CP. In this review, CP will be used to describe the histological manifestations, primarily loss of normal parenchyma, replacement with fibrotic stroma and the presence of inflammation, with or without other clinical criteria. Clinical CP is a disease initiated in pancreatic acinar cells. However, the primary manifestation of CP is due to indirect effects on the stromal PSCs which produce the fibrotic matrix. The specific mechanisms influencing the stroma cells to produce the abundant desmoplastic reaction are not well understood.

3 Observed Relationships Between CP and PDAC

3.1 CP and PDAC Share Histopathological Features

The most obvious relationship between CP and PDAC is that they both develop an extensive fibrotic response often referred to as desmoplasia (❯ *Fig. 11-1c–f*). This desmoplastic response leads to similar histopathological features including abundant and extensive fibrotic stroma, inflammation with infiltration of leucocytes, acinar cell atrophy and distorted and blocked ducts [15,16]. The important histological difference between CP and PDAC is the presence of carcinoma in PDAC. However, cancer cells generally make up only a small proportion (∼10%) of the volume of the tumors [17,18]. The shared fibrotic microenvironment has an important influence over both CP and PDAC and the components and potential contributions of the stromal compartment will be covered in depth below. From the standpoint of causality between the two diseases, it is important to note that focal areas of fibrosis lacking cancer that resemble CP are inevitably present surrounding PDAC. Thus, in terms of histology, PDAC always occurs in the presence of CP. However, this does not indicate whether CP is an effect, a cause, or a different result of a common mechanism compared to PDAC.

3.2 CP is a Risk Factor for PDAC

The strongest evidence suggesting a causal relationship between CP and PDAC is that CP is a major risk factor for PDAC [19–22]. While the vast majority of CP patients do not progress to

□ Fig. 11-1
The histology of normal human pancreas, CP, PDAC and PanIN1. Low magnification (20×) and high (60×) magnification micrographs are shown for normal pancreas (a,b), CP (c,d), PDAC (e,f) and PanIN1 lesions (g,h). The similarity in histology between CP and PDAC are obvious. In the normal pancreas the majority of the organ is occupied with mature pancreatic acinar cells. Normal ducts possess a narrow surrounding of stroma. Islets are also observed. In CP and PDAC the acinar cells are displaced by an abundant stroma. These two diseases can be difficult to distinguish for an untrained person. The PanIN1 lesions display a pronounced increase in stroma compared to normal ducts.

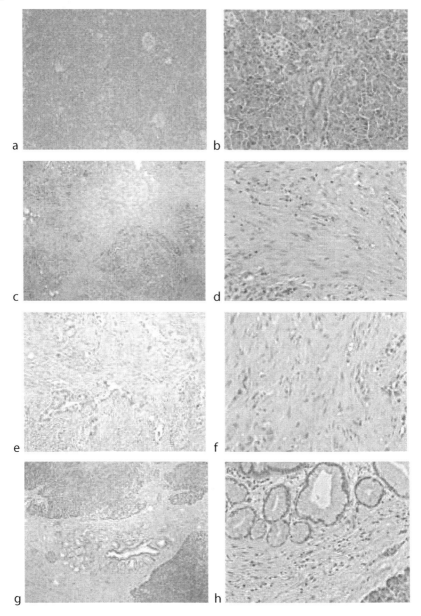

PDAC, the cumulative risk of pancreatic cancer in subjects with CP was reported to be 1.8% after 10 years and 4.0%, after 20 years with an standardized incidence ratio of 14.4 [22]. However, this is at least ten fold greater risk than those without CP. One potential explanation for this might be that both diseases are co-associated with an independent mechanism. CP has several major forms related to their etiologies including alcoholic, gallstone, autoimmune, cystic fibrosis, hereditary, tropical, and idiopathic forms [15]. The major form of CP (70–80%) is associated with alcohol abuse [15]. Thus, one potential explanation for the increased risk associated with CP could be that alcohol might be an independent risk factor for both diseases. However, there is no evidence linking alcohol with increased risk of PDAC [4]. Rather, CP of all forms appears to increase the risk factor of developing PDAC [23]. The highest known risk factor for PDAC is hereditary pancreatitis, a rare form of CP [24]. Hereditary pancreatitis is associated with mutations in the trypsinogen gene that are thought to lead to inappropriate cellular activity of this digestive enzyme [23,25]. Patients with hereditary pancreatitis have been reported to have a 53-times greater risk of PDAC with a cumulative lifetime risk of 40%, which is the highest of any known genetically associated risk factor [26]. However, the mutations associated with hereditary CP are not observed in PDAC from patients without hereditary CP [23]. Furthermore, each of the different forms of CP presents with specific characteristics, but each also has a very similar end phenotype, suggesting a common underlying pathophysiological mechanism. Thus, it is the common underlying mechanism that appears to link CP with PDAC. Nonetheless, the vast majority of patients with CP do not progress to PDAC. Therefore, significant barriers must exist between the mechanisms responsible for CP and the development of PDAC.

3.3   Both CP and PDAC Possess Preneoplastic Lesions

Pathological studies have suggested three important precursors to invasive pancreatic cancer: pancreatic intraepithelial neoplasias (PanIN), intraductal papillary mucinous neoplasm (IPMN), and mucinous cystic neoplasm (MCN) [27,28]. It has become clear that MCNs lead to a specific type of cancer with prominent ductal ectasia, copious mucin and a distinctive ovarian-type stroma. Therefore, it is currently felt that precursors to the more common PDAC include only IPMNs and PanINs. Of these, the better studied are the PanIN lesions [29,30]. PanINs are thought to progress from flat and papillary lesions within small ducts without cytologic atypia, referred to as "low-grade" or "early" PanINs (PanIN-1A and PanIN-1B), to lesions with pseudostratification of nuclei showing mild-to-moderate cytologic atypia (PanIN-2), to dysplastic duct associated lesions showing carcinoma in situ, referred to as "high-grade" or "late" PanINs (PanIN-3) and finally to invasive and metastatic PDAC. Characterization of molecular abnormalities within the PanINs supports the progression model, in that most of the genetic alterations present in invasive ductal adenocarcinoma (covered below) are found in PanINs, and greater numbers of genetic alterations occur in high-grade PanINs compared to low-grade PanINs [30–32].

PanINs are present in most patients with chronic pancreatitis [33–35] and increased proliferation of duct cells has been observed even in dysplastic ducts of CP [35]. It has also been observed that chromosomal instability and genomic damage are present in pancreatic duct cells from patients with CP, similar to what is observed in PDAC [36]. The specific mechanisms responsible for the genetic instability observed in CP are unclear. Nonetheless, these observations provide a potential explanation for the relationship between CP and PDAC (see below).

Another interesting observation is that, even low-grade PanINs are always found associated with a surrounding of fibrotic tissue. Furthermore, the extent of fibrosis increases with the progression of the lesions. At which point, if ever, this fibrosis becomes CP is difficult to define. However, it is clear that activation of PSCs and the resulting fibrosis is associated with the development of PDAC from the very earliest stages. Therefore, it is highly likely that the PSCs and stroma influence the natural course of PDAC development.

3.4   CP and PDAC Share Genetic Alterations

PDAC, like all cancers, appears to develop due to a series of alterations of critical genes [37,38]. Primary among the genetic causes of cancer are increased activity of oncogenes and loss of tumor suppressor genes [37]. In the case of PDAC, the most commonly mutated oncogene is K-Ras [3,6,39]. Alterations in several tumor suppressors are also observed; most commonly p16 (INK4a), p53, and SMAD4 are deleted, mutated, or epigenetically silenced. Later, many genes involved in angiogenesis, invasiveness, survival in the tumor microenvironment and chemoresistance are expressed. Therefore, consideration of the changes in genetics and gene expression in CP and PDAC may provide insights into the relationship between these diseases.

In PDAC, mutations in the proto-oncogene K-Ras are found in nearly all cases [40]. For this reason, this mutation has been extensively explored as a potential diagnostic marker. K-Ras mutations associated with PDAC have been observed in pancreatic duct histological samples [41], duct brushings [42–44], pancreatic-juice [45–50], fine needle aspirates [41], peripheral blood [51,52], and stool [53,54]. Unfortunately for use of K-Ras mutations as a diagnostic aid, K-Ras mutations have also been observed in ~30% of samples from patients with CP. The actual incidence of K-Ras mutations in CP is uncertain, as highly variable levels have been reported [55–58]. This is likely due to differences in sampling, DNA extraction or polymerase chain reaction (PCR) methods. Nonetheless, it is clear that K-Ras mutations are very often found in CP. Furthermore, CP generally contains early PanINs that often possess mutations in K-Ras [59–62]. Therefore, K-Ras mutations are not specific for invasive PDAC and their presence in normal individuals [63] suggest that they can precede CP. This is particularly interesting in light of the observation that elevated levels of K-Ras activity in acinar cells generates CP in a mouse model [64]. Taken together the data indicate that the qualitative presence of K-Ras mutations is not an accurate predictor of pancreatic cancer, as this mutation can clearly precede other required alterations. However, recent evidence suggests that quantitative assays for Ras might be able to distinguish between pancreatic cancers from CP due to the greater number of cells carrying the mutation in tumors [45].

Tumor suppressor genes are also commonly lost in pancreatic cancer. The most common alteration in tumor suppressor gene expression occurs with the p16 (p16INK4a) gene, which is lost in nearly 100% of cases [65]. Loss of expression of p16 has also been observed in preneoplastic lesions and CP [33]. The reported incidence of p16 loss in CP varies from 0 to 50% in different studies [33,47]. The high variability is likely due to sampling issues. Thus, p16 loss appears to be another early event that is not restricted to fully developed PDAC. In contrast, the common tumor suppressor, p53, is much more specific for PDAC. Mutations of the p53 gene have been reported in 40–76% of pancreatic cancers [3,66]. Alterations of p53 (generally mutations) also occur in advanced PanIN lesions later in the progression towards invasive PDAC [30]. Mutation of p53 has also been observed in CP, but much less frequently than in PDAC as assessed by direct measurements of mutations [67,68] or by analyzing p53 over expression as a sign of mutation [69,70]. Thus, alterations in p53 mutation status, a late event in PDAC progression, seem to be more specific for PDAC than either K-ras or p16 mutations, which are early events.

Disruption of TGFβ signaling is common in PDAC and may also occur by alterations of components of the signaling pathway, such as Smad4, or by effects on TGFβ receptor genes [71]. The Smad4 gene (DPC4) is a tumor suppressor member of the Smad family of proteins, which plays a central role in TGFβ signaling. Bi-allelic inactivation of the Smad4 gene is reported in approximately 50% of cases [3,72]. The loss of Smad4 appears to be a late event as it is only detected in advanced PanINs [73]. Relatively few studies have investigated alterations in Smad4 in CP and the observations have been highly variable [33,47,74]. However, the rate of Smad4 alteration in CP appears to be less than that in PDAC.

Taken together the evidence suggests that alterations in genes associated with early precursor lesions such as K-Ras and p16 are common in CP, whereas alterations that occur later in PanIN progression, such as mutations or loss of p53 and Smad4, are less frequently observed in CP. Furthermore, the shared genetic alterations supports a model wherein CP is a precursor for PDAC.

3.5   CP and PDAC Have Similar Patterns of Gene Expression

The development of PDAC is associated with changes in gene expression within at least four tissue compartments (inflamed acinar cells, inflamed ducts, stroma and cancer) (❯ Fig. 11-2). The gene expression in the cancer cells themselves is an important but minor component of the overall signature of cancer. The impact of the cancer on the local microenvironment is dominant, so that expression profiles from bulk tumors primarily reflect the surrounding stroma with its abundance of stromal PSCs and immune cells. Alterations are also observed in gene expression in the surrounding normal parenchymal cells due to the inflammatory environment [36]. Likewise, changes occur in gene expression in duct cells found in the inflammatory stroma of CP and PDAC [75]. Therefore, comparisons of gene expression in bulk tumors versus normal pancreas do not yield tumor or cancer cell specific gene expression. These complications have led to the use of various profiling strategies to isolate the effects of PDAC on different compartments. One method is to utilized the shared characteristics of CP and compared to normal pancreas to identify shared and specific genes [76]. The majority of genes that are commonly more highly expressed in CP and PDAC compared to normal pancreas have been investigated and primarily belong to the stromal compartment [77]. However, CP and PDAC also share similar alterations in acinar and duct cell gene expression caused by the inflammatory stroma. Thus, the difference in gene expression patterns between CP and PDAC has been used to discover genes that are expressed specifically in cancer cells [76] and the shared gene expression pattern between CP and PDAC has been utilized to discover common stromal and other genes reflective of the inflammatory microenvironment [77].

Two other approaches that have been utilized to identify genes expressed specifically in pancreatic cancer cells are laser capture and profiling of cell lines. Laser capture technology should theoretically be capable of avoiding surrounding cells and providing pure samples of pancreatic cancer. However, laser capture is technically difficult and results from laser capture studies of pancreatic cancer have identified as cancer specific genes that belong rather to the

■ Fig. 11-2

Alterations in cellular compartments due to pancreatic disease. The normal pancreas is composed primarily of healthy acinar, duct and islet cells. In CP the pancreas develops areas where acinar cells are displaced by stroma. CP leads to changes in duct and acinar cell gene expression due to the inflammatory and fibrotic microenvironment. PDAC is similar to CP with the addition of pancreatic cancer cells. Therefore, comparisons between normal pancreas and PDAC yield genes belonging to primarily stromal cells but also inflamed ducts and acinar cells as well as cancer cells. A comparison between samples of CP and PDAC shows that the major difference is the gene expression of the cancer as all other alterations are shared.

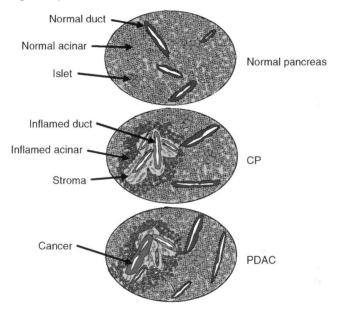

stromal or acinar cell compartments, such as collagens or digestive enzymes [78–80]. Furthermore, the comparisons utilized in the laser capture studies have been between PDAC and normal duct cells, which does not take into account the fact that many changes in gene expression in duct cells in CP and PDAC are similar [75]. Another approach for identification of cancer specific genes is to conduct profiling of pancreatic cancer cell lines [81–83]. Cancer cell lines are technically easy to study and are devoid of confounding cell types. However, there are a number of differences in gene expression between cell lines and the cells present in tumors. Many of these differences are likely due to the differences in the microenvironment. Other differences may be due to the cell lines undergoing changes during long-term adaptation to the in vitro environment. Therefore, differences between gene expression in cancer cells in vivo (identified as genes differentially expressed in PDAC compared to CP) and cancer cell lines in vitro may represent either cancer specific stromal gene expression or the influence of the microenvironment on cancer cells. For the studies available to date it appears that the most successful approach to identify cancer cell specific gene expression remains that of utilizing the similarity between CP and PDAC to identify PDAC specific genes.

3.6　CP and PDAC Mouse Models

One approach to understanding the role of specific molecules and pathways in the development of pancreatic disease is through the development of genetically modified mouse models. Several mouse models have been produced that develop PDAC. These mouse models allow access to early lesions and are able to provide novel insights into the relationship between CP and PDAC.

3.6.1　Genetic Model of Hereditary CP

A mouse model was developed in which the expression of the mouse trypsinogen (PRSS1) mutant R122H was targeted to pancreatic acinar cells by fusion to the elastase promoter [84]. This was meant to mimic the major mutation found in hereditary pancreatitis in humans. The expression of the mutant trypsinogen caused early onset acinar cell injury and inflammatory cell infiltration. With progressing age, the transgenic mice developed focal pancreatic fibrosis and acinar cell dedifferentiation resembling CP. However, at least within the time periods investigated, these animals did not progress to PDAC. Further studies with more of these animals at later times may yield further important insights. Likewise, crossing of these animals with animals possessing deletions or mutations of tumor suppressors has yet to be performed, but may provide an important physiologically relevant model of PDAC.

3.6.2　Mouse Models Involving Inflammatory Mediators

Recently two independent groups have developed mouse models involving cyclooxygenase-2 (COX-2) overexpression in pancreatic cells using a cytokeratin 5 promoter [85,86]. Cytokeratin 5 is expressed in a small subset of adult pancreatic duct cells. However, its expression pattern during pancreatic development is unknown. Cox-2 is an established factor linking chronic inflammation with metaplastic and neoplastic change in various tissues [87]. In both studies, expression of Cox-2 with this promoter was sufficient to cause early development of a CP-like state characterized by acinar-to-ductal metaplasia and fibrotic stroma. In both studies, these changes were prevented by feeding of a cox-2 inhibitor [85,86]. Interestingly, Cox-2 expression was shown to lead to increased Ras activity [86]. Over longer time periods in one study the mice developed serous cystadenoma, intraductal papillary mucinous, and PanINs, but not invasive PDAC [86]. In the other study, the mice over several months developed strongly dysplastic features suggestive of pancreatic ductal adenocarcinoma with increased proliferation, cellular atypia, and loss of normal cell/tissue organization [85]. Despite these alterations, there was only limited evidence of invasion to adjacent tissues and no evidence of distant metastases. However, cell lines derived from spontaneous lesions were aggressively tumorigenic when injected into syngeneic or nude mice. Therefore, this model appears to indicate that CP can be an early outcome of inflammation that is followed by transition from chronic inflammation to neoplasia.

3.6.3　Mouse Models Involving K-Ras Mutations

Mutations in K-Ras are nearly universal in PDAC. Therefore, a number of models based on expression of mutant K-Ras have been developed. Several studies have shown that when mutant K-Ras expression is directed by promoters active during pancreatic development such as PDX1 [12,88], p48 [12], nestin [13], or elastase [9] it results in development of pancreatic intraepithelial neoplasias (PanINs) that progress to invasive PDAC. On the other hand, adult mice were reported to be refractory to adult acinar cell [9] or duct cell [7] expression of mutant K-Ras and did not develop PanINs or PDAC [9]. However, if mice with adult acinar cell expression of mutant K-Ras were challenged with an inflammatory stimulus, then they developed the full spectrum of PanINs and invasive PDAC [9]. These observations have been interpreted to suggest that, during adulthood, PDAC is initiated by a combination of genetic (e.g., somatic K-Ras mutations) and non-genetic (e.g., tissue damage) events [9]. Another interpretation is that stem cells that are more abundant during development, rather than fully differentiated adult cells, may be the most likely candidates for the cells of origin of pancreatic cancer [3]. However, this latter explanation does not seem to account for the fact that PDAC is a disease of the elderly rather than a disease of childhood.

The above models were based on the expression of mutant K-Ras at endogenous levels mediated by knock-in of the mutant version of K-Ras to the normal K-Ras locus [89]. This results in only a minor change in K-Ras activity within the targeted cells [88]. In a very recent mouse model, K-Ras^{G12V} has been expressed in adult acinar cells at either endogenous levels or at higher than endogenous levels [64]. The expression of higher levels of mutant K-Ras were found to be necessary to mimic the levels of K-Ras activity measured in human pancreatic cancer cell lines. Therefore, these high levels closely mimic the level of K-Ras activity observed in human pancreatic cancer cells. In this model, elevated, but not endogenous, mutant K-Ras expression in adult acinar cells caused a rapid development of CP with abundant PanINs and IPMNs that progressed to invasive and metastatic PDAC. Therefore, this model confirms the potential of acinar cells to form PDAC as was previously reported [9] and suggests that at least in mouse models, elevated levels of K-Ras activity are necessary and sufficient to cause both CP and PDAC. It is important to note that in this model increased activity of K-Ras was the cause, rather than the result, of CP. These data suggest that the activity level of the K-Ras pathway, rather than the presence of mutations, is the biologically relevant parameter. Currently nothing is known about the activity level of K-Ras in CP. However, it is known that K-Ras is activated by several stimuli including CCK treatments [90], expression of Cox-2 [86] and expression of TGF-α [91] and each of these has been shown to induce CP-like fibrosis when examined in animal models [85,86,92]. Therefore, these data suggest the possibility that increases of Ras activity in pancreatic acinar cells brought about by various etiological stimulations may mediate fibrosis and inflammation. Whether these concepts apply to human disease will require further investigation.

4   Pancreatic Stellate Cells Link Pancreatitis and Pancreatic Carcinoma

As summarized in the preceding sections, considerable evidence exists for a potential link between chronic pancreatitis (CP) and pancreatic adenocarcinoma (PAC). Perhaps the most striking of these various associations is the obvious shared morphology of CP and PDAC based on the activity of the PSC. In this section we will review the identity and role of PSCs in pancreatic disease.

4.1   Identification of Pancreatic Stellate Cells in CP

A key piece of the puzzle that links CP and PAC was the identification of the PSC as a mediator of fibrosis in both diseases. Earlier studies on liver fibrosis had previously identified the hepatic stellate cell (HSC, also known as Ito cell) as the main cell responsible for the progression of liver fibrosis following chronic tissue injury [93–95]. In an un-activated, quiescent state, HSCs are compact perisinusoidal cells that store vitamin A in lipid droplets. When activated by liver tissue injury, HSCs develop long cytoplasmic extensions which give them a "stellate" appearance, resembling smooth muscle cells. They lose their lipid droplets, become highly proliferative, and elaborate extracellular matrix molecules (ECM), resulting in liver fibrosis [94,96]. In 1998, two groups isolated retinoid-containing cells resembling HSCs in rat pancreas and human chronic pancreatitis samples [97,98] and termed these pancreatic stellate cells (PSCs). Similar to their counterparts in the liver, PSCs change from a quiescent fat-storing phenotype to a myofibroblast-like cell upon activation by primary culture for several days [98].

In the subsequent sections, we will describe the role of PSCs in CP and also summarize the emerging data on their potential role in cancer. Many of the cited studies, particularly on CP, used PSCs that were isolated from rats or humans and were confirmed by expression of stellate cell-specific markers. However, most studies on the stroma associated with PDAC used stromal fibroblasts that were derived from rat or human pancreas, that typically did not contain cancer and in some cases the cells may not have been confirmed to be PSCs by marker expression. In this review, the identity and origin of the stromal cell will be specified whenever possible. The term pancreatic stellate cell will be reserved for cells that are confirmed by stellate cell-specific marker expression; if stellate cell markers were not confirmed, the cells are termed simply "pancreatic fibroblasts." Whether the stromal fibroblasts from CP differ significantly from those in PDAC is not clear, although expression profiling of both suggest that there may be differences in gene expression in the stromal compartments of both diseases [76].

Activated PSCs stain positively for markers such as alpha-smooth muscle actin (α-SMA), desmin, glial fibrillary acidic protein (GFAP) and produce ECM factors such as collagen types I and III, fibronectin and laminin. Quiescent PSCs are also characterized by retinoid-containing lipid droplets in the cytoplasm [97]. None of these markers alone is able to identify PSCs, but the combination of α-SMA and at least one of the other markers listed above is usually considered sufficient for positive identification.

The PSC plays a critical role in pancreatic fibrogenesis and the pathogenesis of chronic pancreatitis. PSCs can be activated by ethanol or acetaldehyde, with increased expression of α-SMA and collagen; these effects are blocked by the antioxidant vitamin E and by vitamin A [99,100]. PSCs can also be activated by various proinflammatory cytokines, such as platelet-derived growth factor (PDGF) or transforming growth factor β (TGF-β). These mediators increase proliferation of PSCs and the expression of α-SMA and collagen [101]. Activation of PSCs by these proinflammatory mediators also increases the expression of matrix metalloproteinases (MMPs), known to degrade ECM proteins, such as MMP2, MMP9, MMP13 as well as tissue inhibitors of metalloproteinases (TIMP1 and TIMP2) [102]. MMP2 secretion by PSCs was induced by exposure to TGF-β1 or interleukin 6 (IL-6) [102]. In a caerulein-induced model of chronic pancreatitis in Wistar rats, vitamin E significantly reduced the number of PSCs, decreased pancreatic weight, and reduced the levels of pancreatic hydroxyproline, and plasma hyaluronic acid and TGF-β [103]. Novel antioxidants such as DA-9601 and troglitazone have also reduced pancreatic fibrosis, expression of α-SMA, collagen and fibronectin in caerulein-induced CP models [104,105]. These results suggest that inhibition of PSCs with these drugs may deter the development of CP, however, the clinical applicability of these studies is not clear since the therapeutic drugs were all administered along with, or prior to the induction of CP in these animal models. Whether these agents will be effective in clinical cases of CP, where the opportunity to provide treatment prior to injury is not available, remains to be confirmed. Nevertheless, there is sufficient evidence to conclude that PSCs play a crucial role in the complex tissue remodeling process that results in the fibrogenesis of CP.

4.2   PSCs are Present in PDAC and Interact with Cancer Cells

A well-recognized hallmark of pancreatic cancer is the dense desmoplastic reaction around tumor cells [17,18]. As mentioned above, this tumor-associated stroma is very similar to the fibrosis present in CP, with abundant connective tissue comprised of collagen and other glycoproteins. As in CP, the cell responsible for ECM synthesis in the stroma associated with pancreatic cancer is the PSC [106]. The stromal areas of human pancreatic cancer stain strongly for PSC-selective markers desmin, GFAP, and α-SMA, whereas adjacent areas of normal pancreas without malignancy contain minimal fibrosis and α-SMA positive cells [106]. Collagen is expressed in the vicinity of α-SMA positive cells [106], supporting the suggestion that stellate cells are the predominant source of collagen production in both CP and PDAC.

The precise role of the PSC in the development of pancreatic cancer is not well understood. However, in many malignancies, there is increasing evidence that carcinoma-associated fibroblasts (CAFs), which may well be similar to PSCs, contribute to tumor progression (reviewed in [107]). Stromal factors such as tenascin C are associated with increased invasiveness in breast and bladder cancer and correlate with poor prognosis [108–110]. In breast cancer, xenograft tumors containing CAFs grew larger than tumors containing normal fibroblasts [111]. Moreover, the nature of the stromal fibroblast can override the epithelial component. When normal prostate epithelial cells were implanted into mice with CAFs derived from prostate carcinoma, the mice developed intraepithelial neoplastic lesions [112]. In contrast, no tumors developed from the combination of normal epithelial cells and normal fibroblasts [112]. In pancreatic cancer, recent studies have begun to examine the contributions of PSCs to tumor progression.

We and others have demonstrated that PSCs have tumor-promoting effects on PDAC in vivo. In a subcutaneous mouse model, the injection of both pancreatic cancer and stromal fibroblasts increased the growth of tumors compared to cancer cells alone [22]. Similarly, in an orthotopic mouse model with MiaPaCa-2 cancer cells, Vonlaufen et al. found that the co-injection of HPSCs resulted in larger primary tumors containing fibrotic bands and increased tumor cell numbers compared to control animals that received MiaPaCa-2 cells alone [23]. These effects of HPSCs appear to be dependent on the ratio of cancer cells. In an orthotopic nude mouse model, mice were injected with various ratios of HPSCs and Bxpc3 cancer cells labeled with firefly luciferase, while control mice received injections of either cancer cells or HPSCs alone [113]. The ratio of tumor-to-stromal cells varied from 1:0 (Bxpc3 cells only), 1:1 (equal number of Bxpc3 and HPSCs), 1:2 and 1:5 (increasing proportions of HPSCs compared to Bxpc3 cells). The mice that received both HPSCs and Bxpc3 developed significantly larger primary tumors and metastatic lesions than control mice, which could be visualized with real-time imaging of the luciferase signal [113] (◉ *Fig. 11-3*). Similar to the in vitro results, the in vivo effects of HPSCs were dose-dependent, with larger tumors developed in mice that received a higher dose of stromal cells. No tumors developed in mice that were injected with HPSCs alone [113]. Since human pancreatic adenocarcinoma typically contains a much higher proportion of stromal cells than cancer cells [17], the mice injected with more stromal than cancer cells may be more analogous to the true clinical situation than traditional orthotopic models that use cancer cells alone.

4.3   Pancreatic Cancer Cells Influence PSCs

The interactions between PSCs and pancreatic cancer cells are not well understood, but the data available indicate that the communication is bi-directional. Likely, much of this communication is in the form of secreted factors. Conditioned media (CM) from pancreatic cancer cells has been found to increase PSC proliferation [106], activation of the MAP kinase pathway [114] and expression of α-SMA [106] and TIMP-1 [114]. Interestingly, the proteoglycans decorin and lumican, which are thought to have tumor-inhibitory effects, were decreased in PSCs treated with supernatant from pancreatic cancer cells [115]. In contrast, expression of versican, a pro-metastatic proteoglycan, was increased when PSCs were exposed to cancer cell supernatants [115]. Several secreted factors derived from pancreatic cancer cells that stimulate PSCs have been identified. For example, pancreatic cancer cells secrete fibroblast growth factor 2 (FGF2), TGFβ1, and platelet-derived growth factor (PDGF), which increase PSC proliferation and synthesis of collagen type I and fibronectin [116]. Thus, these data suggest that the malignant cells can alter the composition of the ECM in their microenvironment by influencing the activity of PSCs to favor tumor progression.

◘ Fig. 11-3

Effects of HPSCs on tumor growth and metastasis in an orthotopic nude mouse model of pancreatic cance. HPSCs were injected with luciferase labeled Bxpc3 cells (0.5 × 10⁶ cells) in varying tumor/stroma ratios. At 8 weeks, mice were sacrificed and primary tumors (a) and metastases (b) were measured by luciferase imaging. The luciferase signal from a representative mouse in each group is shown. *$p < 0.01$ tumor:stroma ratio 1:0 or 0:1 (from [113] with permission).

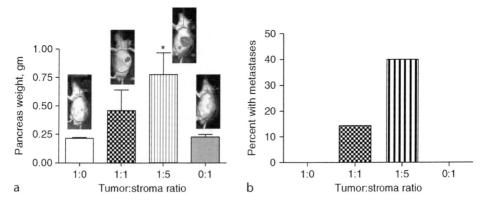

4.4 PSCs Influence Pancreatic Cancer Cells

Several groups have recently shown that PSCs can act in a paracrine fashion to stimulate pancreatic cancer cells. The addition of concentrated CM from human PSCs (HPSC-CM) obtained from surgically resected human pancreatic adenocarcinoma specimens significantly increased proliferation, migration, invasion, and anchorage-independent growth of the pancreatic cancer cells [113]. These effects were dose-dependent with the concentration of HPSC-CM, even surpassing the stimulation induced by the positive control of media with 10% fetal calf serum in some cases [113]. Thus, secretion of soluble factors is one mechanism for PSC modulation of cancer cell biology. Whether other forms of communication occur between PSC and cancer cells remains unknown.

Specific stromal-derived factors have been identified that influence progression of some malignancies but the precise characterization of many of these stromal signaling pathways is not well-described. Since PSCs were first identified in chronic pancreatitis, it is possible that the signaling mechanisms of PSC activation in pancreatitis may also be relevant in pancreatic cancer. Transforming growth factor-β (TGF-β) is known to play a pivotal role in fibrosis in CP. TGF-β1 is highly expressed in human chronic pancreatitis and transgenic mice that over-express TGF-β1 in the pancreas develop destruction of the exocrine pancreas and deposition of ECM that strongly resembles human chronic pancreatitis [117,118]. Inhibition of TGF-β function using a soluble TGF-β receptor decreases pancreatic fibrosis and protects the pancreas against chronic injury by caerulein [119]. Specifically, TGF-β1 is expressed by PSCs and increases collagen production. TGF-β1 also decreased MMP-3 and MMP-9 expression by PSCs and decreased cell proliferation [120]. The net result is that of enhanced fibrogenesis by increased production and reduced degradation of collagen.

The precise role of stromal-derived TGF-β in pancreatic cancer has not been clearly defined. Inactivation of the TGF-β type II receptor (TβRII) gene in mouse fibroblasts results in increased number of stromal cells and carcinoma of the prostate and forestomach [121]. Compared to control fibroblasts, fibroblasts lacking TβRII were able to promote invasion of adjacent carcinoma cells. Although TGF-β1 is tumor suppressive in many epithelial cells, during tumor progression tumor cells often lose their growth-inhibitory response to TGF-β. In advanced cancer cells TGF-β often promotes invasion and metastasis, possibly through the induction of epithelial-mesenchymal transition (EMT) (reviewed in [122]). It is also possible that TGF-β1 may have different roles depending on its source, since fibroblasts from different organs have distinct molecular profiles [123]. Thus, TGF-β signaling in cancer is a complex process, which involves cross-talk between cancer and stromal cells and these relationships change during the course of tumor progression.

Platelet-derived growth factor (PDGF) is also important in tumor-stromal interactions in pancreatic cancer. In culture, L3.6pl pancreatic cancer cells do not express high levels of PDGF-A or −B or the receptors PDGFR-α and -β [124]. However, when L3.6pl cells are implanted in nude mice in an orthotopic model of pancreatic cancer, the resulting tumors expressed PDGF ligands and receptors. Thus, the tumor microenvironment was necessary to induce expression of PDGF receptors in this tumor model. Compared to other mediators such as TGFβ, basic fibroblast growth factor (bFGF) and tumor necrosis factor TNFα, PDGF was found to be the most effective mitogen of PSCs [125] PDGF-induced proliferation of PSCs required activation of the JAK-STAT pathway [126] and could be inhibited by a neutralizing antibody to PDGF [127] or by a derivative of green tea [128].

In addition to cytokines, PSCs produce several other molecules that may also influence tumor progression. Type I collagen increased pancreatic cancer cell proliferation in vitro and protected cells from chemotherapy-induced apoptosis [129]. Connective tissue growth factor (CTGF) is expressed by PSCs [130,131] and enhances pancreatic tumor growth in vitro and in vivo in a mouse model [132,133]. However, high CTGF levels in human pancreatic cancer were associated with increased tumor differentiation and improved survival [130]. Thus, the existing data on the role of CTGF in pancreatic cancer is conflicting and whether CTGF will be a valid target for therapy is unclear. Finally, secreted protein acidic and rich in cysteine (SPARC/osteonectin) is a matricellular glycoprotein that is highly expressed in pancreatic cancer, predominantly in the stromal fibroblasts adjacent to neoplastic epithelium [134]. Treatment of pancreatic cancer cell lines with exogenous SPARC significantly suppressed cell growth by 27–30% [134], suggesting that SPARC may have tumor-suppressive effects.

4.5   PSCs Contribute to Chemo- and Radiation- Resistance

Of particular significance are the observations made in several studies that support the hypothesis that stromal fibroblasts within tumors contribute to resistance of cancer cells to chemotherapy and radiation. Treatment of BxPC3 cancer cells with HPSC-CM protected the cells from apoptosis when exposed to gemcitabine [113]. In addition, caspase activation was decreased in cancer cells treated with HPSC-CM after treatment with 100 Gy of radiation [113]. It was also reported that pancreatic cancer cell lines became much less sensitive toward treatment with etoposide when cultured with mouse pancreas fibroblasts, or their conditioned media [135]. Thus, supernatant from fibroblasts is able to protect cancer cells from chemotherapy or radiation-induced apoptosis.

The mechanisms involved in the protection of cancer cells mediated by the presence of HPSC are not well understood. The resistance-inducing effect of the fibroblasts was abrogated with a specific inhibitor to inducible nitric oxide synthase (iNOS), suggesting that nitric oxide secreted by the fibroblasts contributed to chemoresistance of the cancer cells [135]. Others have found that extracellular matrix proteins laminin, fibronectin, decorin, and collagens type I and IV, which are produced by pancreatic stellate cells, can also protect pancreatic cancer cells from death [136] and may contribute to chemoresistance [136–138]. One study indicated that supernatant from mouse pancreatic fibroblasts was able to confer resistance to etoposide in cancer cells and this was thought to be mediated by epigenetic down-regulation of caspases [139]. In summary, there is considerable evidence that HPSCs may protect pancreatic cancer cells from chemotherapy or radiation through secreted factors and does not require cell to cell contact.

Interestingly, radiation treatment of stromal fibroblasts appears to augment their pro-invasive effect on pancreatic cancer cells. Exposure of cancer cells to conditioned media from irradiated fibroblasts resulted in increased c-Met phosphorylation and stimulation of mitogen-activated protein kinase (MAPK) activity [140]. The increase in invasion was blocked by NK4, an antagonist of hepatocyte growth factor (HGF), which suggests that soluble mediators produced by irradiated stromal fibroblasts in the pancreas further enhance their invasive effects. Thus, HPSCs protect pancreatic cancer cells from both chemotherapy and radiation most likely through secretion of paracrine factors.

4.6   Summary of PSC and Cancer Cell Communication

In summary, a number of secreted molecules have been identified that are derived from PSCs and influence cancer cells and others derived from cancer cells that influence PSCs. Thus, these cell types exist in constant communication such that studies on isolated cells may miss important regulatory features present in tumors. While many of these factors have an overall tumor-promoting effect, others appear to suppress tumorigenesis and some like TGF-β1 can affect cancer in both directions, depending on the context. It is likely that the effects of these stromal derived factors may vary between precursor lesions and PDAC due to genetic changes in the progressing cancer precursor cells. Further understanding of these various factors will be necessary to determine which might be suitable targets for development of anti-fibrotic or anti-cancer therapies.

5   Speculations on the Associations Between CP and PDAC

5.1   Inflammation as the Link Between CP and PDAC

Clearly the most likely explanation for the observed relationships between CP and PDAC involves the common link of inflammation, as has been previously discussed [23,141–144]. Chronic inflammation provides a microenvironment that contains activated leukocytes including macrophages, dendritic cells, neutrophils, mast cells and T cells which secrete a wide variety of cytokines, chemokines and enzymes and lead to increased levels of reactive oxygen species [145]. Specific mechanisms potentially linking inflammation with cancer include NFκB [146] and Cox-2 [87], both of which are present in CP [147,148]. However, the specific roles of these molecules in pancreatitis and pancreatic cancer remain uncertain. The association between inflammation and cancer has been well defined in several organs [149]. For example, several lines of evidence support the suggestion that chronic inflammation of the colon is an important factor in the progression from inflammatory bowel disease to colorectal cancer [150]. In another GI malignancy, gastric cancer, infection with H.pylori and the associated inflammation have been shown to be mechanistically linked to the risk of gastric cancer [151]. Another example is Barretts esophagous which is an inflammatory condition associated with the development of esophageal cancer [152]. Therefore, chronic inflammation is likely to provide the crucial link between CP and PDAC.

5.2   K-Ras Activity may be a Common Cause of Inflammation in CP and PDAC

An important unanswered issue remains the identity of the mechanisms that generate inflammation in CP and PDAC and those that provide the link between these diseases. Interestingly, K-Ras activity itself leads to both NFκB [153] and Cox-2 [154,155] activation. This may help explain the observation that pancreatic cancer cells, which have high levels of Ras activity, also have high levels of constitutive NFκB [156] and Cox2 activity [157]. This would also explain the observation that treatments that increase K-Ras activity levels generate CP-like fibrosis and accelerate PDAC in the presence of low levels of mutant K-Ras [9,85,86] and that high levels of K-Ras activity alone are sufficient to initiate both diseases [64]. K-Ras activity has also been linked with increased levels epigenetic modifications including gene methylations [158]. Therefore, it is possible that K-Ras signal pathway activity is the common denominator in both CP and PDAC. Increased K-Ras activity can be brought about by increased levels of a variety of secreted cytokines, neurotransmitters, growth factors or hormones (extrinsic pathway) or by mutations in a variety of signaling pathways that impinge upon the K-Ras pathway (intrinsic pathway). In particular, mutations in K-Ras itself are likely to alter the characteristics of K-Ras down-stream signaling. However, initially it would not be necessary to have K-Ras mutations in order to achieve high pathological levels of K-Ras signaling pathway activity. Whether or not K-Ras activity is a common underlying mechanism for the inflammation associated with CP, it seems likely that inflammation itself is a crucial aspect of both diseases.

5.3   Modeling the Relationship Between CP and PDAC

With our current understanding of the influence of inflammation on tumorigenesis, we can describe a model that explains many of the known observations (⬡ *Fig. 11-4*). The initial event common to CP and PDAC is inflammation, possibly mediated in both cases by Ras activation. The causes of pancreatic inflammation in CP can be related to the effects of ethanol, or blockage of ducts or hereditary alterations of trypsinogen or a variety of other etiologies [15]. If these stimuli are sufficiently strong, acinar cells are lost and PSCs are recruited and activated which result in the formation of histological CP. Multiple repetitions of this cycle lead to full-blown clinical CP. During this early period, it is likely that increases in Ras activity occur primarily through the extrinsic pathway without the necessity of mutations of K-Ras. However, the chronic inflammatory microenvironment found in CP increases genetic insta-bility [159] and cell proliferation [35]. This accelerates the rate of gene mutation and therefore increases the probability of K-Ras mutations. If K-Ras becomes mutated it results in the development of early PanINs with their surrounding stroma and increases the likelihood of developing PDAC [44]. However, this occurrence has a low probability of occurrence and partially explains why most CP does not lead to PDAC and why CP of longer duration is related to increased incidence of K-Ras mutations and PDAC. It is also likely that in the early stages, the effects of the PSC derived stroma reduce cell proliferation and reduce the inflam-matory response through the secretion of inhibitory factors such as TGFβ. Alternatively, spontaneous pre-existing mutations in K-Ras, or other molecules impinging on the K-Ras signaling pathway, may increase responses to extrinsic factors leading to higher levels of K-Ras signaling pathway activity and resulting inflammation. Genetic instability mediated by increased inflammation also increases the rate of other spontaneous genetic alterations, including silencing of p16 and other genetic and epigenetic changes that bring about the progression to advanced PanINs and eventually invasive carcinoma [3]. It is likely that during this period of increased genetic instability cells are selected with altered responses to the inhibitory mediators generated by PSCs, such that stromal factors now do not inhibit and may may even stimulate cancer cells. However, the process of mutation and selection is slow and the number of mutations to become invasive PDAC is high, such that most PanINs do not progress to PDAC. Thus, CP generated inflammation explains it as a risk factor for PDAC. Increased genetic instability explains the presence of many early genetic mutations found in CP and low-grade PanINs that are shared with PDAC. The common histology between CP and PDAC is explained by the inflammatory influences of both CP and PDAC on the surrounding

□ Fig. 11-4

Model for PDAC development from CP. Extrinsic factors damaging acinar cells lead to increased fibrosis with acinar-ductal metaplasia. This may be related to effects on Ras activity. The inflammatory influence leads to a combination of increased cell turnover and genetic instability. These extrinsic factors increase the probability of developing mutations in key molecules including K-Ras. Alternatively, mutations in K-Ras may occur in the absence of CP leading to acinar ductal metaplasia and the formation of PanIN1 lesions. PSCs are activated early during inflammation and lead to increasing levels of fibrosis that eventually resemble CP. Mutation of K-Ras and loss of p16 occurs early and drives progression of PanINs but is insufficient for PDAC without further loss of tumor suppressors. Eventually some PanINs develop further mutations, for example in the tumor suppressors Smad4 or p53, allowing them to become invasive PDAC. Other molecular changes contribute to metastatic ability and chemoresistance.

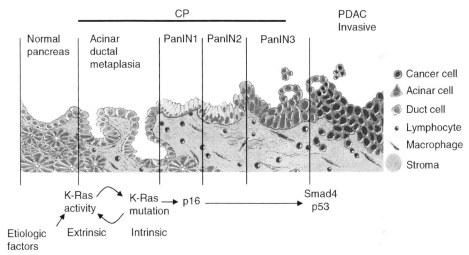

stromal cells. The shared microenvironment explains the commonality in gene expression observed between CP and PDAC. Further understanding of these processes will be necessary for prevention of this deadly cancer and may guide the development of new therapies.

Another observation that needs to be explained is the presence of areas of CP within the PDAC tumors. Some have suggested that CP in the area of the tumors could be caused by the blockage of small ducts by PDAC. Gallstones, which are a common cause of chronic pancreatitis, appear to mediate their effects by blockage of the common duct [160]. Likewise, experimental ligation of the main pancreatic duct causes CP which has been used as a model of pancreatitis [161,162]. However, it is unclear that blockage of small ducts can have the same effects as blockage of these large ducts. Orthotopic models of pancreatic cancer developed by injection of cancer cells into the pancreas of immune compromised mice do not develop CP. Furthermore, CP-like fibrosis is observed in early pre-neoplastic lesions with no apparent blockage of ducts. A different explanation would be that PDAC induces inflammation and fibrosis leading to CP. This would be analogous to the development of CP based on the presence of inflammatory mediators derived from standard CP etiologies. Thus, inflammation could be both a cause and an effect of CP and PDAC. This concept is supported by the observations made with mouse models expressing inflammatory mediators.

This model for the relationship between CP and PDAC does not change greatly based on the cell of origin of PDAC. However, if the cell of origin of PDAC is metaplastic acinar cells, as has been suggested by some [9,163], then both CP and PDAC would originate in the same cell type and these two diseases could be thought of as consequences of the same mechanisms with CP forming a direct precursor stage to PDAC. In this case, there would be a continuum of gene expression changes in the same cell lineage. Alternatively, inflammation initiated in acinar cells could affect proximal duct or progenitor cells, increasing proliferation and genetic instability and leading to increased probability of mutations in K-Ras and the other genes associated with PDAC development. In either case, the key effect is the genetic instability and proliferation generated by inflammatory stimuli.

6   Clinical Implications

6.1   Targeting Stroma as a Therapy for Pancreatic Cancer

Currently, there are no truly effective treatments for pancreatic cancer. The largest randomized trials of adjuvant therapy for resected pancreatic cancer patients have shown a 4.5 month improvement in median survival for 5-fluorouracil (5-FU) compared to no chemotherapy and perhaps only a slight improvement, if any, with the addition of gemcitabine [164]. Despite improved imaging modalities and advances in surgical techniques, there have been no meaningful improvements in survival for patients with resected pancreatic cancer with adjuvant (post-operative) therapy over the past 20 years [164].

The pancreatic tumor stroma provides an exciting new frontier for development of pancreatic cancer therapies. Unlike the cancer cells, stromal cells are reasonably stable genetically. These cells are also more abundant than the cancer cells within a pancreatic tumor. Although the precise mechanisms of tumor-stromal interactions in pancreatic cancer are not well understood, the existing literature demonstrates tumor-promoting properties of cancer-associated fibroblasts and thereby provides strong rationale for stroma-targeted therapies for pancreatic cancer. The selection of the appropriate targets will require further investigation and the development of models that include both cancer cells and PSCs.

One potential target is the TGF-β signaling cascade. However, the dual role of TGF-β as both a tumor promoter and tumor suppressor must be considered carefully in the development of inhibitors of TGF-β for cancer therapy. A perceived risk of TGFβ inhibitors is the acceleration of preneoplastic lesions or cancer in which TGFβ behaves as a tumor suppressor. Deletion of components of the TGF-β signaling pathway accelerates tumor formation in mouse models of pancreatic cancer [165,166]. Yet, transgenic mice expressing a TGF-β antagonist were resistant to the development of metastases from breast cancer without an increase in primary tumorigenesis [167]. Why the mice in the breast cancer study did not develop increased primary tumors is not clear, although the dose of active TGF-β available to normal cells [167]. Other strategies to inhibit TGF-β include blocking antibodies to the ligand and receptor, small molecules that directly block the catalytic activity of TGF-β receptor, and antisense TGFβ-specific oligodeoxynucleotides to inhibit TGF-β2 [168]. None of these approaches have been examined in the context of the tumor microenvironment of pancreatic cancer.

Another candidate for stromal-directed therapy is fibroblast-activation protein (FAP), which is a cell-surface serine protease expressed by activated fibroblasts during wound healing and within tumor stroma. In the liver, FAP is expressed by activated hepatic stellate cells and enhances HSC adhesion, migration and apoptosis [169]. Tumor-specific binding of a humanized antibody to FAP (sibrotuzumab) was observed in a phase I study that included 26 patients with colon and lung cancers, however no objective responses were seen in this limited study [170]. Another group developed an oral DNA vaccine targeting FAP that suppressed primary tumor growth and metastasis of colon and breast cancers in mice [171]. In this model, tumors from FAP-vaccinated mice showed markedly reduced expression of collagen type I and 70% greater uptake of chemotherapeutic drugs [171]. Little is known concerning FAP in CP or PDAC but further research is warranted.

The MMP family of proteases is an obvious therapeutic target in the stroma. MMPs are critical in remodeling of the ECM, thereby facilitating tumor cell migration and metastasis. MMPs are secreted by both PSCs and cancer cells. Unfortunately, the results of clinical trials using MMP inhibitors have been disappointing. Phase III trials of Marimastat, a broad-spectrum MMP inhibitor, in pancreatic cancer have failed to show any survival benefit either alone or or in combination with gemcitabine [172–174]. Further information concerning the specific MMPs and their roles in CP and PDAC should help to guide future efforts toward targeting this family of molecules.

6.2   Modulation of Tumor-associated Stroma to Overcome Resistance to Chemotherapy and Radiation

As described in the preceding sections, several investigators have shown that PSCs protect pancreatic cancer cells from the effects of chemotherapy and radiation through secreted factors [113,135,175]. Although the specific mechanisms involved in stroma-mediated chemo- and radiation-resistance are not well understood, strategies to inhibit such secreted molecules would be a rational approach to improve response to chemotherapy and radiation. In a mouse model of multidrug-resistant colon and breast cancer, Loeffler et al. used an oral DNA vaccine targeting FAP in the tumor associated fibroblasts [171]. FAP-vaccinated mice had significantly less tumor burden with decreased collagen type I and 70% greater uptake of chemotherapeutic drugs [171]. Thus, inhibition of tumor-associated stroma may be an effective approach to the treatment of pancreatic cancer by not only directly inhibiting tumor growth and metastasis, but also by enhancing sensitivity to chemo- and radiation therapy.

6.3   Targeting Stroma as a Chemoprevention Strategy

In this chapter, we have highlighted the critical role that the stroma plays in both chronic pancreatitis and pancreatic cancer. It is clear that the inflammation in CP is a risk factor for pancreatic cancer and the fibrotic response likely precedes the development of cancer. As mentioned previously, even low grade PanINs are almost always associated with fibrosis. Therefore, targeting the stroma at an early stage may be an effective approach to prevent the progression of PanINs to invasive pancreatic cancer. Moreover, the identification of markers specific to activated stroma prior to the development of invasive cancer, and the development of techniques to image these stromal markers, could be an effective approach to early detection of PDAC.

7   Future Scientific Directions

7.1   Further Characterization/development of Mouse Models

Genetic mouse models have provided important insights into the early stages of pancreatic cancer development. However, one criticism of these models is that by directing expression of oncogenes or deletion of tumor suppressors to specific cells the cancer that forms is more likely to be homogeneous than that occurring in patients. Therefore, it will be very valuable to further investigate models based on the generation of an inflammatory microenvironment that can lead to PDAC. Comparison of these various mouse models with the human disease is likely to provide valuable information. Furthermore, new mouse models need to be developed in which gene expression can be manipulated in the PSCs which will allow the dissection of the roles of specific stromal mediators on pancreatic cancer progression. Such models are currently being developed in several laboratories.

7.2   Further Characterization of PSCs

Despite their important roles in CP and PDAC, PSCs remain poorly understood. The origin of these cells remains unclear. There is some data supporting the concept that bone marrow derived cells can differentiated into PSCs in an experimental model of CP [176]. However, after 45 weeks of cerulean treatment the bone derived cells only contributed to around 5% of the PSCs in this model. Therefore, the majority of PSCs do not seem to derive from bone marrow. Further studies need to be undertaken to understand the origins of these cells. Likewise, the influence of these cells on CP and PDAC is only beginning to be explored. The interactions are likely to be complex and may be different during early lesions and during later stages of PDAC.

7.3   Influence of PSC on Immune Responses

PSCs and the stroma that they produce is a prominent feature of PDAC. However, the PSCs are not the only cells found in the stroma. In particular, various leucocytes reside within the stroma of PDAC. It is known that these immune cells to not mount an effective response to PDAC. Whether and how the stroma contributes to the lack of immune responsiveness is unknown. However, PSCs produce TGFβ, which is immunosuppressive [177]. Whether PSC produce other immunosuppressive factors and the overall influence of PSCs on immune responses is unknown. Investigation of these relationships requires new models, as the current orthotopic xenograft models of PDAC do not mimic this interaction and occur in immune compromised animals.

References

1. Mortenson MM, Katz MH, Tamm EP, Bhutani MS, Wang H, Evans DB, Fleming JB: Current diagnosis and management of unusual pancreatic tumors. Am J Surg 2008;196:100–113.

2. Degen L, Wiesner W, Beglinger C: Cystic and solid lesions of the pancreas. Best Pract Res Clin Gastroenterol 2008;22:91–103.

3. Maitra A, Hruban RH: Pancreatic cancer. Annu Rev Pathol 2008;3:157–188.

4. Hart AR, Kennedy H, Harvey I: Pancreatic cancer: a review of the evidence on causation. Clin Gastroenterol Hepatol 2008;6:275–282.

5. Koliopanos A, Avgerinos C, Paraskeva C, Touloumis Z, Kelgiorgi D, Dervenis C: Molecular aspects of carcinogenesis in pancreatic cancer. Hepatobiliary Pancreat Dis Int 2008;7:345–356.

6. Hezel AF, Kimmelman AC, Stanger BZ, Bardeesy N, DePinho RA: Genetics and biology of pancreatic

ductal adenocarcinoma. Genes Dev 2006;20: 1218–1249.

7. Brembeck FH, Schreiber FS, Deramaudt TB, Craig L, Rhoades B, Swain G, Grippo P, Stoffers DA, Silberg DG, Rustgi AK: The mutant K-ras oncogene causes pancreatic periductal lymphocytic infiltration and gastric mucous neck cell hyperplasia in transgenic mice. Cancer Res 2003;63:2005–2009.

8. Grippo PJ, Nowlin PS, Demeure MJ, Longnecker DS, Sandgren EP: Preinvasive pancreatic neoplasia of ductal phenotype induced by acinar cell targeting of mutant Kras in transgenic mice. Cancer Res 2003;63:2016–2019.

9. Guerra C, Schuhmacher AJ, Canamero M, Grippo PJ, Verdaguer L, Perez-Gallego L, Dubus P, Sandgren EP, Barbacid M: Chronic pancreatitis is essential for induction of pancreatic ductal adenocarcinoma by K-Ras oncogenes in adult mice. Cancer Cell 2007;11:291–302.

10. Pour PM, Pandey KK, Batra SK: What is the origin of pancreatic adenocarcinoma? Mol Cancer 2003;2:13.

11. Stanger BZ, Stiles B, Lauwers GY, Bardeesy N, Mendoza M, Wang Y, Greenwood A, Cheng KH, McLaughlin M, Brown D, et al.: Pten constrains centroacinar cell expansion and malignant transformation in the pancreas. Cancer Cell 2005;8:185–195.

12. Hingorani SR, Petricoin EF, Maitra A, Rajapakse V, King C, Jacobetz MA, Ross S, Conrads TP, Veenstra TD, Hitt BA, et al.: Preinvasive and invasive ductal pancreatic cancer and its early detection in the mouse. Cancer Cell 2003;4:437–450.

13. Carriere C, Seeley ES, Goetze T, Longnecker DS, Korc M: The Nestin progenitor lineage is the compartment of origin for pancreatic intraepithelial neoplasia. Proc Natl Acad Sci USA 2007; 104:4437–4442.

14. Otsuki M: Chronic pancreatitis. The problems of diagnostic criteria. Pancreatology 2004;4:28–41.

15. Witt H, Apte MV, Keim V, Wilson JS: Chronic pancreatitis: challenges and advances in pathogenesis, genetics, diagnosis, and therapy. Gastroenterology 2007;132:1557–1573.

16. Steer ML, Waxman I, Freedman S: Chronic pancreatitis. N Engl J Med 1995;332:1482–1490.

17. Seymour AB, Hruban RH, Redston M, Caldas C, Powell SM, Kinzler KW, Yeo CJ, Kern SE: Allelotype of Pancreatic Adenocarcinoma. Cancer res 1994;2761–2764.

18. Mutema G, Fenoglio-Preiser C: Pathology and Natural History of Pancreatic Cancer. In Gastrointestinal Oncology. JL Abbruzzese, (ed.). 2004; New York: Oxford University Press.

19. Ekbom A, McLaughlin JK, Karlsson BM, Nyren O, Gridley G, Adami HO, Fraumeni JF, Jr.: Pancreatitis and pancreatic cancer: a population-based study. J Natl Cancer Inst 1994;86:625–627.

20. Malka D, Hammel P, Maire F, Rufat P, Madeira I, Pessione F, Levy P, Ruszniewski P: Risk of pancreatic adenocarcinoma in chronic pancreatitis. Gut 2002; 51:849–852.

21. Bansal P, Sonnenberg A: Pancreatitis is a risk factor for pancreatic cancer. Gastroenterology 1995; 109:247–251.

22. Lowenfels AB, Maisonneuve P, Cavallini G, Ammann RW, Lankisch PG, Andersen JR, Dimagno EP, Andren-Sandberg A, Domellof L: Pancreatitis and the risk of pancreatic cancer. International Pancreatitis Study Group. N Engl J Med 1993; 328:1433–1437.

23. Whitcomb DC: Inflammation and Cancer V. Chronic pancreatitis and pancreatic cancer. Am J Physiol Gastrointest Liver Physiol 2004;287:G315–G319.

24. Lowenfels AB, Maisonneuve P: Epidemiology and risk factors for pancreatic cancer. Best Pract Res Clin Gastroenterol 2006;20:197–209.

25. Whitcomb DC, Gorry MC, Preston RA, Furey W, Sossenheimer MJ, Ulrich CD, Martin SP, Gates LK, Jr., Amann ST, Toskes PP, et al.: Hereditary pancreatitis is caused by a mutation in the cationic trypsinogen gene. Nat Genet 1996;14:141–145.

26. Lowenfels AB, Maisonneuve P, DiMagno EP, Elitsur Y, Gates LK, Jr., Perrault J, Whitcomb DC: Hereditary pancreatitis and the risk of pancreatic cancer. International Hereditary Pancreatitis Study Group. J Natl Cancer Inst 1997;89:442–446.

27. Takaori K, Hruban RH, Maitra A, Tanigawa N: Current topics on precursors to pancreatic cancer. Adv Med Sci 2006;51:23–30.

28. Maitra A, Fukushima N, Takaori K, Hruban RH: Precursors to invasive pancreatic cancer. Adv Anat Pathol 2005;12:81–91.

29. Hruban RH, Adsay NV, bores-Saavedra J, Compton C, Garrett ES, Goodman SN, Kern SE, Klimstra DS, Kloppel G, Longnecker DS, et al.: Pancreatic intraepithelial neoplasia: a new nomenclature and classification system for pancreatic duct lesions. Am J Surg Pathol 2001;25:579–586.

30. Feldmann G, Beaty R, Hruban RH, Maitra A: Molecular genetics of pancreatic intraepithelial neoplasia. J Hepatobiliary Pancreat Surg 2007; 14:224–232.

31. Wilentz RE, Iacobuzio-Donahue CA, Argani P, McCarthy DM, Parsons JL, Yeo CJ, Kern SE, Hruban RH: Loss of expression of Dpc4 in pancreatic intraepithelial neoplasia: evidence that DPC4 inactivation occurs late in neoplastic progression. Cancer Res 2000;60:2002–2006.

32. Hruban RH, Goggins M, Parsons J, Kern SE: Progression model for pancreatic cancer. Clin Cancer Res 2000;6:2969–2972.

33. Rosty C, Geradts J, Sato N, Wilentz RE, Roberts H, Sohn T, Cameron JL, Yeo CJ, Hruban RH, Goggins M: p16 Inactivation in pancreatic intrae-pithelial neoplasias (PanINs) arising in patients with chronic pancreatitis. Am J Surg Pathol 2003;27:1495–1501.

34. Volkholz H, Stolte M, Becker V: Epithelial dysplasias in chronic pancreatitis. Virchows Arch A Pathol Anat Histol 1982;396:331–349.

35. Hermanova M, Nenutil R, Kren L, Feit J, Pavlovsky Z, Dite P: Proliferative activity in pancreatic intraepithelial neoplasias of chronic pancreatitis resection specimens: detection of a high-risk lesion. Neoplasma 2004;51:400–404.

36. Fukushima N, Koopmann J, Sato N, Prasad N, Carvalho R, Leach SD, Hruban RH, Goggins M: Gene expression alterations in the non-neoplastic parenchyma adjacent to infiltrating pancreatic ductal adenocarcinoma. Mod Pathol 2005;18:779–787.

37. Hanahan D, Weinberg RA: The hallmarks of cancer. Cell 2000;100:57–70.

38. Jones S, Zhang X, Parsons DW, Lin JC, Leary RJ, Angenendt P, Mankoo P, Carter H, Kamiyama H, Jimeno A, et al.: Core signaling pathways in human pancreatic cancers revealed by global genomic analyses. Science 2008;321:1801–1806.

39. Saif MW, Karapanagiotou L, Syrigos K: Genetic alterations in pancreatic cancer. World J Gastroenterol 2007;13:4423–4430.

40. Almoguera C, Shibata D, Forrester K, Martin J, Arnheim N, Perucho M: Most human carcinomas of the exocrine pancreas contain mutant c-K-ras genes. Cell 1988;53:549–554.

41. Ren YX, Xu GM, Li ZS, Song YG: Detection of point mutation in K-ras oncogene at codon 12 in pancreatic diseases. World J Gastroenterol 2004;10:881–884.

42. Sawada Y, Gonda H, Hayashida Y: Combined use of brushing cytology and endoscopic retrograde pancreatography for the early detection of pancreatic cancer. Acta Cytol 1989;33:870–874.

43. Kubota Y, Takaoka M, Tani K, Ogura M, Kin H, Fujimura K, Mizuno T, Inoue K: Endoscopic transpapillary biopsy for diagnosis of patients with pancreaticobiliary ductal strictures. Am J Gastroenterol 1993;88:1700–1704.

44. Arvanitakis M, Van Laethem JL, Parma J, De Maertelaer V, Delhaye M, Deviere J: Predictive factors for pancreatic cancer in patients with chronic pancreatitis in association with K-ras gene mutation. Endoscopy 2004;36:535–542.

45. Shi C, Fukushima N, Abe T, Bian Y, Hua L, Wendelburg BJ, Yeo CJ, Hruban RH, Goggins MG, Eshleman JR: Sensitive and quantitative detection of KRAS2 gene mutations in pancreatic duct juice differentiates patients with pancreatic cancer from

46. Tateishi K, Tada M, Yamagata M, Isayama H, Komatsu Y, Kawabe T, Shiratori Y, Omata M: High proportion of mutant K-ras gene in pancreatic juice of patients with pancreatic cystic lesions. Gut 1999;45:737–740.

47. Costentin L, Pages P, Bouisson M, Berthelemy P, Buscail L, Escourrou J, Pradayrol L, Vaysse N: Frequent deletions of tumor suppressor genes in pure pancreatic juice from patients with tumoral or nontumoral pancreatic diseases. Pancreatology 2002;2:17–25.

48. Furuya N, Kawa S, Akamatsu T, Furihata K: Long-term follow-up of patients with chronic pancreatitis and K-ras gene mutation detected in pancreatic juice. Gastroenterology 1997;113:593–598.

49. Gutierrez AA, Martinez F, Mas-Oliva J: Identification of K-ras mutations in pancreatic juice. Ann Intern Med 1996;124:1014–1015.

50. Kimura W, Zhao B, Futakawa N, Muto T, Makuuchi M: Significance of K-ras codon 12 point mutation in pancreatic juice in the diagnosis of carcinoma of the pancreas. Hepatogastroenterology 1999;46:532–539.

51. Tada M, Omata M, Kawai S, Saisho H, Ohto M, Saiki RK, Sninsky JJ: Detection of ras gene mutations in pancreatic juice and peripheral blood of patients with pancreatic adenocarcinoma. Cancer Res 1993;53:2472–2474.

52. Mulcahy H, Farthing MJ: Diagnosis of pancreaticobiliary malignancy: detection of gene mutations in plasma and stool. Ann Oncol 1999;10:Suppl 4:114–117.

53. Caldas C, Hahn SA, Hruban RH, Redston MS, Yeo CJ, Kern SE: Detection of K-ras mutations in the stool of patients with pancreatic adenocarcinoma and pancreatic ductal hyperplasia. Cancer Res 1994;54:3568–3573.

54. Wu X, Lu XH, Xu T, Qian JM, Zhao P, Guo XZ, Yang XO, Jiang WJ: Evaluation of the diagnostic value of serum tumor markers, and fecal k-ras and p53 gene mutations for pancreatic cancer. Chin J Dig Dis 2006;7:170–174.

55. Lohr M, Maisonneuve P, Lowenfels AB: K-Ras mutations and benign pancreatic disease. Int J Pancreatol 2000;27:93–103.

56. Berthelemy P, Bouisson M, Escourrou J, Vaysse N, Rumeau JL, Pradayrol L: Identification of K-ras mutations in pancreatic juice in the early diagnosis of pancreatic cancer. Ann Intern Med 1995;123:188–191.

57. Hsiang D, Friess H, Buchler MW, Ebert M, Butler J, Korc M: Absence of K-ras mutations in the pancreatic parenchyma of patients with chronic pancreatitis. Am J Surg 1997;174:242–246.

58. Nakaizumi A, Uehara H, Takenaka A, Uedo N, Sakai N, Yano H, Ohigashi H, Ishikawa O, Ishiguro S, Sugano K, et al.: Diagnosis of pancreatic cancer by cytology and measurement of oncogene and tumor markers in pure pancreatic juice aspirated by endoscopy. Hepatogastroenterology 1999;46:31–37.

59. Lohr M, Kloppel G, Maisonneuve P, Lowenfels AB, Luttges J: Frequency of K-ras mutations in pancreatic intraductal neoplasias associated with pancreatic ductal adenocarcinoma and chronic pancreatitis: a meta-analysis. Neoplasia 2005;7:17–23.

60. Deramaudt T, Rustgi AK: Mutant KRAS in the initiation of pancreatic cancer. Biochim Biophys Acta 2005;1756:97–101.

61. Klein WM, Hruban RH, Klein-Szanto AJ, Wilentz RE: Direct correlation between proliferative activity and dysplasia in pancreatic intraepithelial neoplasia (PanIN): additional evidence for a recently proposed model of progression. Mod Pathol 2002; 15:441–447.

62. Klimstra DS, Longnecker DS: K-ras mutations in pancreatic ductal proliferative lesions. Am J Pathol 1994;145:1547–1550.

63. Andea A, Sarkar F, Adsay VN: Clinicopathological correlates of pancreatic intraepithelial neoplasia: a comparative analysis of 82 cases with and 152 cases without pancreatic ductal adenocarcinoma. Mod Pathol 2003;16:996–1006.

64. Ji B, Song J, Tsou L, Logsdon CD: Activation of K-RAS in pancreatic acinar cells causess chronic pancreatitis in transgenic mice. Gastroenterology 2007;132:A116–A117.

65. Schutte M, Hruban RH, Geradts J, Maynard R, Hilgers W, Rabindran SK, Moskaluk CA, Hahn SA, Schwarte-Waldhoff I, Schmiegel W, et al.: Abrogation of the Rb/p16 tumor-suppressive pathway in virtually all pancreatic carcinomas. Cancer Res 1997;57:3126–3130.

66. Kalthoff H, Schmiegel W, Roeder C, Kasche D, Schmidt A, Lauer G, Thiele HG, Honold G, Pantel K, Riethmuller G, et al.: p53 and K-RAS alterations in pancreatic epithelial cell lesions. Oncogene 1993;8:289–298.

67. Bian Y, Matsubayashi H, Li CP, Abe T, Canto M, Murphy KM, Goggins M: Detecting low-abundance p16 and p53 mutations in pancreatic juice using a novel assay: heteroduplex analysis of limiting dilution PCRs. Cancer Biol Ther 2006;5:1392–1399.

68. Talar-Wojnarowska R, Gasiorowska A, Smolarz B, Romanowicz-Makowskal H, Strzelczyk J, Janiak A, Malecka-Panas E: Comparative evaluation of p53 mutation in pancreatic adenocarcinoma and chronic pancreatitis. Hepatogastroenterology 2006;53:608–612.

69. Bhardwaj A, Marsh WL, Jr., Nash JW, Barbacioru CC, Jones S, Frankel WL: Double immunohistochemical staining with MUC4/p53 is useful in the distinction of pancreatic adenocarcinoma from chronic pancreatitis: a tissue microarray-based study. Arch Pathol Lab Med 2007;131:556–562.

70. Itoi T, Takei K, Sofuni A, Itokawa F, Tsuchiya T, Kurihara T, Nakamura K, Moriyasu F, Tsuchida A, Kasuya K: Immunohistochemical analysis of p53 and MIB-1 in tissue specimens obtained from endoscopic ultrasonography-guided fine needle aspiration biopsy for the diagnosis of solid pancreatic masses. Oncol Rep 2005;13:229–234.

71. Truty MJ, Urrutia R: Basics of TGF-beta and pancreatic cancer. Pancreatology 2007;7:423–435.

72. Hahn SA, Schutte M, Hoque AT, Moskaluk CA, da Costa LT, Rozenblum E, Weinstein CL, Fischer A, Yeo CJ, Hruban RH, et al.: DPC4, a candidate tumor suppressor gene at human chromosome 18q21.1. Science 1996;271:350–353.

73. Biankin AV, Kench JG, Biankin SA, Lee CS, Morey AL, Dijkman FP, Coleman MJ, Sutherland RL, Henshall SM: Pancreatic intraepithelial neoplasia in association with intraductal papillary mucinous neoplasms of the pancreas: implications for disease progression and recurrence. Am J Surg Pathol 2004;28:1184–1192.

74. Salek C, Benesova L, Zavoral M, Nosek V, Kasperova L, Ryska M, Strnad R, Traboulsi E, Minarik M: Evaluation of clinical relevance of examining K-ras, p16 and p53 mutations along with allelic losses at 9p and 18q in EUS-guided fine needle aspiration samples of patients with chronic pancreatitis and pancreatic cancer. World J Gastroenterol 2007;13:3714–3720.

75. Farrow B, Sugiyama Y, Chen A, Uffort E, Nealon W, Mark EB: Inflammatory mechanisms contributing to pancreatic cancer development. Ann Surg 2004;239:763–769.

76. Logsdon CD, Simeone DM, Binkley C, Arumugam T, Greenson JK, Giordano TJ, Misek DE, Hanash S: Molecular profiling of pancreatic adenocarcinoma and chronic pancreatitis identifies multiple genes differentially regulated in pancreatic cancer. Cancer Res. 2003;63:2649–2657.

77. Binkley CE, Zhang L, Greenson JK, Giordano TJ, Kuick R, Misek D, Hanash S, Logsdon CD, Simeone DM: The molecular basis of pancreatic fibrosis: common stromal gene expression in chronic pancreatitis and pancreatic adenocarcinoma. Pancreas 2004;29:254–263.

78. Crnogorac-Jurcevic T, Efthimiou E, Nielsen T, Loader J, Terris B, Stamp G, Baron A, Scarpa A, Lemoine NR: Expression profiling of microdissected pancreatic adenocarcinomas. Oncogene 2002;21: 4587–4594.

79. Nakamura T, Furukawa Y, Nakagawa H, Tsunoda T, Ohigashi H, Murata K, Ishikawa O, Ohgaki K,

Kashimura N, Miyamoto M, et al.: Genome-wide cDNA microarray analysis of gene expression profiles in pancreatic cancers using populations of tumor cells and normal ductal epithelial cells selected for purity by laser microdissection. Oncogene 2004;23:2385–2400.

80. Grutzmann R, Pilarsky C, Ammerpohl O, Luttges J, Bohme A, Sipos B, Foerder M, Alldinger I, Jahnke B, Schackert HK, et al.: Gene expression profiling of microdissected pancreatic ductal carcinomas using high-density DNA microarrays. Neoplasia 2004; 6:611–622.

81. Alldinger I, Dittert D, Peiper M, Fusco A, Chiappetta G, Staub E, Lohr M, Jesnowski R, Baretton G, Ockert D, et al.: Gene expression analysis of pancreatic cell lines reveals genes overexpressed in pancreatic cancer. Pancreatology 2005;5:370–379.

82. Missiaglia E, Blaveri E, Terris B, Wang YH, Costello E, Neoptolemos JP, Crnogorac-Jurcevic T, Lemoine NR: Analysis of gene expression in cancer cell lines identifies candidate markers for pancreatic tumorigenesis and metastasis. Int J Cancer 2004; 112:100–112.

83. Domagk D, Schaefer KL, Eisenacher M, Braun Y, Wai DH, Schleicher C, Diallo-Danebrock R, Bojar H, Roeder G, Gabbert HE, et al.: Expression analysis of pancreatic cancer cell lines reveals association of enhanced gene transcription and genomic amplifications at the 8q22.1 and 8q24.22 loci. Oncol Rep 2007;17:399–407.

84. Archer H, Jura N, Keller J, Jacobson M, Bar-Sagi D: A mouse model of hereditary pancreatitis generated by transgenic expression of R122H trypsinogen. Gastroenterology 2006;131:1844–1855.

85. Colby JK, Klein RD, McArthur MJ, Conti CJ, Kiguchi K, Kawamoto T, Riggs PK, Pavone AI, Sawicki J, Fischer SM: Progressive metaplastic and dysplastic changes in mouse pancreas induced by cyclooxygenase-2 overexpression. Neoplasia 2008; 10:782–796.

86. Muller-Decker K, Furstenberger G, Annan N, Kucher D, Pohl-Arnold A, Steinbauer B, Esposito I, Chiblak S, Friess H, Schirmacher P, et al.: Preinvasive duct-derived neoplasms in pancreas of keratin 5-promoter cyclooxygenase-2 transgenic mice. Gastroenterology 2006;130:2165–2178.

87. Harris RE: Cyclooxygenase-2 (cox-2) and the inflammogenesis of cancer. Subcell Biochem 2007; 42:93–126.

88. Aguirre AJ, Bardeesy N, Sinha M, Lopez L, Tuveson DA, Horner J, Redston MS, DePinho RA: Activated Kras and Ink4a/Arf deficiency cooperate to produce metastatic pancreatic ductal adenocarcinoma. Genes Dev 2003;17:3112–3126.

89. Johnson L, Mercer K, Greenbaum D, Bronson RT, Crowley D, Tuveson DA, Jacks T: Somatic activation of the K-ras oncogene causes early onset lung cancer in mice. Nature 2001;410:1111–1116.

90. Duan RD, Zheng CF, Guan KL, Williams JA: Activation of MAP kinase kinase (MEK) and Ras by cholecystokinin in rat pancreatic acini. Am J Physiol 1995;268:G1060–G1065.

91. Wagner M, Greten FR, Weber CK, Koschnick S, Mattfeldt T, Deppert W, Kern H, Adler G, Schmid RM: A murine tumor progression model for pancreatic cancer recapitulating the genetic alterations of the human disease. Genes Dev 2001; 15:286–293.

92. Pandol SJ, Gukovsky I, Satoh A, Lugea A, Gukovskaya AS: Animal and in vitro models of alcoholic pancreatitis: role of cholecystokinin. Pancreas 2003;27:297–300.

93. Blomhoff R, Wake K: Perisinusoidal stellate cells of the liver: important roles in retinol metabolism and fibrosis. FASEB J 1991;5:271–277.

94. Gressner A, Bachem M: Molecular mechanisms of liver fibrogenesis – a homage to the role of activated fat-storing cells. Digestion 1995;56:335–346.

95. de Leeuw A, McCarthy S, Geerts A, Knook D: Purified rat liver fat-storing cells in culture divide and contain collagen. Hepatology 1984;4:392–403.

96. Pinzani M: Novel insights into the biology and physiology of the Ito cell. Pharmacol Ther 1995;66:387–412.

97. Apte M, Haber P, Applegate T, Norton I, McCaughan G, Korsten M, Pirola R, Wilson J: Periacinar stellate shaped cells in rat pancreas: identification, isolation, and culture. Gut 1998;43:128–133.

98. Bachem MG, Schneider E, Grob H, Weidenbach H, Schmid RM, Menke A, Siech M, Beger H, Grunert A, Adler G: Identification, culture, and characterization of pancreatic stellate cells in rats and humans. Gastroenterology 1998;115:421–432.

99. Apte M, Phillips PA, Fahmy R, Darby S, Rodgers S, McGaughan G, Korsten M, Pirola R, Naidoo D, Wilson J: Does alcohol directly stimulate pancreatic fibrogenesis? Studies with rat pancreatic stellate cells. Gastroenterology 2000;118:780–794.

100. McCarroll J, Phillips P, Santucci N, Pirola R, Wilson J, Apte M: Vitamin A inhibits pancreatic stellate cell activation: implications for treatment of pancreatic fibrosis.2005.

101. Apte M, Haber P, Darby S, Rodgers S, McCaughan G, Korsten M, Pirola R, Wilson J: Pancreatic stellate cells are activated by proinflammatory cytokines: implications for pancreatic fibrogenesis. Gut 1999;44:534–541.

102. Phillips PA, McCarroll JA, Park S, Wu M-J, Pirola R, Korsten M, Wilson JS, Apte MV: Rat

pancreatic stellate cells secrete matrix metallopro-teinases: implications for extracellular matrix turn-over. Gut 2003;52:275–282.

103. Gomez JA, Molero X, Vaquero E, Alonso A, Salas A, Malagelada JR: Vitamin E attenuates bio-chemical and morphological features associated with development of chronic pancreatitis. Am J Physiol Gastrointest Liver Physiol 2004;287: G162–169.

104. Yoo B, Oh T, Kim Y, Yeo M, Lee J, Surh Y, Ahn B, Kim W, Sohn S, Kim J, et al.: Novel antioxidant ameliorates the fibrosis and inflammation of cerulein-induced chronic pancreatitis in a mouse model. Pancreatology 2005;5:165–176.

105. Hisada S, Shimizu K, Shiratori K, Kobayashi M: Peroxisome proliferator-activated receptor gamma ligand prevents the development of chronic pancreatitis through modulating NF-kappaB-dependent proinflammatory cytokine production and pancreatic stellate cell activation. Rocz Akad Med Bialymst 2005;50:142–147.

106. Apte M, Park S, Phillips P, Santucci N, Goldstein D, Kumar R, Ramm G, Buchler MW, Friess H, McCarroll J, et al.: Desmoplastic reaction in pan-creatic cancer. Role of pancreatic stellate cells. Pancreas 2004;29:179–187.

107. Kalluri R, Zeisberg M: Fibroblasts in cancer. Nat Rev Cancer 2006;6:392–401.

108. Mackie EJ, Chiquet-Ehrismann R, Pearson CA, Inaguma Y, Taya K, Kawarada Y, Sakakura T: Tenas-cin is a stromal marker for epithelial malignancy in the mammary gland. Proc Natl Acad Sci USA 1987;84:4621–4625.

109. Ishihara A, Yoshida T, Tamaki H, Sakakura T: Tenascin expression in cancer cells and stroma of human breast cancer and its prognostic signifi-cance. Clin Cancer Res 1995;1:1035–1041.

110. Brunner A, Mayerl C, Tzankov A, Verdorfer I, Tschorner I, Rogatsch H, Mikuz G: Prognostic significance of tenascin-C expression in superficial and invasive bladder cancer. J Clin Pathol 2004;57:927–931.

111. Orimo A, Gupta P, Sgroi D, Arenzana-Seisdedos F, Delaunay T, Naeem R, Carey V, Richardson A, Weinberg RA: Stromal fibroblasts present in inva-sive human breast carcinomas promote tumor growth and angiogenesis through elevated SDF-1/CXCL12 secretion. Cell 2005;121:335–348.

112. Olumi Af, Grossfeld GD, Hayward SW, Carroll PR, Tlsty TD, Cunha GR: Carcinoma-associated fibroblasts direct tumor progression of initiated human prostatic epithelium. Cancer Res 1999;59: 5002–5011.

113. Hwang RF, Moore T, Arumugam T, Ramachandran V, Amos K, Rivera A, Ji B, Evans DB, Logsdon C: Cancer-associated stromal

fibroblasts promote pancreatic tumor progression. Cancer Res 2008;68:918–926.

114. Yoshida S, Yokota T, Ujiki M, Ding X-Z, Pelham C, Adrian TE, Talamonti MS, Bell Jr RH, Denham W: Pancreatic cancer stimulates pancreatic stellate cell proliferation and TIMP-1 production through the MAP kinase pathway. Biochem Biophy Res Comm 2004;323:1241–1245.

115. Koninger J, Giese T, di Mola FF, Wente MN, Esposito I, Bachem MG, Giese NA, Buchler MW, Friess H: Pancreatic tumor cells influence the composition of the extracellular matrix. Biochem Biophy Res Comm 2004;322:943–949.

116. Bachem M, Schunemann M, Ramadani M, Siech M, Beger H, Buck A, Zhou S, Schmid-Kotsas A, Adler G: Pancreatic carcinoma cells induce fibrosis by stimulating proliferation and matrix synthesis of stellate cells. Gastroenterology 2005;128: 907–921.

117. Lee M, Gu D, Feng L, Curriden S, Amush M, Krahl T, Gurushanthaiah D, Wilson C, Loskutoff D, Fox H, et al.: Accumulation of extra-cellular matrix and developmental dysregulation in the pancreas by trnasgenic produciton of trans-forming growth factor-B1. Am J Path 1995;147:42–52.

118. Sanvito F, Nichols A, Herrera P, Huarte J, Wohl-wend A, Vassalli J, Orci L: TGF-B1 overexpression in murine pancreas induces chronic pancreatitis and, together with TNF-alpha, triggers insulin-dependent diabetes. Biochem Biophy Res Comm 1995;217:1279–1286.

119. Nagashio Y, Ueno H, Imamura M, Asaumi H, Watanabe S, Yamaguchi T, Taguchi M, Tashiro M, Otsuki M: Inhibition of transforming growth fac-tor B decreases pancreatic fibrosis and protects the pancreas against chronic injury in mice. Lab Invest 2004;84:1610–1618.

120. Shek FW, Benyon RC, Walker FM, McCrudden PR, Pender SL, Williams EJ, Johnson PA, Johnson CD, Bateman AC, Fine DR, et al.: Expression of trans-forming growth factor-beta 1 by pancreatic stellate cells and its implications for matrix secretion and turnover in chronic pancreatitis. Am J Pathol 2002;160:1787–1798.

121. Bhowmick NA, Chytil A, Plieth D, Gorska AE, Dumont N, Shappell S, Washington MK, Neilson EG, Moses HL: TGF-beta signaling in fibroblasts modulates the oncogenic potential of adjacent epithelia. Science 2004;303:848–851.

122. Bierie B, Moses HL: Tumour microenvironment: TGF[beta]: the molecular Jekyll and Hyde of cancer. Nat Rev Cancer 2006;6:506–520.

123. Chang HY, Chi JT, Dudoit S, Bondre C, van de Rijn M, Botstein D, Brown PO: Diversity, topo-graphic differentiation, and positional memory in

human fibroblasts. Proc Natl Acad Sci USA 2002;99:12877–12882.

124. Hwang R, Yokoi K, Bucana C, Tsan R, Killion JJ, Evans DB, Fidler IJ: Inhibition of platelet-derived growth factor receptor phosphorylation by STI571 (Gleevec) reduces growth and metastasis of human pancreatic carcinoma in an orthotopic nude mouse model. Clin Cancer Res 2003;9:6534–6544.

125. Schneider E, Schmid-Kotsas A, Zhao J, Weidenbach H, Schmid RM, Menke A, Adler G, Waltenberger J, Grunert A, Bachem MG: 2001. Identification of mediators stimulating proliferation and matrix synthesis of rat pancreatic stellate cells. C532–C543.

126. Masamune A, Satoh M, Kikuta K, Suzuki N, Shimosegawa T: Activation of JAK-STAT pathway is required for platelet-derived growth factor-induced proliferation of pancratic stellate cells. World J Gastroenterol 2005;11:3385–3391.

127. Vonlaufen A, Joshi S, Qu C, Phillips PA, Xu Z, Parker NR, Toi CS, Pirola RC, Wilson JS, Goldstein D, et al.: Pancreatic Stellate Cells: Partners in Crime with Pancreatic Cancer Cells. Cancer Res 2008;68:2085–2093.

128. Masamune A, Kikuta K, Satoh M, Suzuki N, Shimosegawa T: Green tea polyphenol epigallocatechin-3-gallate blocks PDGF-induced proliferation and migration of rat pancreatic stellate cells. World J Gastroenterol 2005;11:3368–3374.

129. Armstrong T, Packham G, Murphy LB, Bateman AC, Conti JA, Fine DR, Johnson CD, Benyon RC, Iredale JP: Type I Collagen Promotes the Malignant Phenotype of Pancreatic Ductal Adenocarcinoma. Clin Cancer Res 2004;7427–7437.

130. Hartel M, Di Mola F, Gardini A, Zimmerman A, di Sebastiano P, Guweidhi A, Innocenti P, Giese T, Giese NA, Buchler MW, et al.: Desmoplastic reaction influences pancreatic cancer growth behavior. World J Surg 2004;28:818–825.

131. Gao R, Birgstock D: Connective tissue growth factor (CCN2) in rat pancreatic stellate cell function: integrin alpha5 beta1 as a novel CCN2 receptor. Gastroenterology 2005;129:1019–1030.

132. Aikawa T, Gunn J, Spong SM, Klaus SJ, Korc M: Connective tissue growth factor-specific antibody attenuates tumor growth, metastasis, and angiogenesis in an orthotopic mouse model of pancreatic cancer. Mol Cancer Ther 2006;5:1108–1116.

133. Dornhofer N, Spong S, Bennewith K, Salim A, Klaus S, Kambham N, Wong C, Kaper F, Sutphin P, Nacamuli R, et al.: Connective tissue growth factor-specific monoclonal antibody therapy inhibits pancreatic tumor growth and metastasis. Cancer Res 2006;66:5816–5827.

134. Sato N, Fukushima N, Maehara N, Matsubayashi H, Koopmann J, Su G, Hruban RH, Goggins M: SPARC/osteonectin is a frequent target for aberrant methylation in pancreatic adenocarcinoma and a mediator of tumor-stromal interactions. Oncogene 2003;22:5021–5030.

135. Muerkoster S, Wegenhenkel K, Arlt A, Witt M, Sipos B, Kruse M-L, Sebens T, Kloppel G, Kalthoff H, Folsch U, et al.: Tumor stroma interactions induce chemoresistance in pancreatic ductal carcinoma cells involving increased secretion and paracrine efects of nitric oxide and interleukin-1B. Cancer Res 2004;15:1331–1337.

136. Vaquero EC, Edderkaoui M, Nam KJ, Gukovsky I, Pandol SJ, Gukovskaya AS: Extracellular matrix proteins protect pancreatic cancer cells from death via mitochondrial and nonmitochondrial pathways. Gastroenterology 2003;125:1188–1202.

137. Miyamoto H, Murakami T, Tsuchida K, Sugino H, Miyake H, Tashiro S: Tumor-stroma interaction of human pancreatic cancer: acquired resistance to anticancer drugs and proliferation regulation is dependent on extracellular matrix proteins. Pancreas 2004;28:38–44.

138. Koninger J, Giese NA, di Mola F, Berberat P, Giese T, Esposito I, Bachem M, Buchler MW, Friess H: Overexpressed decorin in pancreatic cancer: potential tumor growth inhibition and attneuation of chemotherapeutic action. Clin Cancer Res 2004;10:4776–4783.

139. Muerkoster SS, Werbing V, Koch D, Sipos B, Ammerpohl O, Kalthoff H, Tsao MS, Folsch UR, Schafer H: Role of myofibroblasts in innate chemoresistance of pancreatic carcinoma – epigenetic downregulation of caspases. Int J Cancer 2008;123:1751–1760.

140. Ohuchida K, Mizumoto K, Murakami M, Qian L, Sato N, Nagai E, Matsumoto K, Nakamura T, Tanaka M: Radiation to stromal fibroblasts increases invasiveness of pancreatic cancer cells through tumor-stromal interactions. Cancer Res 2004;64:3215–3222.

141. Jura N, Archer H, Bar-Sagi D: Chronic pancreatitis, pancreatic adenocarcinoma and the black box in-between. Cell Res 2005;15:72–77.

142. Garcea G, Dennison AR, Steward WP, Berry DP: Role of inflammation in pancreatic carcinogenesis and the implications for future therapy. Pancreatology 2005;5:514–529.

143. Farrow B, Evers BM: Inflammation and the development of pancreatic cancer. Surg Oncol 2002; 10:153–169.

144. Algul H, Treiber M, Lesina M, Schmid RM: Mechanisms of disease: chronic inflammation and cancer in the pancreas – a potential role for pancreatic stellate cells? Nat Clin Pract Gastroenterol Hepatol 2007;4:454–462.

145. Pelicano H, Carney D, Huang P: ROS stress in cancer cells and therapeutic implications. Drug Resist Updat 2004;7:97–110.

146. Karin M, Greten FR: NF-kappaB: linking inflammation and immunity to cancer development and progression. Nat Rev Immunol 2005;5:749–759.

147. Schlosser W, Schlosser S, Ramadani M, Gansauge F, Gansauge S, Beger HG: Cyclooxygenase-2 is overexpressed in chronic pancreatitis. Pancreas 2002; 25:26–30.

148. Rakonczay Z, Jr., Hegyi P, Takacs T, McCarroll J, Saluja AK: The role of NF-kappaB activation in the pathogenesis of acute pancreatitis. Gut 2008; 57:259–267.

149. Mantovani A, Allavena P, Sica A, Balkwill F: Cancer-related inflammation. Nature 2008;454: 436–444.

150. Itzkowitz SH, Yio X: Inflammation and cancer IV. Colorectal cancer in inflammatory bowel disease: the role of inflammation. Am J Physiol Gastrointest Liver Physiol 2004;287:G7–G17.

151. Farinati F, Cardin R, Cassaro M, Bortolami M, Nitti D, Tieppo C, Zaninotto G, Rugge M: Helicobacter pylori, inflammation, oxidative damage and gastric cancer: a morphological, biological and molecular pathway. Eur J Cancer Prev 2008; 17:195–200.

152. Pondugula K, Wani S, Sharma P: Barrett's esophagus and esophageal adenocarcinoma in adults: long-term GERD or something else? Curr Gastroenterol Rep 2007;9:468–474.

153. Baumann B, Weber CK, Troppmair J, Whiteside S, Israel A, Rapp UR, Wirth T: Raf induces NF-kappaB by membrane shuttle kinase MEKK1, a signaling pathway critical for transformation. Proc Natl Acad Sci USA 2000;97:4615–4620.

154. Repasky GA, Zhou Y, Morita S, Der CJ: Ras-mediated intestinal epithelial cell transformation requires cyclooxygenase-2-induced prostaglandin E2 signaling. Mol Carcinog 2007;46:958–970.

155. Maciag A, Sithanandam G, Anderson LM: Mutant K-rasV12 increases COX-2, peroxides and DNA damage in lung cells. Carcinogenesis 2004; 25:2231–2237.

156. Wang W, Abbruzzese JL, Evans DB, Larry L, Cleary KR, Chiao PJ: The nuclear factor-kappa B RelA transcription factor is constitutively activated in human pancreatic adenocarcinoma cells. Clin Cancer Res 1999;5:119–127.

157. Merati K, said Siadaty M, Andea A, Sarkar F, Ben-Josef E, Mohammad R, Philip P, Shields AF, Vaitkevicius V, Grignon DJ, et al.: Expression of inflammatory modulator COX-2 in pancreatic ductal adenocarcinoma and its relationship to pathologic and clinical parameters. Am J Clin Oncol 2001;24:447–452.

158. Nagasaka T, Koi M, Kloor M, Gebert J, Vilkin A, Nishida N, Shin SK, Sasamoto H, Tanaka N, Matsubara N, et al.: Mutations in both KRAS and

159. Brentnall TA, Chen R, Lee JG, Kimmey MB, Bronner MP, Haggitt RC, Kowdley KV, Hecker LM, Byrd DR: Microsatellite instability and K-ras mutations associated with pancreatic adenocarcinoma and pancreatitis. Cancer Res 1995; 55:4264–4267.

160. Patti MG, Pellegrini CA: Gallstone pancreatitis. Surg Clin North Am 1990;70:1277–1295.

161. Saluja A, Saluja M, Villa A, Leli U, Rutledge P, Meldolesi J, Steer M: Pancreatic duct obstruction in rabbits causes digestive zymogen and lysosomal enzyme colocalization. J Clin Invest 1989;84: 1260–1266.

162. Lerch MM, Saluja AK, Runzi M, Dawra R, Saluja M, Steer ML: Pancreatic duct obstruction triggers acute necrotizing pancreatitis in the opossum. Gastroenterology 1993;104:853–861.

163. Esposito I, Seiler C, Bergmann F, Kleeff J, Friess H, Schirmacher P: Hypothetical progression model of pancreatic cancer with origin in the centroacinar-acinar compartment. Pancreas 2007;35:212–217.

164. Wolff R, Varadhachary G, Evans D: Adjuvant therapy for adenocarcinooma of the pancreas: analysis of reported trials and recommendations for future progress. Ann Surg Onc 2008;15:2773–2786.

165. Kojima K, Vickers SM, Adsay NV, Jhala NC, Kim HG, Schoeb TR, Grizzle WE, Klug CA: Inactivation of Smad4 accelerates Kras(G12D)-mediated pancreatic neoplasia. Cancer Res 2007;67:8121–8130.

166. Bardeesy N, Cheng KH, Berger JH, Chu GC, Pahler J, Olson P, Hezel AF, Horner J, Lauwers GY, Hanahan D, et al.: Smad4 is dispensable for normal pancreas development yet critical in progression and tumor biology of pancreas cancer. Genes Dev 2006;20:3130–3146.

167. Yang Y, Dukhanina O, Tang B, Mamura M, Letterio J, MacGregor J, Patel S, Khozin S, Liu Z, Green J, et al.: Lifetime exposure to a soluble TGF-B antagonist protects mice against metastasis without adverse side effects. J Clin Invest 2002; 109:1607–1615.

168. Arteaga C: Inhibition of TGF[beta] signaling in cancer therapy. Curr Opin Genet Dev 2006; 16:30–37.

169. Wang XM, Ming D, Yu T, McCaughan GW, Gorrell MD: Fibroblast activation protein increases apoptosis, cell adhesion, and migration by the LX-2 human stellate cell line. Hepatology 2005;42: 935–945.

170. Scott AM, Wiseman G, Welt S, Adjei A, Lee F-T, Hopkins W, Divgi CR, Hanson LH, Mitchell P, Gansen DN, et al.: A Phase I Dose-Escalation Study of Sibrotuzumab in Patients with Advanced

or Metastatic Fibroblast Activation Protein-positive Cancer. Clin Cancer Res 2003;9:1639–1647.

171. Loeffler M, Kruger J, Niethammer A, Reisfeld R: Targeting tumor-associated fibroblasts improves cancer chemotherapy by increasing intratumoral drug uptake. J Clin Invest 2006;116:1955–1962.

172. Bramhall S, Schulz J, Nemunaitis J, Brown P, Baillet M, Buckels J: A double-blind placebo-controlled, randomised study comparing gemcitabine and marimastat with gemcitabine and placebo as first line therapy in patients with advanced pancreatic cancer. Br J Cancer 2002;87:161–167.

173. Bramhall SR, Rosemurgy A, Brown PD, Bowry C, Buckels JAC: Marimastat as First-Line Therapy for Patients With Unresectable Pancreatic Cancer: A Randomized Trial. J Clin Oncol 2001;19: 3447–3455.

174. Evans J, Stark A, Johnson C, Daniel F, Carmichael J, Buckels J, Imrie C, Brown P, Neoptolemos J: A

phase II trial of marimastat in advanced pancreatic cancer. Br J Cancer 2001;85:1865–1870.

175. Müerköster SS, Werbing V, Koch D, Sipos B, Ammerpohl O, Kalthoff H, Tsao M-S, Fölsch UR, Schäfer H: Role of myofibroblasts in innate chemoresistance of pancreatic carcinoma - Epigenetic downregulation of caspases. Int J Cancer 2008; 123:1751–1760.

176. Marrache F, Pendyala S, Bhagat G, Betz KS, Song Z, Wang TC: Role of bone marrow-derived cells in experimental chronic pancreatitis. Gut 2008; 57:1113–1120.

177. Wrzesinski SH, Wan YY, Flavell RA: Transforming growth factor-beta and the immune response: implications for anticancer therapy. Clin Cancer Res 2007;13:5262–5270.

12 Pancreatic Cancer Stem Cells

Chenwei Li · Diane M. Simeone

1 Introduction 318

2 Pancreatic Cancer and Cancer Stem Cells 320

3 Origin of Cancer Stem Cells 323

4 Developmental Signaling Pathways 325

5 Cancer Stem Cells and Metastasis 326

6 Cancer Stem Cells are Resistant to Standard Therapies 326

7 Conclusions 328

J. P. Neoptolemos, R. Urrutia, J. L. Abbruzzese, M. W. Büchler (eds.), *Pancreatic Cancer*,
DOI 10.1007/978-0-387-77498-5_12, © Springer Science+Business Media, LLC 2010

Abstract: The concept of cancer stem cells was first proposed 150 years ago and recent studies have demonstrated the existence of cancer stem cells that have the exclusive capacity for tumor initiation and propagation. Emerging data has been provided to support the existence of cancer stem cells in human blood cell-derived cancers and solid organ tumors of the breast, prostate, brain, pancreas, head and neck, skin, and colon. Furthermore, pathways that regulate self-renewal, such as Bmi-1, Wnt, PTEN, Notch and Hedgehog which are known to regulate self-renewal of normal stem cells, have been implicated in the regulation of cancer stem cell self-renewal in a number of different tumor types. The study of human pancreatic cancers has revealed a unique subpopulation of cancer cells that possess the all characteristics of cancer stem cells. The pancreatic cancer stem cells express the cell surface markers CD44, CD24, and epithelial-specific antigen (ESA), and represent 0.5–1.0% of the total pancreatic cancer cell population. Along with the characteristics of self-renewal and multilineage differentiation, pancreatic cancer stem cells display upregulation of Sonic hedgehog (SHH) and Bmi-1. Aberrant activation of these pathways in cancer stem cells are believed to be responsible for uncontrolled self-renewal of cancer stem cells which generate tumors that are resistant to radiation and chemotherapy. Conventional cancer therapeutics eliminate differentiated tumor cells, but do not target the cancer stem cells. The cancer stem cell concept points to a new direction of cancer therapeutics, which targets cancer stem cells. Pancreatic cancer stem cell research will aid our understanding of the molecular and cellular events leading to the development of pancreatic cancer and may change the therapeutic approach to the treatment of pancreatic cancer.

1 Introduction

The concept that cancers arise from normal stem cells was first hypothesized more than 150 years ago [1], however, only recently have the techniques been developed to test the cancer stem-cell hypothesis in human solid tumors. Scientists first observed that when cancer cells of many different types were assayed for their proliferative potential, only a minority of cells showed extensive proliferation [2]. This observation suggested that malignant neoplasms are comprised of a small subset of distinct cancer stem cells (typically <5% of total cancer cell population based on expression of various cell surface markers) with great proliferative potential, and well-differentiated cancer cells have very limited proliferative potential. The traditional theory about how tumors develop is shown in ❯ *Fig. 12-1a*, in which tumor cells are heterogeneous and most cancer cells can proliferate extensively to form new tumors. In the cancer stem cell theory (❯ *Fig. 12-1b*), tumor cells are also heterogeneous, but only a small portion of cancer cells are able to proliferate extensively and form new tumors. These cells are termed cancer stem cells because like normal stem cells, they can both self-renew and produce differentiated progeny.

Studies in the field of hematopoiesis have provided a powerful means of investigating normal versus malignant stem cell biology, as the cell surface markers that identify a normal stem cell population are well characterized [3]. The isolation of the cancer stem cell was elusive initially due to the absence of a reproducible behavior or surface phenotype. John Dick and colleagues first identified cancer stem cells in acute myeloid leukemia in 1997 [4], showing that the ability to regenerate human leukemia in non-obese diabetic severe combined deficiency (NOD/SCID) mice was retained in a rare subgroup of cancer stem cells. These cancer stem cells, which displayed the cell surface marker phenotype of $CD34^+/CD38-$, represented only

■ Fig. 12-1

The cancer stem cell theory. The traditional theory about how neoplasms develop is shown in (a), where most tumor cells can proliferate extensively and form new tumors. In the cancer stem cell theory (b), tumor cells are heterogenous, but only cancer stem cells are able to proliferate extensively and form new tumors. These cells are termed cancer stem cells because like normal stem cells, they can both self renew and produce differentiated progeny. (Stem cells, cancer, and cancer stem cells. Nature 2001;414:05–11.)

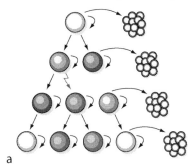 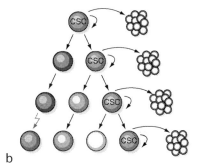

a. Tumour cells are heterogeneous, but most cells can proliferate extensively and form new tumours

b. Tumour cells are heterogeneous and only the cancer stem cell subset (CSC: yellow) has the ability to proliferate extensively and form new tumours

0.1% of the total cancer cell population and regenerated a tumor identical in appearance to the parent neoplasm. In contrast, tens of thousands of leukemic cancer cells lacking this phenotype were not tumorigenic.

Recently, several studies have provided direct evidence for the existence of cancer stem cells in several types of solid tumors. In 2003, Al-Hajj et al. reported that a phenotypically distinct and relatively rare population of tumor-initiating cells (TICs) was responsible for the propagation of tumors from eight of nine human metastatic breast cancer specimens [5]. Primary tumor cells expressing a CD44+/CD24– were shown to initiate tumors upon transplantation into immune-deficient NOD/SCID mice, while all the other tumor cells failed to propagate tumors. Importantly, as few as 100 flow cytometry purified cells could initiate tumor formation and were able to not only undergo self-renewal but also produce a more differentiated cell population in secondary recipient mice. Further evidence in support of a role for cancer stem cells in solid tumors has also come recently from the study of brain tumors. Studies by Singh et al. have shown that the neural stem cell antigen CD133 is expressed on brain-derived TICs from pediatric medulloblastomas and pilocytic astrocytomas [6]. The CD133+ subpopulations from these tumors were able to initiate clonally derived neurospheres in vitro that demonstrated self-renewal, differentiation and proliferative characteristics similar to normal brain stem cells [6–8]. Furthermore, transplantation of CD133+ cells, but not CD133– cells into NOD/SCID mice was sufficient to induce growth of tumors in vivo. Taken together, these findings strongly implicate TICs in at least some forms of brain cancer. In addition, given the similarity of normal neural stem cells and TICs, the data suggest that normal stem cells are the target of transforming events that lead to brain cancer.

The existence of human cancer stem cells in other solid tumor types has since been proven, including glioblastoma [9], multiple myeloma [10], prostate [11], ovarian [12], colon [13,14],

☐ Table 12-1

Cancer stem cells have been identified in several types of human cancer

Cancer type	Surface marker (s)	Reference (s)
Leukemia	$CD34^+/CD38^-$	4
Breast cancer	$CD44^+$ ESA^+ $CD24^-$/low	5
Brain cancer	$CD133^+$	6, 8, 9
Multiple myeloma	$CD138^-$	10
Prostate cancer	$CD44^+$	11
Ovarian cancer	SP cells	12
Colon cancer	$CD133^+$	13, 14
Pancreatic cancer	$CD44^+$ $CD24^+$ ESA^+	15
Liver	$CD133^+$	16
Head and Neck	$CD44^+$	17

liver [15], head and neck [16] and pancreatic cancer [17]. Although some cell surface markers seem to define a cancer stem cell in several cancer types (e.g., CD44 and CD133), it appears that each tumor type possesses a unique combination of cell surface markers that define the cell subpopulation with the highest tumorigenic potential (❯ *Table 12-1*).

2 Pancreatic Cancer and Cancer Stem Cells

Pancreatic adenocarcinoma is a highly lethal disease, which is usually diagnosed in an advanced state for which there are little or no effective therapies. It has the worst prognosis of any major malignancy (3% 5-year survival) and is the fourth most common cause of cancer death yearly in the United States, with an annual incidence rate approximating the annual death rate of 37,000 people [18]. Despite advances in surgical and medical therapy, little effect has been made on the mortality rate of this disease. One of the major hallmarks of pancreatic cancer is its extensive local tumor invasion and early systemic dissemination. The molecular basis for these characteristics of pancreatic cancer is incompletely understood. Attempts to better understand the molecular characteristics of pancreatic cancer have focused on studying gene and protein expression profiles of samples of pancreatic cancer. However, these types of studies have not taken into account the heterogeneity of cancer cells within pancreatic tumor.

A recent study by our group identified a subpopulation of pancreatic cancer cells with a $CD44^+$ $CD24^+$ ESA^+ surface marker expression profile as putative pancreatic cancer stem cells [17]. Primary tumor cells taken directly from patients or obtained from low passage (passage 1 or 2) primary pancreatic tumors expanded as xenografts in NOD-SCID mice were sorted for the markers CD44, CD24, and ESA, either individually or in combination. These sorted cells were injected into NOD/SCID mice and their tumorigenic potential was assessed (❯ *Table 12-2*). Data generated from 10 pancreatic cancers showed that cells expressing all three surface markers $CD44^+$ $CD24^+$ ESA+, comprising only 0.2–0.8% of all human pancreatic cancer cells, had the highest tumorigenic potential. As few as 100 $CD44^+$ $CD24^+$ ESA^+ cells were able to generate tumors in 50% of mice (six of 12 mice), while tumors did not form in mice until 10,000 CD44–CD24–ESA– were injected into NOD/SCID mice (one of

◘ Table 12-2

Tumorigenic pancreatic cancer cells were highly enriched in the CD44$^+$ CD24$^+$ ESA$^+$ population

Cell Number	10^4	10^3	500	100
Unsorted	4/6	0/6	0/3	0/3
CD44$^+$	8/16	7/16	5/16	4/16
CD44$^-$	2/16	1/16	1/16	0/16
ESA$^+$	12/18	13/18	8/18	0/18
ESA$^-$	3/18	1/18	1/18	0/18
CD24$^+$	11/16	10/16	7/16	1/16
CD24$^-$	2/16	1/16	0/16	0/16
CD44$^+$ CD24$^+$ ESA$^+$	10/12	10/12	7/12	6/12
CD44-CD24-ESA-	1/12	0/12	0/12	0/12

12 mice). CD44$^+$ CD24$^+$ ESA$^+$ cells demonstrated at least a 100-fold greater tumor-initiating potential than maker negative cells.

CD44 is a transmembrane glycoprotein, which relates to drug resistance and poor prognosis in many malignancies [19]. In addition to hyaluronic acid, CD44 binds fibrinogen, fibronectin, collagen, laminin, FGF2, other heparin-binding growth factors, and osteopontin, an inflammatory cytokine that is associated with metastasis. The role of CD44 in drug resistance by activating multiple survival pathways via growth factor receptors or integrin-mediated signaling is not known and further study is needed to determine the functional significance of CD44 in cancer stem cell biology. CD24 is a cell adhesion molecule and involved in signaling pathways in cancer cells that are dependent on interactions with P-selectin [20,21]. CD24-mediated binding to P-selectin on endothelial cells may participate in the process of metastasis. Epithelial surface antigen (ESA) is a glycoprotein that is largely confined to human epithelial cells.

The ability of CD44$^+$ CD24$^+$ ESA$^+$ pancreatic cancer stem cells to produce differentiated progeny and recapitulate the phenotype of the primary tumor of origin was verified by histology (◉ Fig. 12-2a). Tumors derived from CD44$^+$ CD24$^+$ ESA$^+$ pancreatic cancer stem cells were almost identical in appearance to the primary tumor of origin and also had similar patterns of expression of the differentiation markers S100P and stratifin, which are expressed in the most human pancreatic adenocarcinomas (◉ Fig. 12-2b). The highly tumorigenic CD44$^+$ CD24$^+$ ESA$^+$ cells gave rise to additional CD44$^+$ CD24$^+$ ESA$^+$ cells as well as phenotypically diverse non-tumorigenic cells, demonstrating the same phenotypic complexity as the primary tumor from which the tumorigenic cells were derived. This data verified that CD44$^+$ CD24$^+$ ESA$^+$ pancreatic cancer cells have the ability to both self-renew and produce differentiated progeny. In addition to in vivo dilutional tumor propagation assays, pancreatic cancer stem cells have also been identified based on in vitro sphere forming assays. It was observed that visually inspected and plated, single CD44$^+$ CD24$^+$ ESA$^+$ cells form pancreatic tumorspheres, while CD44–CD24–ESA– cells do not (◉ Fig. 12-3). These CD44$^+$ CD24$^+$ ESA$^+$ tumorspheres could be passaged multiple times without loss of tumorsphere forming capability, which is reflective of self-renewal capacity in vitro.

Hermann et al. [22] reported that CD133$^+$ cells in primary pancreatic cancers and pancreatic cancer cell lines also discriminate for cells with enhanced proliferative capacity.

■ Fig. 12-2

Tumor formation in NOD/SCID mice injected with highly tumorigenic $CD44^+$ $CD24^+$ ESA^+ pancreatic cancer cells. (a) H & E staining of the tumor generated from $CD44^+$ $CD24^+$ ESA^+cells in NOD/SCID mice (right panel) has similar histologic features to the corresponding patient's primary pancreatic tumor (left panel). Magnification 200X. (b) Expression of the differentiation markers S100P (top two panels) and stratifin (bottom two panels) is similar in tumors derived from $CD44^+$ $CD24^+$ ESA^+pancreatic cancer stem cells in NOD/SCID and the corresponding primary tumor form the patient. Antibody localization was performed using horseradish peroxidase, with dark brown staining indicating the presence of the specific antigen.

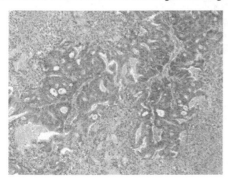

a   Primary tumor   Tumor generated from
                                             CD44⁺ CD24⁺ ESA⁺ cells

              Primary tumor   Tumor generated from
                                             CD44⁺ CD24⁺ ESA⁺ cells

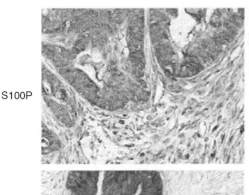
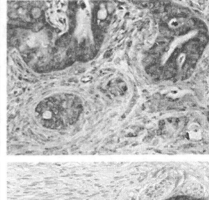
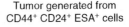

S100P

Stratifin

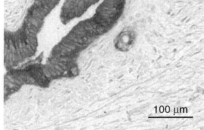
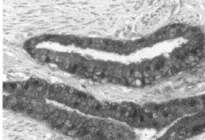

100 μm

b

◘ Fig. 12-3

Tumorsphere formation from a CD44$^+$ CD24$^+$ ESA$^+$ pancreatic cancer cell in vitro.

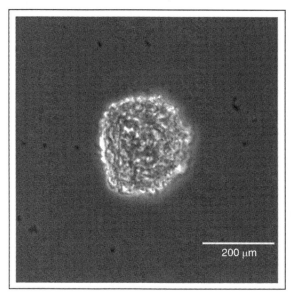

The CD133$^+$ cells comprised 1–3% of pancreatic adenocarcinoma cells analyzed in the study, and as few as 500 CD133$^+$ cells injected in immunocompromised mice generate tumors that recapitulated the primary tumor of origin, but as many as 1 million CD133-tumor cells did not result in any tumor formation. They also reported an overlap of 14% between CD44$^+$ CD24$^+$ ESA$^+$ and CD133$^+$ pancreatic cancer cells. Wright et al. [23] recently reported that there are two distinct phenotypes of stem cells in breast cancer expressing CD44$^+$/CD24– and CD133$^+$ with no overlap of surface marker depending on the tumor that they used to isolate the cancer stem cell populations. Each cancer stem cell population behaved similarly with equal potency for tumor formation. Further experiments will be needed to verify whether CD44$^+$ CD24$^+$ ESA$^+$ and CD133$^+$ pancreatic cancer cells represent two distinct cancer stem cell populations or if overlap of all four cell surface markers identifies a further enriched pancreatic cancer stem cell population.

3   Origin of Cancer Stem Cells

There are two parts to the cancer stem cell hypothesis. The first part of the hypothesis is that cancers are "driven" by cells with stem cell-like properties. Published data discussed above supports this aspect of the cancer stem cell hypothesis for human pancreatic cancer. The second part of the cancer stem cell hypothesis is that cancers arise from tissue stem or progenitor cells. The answer to the second part of the hypothesis with regard to pancreatic cancer remains unclear. It is possible that pancreatic cancer stem cells arise from differentiated cell within the organ that undergoes de-differentiation and adopts a stem cell-like phenotype, or alternatively that pancreatic cancers arise from a normal stem or progenitor cell that undergoes malignant change to become a cancer stem cell. Cancer stem cells possess many

◻ Table 12-3

Common characteristics of normal stem cells and cancer stem cells

Ability to self-renew
Ability to make differentiated progeny
Long-lived
Resistant to damaging agents
Anchorage-independent

◻ Table 12-4

Pathways involved in stem cell self-renewal

Hedgehog
Notch
Bmi-1
Wnt
PTEN

features of normal stem cells, such as the ability to undergo self-renewal and multilineage differentiation, resistance to DNA damaging agents, and anchorage-independent survival (◉ *Table 12-3*). Stem cells are defined by their ability to undergo self-renewal, which is a cell division in which one or both of the daughter cells remain undifferentiated and retain the ability to produce another stem cell with the same capacity to proliferate as the parental cell. Researchers have hypothesized that cancer stem cells arise from their normal stem cell counterparts that gradually undergo accumulation of genetic changes until the cells acquire a malignant phenotype. Normal stem cells are the longest lived cells in tissues, and it is thought that these cells are more likely to accumulate mutations over time and ultimately assume a malignant phenotype. Studies in both hematologic malignancies and breast cancer support the concept that cancer stem cells may arise from self-renewing normal stem cells that are transformed by dysregulation of a self-renewal pathway, resulting in expansion of tumorigenic cancer cells [24,25]. In fact, pathways involved in self renewal in normal stem cells are found to be dysregulated in human malignancies. These pathways include the Wnt, Sonic hedgehog, Bmi-1, PTEN, and Notch (◉ *Table 12-4*). Alternatively, in some cancer types, studies suggest that cancer stem cells may arise from mutated progenitor cells called transit-amplifying cells that develop the capacity for unregulated self-renewal [26,27]. In pancreatic cancer, recent data in a genetically engineered mouse model of pancreatic cancer suggests that pancreatic acinar or centroacinar cells may indeed be the "cell of origin" of pancreatic cancer [28], although this remains quite controversial. Additional studies are currently underway in several laboratories to validate this finding.

The identification of normal pancreatic stem cells has been elusive despite attempts made by research groups to identify this cell. Researchers believe that like other tissues, stem/progenitor cells must also exist in the pancreas and that putative multipotent, adult resident pancreatic stem or progenitor cells are capable of giving arise to the pancreatic ductal epithelial cells, acinar cells and endocrine cells. There is some evidence to suggest that pancreatic stem/progenitor cells reside within pancreatic ductal cells, where they can differentiate and migrate to form new islets during both organogenesis and regeneration [29,30]. In addition, endocrine differentiation has been reported in human pancreatic duct cells [31,32], when these newly generated islets were transplanted into diabetic NOD mice, diabetes was reversed. Furthermore, a recent study demonstrated that fetal pancreatic ductal cells could differentiate into insulin-producing cells [33]. These data suggest that duct cells are a source of pancreatic progenitor cells. There is also some support for the notion that pancreatic stem/progenitor cells reside inside the islet or acinar tissue [34]. A distinct population of nestin-positive cells resides in the rat and human islets and has been reported as hormone-negative immature cells that can proliferate extensively in vitro and appear to be multipotent [35,36]. Although this study does not provide evidence of the proliferation and differentiation potential of these putative stem cells, their immature morphology, their small size and quiescence has lead to the hypothesis that these cells may serve as stem/progenitors contributing to islet growth. Furthermore, Suzuki et al identified a possible pancreatic stem/progenitor cell candidate that expresses the receptor for hepatocyte growth factor (HGF), c-Met, and resides in the developing and adult mouse pancreas. In adults these cells are expressed in the duct as well as in some of the acinar cells. These cells form colonies in vitro and differentiate into multiple pancreatic lineage cells from single cells [37]. Ultimately, identification and characterization of normal pancreatic stem cells will help determine if pancreatic cancers arise from a mutated normal stem cell or from a mutated differentiated cell type.

4 Developmental Signaling Pathways

It has been reported that human pancreatic adenocarcinomas display increased hedgehog pathway activity [38,39]. Transgenic overexpression of SHH within the pancreas results in the development of cancer precursor lesions (PanIN lesions) in a genetically engineered mouse model. To determine if the putative pancreatic cancer stem cell population had enhanced expression of developmental genes, Li et al. examined expression level of SHH, based on previous reports linking hedgehog signaling to pancreatic cancer [17]. Misregulation of hedgehog signaling has also been shown to play a role in other types of cancer, including basal cell carcinoma, breast cancer, and small cell lung cancer [24,40]. Hedgehog pathway activation occurs in a significant number of primary human pancreatic carcinomas [38, 39] and PanIn lesions, precursor lesions of invasive pancreatic cancer. Additionally, transgenic overexpression of SHH within the pancreas results in PanIn lesions and the accumulation of genetic mutations commonly seen in pancreatic cancer, including k-ras mutations and up-regulation of Her2/neu, suggesting that Hedgehog signaling is an early mediator of pancreatic cancer tumorigenesis. Inhibition of hedgehog signaling by cyclopamine inhibited pancreatic cancer growth in vitro and in vivo, suggesting that this signaling pathway has an early and critical role in the genesis of pancreatic cancer [39]. Li et al. reported that expression of the SHH transcript was increased about fourfold in bulk and CD44−CD24−ESA− pancreatic cancer cells when compared with normal pancreatic epithelial cells, but was increased >40 fold in CD44$^+$ CD24$^+$ ESA$^+$ cells (❯ Fig. 12-4), suggesting that SHH is highly up-regulated in pancreatic cancer stem cells, with persistent, albeit lower, expression in their differentiated progeny [17]. Studies are currently underway to assess whether the hedgehog signaling pathway is activated in pancreatic cancer stem cells and to determine the role of hedgehog signaling in pancreatic cancer stem cell function. We also observed that BMI-1, a protein important in mediating self renewal pathways in many types of stem cells, is significantly

■ Fig. 12-4

mRNA expression of Sonic Hedgehog (SHH) and Bmi-1, genes important in developmental signaling pathways, in normal pancreas, nontumorigenic pancreatic cancer cells and highly tumorigenic CD44+ CD24+ ESA+ pancreatic cancer cells. Total RNA was isolated and mRNA was quantitated by real-time RT-PCR. Data are expressed as the mean ±SE. *$P < 0.05$ versus normal pancreas.

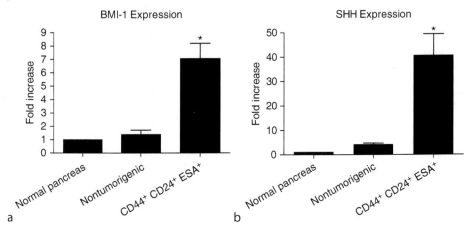

elevated in CD44+ CD24+ ESA+ pancreatic CSCs compared to their differentiated pancreatic cancer cells. This data suggests that BMI-1 may play a role in the maintenance of self-renewal in the pancreatic CSC population (unpublished data).

5 Cancer Stem Cells and Metastasis

Researchers in the cancer stem cell field have theorized that not only are cancer stem cells the "drivers" for cancer formation, but that cancer stem cells are the cells responsible for metastasis. A recent support by Hermann and colleagues suggests that this may indeed be the case. Hermann et al. [22] investigated the relationship between CD133+ pancreatic cancer stem cells, CXCR4 expression, and metastasis. CXCR4 is a chemokine receptor for the ligand stromal derived factor-1, a mediator of cell migration [41,42]. The authors reported that at the invading front of pancreatic tumors, CD133+ pancreatic cancer stem cells also co-express CXCR4. CD133+ CXCR4– and CD133+ CXCR4+ cells were able to form primary tumors equally, but only CD133+ CXCR4+ cells were able to metastasize [22]. The authors found that blockade of CXCR4 function prevented metastasis in this tumor model. These findings may have clinical implications when considering therapies to inhibit metastasis of cancer stem cells.

6 Cancer Stem Cells are Resistant to Standard Therapies

Conventional cancer treatments have been focused on the ability to kill most of the tumor population, but in doing so may miss the cancer stem cells. In several tumor types, cancer stem

◘ Fig. 12-5

Cancer stem cells are resistant to standard therapies. Only treatments that specifically target cancer stem cells will result in cancer cure. (Reya T, Morrison SJ, Clarke MF, et al. Stem cells, cancer, and cancer stem cells. Nature 2001;414:105–11.)

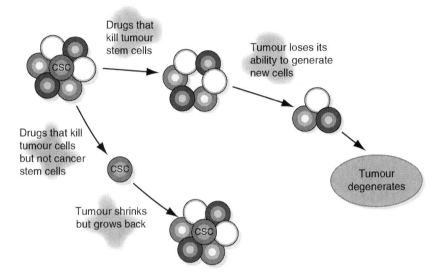

cells have been shown to be more resistant to chemotherapy and radiation. This may explains why conventional treatment may result in tumor shrinkage, but most tumors recur, likely because the cancer stem cell survives and regenerates the neoplasm (● Fig. 12-5). A prediction of the model is that treatments targeted specifically to the cancer stem cell population will be required to result in an effective cure of cancer. Studies in CD34+ CD38– cancer stem cells from leukemia showed that these cancer stem cells were significantly less sensitive to the treatment of daunorubicin or cytarabine than the bulk population of leukemic blast cells [43]. In addition, Matsui et al. [10] have shown that myeloma cancer stem cells are more resistant to standard therapies, including chemotherapy and proteosome inhibitors. It was also reported that the glioblastoma cancer stem cell expressing CD 133+ in both primary tumors and xenografts increased two- to fourfold after ionizing radiation [44]. This enrichment of CD133+ cancer stem cells was due to activation of the DNA damage response, protecting these cells from DNA damaging effects of radiation. Todaro et al. reported that CD133+ colon cancers tem cells were resistant to chemotherapeutic agents oxiplatin and fluorouracil, mediating by expression of interleukin (IL)-4 by the CD133+ colon cancer stem cells. Blocking IL-4 enhanced the antitumor efficacy of these chemotherapeutic agents through selective sensitization of CD133+ cancer stem cells [45].

Recent work on pancreatic cancer suggests that pancreatic cancer stem cells may be also resistant to chemotherapy and radiation. Shah et al. [46] reported that comparing to the parental cells from which they were derived, the gemcitabine-resistant pancreatic cancer cells expressed an increased level of the cell surface proteins CD44, CD24, and ESA. Hermann et al. [22] demonstrated that the CD133+ population in the L3.6p pancreatic cancer cell line was enriched after exposure to gemcitabine. Experiments performed in our laboratory indicate that treatment with ionizing radiation and the chemotherapeutic agent gemcitabine results in enrichment of the CD44$^+$ CD24$^+$ ESA$^+$ population in human primary pancreatic cancer xenografts and that these cells are more resistant to apoptosis induced by chemotherapy and radiation, compared to the non-tumorigenic pancreatic cancer cell population (unpublished observations). The mechanism which is involved in pancreatic cancer stem cell resistance to DNA damage induced by chemotherapy and radiation are unclear. It has been shown that some self-renewal pathways (Wnt, Notch) may contribute to cancer stem cell resistance to chemotherapy and radiation [47–49]. The detail mechanisms involved in the resistance of pancreatic cancer stem cells to chemotherapy and radiation, and the role of self-renewal pathways in mediating this resistance, remains to be elucidated.

Many studies have highlighted the extensive phenotypic and functional similarities between normal stem cells and cancer stem cells. Since cancer stem cells possess many of the features of normal stem cells, it will be important to determine if targeting strategies that may be effective in tackling cancer stem cells will unduly harm normal stem cells. Two recent papers suggest that selective targeting of cancer stem cells may indeed be possible. Yilmaz et al. [24] reported that conditional deletion of PTEN in adult hematopoietic cells lead to expansion of leukemic cancer stem cells and depletion of normal hematopoietic stem cells in a mouse model. Treatment of the mice with rapamycin, which functions to reverse the effects of PTEN deletion, blocked the development of cancer stem cells while not affecting the normal stem-cell population. In a separate study, specific targeting of the leukemic cancer stem cell surface molecule CD44 using a monoclonal antibody resulted in eradication of human acute myeloid leukemic stem cells while sparing normal stem cells in a xenogaft model [50].

7   Conclusions

In conclusion, recent evidence suggests that pancreatic cancer is a cancer stem cell driven disease. Isolation and characterization of pancreatic cancer stem cells reveal that these tumor-initiating cells share important signaling pathways seen in other solid organ cancer stem cells and contribute to resistance to conventional chemotherapy and radiation. Much work needs to be done to better understand the molecular machinery that regulates self-renewal and therapeutic resistance, as well as to better to understand the interactions between these cells and the tumor microenvironment. Such studies will hopefully translate into improved therapeutics and subsequently outcomes in patients with pancreatic cancer.

Key Research Points

- A unique subpopulation in pancreatic cancer cells expressing CD44$^+$ CD24$^+$ ESA$^+$ or CD133$^+$ with high tumorigenic potential are termed pancreatic cancer stem cells.
- These putative pancreatic cancer stem cells can self-renew and give rise to differentiated progeny.
- These putative pancreatic cancer stem cells display aberrant activity of pathways regulating self-renewal, like SHH and Bmi-1.

Future Research Directions

- Study and determine the specific gene expression patterns of pancreatic cancer stem cells.
- Characterize the pancreatic cancer stem cell microenvironment or niche.
- Explore the difference between pancreatic cancer stem cells and normal stem cells.

Clinical Implications

- Pancreatic cancer stem cells may be responsible for resistance to radiation and chemotherapy, cancer metastasis and cancer relapse.
- New therapeutic strategies targeting pancreatic cancer stem cells or their microenvironment, alone or in combination with chemotherapy, may lead to more effective clinical treatment or even a cure of pancreatic cancer.

References

1. Julius Cohnheim: (1839–1884) Experimental pathologist. JAMA 1968;206:1561–1562.
2. Reya T, Morrison SJ, Clarke MF, Weissman IL: Stem cells, cancer, and cancer stem cells. Nature 2001;414:105–111.
3. Jordan CT: Cancer stem cell biology: from leukemia to solid tumors. Curr Opin Cell Biol 2004;16:708–712.
4. Bonnet D, Dick JE: Human acute myeloid leukemia is organized as a hierarchy that originates from a primitive hematopoietic cell. Nat Med 1997;3:730–737.
5. Al-Hajj M, Wicha MS, Benito-Hernandez A, Morrison SJ, Clarke MF: Prospective identification of tumorigenic breast cancer cells. Proc Natl Acad Sci USA 2003;100:3983–3988.
6. Singh SK, Hawkins C, Clarke ID, Squire JA, Bayani J, Hide T, Henkelman RM, Cusimano MD, Dirks PB: Identification of human brain tumour initiating cells. Nature 2004;432:396–401.
7. Singh SK, Clarke ID, Terasaki M, Bonn VE, Hawkins C, Squire J, Dirks PB: Identification of a cancer stem cell in human brain tumors. Cancer Res 2003;63:5821–5828.
8. Hemmati HD, Nakano I, Lazareff JA, Masterman-Smith M, Geschwind DH, Bronner-Fraser M, Kornblum HI: Cancerous stem cells can arise from pediatric brain tumors. Proc Natl Acad Sci USA 2003;100:15178–15183.
9. Galli R, Binda E, Orfanelli U, et al.: Isolation and characterization of tumorigenic, stem-like neural precursors from human glioblastoma. Cancer Res. 2004;64:7011–7021.
10. Matsui W, Huff CA, Wang Q, et al.: Characterization of clonogenic multiple myeloma cells. Blood 2004;103:2332–2336.
11. Patrawala L, Calhoun T, Schneider-Broussard R, et al.: Highly purified CD44+ prostate cancer cells from xenograft human tumors are enriched in tumorigenic and metastatic progenitor cells. Oncogene 2006;25:1696–1708.
12. Szotek PP, Pieretti-Vanmarcke R, Masiakos PT, et al.: Ovarian cancer side population defines cells with stem cell-like characteristics and Mullerian inhibiting substance responsiveness. Proc Natl Acad Sci USA 2006;103:11154–11159.
13. O'Brien CA, Pollett A, Gallinger S, et al.: A human colon cancer cell capable of initiating tumour growth in immunodeficient mice. Nature 2007;445:106–110.
14. Ricci-Vitiani L, Lombardi DG, Pilozzi E, et al.: Identification and expansion of human-colon-cancer-initiating cells. Nature 2007;445:111–115.
15. Ma S, Chan KW, Hu L, et al.: Identification and characterization of tumorigenic liver cancer stem/progenitor cells. Gastroenterology 2007;132:2542–2556.
16. Prince ME, Sivanandan R, Kaczorowski A, et al.: Identification of a subpopulation of cells with cancer stem cell properties in head and neck squamous cell carcinoma. Proc Natl Acad Sci USA 2007;104:973–978.
17. Li C, Heidt DG, Dalerba P, et al.: Identification of pancreatic cancer stem cells. Cancer Res 2007;67:1030–1037.
18. Hoyert DL, Heron MP, Murphy SL, Kung HC: Deaths: final data for 2003. Natl Vital Stat Rep 2006;19:1–120.

19. Naor D, Nedvetzki S, Golan I, Melnik L, Faitelson Y: CD44 in cancer. Crit Rev Clin Lab Sci 2002; 39:527–579.

20. Aigner S, Ruppert M, Hubbe M, Sammar M, Sthoeger Z, Butcher EC, Vestweber D, Altevogt P: Heat stable antigen (mouse CD24) supports myeloid cell binding to endothelial and platelet P-selectin. Int Immunol 1995;7(10):1557–1565.

21. Kristiansen G, Sammar M, Altevogt P: Tumour biological aspects of CD24, a mucin-like adhesion molecule. J Mol Histol 2004;35(3):255–262.

22. Hermann PC, Huber SL, Herrler T, et al.: Distinct populations of cancer stem cells determine tumor growth and metastatic activity in human pancreatic cancer. Cell Stem Cell 2007;1:313–323.

23. Wright MH, Calcagno AM, Salcido CD, et al.: BRCA1 breast tumors contain distinct CD44+/CD24- and CD133+ cells with cancer stem cell characteristics. Breast Cancer Res 2008;10:R10.

24. Yilmaz OH, Valdez R, Theisen BK, et al.: Pten dependence distinguishes hematopoietic stem cells from leukemia-initiating cells. Nature 2006;441:475–482.

25. Ayyanan A, Civenni G, Ciarloni L, et al.: Increased Wnt signaling triggers oncogenic conversion of human breast epithelial cells by a Notch dependent mechanism. Proc Natl Acad Sci USA 2006;103:3799–3804.

26. Huntly BJ, Shigematsu H, Deguchi K, et al.: MOZ-TIF2, but not BCR-ABL, confers properties of leukemic stem cells to committed murine hematopoietic progenitors. Cancer Cell 2004;6:587–596.

27. Jamieson CH, Ailles LE, Dylla SJ, et al.: Granulocyte-macrophage progenitors as candidate leukemic stem cells in blast-crisis CML. N Engl J Med 2004;351:657–667.

28. Guerra C, Schuhmacher AJ, Canamero M, et al.: Chronic pancreatitis is essential for induction of pancreatic ductal adenocarcinoma by K-Ras oncogenes in adult mice. Cancer Cell 2007;11:291–302.

29. Gu D, Sarvetnick N: A transgenic model for studying islet development. Recent Prog Horm Res 1994;49:161–165.

30. Madsen OD, Jensen J, Blume N, Petersen HV, Lund K, Karlsen C, Andersen FG, Jensen PB, Larsson LI, Serup P: Pancreatic development and maturation of the islet B cell. Studies of pluripotent islet cultures. Eur J Biochem 1996;242:435–45.

31. Bonner-Weir S, Taneja M, Weir GC, Tatarkiewicz K, Song KH, Sharma A, O'Neil JJ: In vitro cultivation of human islets from expanded ductal tissue. Proc Natl Acad Sci USA 2000;97:7999–8004.

32. Gao R, Ustinov J, Pulkkinen MA, Lundin K, Korsgren O, Otonkoski T: Characterization of endocrine progenitor cells and critical factors for their differentiation in human adult pancreatic cell culture. Diabetes 2003;52:2007–2015.

33. Ogata T, Park KY, Seno M, Kojima I: Reversal of streptozotocin- induced hyperglycemia by transplantation of pseudoislets consisting of β cells derived from ductal cells. Endocr J 2004;51:381–386.

34. Guz Y, Nasir I, Teitelman G: Regeneration of pancreatic beta cells from intra-islet precursor cells in an experimental model of diabetes. Endocrinology 2001;142:4956–4968.

35. Zulewski H, Abraham EJ, Gerlach MJ, Daniel PB, Moritz W, Muller B, Vallejo M, Thomas MK, Habener JF: Multipotential nestin-positive stem cells isolated from adult pancreatic islets differentiate ex vivo into pancreatic endocrine, exocrine, and hepatic phenotypes. Diabetes 2001;50:521–533.

36. Abraham EJ, Leech CA, Lin JC, Zulewski H, Habener JF: Insulinotropic hormone glucagon-like peptide-1 differentiation of human pancreatic islet-derived progenitor cells into insulin-producing cells. Endocrinology 2002;143:3152–3161.

37. Suzuki A, Nakauchi H, Taniguchi H: Prospective isolation of multipotent pancreatic progenitors using flowcytometric cell sorting. Diabetes 2004;53:2143–2152.

38. Berman DM, Karhadkar SS, Maitra A, et al.: Widespread requirement for Hedgehog ligand stimulation in growth of digestive tract tumours. Nature 2003;425:846–851.

39. Thayer SP, di Magliano MP, Heiser PW, et al.: Hedgehog is an early and late mediator of pancreatic cancer tumorigenesis. Nature 2003;425:851–856.

40. Pasca di Magliano M, Hebrok M: Hedgehog signaling in cancer formation and maintenance. Nat Rev Cancer 2003;3:903–911.

41. Narducci MG, Scala E, Bresin A, et al.: Skin homing of Sezary cells involves SDF-1-CXCR4 signaling and down-regulation of CD26/dipeptidylpeptidase IV. Blood 2006;107:1108–1115.

42. Doitsidou M, Reichman-Fried M, Stebler J, et al.: Guidance of primordial germ cell migration by the chemokine SDF-1. Cell 2002;111:647–659.

43. Costello RT, Mallet F, Gaugler B, Sainty D, Arnoulet C, Gastaut JA, Olive D: Human acute myeloid leukemia CD34+/CD38- progenitor cells have decreased sensitivity to chemotherapy and Fas-induced apoptosis, reduced immunogenicity, and impaired dendritic cell transformation capacities. Cancer Res. 2000;60:4403–4411.

44. Bao S, Wu Q, McLendon RE, et al.: Glioma stem cells promote radioresistance by preferential activation of the DNA damage response. Nature 2006;444:756–760.

45. Todaro M, Alea Mp, Stefano AB, et al.: Colon cancer stem cells dictate tumor growth and resist

cell death by production of interleukin-4. Cell Stem Cell 2007;1:389–402.

46. Shah AN, Summy JM, Zhang J, et al.: Development and characterization of gemcitabine-resistant pancreatic tumor cells. Ann Surg Oncol 2007;14: 3629–3637.

47. Asanuma K, Moriai R, Yajima T, et al.: Survivin as a radioresistance factor in pancreatic cancer. Jpn J Cancer Res 2000;91:1204–1209.

48. Phillips TM, McBride WH, Pajonk F: The response of CD24(-/low)/CD44+ breast cancer-initiating cells to radiation. J Natl Cancer Inst 2006;98:1777–1785.

49. Mungamuri SK, Yang X, Thor AD, et al.: Survival signaling by notch1: Mammalian target of reapamycin (mtor)-dependent inhibition of p53. Cancer Res 2006;66:4715–4724.

50. Jin L, Hope KJ, Zhai Q, et al.: Targeting of CD44 eradicates human acute myeloid leukemic stem cells. Nature Med 2006;12:1167–1174.

13 Cell Cycle Control in Pancreatic Cancer Pathogenesis

Brian Lewis

1	***The Cell Cycle***	**335**
1.1	The Phases of the Cell Cycle	336
1.1.1	G_1	336
1.1.2	S	337
1.1.3	G_2	339
1.1.4	M	339
1.2	Cell Cycle Control	341
1.2.1	Cell Cycle Regulatory Proteins	341
1.2.2	D-Type Cyclins	342
1.2.3	E-Type Cyclins	343
1.2.4	A-Type Cyclins	343
1.2.5	B-Type Cyclins	343
1.2.6	Regulation of Cdks	343
1.2.7	Cdk Inhibitors	344
1.2.8	Regulating the Regulators: Transcription	345
1.2.9	Regulating the Regulators: Proteolytic Degradation	346
1.2.10	Other Regulators	347
1.3	Cell Cycle Checkpoints	348
1.4	The DNA Damage Response	349
2	***The Cell Cycle and Cancer***	**351**
2.1	Self-Sufficiency in Growth Signals	351
2.2	Insensitivity to Anti-Growth Signals	352
2.3	Limitless Replicative Potential	353
2.4	Reduced Apoptosis	353
2.5	Angiogenesis	354
2.6	Consequences of Aberrant Cell Cycle Progression	354
3	***The Cell Cycle and Pancreatic Cancer***	**356**
3.1	KRAS	357
3.2	MYC	358
3.3	INK4A/ARF	359
3.4	TP53	359
3.5	TGF-β Signaling	360
3.6	MicroRNAs	361

J. P. Neoptolemos, R. Urrutia, J. L. Abbruzzese, M. W. Büchler (eds.), *Pancreatic Cancer*,
DOI 10.1007/978-0-387-77498-5_13, © Springer Science+Business Media, LLC 2010

3.7   Hedgehog Signaling 362
3.8   Pancreatic Stellate Cells 362
3.9   Targeting the Cell Cycle During Therapy 362

Abstract: All multicellular organisms arise from the division of a single cell. Thus, to generate a complex living organism, these cell divisions must be performed with extremely high fidelity and reproducibility during the development of the organism. Furthermore, in the mature, or adult, organism, tissue and organismal homeostasis must be maintained, and this requires the coordination of cell division with cell growth and cell death. These needs have led to the evolution of a cell replication process, known as the cell division cycle, that is highly conserved among all eukaryotes from simple single cellular organisms such as budding yeast to complex mammals such as humans.

Pioneering studies by Lee Hartwell, performed in budding yeast, laid the groundwork for the identification and characterization of the key positive and negative regulators of this process. Given the importance of the regulation of the cell division cycle and its high fidelity execution to organismal homeostasis, it is unsurprising that alteration of the cell cycle is a hallmark feature of human malignancies. Importantly, many of the genes encoding key regulators of the cell cycle are mutated in both sporadic and hereditary forms of cancer including pancreatic cancers.

This chapter will provide an overview of the cell division cycle, as well as describe several of the key regulatory mechanisms that promote its high fidelity. The chapter will then illustrate how the cell cycle is altered in cancer cells, and how this contributes to cancer pathogenesis. Finally, the chapter will focus on pancreatic cancer, with an emphasis on understanding how many of the common genetic alterations identified in this tumor type contribute to dysregulation of the cell division cycle and to the malignant phenotype in this disease.

1   The Cell Cycle

Eukaryotic cells reproduce themselves through a highly ordered and regulated series of events that are collectively known as the eukaryotic cell cycle. During cell division, the genetic material and cellular contents of the cell must be faithfully replicated and transmitted to the resulting progeny as this is absolutely required of the viability and evolution of species. Thus, the dual goals of eukaryotic cell division are (1) to replicate the genetic material and other cellular contents with extraordinary conformity, lest the lineage be corrupted, and (2) to appropriately apportion and transmit the copies to progeny. To accomplish these objectives, a highly-ordered, -regulated and -accurate stepwise process has evolved that is conserved across eukaryotic species.

The greatest portion of the cell cycle is spent preparing for the proportionate division of the cellular contents, through a series of processes that involve the replication of the chromosomes that contain the genetic content; the expansion of cellular organelles such as the mitochondria and endoplasmic reticulum; and the production of the machinery required for the faithful transmission of these organelles and the genetic material to the resulting progeny. Thus, the cell division cycle is highly coupled to the growth of a cell, such that a cell approximately doubles in size from the time of its "birth" until the time of its next division.

Progress through the cell cycle is regulated such that each phase occurs only once during each cycle. Thus, the genomic information, DNA, is replicated only once during each cell cycle. Likewise, entry into active division, mitosis, occurs only once (after all of the DNA has been replicated), and the replicated chromosomes are segregated to progeny cells only once per cycle. Such tight control ensures that each daughter cell produced retains a diploid genome. (Meiosis is an exception in which two segregation events occur during a single cycle to produce the haploid gametes required for sexual reproduction.)

The cell cycle can also be regulated or halted at several stages, so-called checkpoints. These checkpoints are activated by a variety of factors including the detection of errors in DNA replication, damage to the existing DNA, and improper alignment of chromosomes before segregation to daughter cells. Of note the cell cycle can also be prevented from beginning, or halted after initiation, in response to external stimuli such as the unavailability of adequate nutrients that are required to produce the energy needed to complete the cell division process.

This section of the chapter will therefore begin by describing the various phases of the cell cycle and the events that occur during each of these phases. It will next focus on several of the key regulatory molecules that govern the cell cycle and their roles in providing appropriate positive or negative signals to the cell during this process.

1.1   The Phases of the Cell Cycle

The cell cycle contains four phases, identified as the G_1, S, G_2, and M phases. During S phase the chromosomes are replicated via DNA synthesis. The replicated chromosomes are then distributed to the progeny cells in M phase, during which active mitosis, the process by which chromosomes are condensed and then distributed to the daughter cells, occurs. The distribution of the chromosomes is followed by a cleavage event that results in the division of other cellular contents. G_1 and G_2 are the so-called gap phases because they occur in the periods that precede DNA replication and mitosis respectively. It was originally believed that the gap phases were relatively unimportant parts of the cell cycle that merely served to bridge the S and M phases. Indeed, in the early Xenopus embryo multiple rounds of DNA replication immediately followed by mitosis take place, such that a single cell embryo matures into a multicellular embryo in a few short hours. However, it is now known that G_1 and G_2 are critical phases of the cell cycle. Much of the cell growth that is a prerequisite for entry and progression through the cell cycle takes place during these parts of the cycle, and it is at these phases that many of the key regulatory factors act to either commit cells to progression through the cell cycle, or to halt progress should errors or unfavorable conditions be detected.

While the organization and coordination of the cell cycle is highly conserved among all eukaryotes, there are differences that occur between species. For example, the timing of cell cycles differs between species such as yeast and humans. Also, while the division of mammalian cells produces progeny of approximately equal size and cellular content, asymmetric division is the rule in budding yeast where, although the genetic content is equally distributed, the cellular contents are not. Also, there is a specialized cell cycle, the meiotic cell cycle, which results in the production of the gametes required for sexual reproduction. However, meiosis will not be discussed in this chapter. Therefore, throughout this chapter, the descriptions provided pertain to the mammalian mitotic cell cycle, unless otherwise specified.

1.1.1 G_1

The G_1 phase prepares the cell for DNA synthesis and execution of other steps in the cell cycle. It is here that the cell commits to, or halts, entry into the cell division cycle. Thus, it is in G_1 that much of the cell growth occurs that increases the size of the cellular organelles. The execution of the cell cycle requires a significant amount of energy. Therefore, the cell also senses whether there are adequate nutrients available in its environment and cellular stores.

A key regulator in this process is the protein kinase mTOR (mammalian target of rapamycin). mTOR couples nutrient sensing to cell growth, principally by regulating the phosphorylation and function of central regulators of the protein translation machinery, eukaryotic initiation factor 4E (eIF4E) and ribosomal S6 kinase (S6K) [1,2]. Significantly, inhibition of mTOR function by the drug rapamycin induces a G_1 phase cell cycle arrest, indicative of the critical role played by this kinase in the G_1 phase of the cell cycle [3]. Also, indicative of the importance of mTOR-regulated signaling in G_1 progression, mitogens, factors that stimulate cell cycle entry, induce signaling cascades that stimulate mTOR activity.

1.1.2 S

The S phase of the cell cycle involves the replication of the genomic content (DNA) and the duplication of the chromosomes. A complete description of the process of DNA replication could occupy an entire chapter, and so only an overview will be provided here. The replication of DNA is performed by a group of enzymes known as DNA polymerases. There are several DNA polymerases encoded in mammalian genomes, and different polymerases typically have different functions – some polymerases are responsible for the replication of genomic DNA, others replicate mitochondrial DNA, and still others act in repair complexes responsible for responding to specific types of DNA damage. All DNA polymerase synthesize DNA in a $5'-3'$ direction. Additionally, some of the polymerases have $5'-3'$ and $3'-5'$ proofreading capabilities. These proofreading activities ensure the high fidelity of DNA replication and result in an error rate of approximately one nucleotide in 10^9.

In mammalian cells, DNA replication is initiated at multiple locations on all chromosomes, at specific regions called origins of replication. While the consensus sequence of replication origins in budding yeast has been defined, the sequences of origins in mammals remain unknown, and published studies suggest that chromatin structure is an important determinant of replication origins in metazoans. However, the specific chromatin modifications that define replication origins in these organisms remain undefined. Importantly, published work analyzing the utilization of replication origins in yeast have demonstrated that not all origins fire during a given round of DNA replication. Furthermore, these studies demonstrated that specific origins were more likely to be utilized than others, and that the timing of origin firing was also regulated, such that specific origins fired early during replication, while others frequently fired later during the process. Of interest, those origins that are near to either the centromeres or the telomeres were commonly among the origins that fired last.

The preparation of origins for DNA replication begins during late mitosis or early G_1 when the prereplicative complex forms at the origins. This complex consists of several proteins that comprise the origin recognition complex (ORC), as well as several proteins of the mini chromosome maintenance (MCM) family [4]. Importantly, the proteins in the ORC are required for recognition of replication origins and the initiation of DNA synthesis, and mutations in core components of the complex prevent binding to origins and DNA replication. The MCM complex is the DNA helicase that unwinds the DNA at the origin of replication, and proceeds along the chromosome unwinding the DNA ahead of the DNA polymerase at the replication fork.

In S phase, the previously inactive prereplicative complex is switched on and converted into the pre-initiation complex, by the dissociation of the MCM complex from the ORC, and by the recruitment of several additional protein subunits. The newly formed complex recruits and binds the DNA polymerase α-primase complex, as well as the processive DNA polymerases δ and ε, a process which requires the activity of the Cdc7 kinase and the cyclin A/Cdk2 complex, the latter only found in S phase. In other words, conversion of the inactive prereplicative complex to the active pre-initiation complex is restricted to S phase, when cyclin A levels (and therefore cyclin A/Cdk2 activity) are high.

Once DNA replication is initiated at an origin, the prereplication complex components dissociate from the origin and their ubiquitin-mediated degradation is stimulated by the anaphase promoting complex (APC). Their reassembly is also inhibited by Cdk kinase activity. In this way, their reassembly at the origin is prevented until late mitosis or early G_1, when the APC is destroyed and cyclin/Cdk activity is at its lowest. Thus, a given origin can be activated only once per cell cycle, ensuring that segments of DNA do not undergo multiple rounds of duplication per cell cycle.

Once the initiation complex is bound at the origin, the DNA is then opened up and unwound by DNA helicase to provide access for the DNA replication machinery. The single-stranded DNA is prevented from reannealing by single strand DNA binding proteins. A DNA polymerase α-primase complex adds a short RNA primer sequence complementary to the template strand, which the DNA polymerase α then extends to a short ∼30 base long oligonucleotide. After the primer is completed, high speed and high fidelity DNA polymerases, polymerase δ or ε, then extend the primer along the leading strand.

DNA replication proceeds bi-directionally from the origin along Y-shaped structures known as the replication forks. Importantly, DNA polymerases can synthesize DNA only in a $5'–3'$ direction. Since the two strands of DNA run in opposite directions, as the replication fork extends away from the origin only one strand, known as the leading strand, can be synthesized in a continuous fashion in the direction of the expanding replication fork. The other, "lagging strand," must therefore be replicated in the opposite direction (away from the expanding replication fork). This occurs via the discontinuous replication of the lagging strand in short segments (about 200 nucleotides), known as Okazaki fragments, which are generated in the same manner as DNA synthesis on the leading strand. These short fragments are then joined together later by DNA ligase. Thus, DNA synthesis is able to proceed on both strands in the same direction as the growing replication fork.

The discontinuous nature of DNA synthesis on the lagging strand presents a problem for the cell during each replication cycle. The ends of the chromosomes cannot be replicated using this mechanism because there is not space to form the Okazaki fragments at the ends of the chromosomes, so the chromosomes inevitably become shorter after each division cycle. This problem is countered by the use of a special enzyme, telomerase, to replicate the telomeric sequences at the ends of the chromosomes. Telomerase is composed of an RNA template that is complementary to the repeat sequence found at the telomeres, and a reverse transcriptase that catalyzes DNA synthesis [5]. However, human somatic cells do not have telomerase activity (the reverse transcriptase is silenced) and so the telomeres shorten after each cell division cycle [6]. This shortening provides a proscribed limit on the number of cell divisions that a normal somatic cell can undergo before the telomeres trigger a phenomenon known as replicative senescence that inhibits further divisions. As will be discussed later, this process is subverted in cancer cells, most of which reactivate telomerase activity.

DNA is present on chromosomes, and the chromosomes are maintained in the form of chromatin, a DNA-protein assembly. In particular, specialized parts of the chromosomes, such as centromeres and telomeres, are maintained in specific chromatin states reflective of their function, and for the maintenance of that function as well as its heritability to the daughter cells, this chromatin state must also be replicated. Thus, during DNA replication in S phase, both the DNA and chromatin must be replicated. This necessitates that histones, the proteins around which DNA is wrapped to form chromatin, must be produced in significant quantities during S phase in concert with the ongoing DNA replication. This occurs via increased transcription of the histone encoding genes, as well as enhanced processing and stability of their mRNAs [7]. The detailed mechanisms of how this is regulated during the cell cycle are not fully elucidated, but the enhanced processing of histone mRNAs is dependent on a protein called SLBP whose levels are highest during S phase [8]. The levels of free histones also seem to serve as a signal that stimulates histone production, with low levels of free histones, resulting from the incorporation of histone proteins onto newly synthesized DNA, serving as a stimulatory signal for histone production.

1.1.3 G_2

Much like the G_1 phase preceding DNA replication, the G_2 phase of the cell cycle serves as a preparatory phase preceding the segregation of the chromosomes during mitosis. During the G_2 phase, the cell ensures that DNA replication is completed, all DNA damage has been repaired, and the chromosomes are ready for mitosis and the subsequent cell cleavage event known as cytokinesis. As discussed below, a critical checkpoint exists in this phase of the cell cycle, the so-called G_2/M checkpoint, that blocks further cell cycle progression if DNA damage, unreplicated DNA, or other cues are detected.

1.1.4 M

The M phase of the cell division cycle involves the separation of the duplicated chromosomes generated during S phase and their equal distribution to the daughter cells. This phase of the cell cycle can be roughly broken into five segments: prophase, during which chromosome condensation occurs; prometaphase, which involves the breakdown of the nuclear envelope and the attachment of the condensed chromosomes to the mitotic spindle; metaphase, during which the attached chromosomes are aligned at the center of the spindle, or metaphase plate; anaphase, during which the sister chromatids are pulled apart and toward opposing poles of the mitotic spindle; and finally, telophase, during which the nuclear envelope reforms around each of the two collections of chromosomes to generate two new nuclei. The events of mitosis are then followed by cytokinesis during which the plasma membrane invaginates and constricts dividing the parent cell into two resulting progeny cells.

The replicated chromosomes generated during S phase are tightly interlinked by catenation of their DNA, and by protein complexes known as cohesins that serve to hold the sister chromatids together. This cohesion of the replicated chromosomes plays a critical role in the ability of the cell to properly align sister chromatids along the metaphase plate. DNA catenation begins as the DNA is replicated during S phase as adjacent replication forks meet, and its untangling, by the enzyme DNA topoisomerase II, begins during S phase and continues during G_2 and M phase, such that by the time of the alignment of the chromosomes during metaphse, catenation contributes a minor fraction of the force holding the chromatids together. The cohesin complex interacts with the replicated DNA during S phase as well, and this interaction continues until the metaphase to anaphase transition during mitosis, when the proteolytic cleavage of key subunits of the complex allows the chromatids to be separated in response to the contractile forces generated by the opposing spindle poles.

The entry into mitosis requires cyclin A/Cdk2 activity, which is induced during S phase and remains high until early in mitosis. Indeed, chromosome condensation is blocked in cells injected with a protein inhibitor of cyclin A/Cdk2. A key suspected target of cyclin A/Cdk2 activity is the condensin protein complex. Condensins are activated early during mitosis and catalyze the condensation of the chromosomes into the rod-like structures seen in metaphase. As cyclin A/Cdk2 activity dissipates during early mitosis, the continued activation of the condensin complexes is performed by cyclin B1/Cdk1 complexes. The condensin complexes are also involved in the resolution of the sister chromatids from each other, so that they can be safely segregated during anaphase. However, the precise mechanisms by which the condensin complexes perform these functions remain unclear.

The condensed and resolved sister chromatids align themselves along the metaphase plate, with the kinetochores of sister chromatids bound to mitotic spindle fibers emanating from opposite spindle poles. The establishment and orientation of the spindle poles is dependent on protein organelles known as centrosomes. After the completion of mitosis, centrosomes are present in single copies in the resulting daughter cells. The centrosomes are then duplicated during the subsequent cell cycle, beginning in G_1. This duplication is complete by the onset of M phase, and the two centrosomes remain associated with each other until entry into mitosis, when they separate and migrate away from each other to establish the opposing spindle poles. As the centrosomes migrate, they elaborate the microtubule arrays that form the mitotic spindle. The establishment of the spindle poles at opposing sides of the mitotic cell is important for the uniform distribution of the chromosomes. Aberrant centrosome number is a commonly identified trait in cancer cells, and has been shown to lead to altered chromosome segregation resulting in aneuploidy, which is itself a key trait of malignant cells.

Once the chromosomes are aligned along the metaphase plate and bipolar spindle attachment is achieved, the cell proceeds through anaphase during which the contracting microtubule spindle pulls sister chromatids to opposing spindle poles. Once anaphase begins, the chromosomes are rapidly distributed to the daughter cells, and so progression to this stage of mitosis is tightly regulated. The anaphase promoting complex (APC) is a key regulator of this transition, and its functions are described in greater detail later in this chapter. Significantly, the presence of unattached chromosomes induces a mitotic arrest, called the spindle checkpoint, that blocks anaphase until all chromosomes have are attached to both spindle poles. After the chromosomes have been segregated, the nuclear envelope reforms during telophase and the two nuclei are separated from each other following cell cleavage or cytokinesis.

The preceding paragraphs described the steps in a stereotypical cell division cycle from the commitment to the cell cycle after transition through START, to the segregation of sister chromatids in mitosis. However, it should be noted that there is an additional cell cycle phase known as G_0. Many of the cells within the body, particularly terminally differentiated cells, enter this phase. It is an extended gap phase between cell cycles from which it is often difficult to reenter active cycling. Cells exit the cell cycle into G_0 from G_1 prior to the restriction point known as START. Frequently, strong stimuli, such as those encountered during significant tissue damage, are required for the reentry of G_0 cells into active cell division. This is a critical mechanism through which the organism maintains homeostasis in various tissue compartments.

1.2 Cell Cycle Control

As mentioned above, progress through the cell cycle is tightly regulated. In pioneering work, Lee Hartwell conducted mutagenesis screens in budding yeast, *Saccharomyces cerevisiae*, to identify mutants that failed to properly execute the cell cycle. These screens identified genes that encode proteins involved at all stages of the cell cycle from DNA replication to cytokinesis, and the mutants were labeled as cell division cycle, or cdc, mutants [9]. While these screens identified mutations that disrupted many of the key regulatory steps of the cell division, the absence of modern molecular biology tools meant that it took later studies to identify the specific genes and their specific regulatory mechanisms. Subsequent studies by Hartwell, Paul Nurse, Tim Hunt, and others, further elucidated many of the genes involved in various stages of the cell cycle, and demonstrated that these genes were conserved across several species from yeast to humans [10,11]. This section reviews the regulatory proteins necessary for the proper execution of the cell cycle.

1.2.1 Cell Cycle Regulatory Proteins

Among the key regulators of the cell cycle transition are the cyclin dependent kinases (Cdks), serine/threonine kinases whose functions are dependent on their interaction with partner proteins called cyclins, that are obligate activators of Cdk activity [12]. Cdks target a large number of proteins that have consensus phosphorylation sequences [S/T]PX[K/R]. In the absence of bound cyclin, the active site of the kinase is blocked by a flexible loop, the T-loop. Binding of appropriate cyclins to the Cdk induces a conformational change that opens up the active site to the target substrate and ATP. While the cyclins are quite divergent from each other in amino acid sequence, they contain a highly conserved region called the cyclin box that is required for Cdk binding and activation. In addition, despite their sequence divergence, all cyclins are thought to form a similar tertiary structure known as the cyclin fold that is important for their interactions with the Cdks.

While the levels of the Cdks remain relatively constant, the levels of their partner cyclins fluctuate significantly during the cell cycle [10]. The cyclin/Cdk complexes, and their periods of action, are shown in ⊘ *Fig. 13-1*. The levels of the cyclins are rapidly induced through transcriptional activation upon receipt of the appropriate signals for movement through the cycle, allowing the formation of appropriate cyclin/Cdk complexes. The cyclin/Cdk complexes then phosphorylate their target proteins to stimulate progression to the next phase of the cell cycle. Once the appropriate target proteins have been phosphorylated, the cyclins are then rapidly degraded by ubiquitin-induced proteasome degradation, and the Cdks returned to an inactive state. Thus, the activity of individual Cdks is restricted to the specific phases of the cell cycle where their partner cyclins are in abundance.

The different cyclin/Cdk complexes regulate the transition through different phases of the cell cycle. The cyclin D/Cdk4 and cyclin D/Cdk6 complexes regulate progression through the G_1 phase of the cell cycle, and are believed to be critical for the initial commitment of the cell to entering the cell division cycle. The cyclin E/Cdk2 and complexes regulate the progression of cells from the G_1 phase to the S phase, the so-called G_1/S transition, while cyclin A/Cdk2 complexes regulate progression through S phase. Finally, cyclin B/Cdk1 complexes regulate the progression through the M phase of the cell cycle. The activity of these

■ Fig. 13-1

The cell cycle. Schematic representation of the cell cycle depicting the points of action of key regulators including the cyclins, cyclin dependent kinases, and cyclin dependent kinase inhibitors.

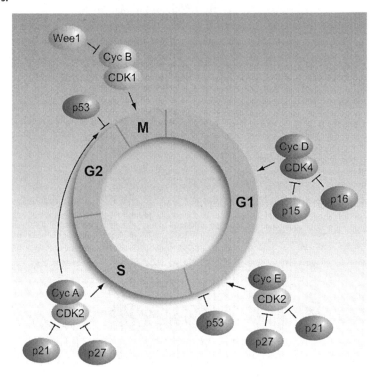

cyclin/Cdk complexes is controlled by several regulatory mechanisms that prevent the premature entry of cells into the cell cycle, and ensure the appropriate progression through the cell cycle.

1.2.2 D-Type Cyclins

In mammalian cells, the D-type cyclins – cyclins D1, D2, and D3 – bind to Cdk4 and Cdk6 stimulating their activity. Unlike the other cyclins, the levels of the D-type cyclins do not oscillate greatly during the cell cycle. Instead their levels respond to external stimulatory cues, such as those provided by mitogens (e.g., epidermal growth factor), that induce cells to enter the cell cycle. In addition, their levels also gradually increase as cells increase in size and prepare for the next division cycle. The function of the cyclin D/Cdk complexes appears to be primarily to regulate the commitment of the cell to progression through the cell cycle. Among the key targets of this kinase complex are the Rb family proteins, that act to constrain commitment of the cell to the cell cycle at a critical juncture of G_1 known as START, primarily by negatively regulating the transcriptional activity of the E2F proteins that are important regulators of the G_1/S transition and DNA replication.

1.2.3   E-Type Cyclins

The E cyclins, cyclin E1 and E2, regulate the G_1/S transition, and cyclin E/Cdk2 activity is required for progression into S phase. During the cell cycle, cyclin E levels increase during G_1 and then fall during S phase after the initiation of DNA replication. As discussed below, cyclin E mRNA levels are induced upon mitogenic stimulation, and published work has demonstrated that the c-Myc transcription factor is a key regulator of cyclin E levels. Among the targets of cyclin E/Cdk2 complexes are members of the Rb protein family, and phosphorylation by cyclin E/Cdk2 impairs the ability of Rb proteins to inhibit the expression of E2F target genes. Cyclin E/Cdk2 has also been shown to phosphorylate the NPAT transcription factor, a key regulator of histone gene expression.

1.2.4   A-Type Cyclins

The levels of cyclin A1 and A2 increase as cells progress into S phase, and cyclin A/Cdk2 activity is increased in S phase and remains elevated until the early stages of mitosis. Cyclin A2 is the predominant A-type cyclin present in human somatic cells, and like cyclin E, cyclin A2 is a transcriptional target of c-Myc, and its levels are induced in response to mitogenic signaling. In S phase, cyclin A/Cdk2 stimulates the conversion of the inactive prereplicative complex into the active pre-initiation complex, stimulating the onset of DNA replication. Cyclin A/Cdk2 also acts during early mitosis where it activates the condensins that initiate of the chromosomes during prophase.

1.2.5   B-Type Cyclins

The activity of the B cyclins is restricted to M phase, where cyclin B/Cdk1 complexes phosphorylate several substrates that are critical for the progression through mitosis, including components of the nuclear envelope, the golgi complex, and the APC. Cyclin B levels are kept low during the late stages of mitosis and G_1 by the activity of the APC ubiquitin ligase complex. Upon inactivation of the APC during late G_1, cyclin B levels rise, however, cyclin B/Cdk1 activity remains low until M phase as a consequence of the activity of the inhibitory kinase Wee1 (discussed in greater detail below). Removal of the inhibitory phosphates by the Cdc25 phosphatase stimulates cyclin B/Cdk1 activity as cells enter M phase.

1.2.6   Regulation of Cdks

In addition to activating the Cdks by binding to them, the cyclins also regulate the activity of Cdks by targeting them to their specific substrates. For example, cyclin A/Cdk2 binds to and phosphorylates the retinoblastoma protein family member p107, whereas cyclin B/Cdk1 complexes fail to interact with p107. Cyclins also regulate the activity of Cdks by regulating their subcellular location. For instance, cyclin B1/Cdk1 complexes are maintained in the cytoplasm until late prophase when they are rapidly translocated to the nucleus, upon which the complex phosphorylates its targets leading to nuclear envelope breakdown. The nuclear translocation of this complex is dependent on sequences in the amino terminal region of cyclin B1, outside the Cdk binding domain. Similarly, cyclin B2/Cdk1 complexes are targeted to the golgi during mitosis where phosphorylation leads to the fragmentation of that organelle allowing its redistribution to the resulting daughter cells. As was the case with the cyclin B1/Cdk1 complexes, targeting to the golgi is dependent on sequences outside the Cdk binding domain.

Cyclin Cdk complexes are also regulated by phosphorylation events. A trimeric enzyme, Cdk activating kinase (CAK), composed of Cdk7, cyclin H, and Mat1, phosphorylates and activates Cdks [13–15]. The phosphorylation of Cdks by CAK is required for the activation of the kinase activity of the targeted Cdk. While the activity of CAK is not regulated during the cell cycle and remains high throughout, phosphorylation of Cdks by CAK requires prior binding of the appropriate cyclin to the targeted Cdk. For example, CAK cannot phosphorylate Cdk2 before cyclin E is bound to Cdk2, thus ensuring that Cdk2 is not prematurely activated.

Unlike CAK-mediated phosphorylation, two inhibitory phosphorylation events on Cdks are tightly regulated. These are phosphorylations at tyrosine 15 and threonine 14. The phosphorylation event at tyrosine 15 is conserved across all eukaryotes and is carried out by the conserved kinase Wee1 [16]. The phosphorylation event at threonine 14 is specific to animals and is performed by the kinase Myt1. Thus, Wee1 and Myt1 act as inhibitors of cell cycle progression. The three members of the Cdc25 family of protein phosphatases – Cdc25a, b, and c – which remove these inhibitory phosphate groups, oppose the actions of the Myt1 and Wee1 kinases [17]. Both Wee1 and cdc25 are phosphorylation substrates of cyclin/Cdk complexes, with Wee1 activity inhibited as a consequence, and Cdc25 being activated. Thus, cyclin/Cdk complexes inhibit their inhibitor and activate their activator, establishing an important regulatory feedback mechanism. This effect is especially robust in M phase where the cyclin B/Cdk1 complex phosphorylates and inhibits Wee1 and phosphorylates and activates cdc25, and provides for a switch-like (on/off) activity of cyclin B/Cdk1 complexes and a rapid and irreversible commitment to progression through mitosis.

1.2.7 Cdk Inhibitors

The activity of Cdks is also regulated by the binding of another class of proteins, called the Cdk inhibitors or CKIs, that act as allosteric inhibitors of the Cdks and block their kinase activity [18–20]. There are two groups of CKIs – the Ink4 family that binds to cyclin D/Cdk complexes, and the Cip/Kip family that binds and inhibits cyclin/Cdk2 complexes. Of the four Ink4 proteins, p15 and p16 are widely expressed while p18 and p19 have more restricted expression patterns. Members of this family bind the Cdk subunit and impair cyclin D binding. Ink4 protein levels are low in actively cycling cells, but are induced by growth arrest signals, such as those produced by nutrient deprivation, that block cell cycle progression in G_1. Cip/Kip proteins bind to both the cyclin and Cdk subunits to induce both G_1 and G_2 cell cycle arrest. Like the Ink4 proteins, the levels of Cip/Kip proteins are low in dividing cells, but are induced by growth arrest signals. Interestingly, Cip/Kip proteins are involved in the assembly of cyclin D/Cdk complexes, and are associated with active Cdk4 complexes. Thus, high cyclin D levels additionally lead not only to increased Cdk4 and Cdk6 activity, but also to the sequestration of Cip/Kip proteins away from cyclin E/Cdk2 and cyclin A/Cdk2 complexes, and therefore their stimulation. Conversely, high Ink4 levels lead to the displacement of Cip/Kip proteins from Cdk4 complexes and their redistribution to Cdk2 complexes, reinforcing the Ink4-induced cell cycle arrest.

As the above paragraphs illustrate, the cell division cycle is a complicated meta-system containing simultaneous activation and/or inhibition of multiple proteins and mechanisms. This complex and interdependent web provides many opportunities for error, and so there are many layers of control, including those provided by the non-cyclin regulators described next.

1.2.8 Regulating the Regulators: Transcription

The levels of the cyclins that regulate progression through the cell cycle are actively regulated both by transcriptional induction in response to appropriate signals, and by proteolytic degradation. Likewise, the levels of other proteins involved in the various stages of cell cycle progression are similarly regulated. Members of the E2F family of transcription factors, which act as heterodimers with proteins of the DP1 class of DNA binding proteins, are key transcriptional regulators of the cell cycle [21,22]. The targets of the E2F-DP1 complexes include several genes critical for the G_1/S transition and the initiation of DNA synthesis. Importantly, the activity of E2F factors is negatively regulated by the members of the Rb protein family that act through multiple ways to impair the ability of E2F family members to stimulate the expression of their target genes (and sometimes repress them). Interestingly, the Rb family proteins are targets of the cyclin D/Cdk complexes, and phosphorylation of the Rb proteins by these kinases reduces their affinity for the E2F transcription factors, alleviating the negative regulation of critical G_1/S transcription.

Another key transcriptional regulator of the cell cycle is the basic helix-loop-helix transcription factor c-Myc. Myc was originally identified as the cellular gene activated by integration of an avian leukosis virus [23]. It is also one of a handful of genes known as immediate early genes, so named because their mRNA and protein levels increase rapidly after the stimulation of G_1 arrested cells by mitogens. Among the transcriptional targets of c-Myc are E2F1, cyclin E, and cyclin A [24]. Thus, c-Myc acts to stimulate the expression of several important regulators of the G_1/S transition, including E2F1, itself a master regulator of the transition, and this concerted regulation by c-Myc and E2F propels cells through G_1 and into S phase. Interestingly, c-Myc also induces the expression of microRNAs that act as negative regulators of itself and E2F1. Thus, by this mechanism, c-Myc activity can be very tightly regulated. Global mRNA profiling studies have also demonstrated that c-Myc regulates several genes involved in ribosomal biogenesis, and that c-Myc activity is required for proper mitochondria biogenesis. Thus, c-Myc activity links together several activities involved in cell growth with those involved in cell cycle progression.

Like the activity of the cyclin/Cdk complexes, the activities of the important transcriptional regulators are also very tightly regulated. c-Myc works as part of a heterodimer with its binding partner Max. While Max levels remain stable throughout the cell cycle, the levels of c-Myc are rapidly induced as cells enter the cell cycle in G_1, and the mRNA and protein levels decrease rapidly after cells commit to the G_1/S transition. Importantly, c-Myc activity is also negatively affected by the functions of a series of Max-interacting proteins, including the Mad family of transcription factors, which act to repress the expression of c-Myc activated genes. Thus, as c-Myc levels fall, Myc/Max heterodimers are replaced by Max/Mad heterodimers that repress the expression of c-Myc target genes. Consistent with this, while c-Myc acts to promote cell cycle progression, Mad transcription factors promote terminal cell differentiation and cell cycle exit.

Intrinsic mechanisms render normal cells sensitive to the inappropriate activation of these transcriptional regulators. Inappropriate activation of c-Myc sensitizes cells to p53-dependent and -independent apoptosis. Similarly, ectopic activation of the E2F1 transcription factor stimulates the formation of DNA double strand breaks and the consequent activation of the DNA damage checkpoint (discussed later in this chapter), halting the cell cycle. This is an intrinsic cellular response, as deletion or inactivation of pRb results in a similar phenotype. Inappropriate E2F1 activation also stimulates cell death via the induction of apoptosis. These mechanisms serve as checks to eliminate cells that have inappropriately entered the cell cycle. Interestingly, deletion of E2F1 in the mouse results in enhanced tumor susceptibility as a consequence of reduced apoptosis. This finding suggests that the induction of apoptosis is a critical normal function of E2F proteins in regulating the balance between cell proliferation and cell death required for proper tissue and organismal homeostasis.

1.2.9   Regulating the Regulators: Proteolytic Degradation

In addition to transcriptional regulation, several key controllers of the cell cycle are regulated by proteolysis. The key mediator of protein turnover during mitosis is the anaphase promoting complex or APC [25]. The APC is a multi-subunit ubiquitin ligase complex consisting of several core subunits, and one of two activating subunits – Cdc20 and Cdh1 – that govern APC activity during mitosis and G_1 respectively. The APC recognizes the destruction box (D-box) and KEN-box motifs in its target substrates. Among the targets for APC are the M phase cyclins, as well as the protein securin that regulates the separation of sister chromatids. Destruction of securin leads to the activation of the enzyme separase, allowing the movement of sister chromatids to opposite poles of the mitotic spindle, and the onset of the metaphase to anaphase transition. APC components are present throughout the cell cycle, however, the complex remains inactive until cyclin B/Cdk1 phosphorylates core APC subunits, enhancing the affinity of the activator subunit Cdc20 for the APC core subunits. Interestingly, cyclin B is a substrate of the APC, so activation of the APC by cyclin B/Cdk1 establishes a negative feedback loop. This feedback loop works both ways, since APC activation by Cdc20 requires phosphorylation of the APC core subunits by cyclin B/Cdk1. Thus, the APC also stimulates its own inactivation.

In addition to its function during the metaphase to anaphase transition, the APC also acts during G_1 to prevent the premature activation of S and M phase cyclin/Cdk complexes. Here, Cdh1 is the activator subunit of the APC. Cdh1 function is not dependent on phosphorylation of the APC core subunits by Cdks, but rather, phosphorylation of Cdh1 by Cdks results in its inactivation. Importantly, cyclin E is not a target of Cdh1, thus as cyclin E/Cdk2 activity rises, the APC is inactivated allowing the induction of S phase cyclin activity. The APC then remains inactive until M phase when phosphorylation of APC core subunits triggers binding by Cdc20.

Feedback regulation restricts the activity of the APC to mitosis and G_1, however proteolytic-based regulation of progression through the cell cycle occurs at all stages. Much of this regulation is performed by a group of ubiquitin ligases known as Skp1-Cul1-F-box (SCF) complexes, composed of the core subunits Skp1 and Cul1, together with one of over 70 F-box-containing subunits [26]. The F-box subunit provides the target specificity to the SCF complex. In most cases, SCF complexes recognize their substrates only when the target protein is phosphorylated, however, binding is not dependent on the presence of specific "destruction motifs" such as the D-box or KEN-box. SCF complexes target several integral regulators of the cell cycle, including both positive and negative regulators of cell cycle progression.

For example, Skp2 containing SCF complexes target the CKI p27 for degradation. Consistent with this, published studies have demonstrated that ectopic expression of Skp2 induces DNA synthesis and enhances cellular transformation. By contrast, the F-box protein Fbw7 binds (among others) cyclin E, c-Myc. c-Jun, and Notch1, and targets these proteins for degradation via the proteosome. Thus, Fbw7 acts to constrain progression through the cell cycle, and inactivating mutations in *FBW7* are found in human tumors. Thus, strict regulation of protein turnover is critical for appropriate cell cycle progression, and its alteration is implicated in tumorigenesis.

1.2.10 Other Regulators

As mentioned previously, cells require positive signals to commit to progression through the cell cycle. One of the mechanisms through which this is achieved is by the stimulation of receptor-mediated cell signaling by mitogens. Mitogens are growth factors, such as platelet derived growth factor (PDGF) or epidermal growth factor (EGF), that are secreted from neighboring cells and bind their cognate receptors on the surface of responding cells. Binding of the mitogens activates their receptors and stimulates signaling cascades downstream. Among the signaling pathways activated downstream of the activated receptor tyrosine kinases are the mitogen activated protein kinase (MAPK) and phosphotidylinositol trisphosphate kinase (PI3K) signaling cascades. Activation of these signaling pathways influences many cellular phenotypes, but both of these pathways stimulate progression through the cell cycle. For example, a key target of the MAPK signaling pathway is the AP-1 transcription factor, a key regulator of proliferation related genes. Likewise, the PI3K signaling pathway stimulates the activity of molecules involved in cell proliferation, cell survival, and cell growth. A key downstream target in the PI3K signaling pathway is the kinase mTOR, which, as mentioned earlier in this chapter, acts to promote cell growth. Thus, mitogen-induced signaling promotes entry into the cell division cycle, and coordinates cell growth, cell survival, and progression through the cell cycle.

Additional regulators act at later stages of the cell cycle as well. Among these are the polo-like kinase (Plk) and the aurora A and aurora B kinases that stimulate progression through mitosis. Plk plays important roles in the separation of the duplicated centrosomes and the establishment of the bipolar mitotic spindle. Indeed, blockade of Plk activity results in monopolar or otherwise abnormal spindles. Plk also functions after the completion of mitosis to regulate cytokinesis. The aurora A kinase is present at the centromere and along the spindle, and its function is important for the assembly and stability of the bipolar spindle. The aurora B kinase displays a different localization and is present along the chromosome arms and is involved in the condensation of the chromatids during early mitosis. During later stages of mitosis it is present primarily at the kinetochore, the site on the chromosome to which the spindle attaches. Thus, each of these kinases plays important roles in regulating mitosis. However, the identities of their target proteins are just beginning to emerge, and the precise mechanisms through which they contribute to mitotic regulation remain to be fully elucidated. Importantly, as is the case with other important cell cycle regulators, the aurora and polo-like kinases are misexpressed in human cancers, and contribute to disease pathogenesis.

Given the multiple mechanisms that have evolved to regulate their activity, it is unsurprising that many of the genes encoding cyclins, Cdks, and CKIs are altered in human cancers. For example, cyclin D and cyclin E levels are elevated in many human cancers, and amplification of these genes is observed in a subset of human malignancies including gastric, ovarian, and head and neck cancers. Likewise, activating mutations in Cdk4 that prevent binding of the CKI p16 are found in families with inherited predisposition to melanoma. These mutations induce enhanced cellular proliferation in cultured cells, and mice expressing mutant Cdk4 have enhanced susceptibility to tumor formation. Consistent with this, inactivation of the p16 protein, by a variety of mechanisms, is found in several malignancies including pancreatic cancer, and the tumor associated mutations have been demonstrated to result in increased cellular proliferation and tumorigenicity in vivo.

1.3   Cell Cycle Checkpoints

There are several checkpoints at which progress through the cell cycle can be halted if the cell senses that conditions are not appropriate for the faithful execution of the cell cycle [27]. These checkpoints are present at each of the phases of the cell cycle. The first of these, frequently referred to as START, occurs at the G_1/S transition, and progression through this checkpoint commits the cell to the cell cycle. In mammalian cells, a critical event at this checkpoint is the phosphorylation of the retinoblastoma (Rb) family proteins by cyclin D/Cdk complexes. As discussed previously, the Rb proteins inhibit the transcription activation function of members of the E2F family of transcription factors that regulate the expression of several genes important for cell cycle progression, and cyclin D/Cdk-mediated phosphorylation of Rb blocks its ability to repress E2F-mediated transcription. Other integral components of the G_1/S checkpoint in mammalian cells, are members of the Ink4 family of CKIs that block the function of cyclin D/Cdk complexes if the G_1/S checkpoint is activated. The pRb and Ink4 proteins prevent activation of the S-phase cyclins, as well as other factors important for DNA synthesis, and therefore serve as a brake on cell cycle progression. Unsurprisingly, the p16-cylin D/Cdk4-Rb axis is among the most frequently altered in human cancers.

Another key inducer of the G_1 cell cycle checkpoint is the p53 tumor suppressor protein, which induces growth arrest through the transcriptional activation of the CKI p21, a member of the Cip/Kip family of CKIs [28]. p21 binds to and inhibits the functions of cyclin E/Cdk2 and cyclin A/Cdk2 complexes, preventing progression of cells through the G_1/S transition. p53 is also a key component of the DNA damage response described below, as well as an important regulator of cell death through its induction of a number of pro-apoptotic genes. Notably, the p53 protein is usually unstable, however, signals such as those manifested by aberrant oncogene activation or DNA damage induce its stabilization. The stabilized protein then stimulates the transcription of its target genes, including its negative regulator Hdm2. Underscoring the importance of p53 in mediating cell cycle arrest, inactivating p53 gene mutations are among the most common genetic alterations in human cancers, including pancreatic cancer.

The second checkpoint occurs at the G_2/M transition. The S-phase cyclins act to push cells through this transition by activating the M-phase cyclins, but progression through this checkpoint is dependent on several factors, including the completion of DNA replication. The CKIs of the Cip/Kip family serve to block progression through this phase of the cell cycle should DNA replication not be completed, or DNA damage is detected. As was true for the G_1 cell cycle checkpoint, p53 is a key inducer of cell cycle arrest at this checkpoint, through its transcriptional activation of p21, Gadd45, and other genes.

The third checkpoint, referred to as the spindle checkpoint, occurs at the metaphase to anaphase transition during mitosis. At this stage, the sister chromatids are aligned along the metaphase plate, leading to their separation and distribution to opposing poles of the spindle apparatus. Progression through this critical transition point requires the activity of cyclin B/Cdk1 complexes, which activate the multi-subunit APC ubiquitin ligase. The APC stimulates the destruction of the B cyclins, as well as proteins that hold the sister chromatids together. This action stimulates the separation and segregation of the sister chromatids noted above, and moves cells into anaphase. As with the other major transition points, movement through this phase is tightly regulated by negative regulatory factors that ensure that the mitotic spindle is properly assembled, and sister chromatids are properly aligned, before anaphase can proceed. Failure of a chromosome to attach properly to the spindle apparatus stimulates activation of this checkpoint.

Several of the key components of this checkpoint were originally identified in budding yeast, in screens to detect cells that failed to undergo arrest when treated with mitotic poisons that blocked spindle assembly [29,30]. These genes, designated as Bub (budding uninhibited by benomyl) and Mad (mitotic arrest defective) mutants, were subsequently shown to encode kinetochore binding proteins that sense attachment of the spindle to the kinetochore. The Bub and Mad proteins form a multi-protein complex along with other kinetochore proteins, which is bound to the kinetochore in the absence of bipolar spindle attachment. In the absence of proper attachment, these proteins block progression to anaphase, but upon bipolar attachment these proteins dissociate from the kinetochore allowing the onset of anaphase. Significantly, failure of a single chromosome to achieve bipolar attachment triggers the checkpoint and mitotic arrest. The precise nature of the signals detected by this complex are unclear, but they potentially include the sensing of increased tension at the kinetochore induced by retracting forces from the opposing spindle poles. Importantly, the Bub and Mad genes have mammalian homologs, and loss of these genes stimulates chromosome missegregation and the development of aneuploidy. Given that aneuploidy is a cardinal feature of human cancer cells, the compromise of this checkpoint appears to be a significant event during tumor development.

1.4 The DNA Damage Response

The sustained viability of a cell or multi-cellular organism depends on the faithful replication and segregation of its genomic content. Cells have therefore evolved very high fidelity systems for the replication and segregation of the chromosomes during S phase and mitosis. However, despite the fidelity of these systems, errors are still generated at a low but measurable rate. Perhaps more importantly, molecules and radiation that frequently induce changes in the DNA constantly bombard the DNA within a eukaryotic cell. Within multi-cellular organisms such as humans, these changes can lead to altered phenotypes, giving rise to various disease states including cancer. To counter this, eukaryotic cells have evolved a series of mechanisms, known collectively as the DNA damage response, to detect and correct the damaged DNA and to halt cell cycle progression in the presence of significant DNA damage [31]. Unlike the checkpoints discussed above, which are activated at specific phases of the cell cycle, the DNA damage response can induce cell cycle arrest at any phase of the cell cycle, requiring only the presence of sufficient DNA damage to trigger the response. This arrest is maintained until the damaged DNA is repaired; if the cell cannot repair the damage, it either enters into permanent cell cycle arrest or undergoes cell death via apoptosis.

There are several modes of DNA repair, depending on the type of lesion. Damage present on a single DNA strand is repaired either by base excision repair or nucleotide excision repair.

Base excision repair is utilized to repair relatively minor alterations in base structure, such as deaminated nucleotides. When damage of this sort is found, the altered base is excised from the sugar-phosphate backbone, the sugar-phosphate backbone is excised at the site of the damaged nucleotide, and the correct nucleotide inserted by DNA polymerase. When bulky DNA lesions occur that affect the conformation of the double helix, the nucleotide excision pathway is used. In this repair mode, a short stretch of DNA including the damaged nucleotides is removed. The undamaged DNA strand is then used as a template to synthesize a new strand.

DNA double strand breaks are repaired using one of two mechanisms – homologous recombination or non-homologous end joining. Homologous recombination is the preferred mode of repair as it utilizes a complementary DNA strand as a template and can thus faithfully restore the DNA segment to its original sequence. However, this repair mechanism can lead to the loss of heterozygosity at a gene locus. For example, if the wild-type allele of gene X is damaged, its sequence may be replaced by that of a mutant allele on the homologous chromosome. Thus, repair by homologous recombination is activated only during those phases of the cell cycle when a sister chromatid is present. During G_1, before the DNA has been replicated, the preferred mode of repair is non-homologous end joining. In this mode of repair, the damaged DNA is resected and the two exposed ends of DNA reconnected by DNA ligase. This mode of repair is tolerated in higher eukaryotes where much of the DNA does not contain protein-coding sequences.

While minor DNA damage is repaired without stimulating the DNA damage response, extensive damage that is more difficult to repair induces the damage response and cell cycle arrest. The presence of extensive DNA damage is sensed by a pair of conserved kinases, ataxia telangiectasia mutated (ATM) and ATM-related (ATR). ATR is responsible for the response to multiple forms of DNA damage, while ATM appears to be specialized for the response to DNA damage that induces double strand breaks. Binding of ATR and ATM to sites of DNA damage induces their activation and the resulting recruitment and phosphorylation of the downstream kinases Chk1 and Chk2. Chk1 and Chk2 themselves phosphorylate several key substrates, including the p53 transcription factor that induces cell cycle arrest in response to DNA damage. The p53 interacting protein Hdm2 is an E3 ubiquitin ligase that mediates the rapid turnover of p53. In response to damage, the ATM, ATR, and Chk2 kinases all phosphorylate p53 on target serine residues, reducing the affinity of Hdm2 for p53 resulting in p53 stabilization. These kinases also phosphorylate Hdm2 as well to further reduce its affinity for p53. The stabilized p53 protein then forms an active tetramer that regulates the transcription of target genes.

Consistent with the importance of the DNA damage response to the prevention of cancer development, many of the genes encoding key components of the response are mutated in human malignancies, including various cancer predisposition syndromes. For example, the ATM kinase is mutated in the hereditary cancer syndrome ataxia telangiectasia [32]. Likewise the Chk2 kinase, which is activated by ATM and ATR, and the p53 tumor suppressor gene are mutated in the Li-Fraumeni cancer predisposition syndrome [33,34]. Other examples, notably the Fanconi Anemia genes and the breast cancer susceptibility genes BRCA1 and BRCA2, abound in the literature. Importantly, not only are genes involved in the checkpoint mutated in human cancer, but genes involved in repairing the damaged DNA, and DNA replication errors, are also mutated in human malignancies. For example, components of the DNA mismatch repair system are commonly mutated in the Hereditary Non-Polyposis Colorectal Cancer (HNPCC) syndrome, as well as sporadic colorectal cancers [35–37]. Mutations in these genes are also present in a small but significant fraction of human pancreatic cancers.

2   The Cell Cycle and Cancer

The human body is comprised of multiple organs and tissues, each of which is maintained in homeostasis through the tight regulation of cell growth, cell proliferation, cell differentiation, and cell death. Perturbation of any of these intricately interwoven features can result in the formation of a tumor. Many of these processes, such as programmed cell death, or apoptosis, are covered in other chapters in this book. Therefore, this segment focuses on how dysregulated cell cycle progression contributes to the pathogenesis of human cancers.

In an elegant 2000 review, Hanahan and Weinberg outlined six hallmarks of cancer, namely: self-sufficiency in growth signals, insensitivity to anti-growth signals, limitless replicative potential, reduced apoptosis, sustained angiogenesis, and tissue invasion and metastasis [38]. All of these hallmarks, with the exception of tissue invasion and metastasis, influence the proliferative capacity (and therefore cell cycle) of cancer cells, though the first two are most obviously relevant and will be discussed first. How these "hallmarks" influence cell proliferation is illustrated in ❯ *Fig. 13-2*.

2.1   Self-Sufficiency in Growth Signals

As mentioned previously, many cells within the body enter an extended "rest" phase, G_0, and only reenter the cell cycle upon the receipt of appropriate growth stimulatory signals initiated by mitogens. Mitogens are frequently secreted by surrounding cells; thus, proliferation of an individual cell is largely controlled by its neighbors – that is, the surrounding

◻ Fig. 13-2

The hallmarks of cancer. Diagrammatic representation of the hallmarks of cancer illustrating their influence on cell proliferation.

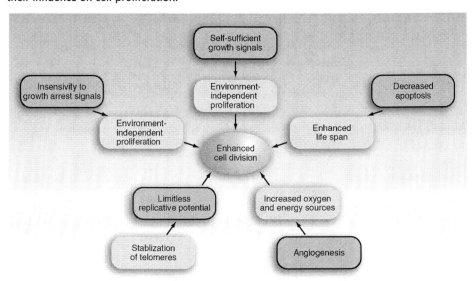

tissue – thereby ensuring that proliferation is controlled to serve the best interests of the tissue and the organism.

In cancer cells, the need for the production of mitogens by neighboring cells or other tissues is subverted by a variety of mechanisms, including the upregulation of mitogenic growth factors – such as those belonging to the epidermal growth factor (EGF), platelet-derived growth factor (PDGF) or insulin-like growth factor (IGF) families – by the cancer cells themselves, the upregulation of the growth factor receptors, or the mutational activation of the receptors such that they no longer require the binding of their cognate ligands for activation and the propagation of signals downstream. An example of this is the mutated EGF receptor in non-small cell lung cancer.

Downstream mediators of pro-mitogenic signaling, including proteins that bind to activated growth factor receptors, or transcriptional regulators that are the terminal targets of these signaling cascades, can also serve to imbue upon cells self-sufficiency regarding growth promoting signals. Indeed, several of the earliest identified oncogenes were genes encoding molecules of this sort, including c-Src, c-Jun, and c-Myc. In addition, human cancers frequently display elevated levels of the cell cycle regulatory factors that promote progression through the cell cycle including the cyclins and Cdks. In fact, numerous studies have identified cyclin D as a causative agent in hepatocellular carcinoma, and the gene is frequently amplified in this malignancy, leading to a pro-proliferation phenotype.

2.2   Insensitivity to Anti-Growth Signals

Cancer cells also frequently inactivate molecules that serve to constrain progression through the cell cycle. The first identified tumor suppressor, the retinoblastoma gene product pRb, acts to block progression through the G_1/S transition. And as discussed earlier, members of the INK4 family act to inhibit the kinase activity of cyclin D/Cdk complexes that inhibit Rb function. Significantly, the *INK4A* tumor suppressor locus that encodes the p16 tumor suppressor is frequently inactivated in human malignancies, including pancreatic cancer, by a variety of mechanisms, and other members of the family are mutated in human cancer as well. Together, these findings demonstrate that bypassing the G_1/S checkpoint is a critical step in tumorigenesis. Importantly, while the genes encoding the Cip/Kip family of CKIs are not frequently mutated in human cancers, the expression of these genes is frequently reduced in tumors resulting in increased activity of cyclin E- and cyclin A-Cdk2 complexes and cell cycle progression. Collectively these changes generate cells in which critical negative regulators of cell cycle progression are inactive, resulting in aberrant cell cycle progression.

Another important anti-growth signal is oncogene-induced senescence. This phenomenon, first described approximately a decade ago by Serrano and colleagues, involves the induction of an irreversible growth arrest after the inappropriate activation of an oncogenic signaling pathway [39]. Most potent transforming genes induce this phenomenon, detectable in vivo by the presence of cells positive for senescence associated beta galactosidase (SA-β-gal) staining. SA-β-gal positive cells are frequently observed in precursor lesions that serve as progenitors for invasive carcinomas. For example, in a mouse model of pancreatic cancer, SA-β-gal positive cells are present within PanIN lesions. Recent data also suggest that oncogene-induced senescence may involve the activation of the DNA damage response described earlier in the chapter. The current belief is that the oncogene-induced senescence pathway acts as a safety mechanism in normal cells to prevent tumorigenesis. Thus, cells must circumvent this mechanism before tumor progression can occur. Interestingly, while overexpression of activated Ras proteins in murine embryonic fibroblasts induces senescence, expression of an activated Kras allele from the endogenous locus does not. This finding suggests that in certain contexts, activated oncogenes do not effectively stimulate this safety mechanism. Nonetheless, the prevailing data indicate that oncogene-induced senescence must be bypassed in order for neoplastic transformation to occur.

2.3   Limitless Replicative Potential

All cells have a proscribed limit to the number of times that they can divide. In somatic cells in the body, the length of the telomeres that protect the ends of the chromosomes commonly determines this limit. Because of the end replication problem and the absence of telomerase enzyme activity in human somatic cells, the telomeres become progressively shorter after each cell division. When the telomeres become excessively shortened they fail to protect the ends of the chromosomes from damage and chromosome rearrangements, so to prevent genomic catastrophe, cells with critically short telomeres block further cell divisions and enter replication-induced senescence.

Cancer cells frequently reactivate the reverse transcriptase component of the telomerase enzyme, and this reactivation allows them to stabilize their chromosome ends, permitting additional rounds of cell division without further telomere attrition [40,41]. Telomerase reactivation occurs in approximately 90% of human cancers, and in the other 10% the telomeres are maintained through alternate mechanisms, and as a result, telomere length is maintained in all human solid tumors.

The current model is that telomere erosion occurs during the transformation of normal cells into cancer cells, resulting in critically short telomeres that induce non-reciprocal chromosomal translocations and other genomic rearrangements that are commonly found in cancer cells. Thus, telomere attrition allows the generation of additional genetic lesions that may provide selective advantage to cancer cells. If the induced gross genomic instability remained unchecked, these cells would likely die. Thus, the subsequent reactivation of telomerase activity in human tumors prevents genomic catastrophe, stabilizes the advantageous genomic alterations, and provides the capability for limitless cell replication.

Consistent with telomere attrition contributing to genomic instability and cancer, aged mice deficient for telomerase activity are more susceptible to tumor formation than their telomerase proficient counterparts [42]. Interestingly, telomerase deficient animals that are deficient at the *Ink4a/Arf* tumor suppressor locus have reduced tumor development compared with *Ink4a/Arf* null mice with intact telomeres [43]. However, p53 deficient animals with defective telomeres display enhanced tumor development when compared to p53 deficient animals with intact telomeres [44]. These studies suggest that critically short telomeres activate a p53-dependent DNA damage response that acts to constrain tumor development. Thus, inactivation of this response would appear to be a critical step in tumor development.

2.4   Reduced Apoptosis

Apoptosis is an integral mechanism through which tissue homeostasis is maintained. When cells sustain irreparable damage or receive external pro-death cues, they execute a cell autonomous death program, a sacrifice that usually preserves the health of the tissue or organism. (Cells may also die through an alternate process known as autophagy.) Among the key pro-apoptotic regulators is p53, a protein that is integrally involved in the DNA damage response. When a tumor cell becomes insensitive to apoptotic cues it fails to undergo cell death. Thus, the evasion of apoptosis results in the continued proliferation of cells, even those with damaged DNA and pro-tumorigenic genetic lesions.

2.5   Angiogenesis

The pioneering work of Judah Folkman and others has made clear the importance of angiogenesis in tumor progression [45]. Because tumor masses rapidly outgrow their available blood supply, their local environment becomes hypoxic and low in necessary nutrients. Thus, to survive, tumors must stimulate the formation of new blood vessels. Since cell proliferation is tightly linked to external cues and to nutrient sensing, the formation of new blood vessels, and the consequent elevation in oxygen tension and nutrient levels, supports the continued proliferation of cancer cells.

However, blood vessels formed during angiogenesis are often leaky, and the observation of regions of hemorrhage is common in human tumors. Also, this new blood vessel formation is frequently inadequate to support the entire tumor, and regions of necrosis are also frequently observed within solid tumors. As a consequence, despite the presence of the new blood vessels, many regions within a tumor remain hypoxic. Under these conditions, normal cells would receive signals preventing cell cycle entry. However, in tumor cells, this signal is circumvented and the cells continue to proliferate. The interplay between the hypoxia induced factor, HIF1α, and c-Myc, and their coordinated regulation of several genes involved in metabolism is a central cause of this sustained proliferation in the presence of limiting oxygen.

2.6   Consequences of Aberrant Cell Cycle Progression

What are the consequences of the aberrant entry and progression through the cell cycle that is a hallmark of cancer cells? At their core, cancers are genetic diseases, marked by a collection of gene mutations that provide selective advantages for cell proliferation, cell survival, and invasion and metastasis. For example, tumor-promoting genes such as *MYC* are frequently amplified leading to increased gene expression and activity of the encoded protein. Indeed global gene copy number analyses of human tumors indicate that individual tumors harbor multiple regions of chromosomal amplification that contain genes, such as *MYC* and *CCND1* (which encodes cyclin D1), that promote cell cycle entry and progression. Likewise, the converse is often true. Tumors also contain several deleted chromosome regions that contain genes encoding negative regulators of the cell cycle such as p16 and p53. These regions are lost via a variety of mechanisms including loss of entire chromosomes or chromosome arms, indicating that proper chromosome alignment on the mitotic spindle and/or movement toward the spindle poles is lost in cancer cells. This chromosome missegregation results in aneuploidy – the presence of an abnormal number of chromosomes.

In addition to chromosomal alterations that commonly affect multiple genes simultaneously, tumor-related genes are also commonly altered by point mutations that either confer gain- or loss-of function properties to the encoded protein. The presence of these mutations suggests the occurrence of errors that are not corrected by the DNA repair system.

On the whole, the accumulation of genetic alterations indicates the inactivation of critical cell cycle checkpoints in cancer cells, and/or the ability of cancer cells to override these checkpoints once they have been activated.

A common feature of human cancers is the presence of abnormal numbers of centrosomes. Normally, there is one centrosome per cell, and this organelle replicates during the early phases of the cell cycle such that during mitosis there are two centrosomes that establish the opposing poles of the spindle apparatus. However, cancer cells frequently contain multiple centrosomes, resulting in the formation of multi-polar spindles during mitosis, and the unequal segregation of chromosomes to the daughter cells after completion of the cell division cycle. Thus, abnormal centrosome numbers is another mechanism through which aneuploidy is generated in cancer cells.

Whether aneuploidy is a cause of tumor development, or simply a consequence reflective of the properties displayed by cancer cells, such as inappropriate cell cycle entry and progression, continues to be debated. However, the emerging consensus appears to be that both are true. Evidence indicates that many of the proteins that are involved in tumor initiation and progression, such as c-Myc and p53, cause genomic instability when they are overexpressed or mutated respectively.

For example, transient expression of c-Myc in rodent and human fibroblasts induces the accumulation of genomic alterations in these cells, including karyotypic abnormalities and gene amplifications. Likewise, several mouse models in which p53 function is abrogated demonstrate elevated levels of genomic alterations relative to p53 wild-type controls, indicative of a role for p53 loss in the induction of genomic instability. These data indicate that gene alterations commonly found in human cancers stimulate genomic instability, suggesting that genomic instability may be a consequence of the tumor phenotype.

Yet, it is also clear that human cancers contain multiple genetic alterations that play causative roles in the development of the malignancy. Based on the normal error rate of chromosome missegregation and error generation during DNA replication, it is clear that accelerated generation of errors of these kinds must occur in cancer cells to induce the required number of changes needed for tumor development. This suggests that genomic instability is a key component of tumor development and plays a causative role.

Confirmatory evidence for this view comes from recent studies performed by Don Cleveland and colleagues in which they generated mice null for the gene encoding CENP-E, a kinetochore associated protein that is important for proper chromosome segregation during mitosis [46]. In aged mice, CENP-E deficiency induced aneuploidy and tumor development. However, in chemical carcinogenesis models, CENP-E deficiency impaired tumor progression. A potential explanation for these conflicting results is that in the chemical carcinogenesis model, the mitotic checkpoint remained intact leading to the elimination of aneuploid cells, whereas in the spontaneous tumor development models, where tumor initiation occurs more slowly, cells defective for the spindle checkpoint arose and conferred a selective advantage on aneuploid cells allowing their expansion and subsequent tumor development. These results are consistent with the findings in telomerase deficient mice that were discussed earlier in this chapter; namely that critical cell cycle checkpoints must be inactivated before genetic alterations that induce gross genomic changes can confer a selective advantage leading to tumorigenesis. In addition, consistent with this idea, regulators of mitosis and the spindle checkpoint such as Bub1, Mad2, Aurora kinase, and polo like kinase, display altered expression in human tumors, and animal models demonstrate that the observed alterations confer tumorigenic phenotypes in vivo.

Thus, through a variety of means, cancer cells have developed mechanisms that lead to increased survival and enhanced cell cycle entry and progression, resulting in elevated proliferative capacity. While the alterations that lead to enhanced proliferation also impact other critical properties of cancer cells, the effects on the cell cycle have a profound impact on the formation and growth of the tumor. This is underscored by the presence in human tumors of alterations that impact each of the phases of the cell cycle, as well as each of the checkpoints that serve to regulate the entry and progression of cells through the cell cycle.

3   The Cell Cycle and Pancreatic Cancer

The normal adult pancreas is a quiescent organ, with less than 1% of all cells actively undergoing proliferation at any given time. However, pancreatic cancers display highly elevated levels of proliferating cells, observable even in early precursor PanIN lesions. Importantly, in a mouse model of PDAC, Tuveson and colleagues were able to carefully quantify the proliferation levels in PanINs relative to normal duct epithelium. They found that the proliferation rate, as assessed by PCNA staining, was increased by over 18-fold in early PanIN lesions relative to normal pancreatic ducts [47]. Thus, enhanced proliferation, indicative of altered cell cycle regulation is present in the earliest precursor lesions for the disease.

Pancreatic ductal adenocarcinomas (PDAC) display a wide spectrum of genetic alterations. Recent large-scale genome sequencing efforts and genome copy number analyses have provided even greater detail about the pancreatic cancer genome [48,49]. Yet, despite the presence of a large number of genomic alterations in pancreatic cancer, several signature alterations, highlighted in ◗ *Fig. 13-3* can be identified. Principal among these are activating mutations in the *KRAS* oncogene that result in a constitutively active Kras protein. These mutations are present in a significant fraction of PanIN1 lesions, indicating the involvement of activated Kras in the initiation of pancreatic tumorigenesis [50]. Inactivating mutations in the *INK4A* tumor suppressor gene encoding the cyclin dependent kinase inhibitor p16 are also commonly found in PDAC. Indeed, p16 function is lost in almost all PDAC through a variety of mechanisms including gene mutation, gene deletion, and gene silencing via DNA

◘ Fig. 13-3

Genetic alterations in pancreatic cancer. A schematic illustration of how genes commonly altered in pancreatic cancer influence cell cycle progression.

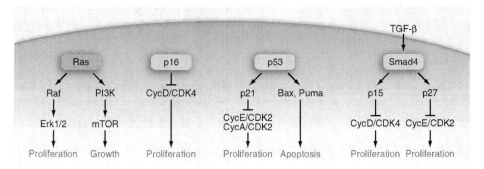

methylation. Importantly, *INK4A* gene alterations are also present in early PanIN lesions, indicating an important role for loss of this tumor suppressor in early pancreatic tumor development [50]. Other commonly identified genetic alterations in PDAC include loss of the p53 and Smad4 tumor suppressor proteins. This section of the chapter will look at how each of these alterations alters cell cycle regulation in pancreatic cells and contributes to malignant transformation in the pancreas.

3.1 KRAS

The *KRAS* oncogene is mutationally activated in over 90% of pancreatic ductal adenocarcinomas, and these mutations are frequently present in early precursor PanIN lesions, indicative of a role for activated Kras in the initiation of pancreatic tumorigenesis in vivo. Consistent with a role for activated Kras in tumor initiation, mice engineered to express an activated Kras allele in the pancreas develop PanIN lesions that progress to invasive adenocarcinoma [47].

Kras is a member of a family of small GTPases that recruit target proteins to cellular membranes resulting in their activation. Tumor-associated mutations block Kras GTPase activity, locking the protein in a GTP-bound, or active, state. Three members of the family – Hras, Kras, and Nras – are very closely related in terms of sequence and function. Ras proteins activate signaling through several downstream effector pathways, the best studied of which are the Raf-MAP kinase, PI3 kinase-Akt, and Ral signaling cascades [51]. These signaling cascades are associated with enhanced proliferation, survival, and cell growth in several experimental settings. Thus, activated Ras proteins integrate cellular proliferation with cellular growth and enhanced cell survival. Importantly, each of these signaling cascades has been demonstrated to be important for the ability of activated Ras oncoproteins to induce cellular transformation and oncogenesis in various settings, both in cell culture systems and in vivo.

The Raf-MAP kinase signaling cascade has been linked to cellular proliferation in many contexts. Indicative of the importance of this signaling pathway, activating mutations in the *BRAF* gene are found in several human malignancies, including a subset of the pancreatic cancers lacking activating mutations in *KRAS* [52]. Stimulation of Raf proteins by Ras leads to the activation of the extracellular-signal regulated kinases Erk1 and Erk2. These kinases then phosphorylate their targets to regulate their cellular function, among them ETS family transcription factors, and the c-Jun DNA binding protein that is part of the AP-1 transcription factor. As discussed earlier in this chapter, the AP-1 transcription factor is an important regulator of genes involved in cell cycle progression, including cyclin D, and is a key effector of mitogenic signaling.

The second pathway stimulated by activated Kras is the PI3kinase-Akt signaling cascade. This signaling pathway has been linked to increased cell proliferation, and is also an important regulatory input for cell growth and cell survival. One of the downstream targets of this signaling cascade is the mTOR kinase, a key regulator of cell growth that links nutrient sensing with cell growth and cell proliferation, in large part by regulating protein translation. As seen earlier in this chapter, cell growth is required for normal cells to commit to cell cycle progression. Thus, through its activation of the PI3 kinase signaling axis, activated Kras links, and stimulates, enhanced cell growth and cell proliferation. The PI3 kinase signaling axis also provides a potent anti-apoptotic signal. Aberrant cell cycle entry, such as that induced by the Kras and c-Myc oncoproteins, can stimulate apoptotic cell death, therefore by activating an anti-apoptotic signal, Kras inhibits cell death that might otherwise occur as a consequence of its enhanced cell proliferation.

Signaling through the RalA and RalB proteins influences several cellular processes including cellular trafficking, cell proliferation, and cell survival. In addition, recent work has demonstrated that Ral-mediated signaling is sufficient to induce the transformation of immortalized human fibroblasts, underscoring the importance of this signaling axis in Ras-induced cellular transformation and tumorigenesis. While the precise mechanisms underlying some of these phenotypes remain unclear, Ral-mediated signaling has been shown to activate several growth promoting genes including those encoding c-Src and cyclin D1. RalB has also recently been shown to enhance the survival of cancer cells through its activation of the kinase TBK1, thereby blocking the initiation of apoptosis in response to oncogene-induced stress.

Does activated Kras induce proliferation in primary pancreatic cells, and if so, through which pathways? The increased proliferation of PanIN lesions in the Kras-induced pancreatic cancer mouse model suggests that this is the case. Consistent with this, activated Kras enhances the proliferation and survival of isolated pancreatic duct epithelial cells in culture [53]. Thus, the existing evidence demonstrates that activated Kras enhances proliferation in pancreatic epithelial cells; however, the roles of the various Kras-induced signaling pathways in this phenotype remain to be determined. Recent work has shown that the activation of Ras proteins may have different consequences in different cell types, and that these effects may reflect the localization of different Ras proteins to different membrane compartments. Indeed, activated Nras, but not activated Kras, stimulates the proliferation of isolated primary melanocytes. Therefore, it will be interesting to determine whether other Ras proteins can elicit similar phenotypes in pancreatic epithelial cells.

3.2   MYC

The *MYC* oncogene is frequently overexpressed in human cancers by a variety of mechanisms. Published reports have demonstrated elevated *MYC* gene expression in a majority of pancreatic cancers, and consistent with this, the *MYC* locus is amplified in a subset of pancreatic cancers.

MYC is an immediate early gene whose expression is stimulated by mitogenic signaling, and the encoded protein is an important transcriptional regulator of several cell cycle regulatory genes, including those encoding cyclin D2, cyclin A2, and cyclin E1. Thus, c-Myc overexpression promotes progression through the G_1/S transition. Also among the c-Myc target genes are members of the E2F family of transcription factors that are themselves key transcriptional regulators of the cell cycle. c-Myc also induces the expression of the mir17–92 and mir106 microRNA clusters that have been demonstrated to enhance cell proliferation and tumorigenesis. Interestingly, these miRNAs also target E2F1 and c-Myc, establishing a regulatory feedback loop.

c-Myc also interacts with the Miz-1 transcription factor to repress the expression of several genes, among them the genes encoding the cell cycle inhibitors p15, p21, and p27. Thus, in addition to stimulating the expression of cell cycle promoting genes, c-Myc also represses the expression of cell cycle inhibitory genes. Further, the stimulation of cyclin D2 gene expression by c-Myc induces the sequestration of p21 and p27 into cyclin D/Cdk complexes, and away from the cyclin E and cyclin A containing Cdk2 complexes, further stimulating progression through the G_1/S transition and the S phase of the cell cycle. Thus, c-Myc provides a multifaceted punch in favor of cell cycle progression and cellular proliferation.

c-Myc also induces the expression of several genes important for mitochondrial development, and function, as well as several ribosomal genes. Importantly, c-Myc functionally cooperates with the hypoxia inducible factor (HIF1-α) to induce the expression of hexokinase 2 and pyruvate dehydrogenase kinase 1 [54]. These factors are important for the switch from aerobic to anaerobic metabolism, allow cancer cells to undergo effective metabolism and meet their energy needs while exposed to low oxygen concentrations, and are important for the sustained proliferation and viability of cancer cells under hypoxic conditions. Thus, c-Myc function links cellular proliferation to cell metabolism and cell growth.

3.3   INK4A/ARF

The *INK4A/ARF* tumor suppressor locus encodes two tumor suppressor proteins, p16^{Ink4a} and p14^{Arf} (p19^{Arf} in mice) [55,56]. p16 loss of function occurs in almost all pancreatic cancers by a variety of mechanisms including homozygous deletion, point mutation, and gene silencing via DNA methylation [57]. The loss of p16 function occurs early in the development of PDAC and can be identified in early PanIN lesions, indicating that p16 loss is a signature event in PDAC development, and is likely involved in initiation of tumorigenesis. Underscoring the importance of p16 loss in pancreatic tumorigenesis, inherited loss of *INK4A* predisposes patients to pancreatic cancer development.

p16 is a CKI that binds and inhibits cyclin D/Cdk complexes. As discussed earlier in this chapter, a primary function of cyclin D/Cdk complexes is the phosphorylation and inhibition of Rb family proteins, resulting in increased E2F transcription activity and progression through the G$_1$/S cell cycle checkpoint. Therefore, loss of p16 results in the elimination of a key negative regulator of transition through this checkpoint. Interestingly, the *INK4B* locus – encoding p15, another CKI that targets cyclin D/Cdk complexes – is commonly co-deleted with the *INK4A* locus in pancreatic tumors, further underscoring the importance of inactivating this cell cycle checkpoint during pancreatic tumor development.

As discussed earlier in the chapter, oncogene-induced senescence is an important anti-tumor safety mechanism. Experimental data demonstrated that loss of p16 impairs oncogene-induced senescence, indicating a critical role for p16 in this phenomenon. Given the early occurrence of activating *KRAS* mutations in PanIN lesions that may induce this response, loss of p16 function may act to remove an important barrier to tumor development. Therefore, p16 gene loss may enhance pancreatic tumorigenesis through multiple mechanisms.

Homozygous deletion of the *INK4A/ARF* locus occurs in approximately 40% of pancreatic cancers, resulting in loss of both p16 and p14^{Arf} function. Arf is an important activator of p53 function in response to certain cellular stresses including aberrant oncogene activation. Arf acts by inhibiting Hdm2 function, alleviating the ubiquitination and destruction of p53 [58]. Once stabilized, p53 acts to regulate the transcription of genes involved in cell cycle arrest and apoptosis. Thus, Arf loss enhances aberrant cell cycle progression induced by oncogene activation.

3.4   TP53

Mutation of the TP53 tumor suppressor gene is among the most common genetic alterations in human cancers, including PDAC where it is mutated in approximately 50–75% of cases [59]. The p53 protein acts as a tetrameric DNA binding protein and transcriptional regulator that controls the expression of multiple genes involved in cell cycle arrest and apoptosis. As indicated earlier in this chapter, p53 levels are kept low through Hdm2-mediated ubiquitination and protein degradation; however, p53 protein levels are rapidly stabilized in response to several cellular stresses including DNA damage and oncogene activation, and induces cell cycle arrest or apoptosis. Underscoring the significance of p53 in cell cycle arrest and apoptosis, p53 function is conserved in organisms from flies to humans, and loss of p53 impairs cell death in response to apoptotic stimuli, blocks the induction of oncogene-induced senescence, and enhances the transformation of cells by oncoproteins such as Kras. Further, p53 deficient mice are susceptible to spontaneous and carcinogen-induced tumors, and mutation of p53 accelerates the development of PDAC, and metastatic spread, in a mouse model of the disease [60].

DNA damage stabilizes p53 through a series of phosphorylation events mediated by the ATM, ATR, and Chk2 kinases, whereas aberrant oncogene activation stimulates Arf-mediated inhibition of Hdm2 to stabilize p53 [58,61]. Studies of p53 deficient animals, and cells derived from these animals, demonstrated that p53 is required for efficient growth arrest in vitro and in vivo, and for the induction of apoptosis after DNA damage.

Among the p53 target genes is the CKI p21 that binds and inhibits cyclin E/Cdk2 and cyclin A/Cdk2 complexes. Studies of p21 deficient cells and animals demonstrated an impaired G_1 cell cycle arrest, indicative of its importance in p53-mediated cell cycle arrest. p53 also plays important roles in maintaining arrest at the G_2/M checkpoint through its induction of growth arrest genes such as p21 and gadd45. p53 also regulates the expression of several genes involved in apoptosis including Bax, PUMA, and Noxa, and deletion of these genes impairs p53-mediated apoptosis in response to several apoptotic stimuli.

3.5   TGF-β Signaling

The transforming growth factor beta (TGF-β) signaling cascade is a complex signaling network that regulates cellular proliferation, apoptosis, and cell migration and invasion. TGF-β ligands bind to their cognate type I and type II receptors on the cell surface, inducing their dimerization and activation. The activated receptors recruit adapter Smads such as Smad2 and Smad3, which then bind Smad4 and translocate to the nucleus. Translocation of the Smad complex into the nucleus induces the regulation of target genes.

In most normal cells, TGF-β induced signaling acts to constrain cellular proliferation through several mechanisms. First, TGF-β signaling stimulates the expression of the genes encoding the p15 and p27 CKIs, as well as other target genes implicated in negative regulation of the cell cycle [62,63]. The TGF-β pathway also acts in a Smad4-independent fashion to inhibit c-Myc function, both by inhibiting *MYC* expression and by impairing the interaction of c-Myc with its partner Miz-1 [64]. As mentioned earlier, the interaction of c-Myc with Miz-1 is required for c-Myc-mediated inhibition of p15 and p27 gene expression. Thus, through multiple mechanisms, TGF-β signaling acts to induce the expression of these cell cycle inhibitors.

The significance of TGF-β signaling in constraining the growth of pancreatic cells is demonstrated by its frequent inactivation in pancreatic cancer. Approximately, half of all PDACs display loss of Smad4, while a small but measurable fraction have inactivation of the TGF-β receptor [65]. *SMAD4* gene mutations are not present in early PanIN lesions, but appear in PanIN3 lesions (the equivalent of carcinoma in situ), suggesting a role in the malignant conversion of precursor lesions into adenocarcinoma.

3.6   MicroRNAs

First discovered in the model organism *C. elegans*, microRNAs (miRNAs) are short non-coding RNAs that bind complementary sequences, primarily within the 3′ untranslated region, in target mRNAs, and inhibit their translation [66]. Recent studies have suggested that miRNAs may also enhance the translation of target mRNAs in some instances. miRNAs have recently emerged as important players in human cancer. Expression profiling studies have demonstrated altered levels of several miRNAs in human cancers including pancreatic cancer [67–69]. These profiling studies demonstrated that miRNA expression signatures are useful prognostic tools, and that serum miRNAs may potentially be useful biomarkers. In addition, depletion of miRNAs, through the inhibition of key processing enzymes in the miRNA maturation pathway, enhanced the tumorigenicity of a lung cancer cell line, highlighting the importance of miRNAs in regulating cancer phenotypes.

Studies of individual miRNAs and miRNA clusters have begun to reveal clues to their regulation and mechanisms of action in tumorigenesis. For example, the mir17–92 cluster is induced by c-Myc, and these miRNAs target E2F1 and c-Myc, establishing a regulatory feedback loop [70]. Significantly, this miRNA cluster is highly expressed in several human cancers, including as a consequence of gene amplification, and inhibition of these miRNAs impairs the proliferation of cancer cell lines. Furthermore, ectopic expression of this miRNA cluster enhances cell proliferation and tumorigenesis in mouse models, underscoring its role in cell transformation [71]. Importantly, the mir17–92 miRNA cluster is required for proliferation of several cell types, and deletion of this miRNA cluster leads to lung hypoplasia and increased apoptosis in the B-cell lineage, suggesting a broad role for these miRNAs in cell proliferation and apoptosis. Could these miRNAs play a similar role in pancreatic cancer? Profiling studies demonstrate that the mir17–92 cluster is overexpressed in pancreatic cancer, and its transcriptional regulator c-Myc, is also overexpressed in this disease, suggesting a potential role for this miRNA cluster in PDAC pathogenesis. Currently, functional studies of these miRNAs are needed to validate their potential oncogenic role during pancreatic tumorigenesis.

Other studies have demonstrated the importance of mir34a-c in mediating p53-regulated phenotypes including cell cycle arrest and apoptosis [72,73]. These miRNAs are transcriptional targets of p53, and their induction after stimuli such as DNA damage requires p53. Given the frequency of *TP53* gene mutations in pancreatic cancer, mir34a-c could potentially play important roles in disease pathogenesis.

Could miRNAs play a similar role in influencing Kras-mediated phenotypes? Published studies have demonstrated that the let-7 miRNA regulates Ras activity, and recent work has suggested that stimulation of Hras activity as a consequence of reduced let-7 expression is important for the phenotype of tumor initiating cells in breast cancer [74]. However, it remains to be determined whether similar mechanisms are at work in pancreatic cancer cells.

While the studies mentioned above demonstrate that miRNAs regulate Ras levels and activity, the regulation of specific miRNAs by activated Kras has not yet been shown. However, given the demonstrated roles of several miRNAs in regulating cell proliferation and apoptosis, their involvement in Kras-mediated phenotypes in pancreatic epithelial cells is an intriguing prospect. Of additional interest would be the determination of the Kras-stimulated cascades involved in regulating these miRNAs.

3.7   Hedgehog Signaling

The hedgehog signaling pathway plays critical roles during embryonic development, and its aberrant activation underlies Gorlin syndrome, an inherited syndrome that includes predisposition to cancer development. Activation of the hedgehog signaling pathway has been demonstrated in several cancer types including medulloblastoma and pancreatic cancer. Elevated expression of pathway components is present in early precursor lesions, suggesting a role for the hedgehog signaling pathway in the initiation of pancreatic tumorigenesis, and mouse models demonstrated that activation of the hedgehog pathway in the pancreas stimulates pancreatic tumorigenesis, either by itself or in collaboration with activated Kras [75–77].

Experiments performed in isolated pancreatic epithelial cells showed that activation of hedgehog signaling enhanced cell proliferation, and simultaneous activation of Kras and hedgehog signaling had an additive effect on cell proliferation. Interestingly, hedgehog induced proliferation depended on the activation of signaling through the MAP kinase and PI3 kinase signaling cascades, confirming the importance of these signaling pathways in this phenotype. Hedgehog signaling also enhanced the survival of pancreatic epithelial cells after exposure to apoptotic stress, in a manner dependent on PI3 kinase signaling, but not the MAP kinase signaling pathway. Combined with the effect of hedgehog signaling on proliferation, these findings suggest a direct role for hedgehog signaling in cell cycle progression during pancreatic tumorigenesis.

3.8   Pancreatic Stellate Cells

Pancreatic ductal adenocarcinoma is characterized by a strong stromal reaction or desmoplastic response, such that stromal elements commonly comprise the majority of the bulk tumor. The causes of this response remain poorly understood, yet its universal occurrence in PDAC underscores its importance to the disease pathology. Recently, published evidence has suggested that activated pancreatic stellate cells (PSCs) are the source of the desmoplastic response in PDAC: Immunostaining of PDAC tissue sections demonstrated the presence of activated PSCs that were actively producing collagen, suggesting that PSCs are the source of the desmoplastic response [78]. Furthermore, subcutaneous and orthotopic mouse models demonstrated that co-injection of pancreatic cancer cell lines with PSCs increased tumor growth [79]. Interestingly, the tumors that developed in the presence of PSCs had more proliferating cells than those formed in the absence of co-injected PSCs. Consistent with this, conditioned medium from activated PSCs enhances the proliferation of cancer cells in culture, suggesting that factors secreted by PSCs stimulate cell cycle progression in pancreatic cancer cells. Interestingly, blocking antibodies against platelet-derived growth factor (PDGF) reduced this proliferation, suggesting that PDGF was an important player in this process. These results are consistent with prior findings that pancreatic cancer cells have enhanced expression of the PDGF receptors. Thus, pancreatic stellate cells stimulate the proliferation of pancreatic cancer cells through the secretion of growth factors including PDGF.

3.9   Targeting the Cell Cycle During Therapy

The use of the current therapeutic approaches employed against pancreatic cancer – cytotoxic compounds such as gemcitabine, and radiation – is based on the premise that the enhanced proliferation of PDAC cells sensitizes them to these approaches. Yet, these strategies have minimal efficacy in PDAC patients. Strategies that target the underlying causes of the enhanced cell proliferation, and altered cell cycle, in PDAC may be more effective.

Given the prevalence of activating *KRAS* gene mutations in PDAC, and its demonstrated role in cell proliferation, Kras and its downstream signaling cascades are attractive therapeutic targets. Indeed, previous studies have demonstrated that, in certain contexts, Ras-induced proliferation and transformation are inhibited by the blockade of downstream signaling cascades. Yet, it is unknown whether pancreatic cancers in vivo remain dependent on Kras and the activation of its downstream signaling cascades. Indeed, experiments in cell culture suggest that the presence of additional genetic perturbations, such as the activation of hedgehog signaling, lead to sustained cell cycle progression in the face of MAP kinase or PI3 kinase pathway inhibition. Thus, it is important to model Kras dependence using inducible mouse models to determine whether pancreatic cancers remain dependent on Kras, and to identify the events that might lessen this dependence. Combinatorial targeting of Kras and additional pathways, such as hedgehog signaling, may be required to halt the proliferation of PDAC cells in vivo.

As discussed previously, many of the genetic alterations found in PDAC coordinately influence cell growth, cell metabolism, and cell proliferation, suggesting their interdependence in the cancer cell. Prior studies in culture have demonstrated that inhibition of c-Myc-induced expression of lactate dehydrogenase A (LDH-A) impairs cell transformation [80]. Importantly, inhibition of LDH-A also sensitizes cells to certain apoptotic stimuli, indicating that decoupling cell metabolism and cell proliferation may be an effective therapeutic approach in combination with cytotoxic agents or targeted agents [81].

The stroma represents an additional attractive therapeutic target. Pancreatic stellate cells stimulate the proliferation of PDAC cells via PDGF-stimulated signaling, and other undetermined mechanisms. Targeting the stromal cells may represent a novel approach to inhibit PDAC cell proliferation. The reactive stroma may also provide a physical barrier preventing effective delivery of therapeutics to PDAC cells. Therefore targeting the stroma may have additional therapeutic benefits.

In summary, pancreatic cancers harbor multiple genetic lesions, and elicit microenvironment changes that alter cell proliferation, growth, and metabolism. These changes render pancreatic cancers resistant to conventional chemotherapeutic approaches, but may also provide new opportunities for therapeutic intervention.

Key Research Points

- The cell cycle is highly ordered and tightly regulated. Cell cycle progression is tightly controlled through gene transcription and protein degradation; multiple layers of regulatory molecules and intricate feedback loops; as well as several checkpoints at which the cell determines whether to move forward or to halt progression.
- Cancer-associated changes lead to alterations in the cell cycle. Many of the hallmark features of cancer cells – such as sufficiency in growth signals, limitless replicative potential, and induction of angiogenesis – alter their own cell division cycle activity, often resulting in tumors.
- Key genes altered in pancreatic cancer affect the cell cycle. For example, the Kras and c-Myc oncoproteins work together to regulate cell growth and cell metabolism, processes vital to

enhanced cell proliferation. Likewise, many of the tumor suppressor genes mutated in pancreatic cancer encode either cell cycle inhibitory proteins, such as p16, or the proteins that are responsible for their activation, such as p53 and Smad4, so that the cell is no longer able to check its own division.

Future Scientific Directions

- How do specific genetic alterations influence the division cycle in pancreatic cells? Activation of Kras (in mice) results in precursor PanIN lesions, yet the majority of pancreatic cells retain normal cell cycle regulatory control. So, what cellular changes induced by Kras are required to stimulate cell proliferation? What are the signaling pathways required for these changes? What additional activities are necessary to convert PanIN lesions into cancer?
- What changes result from activating Kras gene mutations that alter the cell cycle of pancreatic epithelial cells? Does activation of Kras imbue cells with stem cell- or progenitor-like properties, such as limitless replicative potential? What gene expression changes are induced in pancreatic cells in response to Kras activation? Does Kras stimulate changes in the microRNA expression profile of pancreatic cells, and if so, do these changes contribute to tumorigenesis?
- Are pancreatic cancer cells "addicted" to specific alterations in the cell cycle? Are pancreatic cancer cells addicted to activated Kras, just as some non-small cell lung cancers are addicted to the EGF receptor? Is impairment of specific cell cycle checkpoints required for tumor viability – and can this be exploited therapeutically?

Clinical Implications

- Target therapies to the deregulated cell cycle. Many of the signature genetic alterations in pancreatic cancer enhance cell cycle progression or impair cell cycle checkpoints. Can therapies targeting specific molecules at these checkpoints be effective in this disease?
- Therapeutic decoupling of cell growth, metabolism, and proliferation. Activation of Kras and c-Myc leads to unchecked cell proliferation, and changes in cell growth and metabolism that in turn support increased proliferation. Can these properties be targeted to enhance the efficacy of cytotoxic or targeted therapies in pancreatic cancer?
- Aim for the stroma. Pancreatic cancers elicit a strong stromal response; stromal cells enhance the proliferation and survival of pancreatic cancer cells. Can therapies that effectively target the stroma, enhance the efficacy of cytotoxic chemotherapies or targeted agents?

Acknowledgments

The author thanks Kirsten A. Hubbard for editorial assistance with the chapter, and Sara K. Evans for providing the figures. Work in the author's lab is supported by grants from the National Institutes of Health.

References

1. Chung J, et al.: Rapamycin-FKBP specifically blocks growth-dependent activation of and signaling by the 70 kd S6 protein kinases. Cell 1992;69(7): 1227–1236.

2. Peng T, Golub TR, Sabatini DM: The immunosuppressant rapamycin mimics a starvation-like signal distinct from amino acid and glucose deprivation. Mol Cell Biol 2002;22(15):5575–5584.

3. Fingar DC, et al.: mtor controls cell cycle progression through its cell growth effectors S6K1 and 4E-BP1/eukaryotic translation initiation factor 4E. Mol Cell Biol 2004;24(1):200–216.

4. Bell SP, Dutta A: DNA replication in eukaryotic cells. Annu Rev Biochem 2002;71:333–374.

5. Greider CW, Blackburn EH: Identification of a specific telomere terminal transferase activity in Tetrahymena extracts. Cell 1985;43(2 Pt 1):405–413.

6. Harley CB, Futcher AB, Greider CW: Telomeres shorten during ageing of human fibroblasts. Nature 1990;345(6274):458–460.

7. Stein G, et al.: Regulation of cell cycle stage-specific transcription of histone genes from chromatin by non-histone chromosomal proteins. Nature 1975; 257(5529):764–767.

8. Wang ZF, et al.: The protein that binds the $3'$ end of histone mrna: a novel RNA-binding protein required for histone pre-mrna processing. Genes Dev 1996;10(23):3028–3040.

9. Hartwell LH, Culotti J, Reid B: Genetic control of the cell-division cycle in yeast. I. Detection of mutants. Proc Natl Acad Sci USA 1970; 66(2):352–359.

10. Evans T, et al.: Cyclin: a protein specified by maternal mrna in sea urchin eggs that is destroyed at each cleavage division. Cell 1983;33(2):389–396.

11. Nurse P, Thuriaux P, Nasmyth K: Genetic control of the cell division cycle in the fission yeast Schizosaccharomyces pombe. Mol Gen Genet 1976;146 (2):167–178.

12. Reed SI, Hadwiger JA, Lorincz AT: Protein kinase activity associated with the product of the yeast cell division cycle gene CDC28. Proc Natl Acad Sci USA 1985;82(12):4055–4059.

13. Fesquet D, et al.: The MO15 gene encodes the catalytic subunit of a protein kinase that activates cdc2 and other cyclin-dependent kinases (cdks) through phosphorylation of Thr161 and its homologues. Embo J 1993;12(8):3111–3121.

14. Poon RY, et al.: The cdc2-related protein p40mo15 is the catalytic subunit of a protein kinase that can activate p33cdk2 and p34cdc2. Embo J 1993;12 (8):3123–3132.

15. Solomon MJ, Harper JW, Shuttleworth J: CAK, the p34cdc2 activating kinase, contains a protein identical or closely related to p40mo15. Embo J 1993; 12(8):3133–3142.

16. Gould KL, Nurse P: Tyrosine phosphorylation of the fission yeast cdc2+ protein kinase regulates entry into mitosis. Nature 1989;342(6245):39–45.

17. Fantes P: Epistatic gene interactions in the control of division in fission yeast. Nature 1979;279(5712): 428–430.

18. Harper JW, et al.: The p21 Cdk-interacting protein Cip1 is a potent inhibitor of G_1 cyclin-dependent kinases. Cell 1993;75(4):805–816.

19. Serrano M, Hannon GJ, Beach D: A new regulatory motif in cell-cycle control causing specific inhibition of cyclin D/CDK4. Nature 1993;366(6456):704–707.

20. Xiong Y, et al.: p21 is a universal inhibitor of cyclin kinases. Nature 1993;366(6456):701–704.

21. Kovesdi I, Reichel R, Nevins JR: Role of an adenovirus E2 promoter binding factor in E1A-mediated coordinate gene control. Proc Natl Acad Sci USA 1987;84(8):2180–2184.

22. Nevins JR: The Rb/E2F pathway and cancer. Hum Mol Genet 2001;10(7):699–703.

23. Hayward WS, Neel BG, Astrin SM: Activation of a cellular onc gene by promoter insertion in ALV-induced lymphoid leukosis. Nature 1981;290 (5806):475–480.

24. Myc Cancer Gene. Available from: http://www.myc-cancergene.org.

25. Peters JM: The anaphase promoting complex/cyclosome: a machine designed to destroy. Nat Rev Mol Cell Biol 2006;7(9):644–656.

26. Yamasaki L, Pagano M: Cell cycle, proteolysis and cancer. Curr Opin Cell Biol 2004;16(6):623–628.

27. Elledge SJ: Cell cycle checkpoints: preventing an identity crisis. Science 1996;274(5293):1664–1672.

28. el-Deiry WS, et al.: WAF1, a potential mediator of p53 tumor suppression. Cell 1993;75(4):817–825.

29. Hoyt MA, Totis L, Roberts BT: S. Cerevisiae genes required for cell cycle arrest in response to loss of microtubule function. Cell 1991;66(3):507–517.

30. Li R, Murray AW: Feedback control of mitosis in budding yeast. Cell 1991;66(3):519–531.

31. Lou Z, Chen J: Mammalian DNA damage response pathway. Adv Exp Med Biol 2005;570:425–455.

32. Savitsky K, et al.: A single ataxia telangiectasia gene with a product similar to PI-3 kinase. Science 1995;268(5218):1749–1753.

33. Bell DW, et al.: Heterozygous germ line hchk2 mutations in Li-Fraumeni syndrome. Science 1999;286 (5449):2528–2531.

34. Malkin D, et al.: Germ line p53 mutations in a familial syndrome of breast cancer, sarcomas, and other neoplasms. Science 1990;250(4985):1233–1238.

35. Leach FS, et al.: Mutations of a muts homolog in hereditary nonpolyposis colorectal cancer. Cell 1993;75(6):1215–1225.

36. Nicolaides NC, et al.: Mutations of two PMS homologues in hereditary nonpolyposis colon cancer. Nature 1994;371(6492):75–80.

37. Papadopoulos N, et al.: Mutation of a mutl homolog in hereditary colon cancer. Science 1994;263(5153):1625–1629.

38. Hanahan D, Weinberg RA: The Hallmarks of Cancer. Cell 2000;100(1):57–70.

39. Serrano M, et al.: Oncogenic ras provokes premature cell senescence associated with accumulation of p53 and p16ink4a. Cell 1997;88(5):593–602.

40. Counter CM, et al.: Telomere shortening associated with chromosome instability is arrested in immortal cells which express telomerase activity. Embo J 1992;11(5):1921–1929.

41. Kim NW, et al.: Specific association of human telomerase activity with immortal cells and cancer. Science 1994;266(5193):2011–2015.

42. Rudolph KL, et al.: Longevity, stress response, and cancer in aging telomerase-deficient mice. Cell 1999;96(5):701–712.

43. Greenberg RA, et al.: Short dysfunctional telomeres impair tumorigenesis in the INK4a(delta2/3) cancer-prone mouse. Cell 1999;97(4):515–525.

44. Chin L, et al.: p53 deficiency rescues the adverse effects of telomere loss and cooperates with telomere dysfunction to accelerate carcinogenesis. Cell 1999;97(4):527–538.

45. Folkman J: Tumor angiogenesis: therapeutic implications. N Engl J Med 1971;285(21):1182–1186.

46. Weaver BA, et al.: Aneuploidy acts both oncogenically and as a tumor suppressor. Cancer Cell 2007;11(1):25–36.

47. Hingorani SR, et al.: Preinvasive and invasive ductal pancreatic cancer and its early detection in the mouse. Cancer Cell 2003;4(6):437–450.

48. Aguirre AJ, et al.: High-resolution characterization of the pancreatic adenocarcinoma genome. Proc Natl Acad Sci USA 2004;101(24):9067–9072.

49. Jones S, et al.: Core signaling pathways in human pancreatic cancers revealed by global genomic analyses. Science 2008;321(5897):1801–1806.

50. Moskaluk CA, Hruban RH, Kern SE: p16 and K-ras gene mutations in the intraductal precursors of human pancreatic adenocarcinoma. Cancer Res 1997;57(11):2140–2143.

51. Downward J: Targeting RAS signalling pathways in cancer therapy. Nat Rev Cancer 2003;3(1):11–22.

52. Calhoun ES, et al.: BRAF and FBXW7 (CDC4, FBW7, AGO, SEL10) mutations in distinct subsets of pancreatic cancer: potential therapeutic targets. Am J Pathol 2003;163(4):1255–1260.

53. Morton JP, et al.: Sonic hedgehog acts at multiple stages during pancreatic tumorigenesis. Proc Natl Acad Sci USA 2007;104(12):5103–5108.

54. Kim JW, et al.: Hypoxia-inducible factor 1 and dysregulated c-Myc cooperatively induce vascular endothelial growth factor and metabolic switches hexokinase 2 and pyruvate dehydrogenase kinase 1. Mol Cell Biol 2007;27(21):7381–7393.

55. Kamb A, et al.: A cell cycle regulator potentially involved in genesis of many tumor types. Science 1994;264(5157):436–440.

56. Kamijo T, et al.: Tumor suppression at the mouse INK4a locus mediated by the alternative reading frame product p19arf. Cell 1997;91(5):649–659.

57. Caldas C, et al.: Frequent somatic mutations and homozygous deletions of the p16 (MTS1) gene in pancreatic adenocarcinoma. Nat Genet 1994;8(1):27–32.

58. Zhang Y, Xiong Y, Yarbrough WG: ARF promotes MDM2 degradation and stabilizes p53: ARF-INK4a locus deletion impairs both the Rb and p53 tumor suppression pathways. Cell 1998;92(6):725–734.

59. Barton CM, et al.: Abnormalities of the p53 tumour suppressor gene in human pancreatic cancer. Br J Cancer 1991;64(6):1076–1082.

60. Hingorani SR, et al.: Trp53R172H and krasg12d cooperate to promote chromosomal instability and widely metastatic pancreatic ductal adenocarcinoma in mice. Cancer Cell 2005;7(5):469–483.

61. Canman CE, et al.: Activation of the ATM kinase by ionizing radiation and phosphorylation of p53. Science 1998;281(5383):1677–1679.

62. Hannon GJ, Beach D: p15ink4b is a potential effector of TGF-beta-induced cell cycle arrest. Nature 1994;371(6494):257–261.

63. Polyak K, et al.: p27Kip1, a cyclin-Cdk inhibitor, links transforming growth factor-beta and contact inhibition to cell cycle arrest. Genes Dev 1994;8(1):9–22.

64. Seoane J, et al.: tgfbeta influences Myc, Miz-1 and Smad to control the CDK inhibitor p15ink4b. Nat Cell Biol 2001;3(4):400–408.

65. Hahn SA, et al.: DPC4, a candidate tumor suppressor gene at human chromosome 18q21.1. Science 1996;271(5247):350–353.

66. Lee RC, Feinbaum RL, Ambros V: The C. Elegans heterochronic gene lin-4 encodes small rnas with antisense complementarity to lin-14. Cell 1993;75(5):843–854.

67. Bloomston M, et al.: microrna expression patterns to differentiate pancreatic adenocarcinoma from

normal pancreas and chronic pancreatitis. Jama 2007;297(17):1901–1908.

68. Calin GA, et al.: A microrna signature associated with prognosis and progression in chronic lymphocytic leukemia. N Engl J Med 2005;353(17): 1793–1801.

69. Volinia S, et al.: A microrna expression signature of human solid tumors defines cancer gene targets. Proc Natl Acad Sci USA 2006;103(7):2257–2261.

70. O'Donnell KA, et al.: c-Myc-regulated micrornas modulate E2F1 expression. Nature 2005;435 (7043):839–843.

71. He L, et al.: A microrna polycistron as a potential human oncogene. Nature 2005;435(7043):828–833.

72. Chang TC, et al.: Transactivation of mir-34a by p53 broadly influences gene expression and promotes apoptosis. Mol Cell 2007;26(5):745–752.

73. He L, et al.: A microrna component of the p53 tumour suppressor network. Nature 2007;447 (7148):1130–1134.

74. Yu F, et al.: let-7 regulates self renewal and tumorigenicity of breast cancer cells. Cell 2007;131 (6):1109–1123.

75. Berman DM, et al.: Widespread requirement for Hedgehog ligand stimulation in growth of digestive tract tumours. Nature 2003;425(6960):846–851.

76. Pasca di Magliano M, et al.: Hedgehog/Ras interactions regulate early stages of pancreatic cancer. Genes Dev 2006;20(22):3161–3173.

77. Thayer SP, et al.: Hedgehog is an early and late mediator of pancreatic cancer tumorigenesis. Nature 2003;425(6960):851–856.

78. Apte MV, et al.: Desmoplastic reaction in pancreatic cancer: role of pancreatic stellate cells. Pancreas 2004;29(3):179–187.

79. Vonlaufen A, et al.: Pancreatic stellate cells: partners in crime with pancreatic cancer cells. Cancer Res 2008;68(7):2085–2093.

80. Shim H, et al.: c-Myc transactivation of LDH-A: implications for tumor metabolism and growth. Proc Natl Acad Sci USA 1997;94(13):6658–6663.

81. Shim H, et al.: A unique glucose-dependent apoptotic pathway induced by c-Myc. Proc Natl Acad Sci USA 1998;95(4):1511–1516.

Other Resources

Morgan, DO: The Cell Cycle: Principles of Control. 2007. London: New Science Press.

14 Apoptosis Signaling Pathways in Pancreatic Cancer Pathogenesis

David J. McConkey

1   Drug Resistance in Pancreatic Cancer 370

2   Role of Apoptosis in the Outcome of Cancer Therapy 370

3   Molecular Control of Apoptosis 372

4   Expression of Canonical Apoptosis Regulators in Pancreatic Cancer 373

5   Effects of the Major Genetic Alterations Observed in Pancreatic Cancer on Apoptosis 374

6   Role of NFκB Activation 376

7   Role of EMT 377

8   Tumor-Stromal Interactions and Drug Resistance 378

9   Role of Wnt 378

10 Role of Sonic Hedgehog 379

11 Role of Notch 379

12 Summary and Conclusions 379

J. P. Neoptolemos, R. Urrutia, J. L. Abbruzzese, M. W. Büchler (eds.), *Pancreatic Cancer*,
DOI 10.1007/978-0-387-77498-5_14, © Springer Science+Business Media, LLC 2010

Abstract: Conventional and investigational cancer therapies have had little to no effect on the course of pancreatic cancer disease progression. Induction of apoptosis plays a major role in the anti-tumoral effects of conventional chemo and radiotherapy, leading to the conclusion that apoptotic pathways must be more dysfunctional in pancreatic cancer than they are in other solid malignancies. However, in vitro and preclinical in vivo studies indicate that human pancreatic cancer cell lines display remarkable heterogeneity in their sensitivities to conventional and investigational therapeutic agents, and some of the "rules" governing sensitivity and resistance are being identified. More importantly, pancreatic cancer is characterized by the presence of a large inflammatory stromal component, and emerging evidence indicates that tumor-stromal interactions further reinforce drug resistance in vivo. Here we will review what is known about the signaling pathways that mediate apoptosis resistance in pancreatic cancer cells and promising therapeutic strategies to reverse them. We will also discuss growing evidence for the idea that the unique tumor-stromal interactions that occur in pancreatic cancer contribute to the daunting therapeutic resistance observed in patients.

1 Drug Resistance in Pancreatic Cancer

Pancreatic cancer is among the most deadly of malignancies, with median survival rates of approximately 6 months [1]. There is general consensus that the reason for this dismal prognosis is therapeutic resistance. Gemcitabine-based regimens are the gold standard for neoadjuvant and adjuvant therapy, yet most studies agree that any benefit obtained with gemcitabine is palliative and clinical "responses" are modest if they can be demonstrated at all [1]. (For example, gemcitabine is used routinely in the neoadjuvant setting at our institution to make more patients candidates for surgical resection.) Even investigational agents that have exciting activity in other solid tumors (i.e., avastin) have performed relatively poorly in pancreatic cancer patients [1,2]. Thus, there is a great deal of ongoing dialog about the possible biological basis for therapeutic resistance in pancreatic cancer.

Apoptosis is an internally programmed, evolutionarily conserved pathway of cell death [3] that appears to mediate the cytoxic effects of radiotherapy and a variety of different cancer chemotherapeutic agents [4]. Therefore, one likely possibility is that the therapeutic resistance that is such a characteristic feature of pancreatic cancer is due (at least in part) to apoptosis resistance. Aspects of this resistance appear to be due to intrinsic, cell-autonomous mechanisms (Kras mutations, NFκB activation, epithelial-to-mesenchymal transition), but what may really distinguish the apoptosis resistance in pancreatic cancer from resistance in other solid tumors is the extent to which tumor-stromal interactions impart even greater resistance. Here we will review some of the more attractive intrinsic and extrinsic mechanisms of apoptosis resistance in pancreatic cancer and discuss how they might be targeted by novel therapeutic approaches (❍ *Figs. 14-1* and ❍ *14-2*).

2 Role of Apoptosis in the Outcome of Cancer Therapy

Many early studies used immature thymocytes as a model system to study the biochemical mechanisms involved in apoptosis. Early work by Wyllie showed that glucocorticoid hormones trigger thymocyte apoptosis and that this process was associated with oligonucleosomal DNA fragmentation [5]. Because glucocorticoids are commonly used in the treatment

☐ Fig. 14-1

Intrinsic resistance mechanisms

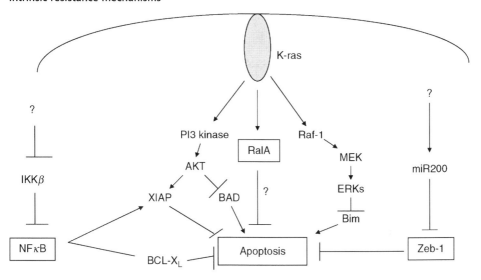

☐ Fig. 14-2

Extrinsic resistance mechanisms

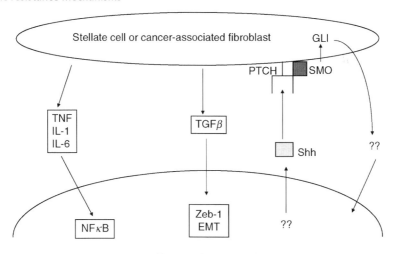

of T and B cell leukemias, it was fairly straightforward to investigate whether or not gluco-corticoids also killed leukemic cells via induction of apoptosis [6,7], and the idea that effective cancer therapy might be mediated by apoptosis was advanced. There is now a wealth of evidence showing that apoptosis mediates the effects of conventional and investigational agents in preclinical models (cell lines and model tumors in mice) [4].

Because ionizing radiation and chemical DNA damaging agents are still among the most effective cancer therapies, there has been considerable attention paid to understanding how DNA damage triggers apoptosis. Experiments comparing the responses of wild-type and $p53^{-/-}$ mice demonstrated that p53 is required for radiation-induced thymocyte cell death [8,9]. Subsequent studies showed that oncogenes like Myc and adenovirus E1A can dramatically increase sensitivity to apoptosis in normal cells [10] and that this sensitivity is lost in cells that lack p53, Apaf-1, or caspase-9 [11,12]. This oncogene-mediated sensitization to apoptosis involves the p19ARF protein, which is activated by oncogenes [13] and functions to shuttle p53's physiological inhibitor (mdm2) to the nucleolus [14]. Many of the proapoptotic transcriptional targets of p53 have been identified, including Bax, several BH3-only proteins (Bid, Puma, and Noxa), Fas, and DR5 [15].

3　Molecular Control of Apoptosis

"Apoptosis" was a term that was coined by Andrew Wyllie, John Kerr, and Alistair Currie in 1972 to describe a series of stereotyped morphological alterations that they noticed were associated with most physiological cell deaths, including programmed cell death during development [16]. These changes included chromatin condensation, nuclear and plasma membrane blebbing, cell shrinkage and detachment from neighboring cells, and specific recognition and engulfment by tissue macrophages. Subsequent biochemical studies led Wyllie to conclude in 1980 that apoptosis was associated with endogenous endonuclease activation, resulting in the formation of oligonucleosome-length DNA fragments ("DNA ladders") that remain diagnostic for this form of cell death to this day [5]. Then Robert Horvitz and his group used chemical mutagenesis in Caenorhabditis elegans embryos to show that developmentally programmed cell death requires two genes, termed ced-3 and ced-4 [17], and they subsequently showed that ced-3 encodes a cysteine protease (the first "caspase") [18]. Subsequent research has confirmed that caspases are required for apoptosis in mammalian cells [3] and that they trigger the DNA fragmentation associated with the response [19,20].

Major insights into the biochemical mechanisms involved in caspase activation were provided by studies from Xiaodong Wang's laboratory. Using large volumes of HeLa cell extracts, they isolated 3 proteins ("apoptosis protease activating factors," or Apafs) that they found could promote activation of recombinant caspase-3 (when the extracts were supplemented with ATP) [21,22]. Microsequencing revealed that one of the proteins was a caspase (caspase-9) and another was the mitochondrial electron transport chain intermediate, cytochrome c. The third (termed Apaf-1) turned out to be the mammalian homolog of ced-4. Functional studies revealed that Apaf-1 functions as an adaptor protein, promoting the cytochrome c- and ATP-dependent oligomerization and activation of caspase-9 [23]. Active caspase-9 then cleaves and activates caspases 3 and 7, the two major mammalian "effector" caspases that initiate cell death [3].

Wang's observations catalyzed an aggressive search for the biochemical mechanisms that control cytochrome c release from mitochondria during apoptosis. Work from several laboratories demonstrated that pro- and anti-apoptotic members of the BCL-2 family are centrally involved [24,25]. BCL-2 was originally cloned as the gene present at the t[14,18] translocation that is a hallmark feature of follicular non-Hodgkins B cell lymphomas [26,27]. Subsequent work revealed that BCL-2 is a functionally novel oncogene, acting to suppress apoptosis without promoting cell division [28], and that it is structurally and functionally related to another molecule (BCL-X$_L$) that also inhibits apoptosis [29]. Korsmeyer's group and others then showed that the protein localizes to mitochondria [30] and that it binds to structurally similar polypeptides (including Bax, Bak, and Bad) that promote cell death [31–33]. It is now appreciated that the BCL-2 family consists of death inhibitors (i.e., BCL-2, BCL-X$_L$, MCL-1) and death promoters (Bax, Bak, Bad, Bid, Bim, etc.), and that the latter can be further divided into "multidomain" and "BH3-only" subfamilies based on the number of domains they share with BCL-2 and the other death inhibitors [34,35]. Cytochrome c release occurs when a BH3-only protein induces Bax and/or Bak to form pores in the outer mitochondrial membrane [36], and the anti-apoptotic members of the family inhibit cytochrome c release by binding to and neutralizing the pro-apoptotic members of the family [34].

A second family of proteins that appears to play a central role in regulating caspase activation is the inhibitor of apoptosis proteins (IAPs) [37]. Originally identified in baculoviruses [38], the IAPs can directly bind to and inhibit certain caspases, thereby preventing cell death [37]. There is reasonably good consensus that X-linked inhibitor of apoptosis protein (XIAP) is the most potent direct inhibitor of caspases, although others (including survivin and the cIAPs) can also block cell death [37]. Parallel studies in *Drosophila* and mammalian cells showed that the death inhibitory activities of the IAPs are under the control of another family of proteins. These polypeptides, including Reaper, Hid, and Grim in *Drosophila* [39–42] and Second Mitochondrial Activator of Caspases (SMAC) in mammals [43,44], directly bind to and neutralize the IAPs, releasing bound caspases to allow them to participate in induction of apoptosis [37].

Apoptosis can be initiated by intracellular stress originating from the mitochondria, endoplasmic reticulum, or nucleus [45]. In addition, apoptosis can be induced by engagement of a family of cell surface receptors (known as "death receptors") [46]. The most familiar death receptors are the type 1 receptor for tumor necrosis factor, Fas, and the receptors for tumor necrosis factor-related apoptosis-inducing ligand (TRAIL), which are known as death receptors 4 and 5 (DR4 and DR5). Following ligand-induced trimerization, death receptors recruit an adaptor protein known as Fas-associated death domain (FADD) [47,48], which binds to and activates caspases 8 and 10 by oligomerizing them [49]. In most cells active caspase-8 then cleaves the BH3-only protein Bid, producing a functionally active form of the protein (tBid) that translocates to the mitochondria and promotes Bax/Bak activation and cytochrome c release [50]. Although its name implies otherwise, few cancer cells are actually sensitive to TNF-induced apoptosis because TNF usually activates pro- and anti-apoptotic signals simultaneously. The anti-apoptotic signal is dependent on the transcription factor nuclear factor kappa B (NFκB), and inhibitors of NFκB are powerful sensitizers to TNF-induced apoptosis [51,52].

4 Expression of Canonical Apoptosis Regulators in Pancreatic Cancer

Early immunohistochemical studies assessed the possible relationship between expression of BCL-2 family polypeptides and outcome in primary pancreatic tumors. In the first of these studies Sinacrope showed that BCL-2 tended to be expressed by well-differentiated tumors, a finding that was confirmed later by Makinen and colleagues [53,54]. Neither group observed a relationship between BCL-2 expression and outcome (resectabily, survival), but these results suggest that BCL-2 is probably not associated with progression. These findings are consistent with results in breast cancer, where BCL-2 is expressed in well-differentiated, estrogen receptor-positive tumors [55]. Fewer studies have been published describing the patterns of BCL-X$_L$ expression in primary tumors, but it appears that increased expression is associated with lower rates of spontaneous apoptosis [56] and may portend a worse prognosis [57–59]. This observation is consistent with mechanistic data showing that NFκB is one of the transcription factors that drives BCL-X$_L$ expression in pancreatic cancer cells. Likewise, more work needs to be performed to determine the role of MCL-1 in pancreatic cancer progression, but the results obtained to date do not support the idea that MCL-1 overexpression plays a major role in cancer progression [60,61]. Proapoptotic members of the BCL-2 family also appear to be differentially expressed in pancreatic cancer. For example, there appears to be a correlation between loss of Bax expression and poor survival [62,63].

A handful of studies have also characterized the expression of IAPs in primary pancreatic cancers, and there is a suggestion that several of them (including XIAP and survivin) may be upregulated [64]. Finally, death receptors appear to be generally upregulated in pancreatic cancers as compared to normal controls [65], perhaps because these cytokine pathways are intimately involved in inflammation [66] and pancreatic cancer is exemplified by a highly reactive stroma.

5 Effects of the Major Genetic Alterations Observed in Pancreatic Cancer on Apoptosis

As discussed throughout this volume, pancreatic cancer progression involves a stereotyped sequence of molecular alterations involving mutational activation of Kras and loss of the p16/ARF, SMAD4, and p53 tumor suppressors. Indeed, one of the major conclusions in a recent high profile study that employed "deep sequencing" to study all of the genetic alterations present in a large set of human pancreatic cancer cell lines and primary xenografts was that these core pathways stand out as the most common features associated with cancer [67]. Thus, it seems reasonable to assume that these core defects contribute to apoptosis resistance. However, among these defects only Kras really stands out as being relatively unique to pancreatic cancer, as defects in the p16/Rb, p53, and TGFβ pathways are almost ubiquitously involved in solid tumor progression in general [68], and mutant Kras is being implicated as a marker of drug resistance (particularly in patients treated with EGFR inhibitors) and poor prognosis in other cancers. This does not diminish the importance of p53 loss in therapeutic resistance – as discussed above, there is outstanding evidence tying p53 to DNA damage-induced apoptosis in model systems. However, p53 loss does not distinguish pancreatic cancer from other malignancies, and it is therefore unlikely to solely account for the unique therapeutic resistance observed.

One clear effect of mutant Kras in tissue culture and in transgenic mouse models is to promote cell proliferation. This is not surprising given that Ras family activation has been shown to activate a large number of mitogenic pathways, including the Raf-MEK-ERK, PI3 kinase-AKT-mTOR, and JAK-STAT3 pathways, among others. Thus, normal human pancreatic cells expressing mutant Kras grow better under normal tissue culture and anchorage-independent conditions [69–71], whereas knockdown of Kras in pancreatic cancer cells inhibits growth [70]. Inhibitors of Raf-ERK and PI-3 kinase pathways blocked the effects of Kras on cell growth, consistent with expectations.

Surprisingly, however, Kras-mediated transformation is not always tightly associated with constitutive ERK or AKT pathway activation. Rather, emerging evidence suggests that the RalGEFs may be more important targets of active Kras in pancreatic cancer cells [71–73].

Knockdown of RalA results in suppression of Kras-mediated anchorage-independent growth, whereas knockdown of RalB does not [72,73]. Instead, Kras-mediated activation of RalB appears to be very important for Kras-mediated invasion in vitro and metastasis in vivo [73]. Interference with RalA or RalB induces some apoptosis in pancreatic cancer cells [74], although the magnitudes of these increases are not tremendously large and the downstream mechanisms involved have not been defined.

Expression of mutant K-ras may also uncouple cell cycle progression through the G_1/S transition from the control of epithelial growth factor receptors, including the epidermal growth factor receptor (EGFR). The best evidence for this comes from recent clinical trials with EGFR inhibitors in patients with non-small cell lung cancer and colon cancer, where the drugs showed absolutely no benefit in patients whose tumors contained activating Kras mutations [75–77]. Even though EGFR inhibitors do have promising growth-inhibitory effects in some human pancreatic cancer cell lines and xenografts that express mutant Kras [78], and the EGFR inhibitor erlotinib is now FDA approved in combination with gemcitabine for pancreatic cancer therapy [79], the emerging evidence that mutant Kras limits the effects of EGFR raises a strong cautionary note.

Tissue-specific expression of mutant Kras in conjunction with mutational inactivation of p16 or p53 leads to a higher penetrance of PanIN lesions that progress more rapidly to invasive cancer [80–82]. Loss of p16 probably contributes to Kras-mediated deregulation of cell cycle progression through the G1/S checkpoint, and p15/19ARF, which is encoded within the same locus, has been implicated in oncogene-mediated activation of p53 [14], so genetic inactivation of the locus disrupts oncogene-mediated activation of the p53 pathway. Gerard Evan was among the first to recognize that oncogenes that deregulate cell cycle checkpoints tend to predispose cells to apoptosis, and that these effects must be compensated for by acquisition of a genetic defect that undermines apoptosis resistance [83]. Indeed, in recent work his group showed that tumor progression selects for loss of oncogene-mediated p53 activation and that the other well-known function of p53 in the DNA damage response appears to be less important [13]. This provides an attractive explanation for why loss of p16/ARF and/or p53 synergizes with mutant Kras to promote tumorigenesis and metastatic progression in transgenic mouse models and why Kras mutations are usually associated with loss of p16/ARF and/or p53 in primary tumors. Adenovirus-mediated overexpression of p16 into pancreatic cancer cells induces mostly cell cycle arrest, although responses are heterogeneous in different cell models [84,85] in a manner that may depend upon whether the p16 that is introduced inhibits cyclin-dependent kinases: cells that display downregulation of cdk activity undergo growth arrest, whereas cells that fail to do so die [86]. Adenoviral p16 delivery can also enhance the pro-apoptotic effects of chemotherapy [87]. However, whether or not loss of endogenous p16 contributes to apoptosis resistance is not clear.

Genetic inactivation of SMAD4 in the mouse leads to lethality by embryonic day 7.5 associated with defects in differentiation with no measurable effects on apoptosis [88]. Similarly, reintroduction of SMAD4 into SMAD4-deficient human BxPC-3 pancreatic cancer cells leads to cell flattening, increased sensitivity to TGFβ-induced inhibition of proliferation, and inhibition of tumorigenicity in vivo without altering rates of apoptosis or angiogenesis [89]. Overexpression of SMAD4 can trigger apoptosis in MDCK cells via a JNK-dependent mechanism [90], but the relevance of these observations to the effects of endogenous levels of SMAD4 can be questioned. Thus, the bulk of the evidence suggests that loss of SMAD4 probably has more to do with uncoupling TGFβ-mediated growth inhibition rather than resistance to apoptosis.

6   Role of NFκB Activation

Nuclear factor kappa B (NFκB) is an inflammation-associated transcription factor that has been implicated in the maintenance of cell survival [91]. Early work by Chiao's laboratory demonstrated that NFκB is constitutively active in a majority of human pancreatic cancer cell lines and primary tumors [92], and subsequent work has shown that NFκB inhibitors sensitize pancreatic cancer cells to chemotherapy-induced apoptosis [93–97]. The molecular mechanisms that drive NFκB activation appear to be complex and probably involve autocrine cytokine production [98], Kras activation [99], and constitutive PI3 kinase/AKT pathway activation [100]. Anti-apoptotic genes downstream of NFκB include BCL-X$_L$ [93,101,102] and XIAP [102,103].

These observations generated enthusiasm for the use of NFκB inhibitors in pancreatic cancer therapy. Unfortunately, no inhibitors are available yet that specifically target the transcription factor or its upstream activators. The first NFκB inhibitor to enter clinical trials was the proteasome inhibitor bortezomib (Velcade, formerly known as PS-341). In preclinical studies PS-341 inhibited the growth of some [104–107] (but not all) [108] pancreatic cancer xenografts, effects that were associated with induction of apoptosis and inhibition of angiogenesis. However, combination therapy with bortezomib plus gemcitabine [109] or carboplatin (G. Varadhachary, personal communication) has produced no detectable clinical benefit in the second line in patients, although similar combinations appear to have activity in non-small cell lung cancer (NSCLC) [110,111]. Furthermore, whether or not any of the anti-tumoral effects are truly linked to NFκB inhibition is not clear. Proteasome inhibitors have a variety of other pro- and anti-apoptotic effects, including stabilization of proapoptotic proteins such as Noxa and Bim, accumulation of heat shock proteins and other protein chaperones, induction of endoplasmic reticular (ER) stress, and activation of autophagy [112]. Thus, whether or not a cell dies in response to proteasome inhibition is controlled by complex mechanisms, and NFκB inhibition is no longer considered a dominant component of the effects of proteasome inhibitors.

Curcumin is a natural product NFκB inhibitor that also displayed promising activity in preclinical models of human pancreatic cancer [92, 94, 113, 114]. Excitingly, in a recent Phase II trial of oral curcumin in patients with advanced pancreatic cancer, 2/25 patients had clear evidence of clinical biological activity [115]. One tumor displayed a short-lived but impressive 73% reduction in volume, and another displayed prolonged stabilization of growth [115]. One likely limitation of the oral formulation was its limited bioavailability, and a liposome-encapsulated formulation with improved in vivo properties has been developed [113]. This new reagent is slated to enter clinical trials in pancreatic cancer patients soon.

The exciting results with curcumin raise new enthusiasm for targeting NFκB in pancreatic cancer. Thus, Logsdon's group recently characterized the effects of siRNA-mediated knockdown of one of NFκB's subunits (p65) to more specifically study its role in regulating cell death in a panel of human pancreatic cancer cell lines and orthotopic xenografts [116]. This panel included cells that were sensitive (BxPC-3, L3.6pl, CFPAC-1) or resistant (mPANC96, Panc-1, MiaPaCa2) to gemcitabine-induced apoptosis [116]. Strikingly, p65 knockdown induced basal apoptosis and increased gemcitabine-induced apoptosis only in the three cell lines that were sensitive to gemcitabine at baseline. In contrast, p65 knockdown had no effect on basal or gemcitabine-induced apoptosis in the gemcitabine-resistant cells in vitro or in vivo [116]. Importantly, p65 silencing can render some gemcitabine-resistant cells (i.e., Panc-1) sensitive to TRAIL [102,103]. Because TRAIL and agonistic anti-TRAIL receptor antibodies are now being evaluated in cancer patients [117], combination therapy with NFκB inhibitors like curcumin plus TRAIL receptor agonists could be an attractive approach to circumventing gemcitabine resistance if the molecular properties of the tumors that are vulnerable to this approach can be identified prior to therapy.

7   Role of EMT

Epithelial-to-mesenchymal transition (EMT) is an important process during normal development that appears to be reactivated in epithelial tumors as they progress and become metastatic [118–123]. The hallmark feature of EMT is loss of the homotypic adhesion due to downregulation of E-cadherin, accompanied by other changes such as loss of cell polarity genes and increased motility and invasion [119]. Loss of E-cadherin and presumably many of the other genes that are repressed during EMT is mediated by a group of transcriptional repressors (Twist, Snail, Slug, Zeb-1, Zeb-2) that recruit histone deacetylases to E-box elements within the E-cadherin promoter [119]. Members of the micro RNA (miR) 200 family, which maintain E-cadherin expression by repressing Zeb-1 and Zeb-2 [124–128], also play important roles in regulating EMT. Recent work has also demonstrated that these transcription factors can drive some of the canonical epigenetic changes (DNA methylation) that are observed during the progression of solid tumors [129], and cells that have undergone EMT share important properties with cancer stem cells [130,131].

We recently compared baseline gene expression profiles in a panel of 10 human pancreatic cancer cell lines selected on the basis of sensitivity or resistance to gemcitabine-induced apoptosis (Arumugam et al., Cancer Research, in press). The results demonstrated that markers of EMT, and in particular expression of Zeb-1, closely correlated with gemcitabine resistance and cross-resistance to cisplatin and 5-fluorouracil. Knockdown of Zeb-1 not only restored E-cadherin expression but also sensitivity to all three drugs. Interestingly, gemcitabine-resistant cells tended to be cross-resistant to TRAIL, but the EMT signature did not correlate as closely with sensitivity to taxanes, suggesting that it may be possible to identify chemotherapeutic agents that are active in subpopulations of these cells. The conclusion that EMT contributes to intrinsic drug resistance is consistent with the similarities between EMT and cancer stem cells and the idea that the latter are more generally responsible for drug resistance in solid tumors.

The role of EMT in resistance to EGFR inhibitors is even clearer. Several studies have now shown that loss of E-cadherin is associated with resistance to gefitinib and erlotinib in NSCLC, colon cancer, pancreatic cancer, and head and neck squamous cell carcinoma lines [132–135]. As was true for the chemotherapeutics listed above, knockdown of Zeb-1 restored EGFR inhibitor sensitivity in HNSCC [132] and pancreatic cancer cells (K. Fournier, A. Kwan, manuscript in preparation). Zeb-1 knockdown also decreased tumor cell invasion and migration [132], indicating that the EMT phenotype is probably intimately involved in metastasis as well.

It would clearly be desirable to be able to pharmacologically reverse EMT in an attempt to restore drug sensitivity in vivo. Given that Zeb-1 and the other modulators of the process act by recruiting histone deacetylases to promoters, it might be possible to do this with clinically available HDAC inhibitors such as vorinostat [136] or SNDX-275 [137]. Indeed, recent work has shown that HDAC inhibitors can in fact restore E-cadherin expression and EGFR inhibitor sensitivity in "mesenchymal" tumor cells [138]. However, HDAC inhibitors promote p21-associated cell cycle arrest [139], and this may not be desirable when these agents are combined with conventional chemotherapeutic agents that are more active in cycling cells. We are attempting to use sequential drug scheduling to obtain the EMT-reversing benefits of HDAC inhibitors while avoiding their potentially undesirable effects on cell cycle progression.

8   Tumor-Stromal Interactions and Drug Resistance

Although even fewer details about how they do so are available, it seems quite likely that cell – extrinsic rather than – intrinsic mechanisms are largely responsible for the remarkable therapeutic resistance that is observed in pancreatic cancer patients. Pancreatic cancers are characterized by an extensive inflammatory stromal compartment that must play important roles in cancer biology. Once tumors have adapted to them (possibly in part by disabling the TGFβ pathway), inflammatory cytokines and other factors secreted by host cells probably promote activation of the NFκB [140] and cyclooxygenase-2 [141] pathways to enhance tumor cell cytoprotection. Targeting these interactions provides a new opportunity to disrupt drug resistance.

One of the challenges facing researchers interested in tumor-stromal interactions has been the inaccessibility of good preclinical models to study them. Pancreatic stellate cells are myofibro-blast-like cells that are a major constituent of the inflammatory stroma in pancreatic cancer [142]. These cells have now been successfully isolated from rodent models [143–145] and primary human tumors [146], and coculture experiments have shown that they promote resistance to gemcitabine and radiation in vitro and tumorigenicity in orthotopic xenografts in vivo [146], establishing direct proof-of-principle evidence for the idea that tumor-stromal interactions contribute to overall drug resistance. Thus, defining the molecular mechanisms involved in cell-cell communication between pancreatic cancer cells and their microenvironment should reveal strategies to reverse drug resistance. Recent studies have implicated reactivation of pathways involved in pancreas development [147, 148], including the Wnt, Notch, and Sonic Hedgehog pathways [149], in these interactions, and small molecule inhibitors of them are currently being tested in clinical trials or are under development. What is known about their contributions to suppression of apoptosis will be summarized below.

9   Role of Wnt

E-cadherin forms a signaling complex at the cell surface with β-catenin. Loss of E-cadherin or activation of the Wnt pathway causes translocation of β-catenin from the plasma membrane to the nucleus, where it regulates gene expression pathways that are involved in the control of proliferation and differentiation. Therefore, their mutual involvement of β-catenin translocation establishes a close mechanistic connection between EMT and activation of the Wnt pathway.

Recent work by Hebrok and a variety of other investigators has demonstrated that the Wnt pathway is constitutively active in primary pancreatic tumors, mouse models of pancreatic cancer, and pancreatic cancer cell lines [150]. They selected four cell lines (CFPAC, BxPC3, L3.6sl, and Panc4.21) and carried out functional studies using various molecular inhibitors of the pathway to determine what role pathway activation played in cell proliferation and survival. Transfection with an inhibitor of β-catenin (Icat), a dominant negative form of the transcription factor that is activated by nuclear β-catenin (TCF-Lef), or an siRNA construct specific for β-catenin reduced rates of cell proliferation and induced significant increases in apoptosis [150]. Precisely how the Wnt pathway suppresses apoptosis was not determined.

Interestingly, CFPAC, L3.6sl, and BxPC-3 cells are all E-cadherin-positive, gemcitabine-sensitive, and display an "epithelial" phenotypic and molecular phenotype (T. Arumugam et al., manuscript under revision). Therefore, Wnt pathway activation in these cells is not due to loss of E-cadherin, as is often true in "mesenchymal" gastrointestinal tumor cells. In addition, whether Wnt pathway disruption will directly promote apoptosis or enhance sensitivity to apoptosis induced by other agents in gemcitabine-resistant cells needs to be determined.

10 Role of Sonic Hedgehog

Many reports have documented that the sonic hedgehog pathway is constitutively active in pancreatic cancer [151]. However, whether the pathway is usually activated in an autocrine or paracine manner remains controversial. Earlier work demonstrated that ligand, receptor, and target genes were all co-expressed in most pancreatic cancer cell lines, and chemically active (but not structurally related inactive) analogs of cyclopamine, a chemical inhibitor of the hedgehog pathway, induced growth inhibition and cell death [152]. However, although subsequent studies have confirmed that the pathway is active and biologically important [153], the newer data strongly suggest that pathway activation more often involves paracrine interactions between ligand expressed by the tumor cell and receptor on the stroma [154,155]. Work in primary xenografts demonstrated that a chemical pathway inhibitor had very promising effects on tumor growth [154], although how pathway inhibition affected proliferation and apoptosis still needs to be characterized further. Overall, there is very high enthusiasm for developing strategies to identify hedgehog-dependent pancreatic cancers and assess the toxicity and activity of pathway inhibitors in clinical trials in patients. In addition, it will be important to determine how pathway inhibition affects tumor sensitivity to gemcitabine and other conventional therapeutic approaches.

11 Role of Notch

Accumulating evidence implicates reactivation of the Notch pathway in pancreatic cancer development and progression [156]. Recent studies led by Sarkar and collaborators suggest that there is a link between NFκB and Notch pathway activation in pancreatic cancer cells [157]. They have also shown that siRNA-mediated inhibition of the Notch pathway induces apoptosis in pancreatic cancer cells [158] and that Notch pathway activation is linked to EMT (F. Sarkar, personal communication). Whether or not paracrine mechanisms also collaborate to promote cancer cell apoptosis resistance will need to be determined in appropriate preclinical models, and the impact of Notch inhibition on gemcitabine sensitivity will also have to be assessed.

12 Summary and Conclusions

In the aftermath of many false preclinical leads, it is easy to understand why medical oncologists may be skeptical about the ability of laboratory science to inform clinical trial design in pancreatic cancer patients. The facts indicate that we have made very little progress in our attempts to design more effective treatments for this disease, even though many mice have been "cured" of pancreatic cancer in the laboratory. Clearly, one of the most important goals for ongoing laboratory research is to do a better job of validating our preclinical models, at the molecular and biological levels, so that they can be better used as screening tools to predict drug activity in patients. Our own group has unfortunately discovered that the models we relied on most heavily (i.e., L3.6pl) are actually among the most gemcitabine-sensitive ones available. The appreciation that other models (Panc-1, mPANC96, etc.) are extremely drug resistant in vitro and in vivo, along with the new appreciation for the importance of developing preclinical regimens that promote overt tumor cell apoptosis and regression (as opposed to disease stabilization), represents one major step in the right direction. Incorporation of other models, most notably primary xenografts and transgenic mice, should greatly improve the predictive power of laboratory studies in general.

Accumulating laboratory evidence indicates that tumor-stromal interactions cooperate with intrinsic tumor cell defects to produce drug-sensitive and drug-resistant phenotypes. Although there is the concern that drug delivery into pancreatic cancers may be challenging in general due to poor vascularization, interstitial pressure, and/or other physical constraints, it is growing clearer that the most effective therapeutic approach will target both the tumor cells themselves as well as interactions between tumor cells and the stroma. Further effort is needed to define the biological effects of tumor-stromal interactions on cancer cell survival and to develop strategies to identify tumors that are dependent upon particular tumor-stromal pathways prospectively. Ongoing clinical trials with sonic hedgehog pathway inhibitors should provide us with some indication about whether this therapeutic paradigm shift produces a real change in the course of disease progression in at least a significant subset of tumors in patients.

Key Research Points

- Intrinsic and extrinsic mechanisms contribute to apoptosis resistance in pancreatic cancer
- Kras-mediated mechanisms appear to be important, and they involve novel downstream pathways (RalA, RalB, etc.)
- Epithelial-to-mesenchymal transition (EMT) and tumor "stemness" also appear to contribute to intrinsic resistance
- Tumor-stromal interactions involving developmental pathways are almost certainly involved

Future Scientific Directions

- A better definition of the downstream targets of Kras and their effects on apoptosis is greatly needed
- The relationship between EMT and "stemness" and the molecular mechanisms that underlie these phenotypes requires further exploration
- A comprehensive understanding of the tumor-stromal interactions, the cell types involved, and methods to detect them should be obtained

Clinical Implications

- Kras imparts clinically relevant drug resistance in other solid tumors, strongly suggesting that it also does so in pancreatic cancer
- Therapeutic approaches that target or bypass mutant Kras should be developed

- Therapeutic approaches that target tumor-stromal interactions should be explored aggressively
- Optimal therapy will almost certainly require that regimens be designed on a patient-by-patient basis and will require a better understanding of the basic biology of apoptosis resistance
- There is a great need to develop and validate preclinical models that better predict drug activity in patients so that new targets and drugs can be prioritized better prior to clinical evaluation

References

1. Cartwright T, Richards DA, Boehm KA: Cancer of the pancreas: are we making progress? A review of studies in the US oncology research network. Cancer Control 2008;15:308–313.

2. Ko AH, Dito E, Schillinger B, et al.: A phase II study evaluating bevacizumab in combination with fixed-dose rate gemcitabine and low-dose cisplatin for metastatic pancreatic cancer: is an anti-VEGF strategy still applicable? Invest New Drugs 2008;26:463–471.

3. Hengartner MO: The biochemistry of apoptosis. Nature 2000;407:770–776.

4. Schmitt CA, Lowe SW: Apoptosis is critical for drug response in vivo. Drug Resist Updat 2001;4:132–134.

5. Wyllie AH: Glucocorticoid-induced thymocyte apoptosis is associated with endogenous endonuclease activation. Nature 1980;284:555–556.

6. Distelhorst CW: Glucocorticosteroids induce DNA fragmentation in human lymphoid leukemia cells. Blood 1988;72:1305–1309.

7. McConkey DJ, Aguilar-Santelises M, Hartzell P, et al.: Induction of DNA fragmentation in chronic B-lymphocytic leukemia cells. J Immunol 1991;146: 1072–1076.

8. Clarke AR, Purdie CA, Harrison DJ, et al.: Thymocyte apoptosis induced by p53-dependent and independent pathways. Nature 1993;362:849–852.

9. Lowe SW, Schmitt EM, Smith SW, Osborne BA, Jacks T: p53 is required for radiation-induced apoptosis in mouse thymocytes. Nature 1993;362:847–849.

10. Evan GI, Wyllie AH, Gilbert CS, et al.: Induction of apoptosis in fibroblasts by c-myc protein. Cell 1992;69:119–128.

11. Lowe SW, Ruley HE, Jacks T, Housman DE: p53-dependent apoptosis modulates the cytotoxicity of anticancer agents. Cell 1993;74:957–967.

12. Symonds H, Krall L, Remington L, et al.: p53-dependent apoptosis suppresses tumor growth and progression in vivo. Cell 1994;78:703–711.

13. Christophorou MA, Ringshausen I, Finch AJ, Swigart LB, Evan GI: The pathological response to DNA damage does not contribute to p53-mediated tumour suppression. Nature 2006;443:214–217.

14. Sherr CJ, Weber JD: The ARF/p53 pathway. Curr Opin Genet Dev 2000;10:94–99.

15. Kuribayashi K, El-Deiry WS: Regulation of programmed cell death by the p53 pathway. Adv Exp Med Biol 2008;615:201–221.

16. Kerr JF, Wyllie AH, Currie AR: Apoptosis: a basic biological phenomenon with wide-ranging implications in tissue kinetics. Br J Cancer 1972; 26:239–257.

17. Ellis HM, Horvitz HR: Genetic control of programmed cell death in the nematode C. elegans. Cell 1986;44:817–829.

18. Yuan J, Shaham S, Ledoux S, Ellis HM, Horvitz HR: The C. elegans cell death gene ced-3 encodes a protein similar to mammalian interleukin-1 beta-converting enzyme. Cell 1993;75:641–652.

19. Liu X, Zou H, Slaughter C, Wang X: DFF, a heterodimeric protein that functions downstream of caspase-3 to trigger DNA fragmentation during apoptosis. Cell 1997;89:175–184.

20. Enari M, Sakahira H, Yokoyama H, Okawa K, Iwamatsu A, Nagata S: A caspase-activated DNase that degrades DNA during apoptosis, and its inhibitor ICAD. Nature 1998;391:43–50.

21. Li P, Nijhawan D, Budihardjo I, et al.: Cytochrome c and dATP-dependent formation of Apaf-1/caspase-9 complex initiates an apoptotic protease cascade. Cell 1997;91:479–489.

22. Zou H, Henzel WJ, Liu X, Lutschg A, Wang X: Apaf-1, a human protein homologous to C. elegans-CED-4, participates in cytochrome c-dependent activation of caspase-3. Cell 1997;90:405–413.

23. Zou H, Li Y, Liu X, Wang X: An APAF-1.cytochrome c multimeric complex is a functional apoptosome

that activates procaspase-9. J Biol Chem 1999;274: 11549–11556.

24. Danial NN, Korsmeyer SJ: Cell death: critical control points. Cell 2004;116:205–219.

25. Scorrano L, Korsmeyer SJ: Mechanisms of cytochrome c release by proapoptotic BCL-2 family members. Biochem Biophys Res Commun 2003;304: 437–444.

26. Tsujimoto Y, Cossman J, Jaffe E, Croce CM: Involvement of the bcl-2 gene in human follicular lymphoma. Science 1985;228:1440–1443.

27. Bakhshi A, Jensen JP, Goldman P, et al.: Cloning the chromosomal breakpoint of t(14;18) human lymphomas: clustering around JH on chromosome 14 and near a transcriptional unit on 18. Cell 1985; 41:899–906.

28. McDonnell TJ, Deane N, Platt FM, et al.: bcl-2-immunoglobulin transgenic mice demonstrate extended B cell survival and follicular lymphoproliferation. Cell 1989;57:79–88.

29. Boise LH, Gonzalez-Garcia M, Postema CE, et al.: bcl-x, a bcl-2-related gene that functions as a dominant regulator of apoptotic cell death. Cell 1993; 74:597–608.

30. Hockenbery D, Nunez G, Milliman C, Schreiber RD, Korsmeyer SJ: Bcl-2 is an inner mitochondrial membrane protein that blocks programmed cell death. Nature 1990;348:334–336.

31. Oltvai ZN, Milliman CL, Korsmeyer SJ: Bcl-2 heterodimerizes in vivo with a conserved homolog, Bax, that accelerates programmed cell death. Cell 1993; 74:609–619.

32. Yang E, Zha J, Jockel J, Boise LH, Thompson CB, Korsmeyer SJ: Bad, a heterodimeric partner for Bcl-XL and Bcl-2, displaces Bax and promotes cell death. Cell 1995;80:285–291.

33. Farrow SN, White JH, Martinou I, et al.: Cloning of a bcl-2 homologue by interaction with adenovirus E1B 19K. Nature 1995;374:731–733.

34. Adams JM, Cory S: The Bcl-2 apoptotic switch in cancer development and therapy. Oncogene 2007; 26:1324–1337.

35. Willis SN, Adams JM: Life in the balance: how BH3-only proteins induce apoptosis. Curr Opin Cell Biol 2005;17:617–625.

36. Antignani A, Youle RJ: How do Bax and Bak lead to permeabilization of the outer mitochondrial membrane? Curr Opin Cell Biol 2006;18:685–689.

37. Eckelman BP, Salvesen GS, Scott FL: Human inhibitor of apoptosis proteins: why XIAP is the black sheep of the family. EMBO Rep 2006;7:988–994.

38. Crook NE, Clem RJ, Miller LK: An apoptosis-inhibiting baculovirus gene with a zinc finger-like motif. J Virol 1993;67:2168–2174.

39. Chen P, Nordstrom W, Gish B, Abrams JM: grim, a novel cell death gene in Drosophila. Genes Dev 1996;10:1773–1782.

40. Grether ME, Abrams JM, Agapite J, White K, Steller H: The head involution defective gene of Drosophila melanogaster functions in programmed cell death. Genes Dev 1995;9:1694–1708.

41. White K, Grether ME, Abrams JM, Young L, Farrell K, Steller H: Genetic control of programmed cell death in Drosophila. Science 1994; 264:677–683.

42. Steller H: Regulation of apoptosis in Drosophila. Cell Death Differ 2008;15:1132–1138.

43. Du C, Fang M, Li Y, Li L, Wang X: Smac, a mitochondrial protein that promotes cytochrome c-dependent caspase activation by eliminating IAP inhibition. Cell 2000;102:33–42.

44. Verhagen AM, Ekert PG, Pakusch M, et al.: Identification of DIABLO, a mammalian protein that promotes apoptosis by binding to and antagonizing IAP proteins. Cell 2000;102:43–53.

45. Oberst A, Bender C, Green DR: Living with death: the evolution of the mitochondrial pathway of apoptosis in animals. Cell Death Differ 2008; 15:1139–1146.

46. Wang S, El-Deiry WS: TRAIL and apoptosis induction by TNF-family death receptors. Oncogene 2003;22:8628–8633.

47. Kischkel FC, Hellbardt S, Behrmann I, et al.: Cytotoxicity-dependent APO-1 (Fas/CD95)-associated proteins form a death-inducing signaling complex (DISC) with the receptor. Embo J 1995; 14:5579–5588.

48. Chinnaiyan AM, O'Rourke K, Tewari M, Dixit VM: FADD, a novel death domain-containing protein, interacts with the death domain of Fas and initiates apoptosis. Cell 1995;81:505–512.

49. Ashkenazi A, Dixit VM: Apoptosis control by death and decoy receptors. Curr Opin Cell Biol 1999; 11:255–260.

50. Li H, Zhu H, Xu CJ, Yuan J: Cleavage of BID by caspase 8 mediates the mitochondrial damage in the Fas pathway of apoptosis. Cell 1998;94:491–501.

51. Beg AA, Baltimore D: An essential role for NF-kappaB in preventing TNF-alpha-induced cell death. Science 1996;274:782–784.

52. Wang CY, Mayo MW, Baldwin AS, Jr.: TNF- and cancer therapy-induced apoptosis: potentiation by inhibition of NF-kappaB. Science 1996;274: 784–787.

53. Makinen K, Hakala T, Lipponen P, Alhava E, Eskelinen M: Clinical contribution of bcl-2, p53 and Ki-67 proteins in pancreatic ductal adenocarcinoma. Anticancer Res 1998;18:615–618.

54. Sinicrope FA, Evans DB, Leach SD, et al.: bcl-2 and p53 expression in resectable pancreatic adenocarcinomas: association with clinical outcome. Clin Cancer Res 1996;2:2015–2022.

55. Leek RD, Kaklamanis L, Pezzella F, Gatter KC, Harris AL: bcl-2 in normal human breast and

carcinoma, association with oestrogen receptor-positive, epidermal growth factor receptor-negative tumours and in situ cancer. Br J Cancer 1994;69: 135–139.

56. Sharma J, Srinivasan R, Majumdar S, Mir S, Radotra BD, Wig JD: Bcl-XL protein levels determine apoptotic index in pancreatic carcinoma. Pancreas 2005;30:337–342.

57. Friess H, Lu Z, Andren-Sandberg A, et al.: Moderate activation of the apoptosis inhibitor bcl-xL worsens the prognosis in pancreatic cancer. Ann Surg 1998;228:780–787.

58. Ghaneh P, Kawesha A, Evans JD, Neoptolemos JP: Molecular prognostic markers in pancreatic cancer. J Hepatobiliary Pancreat Surg 2002;9:1–11.

59. Evans JD, Cornford PA, Dodson A, Greenhalf W, Foster CS, Neoptolemos JP: Detailed tissue expression of bcl-2, bax, bak and bcl-x in the normal human pancreas and in chronic pancreatitis, ampullary and pancreatic ductal adenocarcinomas. Pancreatology 2001;1:254–262.

60. Miyamoto Y, Hosotani R, Wada M, et al.: Immunohistochemical analysis of Bcl-2, Bax, Bcl-X, and Mcl-1 expression in pancreatic cancers. Oncology 1999;56:73–82.

61. Virkajarvi N, Paakko P, Soini Y: Apoptotic index and apoptosis influencing proteins bcl-2, mcl-1, bax and caspases 3, 6 and 8 in pancreatic carcinoma. Histopathology 1998;33:432–439.

62. Friess H, Lu Z, Graber HU, et al.: bax, but not bcl-2, influences the prognosis of human pancreatic cancer. Gut 1998;43:414–421.

63. Magistrelli P, Coppola R, Tonini G, et al.: Apoptotic index or a combination of Bax/Bcl-2 expression correlate with survival after resection of pancreatic adenocarcinoma. J Cell Biochem 2006;97:98–108.

64. Lopes RB, Gangeswaran R, McNeish IA, Wang Y, Lemoine NR: Expression of the IAP protein family is dysregulated in pancreatic cancer cells and is important for resistance to chemotherapy. Int J Cancer 2007;120:2344–2352.

65. Ozawa F, Friess H, Kleeff J, et al.: Effects and expression of TRAIL and its apoptosis-promoting receptors in human pancreatic cancer. Cancer Lett 2001;163:71–81.

66. Whiteside TL: The role of death receptor ligands in shaping tumor microenvironment. Immunol Invest 2007;36:25–46.

67. Jones S, Zhang X, Parsons DW, et al.: Core signaling pathways in human pancreatic cancers revealed by global genomic analyses. Science 2008;321: 1801–1806.

68. Hanahan D, Weinberg RA: The hallmarks of cancer. Cell 2000;100:57–70.

69. Agbunag C, Bar-Sagi D: Oncogenic K-ras drives cell cycle progression and phenotypic conversion of primary pancreatic duct epithelial cells. Cancer Res 2004;64:5659–5663.

70. Campbell PM, Lee KM, Ouellette MM, et al.: Ras-driven transformation of human nestin-positive pancreatic epithelial cells. Methods Enzymol 2008; 439:451–465.

71. Campbell PM, Groehler AL, Lee KM, Ouellette MM, Khazak V, Der CJ: K-Ras promotes growth transformation and invasion of immortalized human pancreatic cells by Raf and phosphatidylinositol 3-kinase signaling. Cancer Res 2007;67:2098–2106.

72. Lim KH, Baines AT, Fiordalisi JJ, et al.: Activation of RalA is critical for Ras-induced tumorigenesis of human cells. Cancer Cell 2005;7:533–545.

73. Lim KH, O'Hayer K, Adam SJ, et al.: Divergent roles for RalA and RalB in malignant growth of human pancreatic carcinoma cells. Curr Biol 2006;16: 2385–2394.

74. Falsetti SC, Wang DA, Peng H, et al.: Geranylgeranyltransferase I inhibitors target RalB to inhibit anchorage-dependent growth and induce apoptosis and RalA to inhibit anchorage-independent growth. Mol Cell Biol 2007;27:8003–8014.

75. Eberhard DA, Johnson BE, Amler LC, et al.: Mutations in the epidermal growth factor receptor and in KRAS are predictive and prognostic indicators in patients with non-small-cell lung cancer treated with chemotherapy alone and in combination with erlotinib. J Clin Oncol 2005;23: 5900–5909.

76. Pao W, Wang TY, Riely GJ, et al.: KRAS mutations and primary resistance of lung adenocarcinomas to gefitinib or erlotinib. PLoS Med 2005;2:e17.

77. Amado RG, Wolf M, Peeters M, et al.: Wild-type KRAS is required for panitumumab efficacy in patients with metastatic colorectal cancer. J Clin Oncol 2008;26:1626–1634.

78. Pino MS, Shrader M, Baker CH, et al.: Transforming growth factor alpha expression drives constitutive epidermal growth factor receptor pathway activation and sensitivity to gefitinib (Iressa) in human pancreatic cancer cell lines. Cancer Res 2006;66: 3802–3812.

79. Senderowicz AM, Johnson JR, Sridhara R, Zimmerman P, Justice R, Pazdur R: Erlotinib/gemcitabine for first-line treatment of locally advanced or metastatic adenocarcinoma of the pancreas. Oncology (Williston Park) 2007;21: 1696–1706; discussion 706–709, 712, 715.

80. Hingorani SR, Petricoin EF, Maitra A, et al.: Preinvasive and invasive ductal pancreatic cancer and its early detection in the mouse. Cancer Cell 2003; 4:437–450.

81. Aguirre AJ, Bardeesy N, Sinha M, et al.: Activated Kras and Ink4a/Arf deficiency cooperate to produce metastatic pancreatic ductal adenocarcinoma. Genes Dev 2003;17:3112–3126.

82. Hingorani SR, Wang L, Multani AS, et al.: Trp53R172H and KrasG12D cooperate to promote chromosomal instability and widely metastatic pancreatic ductal adenocarcinoma in mice. Cancer Cell 2005;7:469–483.

83. Harrington EA, Fanidi A, Evan GI: Oncogenes and cell death. Curr Opin Genet Dev 1994;4:120–129.

84. Calbo J, Marotta M, Cascallo M, et al.: Adenovirus-mediated wt-p16 reintroduction induces cell cycle arrest or apoptosis in pancreatic cancer. Cancer Gene Ther 2001;8:740–750.

85. Ghaneh P, Greenhalf W, Humphreys M, et al.: Adenovirus-mediated transfer of p53 and p16 (INK4a) results in pancreatic cancer regression in vitro and in vivo. Gene Ther 2001;8:199–208.

86. Calbo J, Serna C, Garriga J, Grana X, Mazo A: The fate of pancreatic tumor cell lines following p16 overexpression depends on the modulation of CDK2 activity. Cell Death Differ 2004;11:1055–1065.

87. Halloran CM, Ghaneh P, Shore S, et al.: 5-Fluorouracil or gemcitabine combined with adenoviral-mediated reintroduction of p16INK4A greatly enhanced cytotoxicity in Panc-1 pancreatic adenocarcinoma cells. J Gene Med 2004;6:514–525.

88. Sirard C, de la Pompa JL, Elia A, et al.: The tumor suppressor gene Smad4/Dpc4 is required for gastrulation and later for anterior development of the mouse embryo. Genes Dev 1998;12:107–119.

89. Yasutome M, Gunn J, Korc M: Restoration of Smad4 in BxPC3 pancreatic cancer cells attenuates proliferation without altering angiogenesis. Clin Exp Metastasis 2005;22:461–473.

90. Atfi A, Buisine M, Mazars A, Gespach C: Induction of apoptosis by DPC4, a transcriptional factor regulated by transforming growth factor-beta through stress-activated protein kinase/c-Jun N-terminal kinase (SAPK/JNK) signaling pathway. J Biol Chem 1997;272:24731–24734.

91. Basseres DS, Baldwin AS: Nuclear factor-kappaB and inhibitor of kappaB kinase pathways in oncogenic initiation and progression. Oncogene 2006;25:6817–6830.

92. Wang W, Abbruzzese JL, Evans DB, Larry L, Cleary KR, Chiao PJ: The nuclear factor-kappa B RelA transcription factor is constitutively activated in human pancreatic adenocarcinoma cells. Clin Cancer Res 1999;5:119–127.

93. Kunnumakkara AB, Guha S, Krishnan S, Diagaradjane P, Gelovani J, Aggarwal BB: Curcumin potentiates antitumor activity of gemcitabine in an orthotopic model of pancreatic cancer through suppression of proliferation, angiogenesis, and inhibition of nuclear factor-kappaB-regulated gene products. Cancer Res 2007;67:3853–3861.

94. Li L, Aggarwal BB, Shishodia S, Abbruzzese J, Kurzrock R: Nuclear factor-kappaB and IkappaB kinase are constitutively active in human pancreatic cells, and their down-regulation by curcumin (diferuloylmethane) is associated with the suppression of proliferation and the induction of apoptosis. Cancer 2004;101:2351–2362.

95. Dong QG, Sclabas GM, Fujioka S, et al.: The function of multiple IkappaB: NF-kappaB complexes in the resistance of cancer cells to Taxol-induced apoptosis. Oncogene 2002;21:6510–6519.

96. Bold RJ, Virudachalam S, McConkey DJ: Chemosensitization of pancreatic cancer by inhibition of the 26S proteasome. J Surg Res 2001;100:11–17.

97. Fahy BN, Schlieman MG, Virudachalam S, Bold RJ: Schedule-dependent molecular effects of the proteasome inhibitor bortezomib and gemcitabine in pancreatic cancer. J Surg Res 2003;113:88–95.

98. Arlt A, Vorndamm J, Muerkoster S, et al.: Autocrine production of interleukin 1beta confers constitutive nuclear factor kappaB activity and chemoresistance in pancreatic carcinoma cell lines. Cancer Res 2002;62:910–916.

99. Finco TS, Westwick JK, Norris JL, Beg AA, Der CJ, Baldwin AS, Jr.: Oncogenic Ha-Ras-induced signaling activates NF-kappaB transcriptional activity, which is required for cellular transformation. J Biol Chem 1997;272:24113–24116.

100. Shah SA, Potter MW, Hedeshian MH, Kim RD, Chari RS, Callery MP: PI-3' kinase and NF-kappaB cross-signaling in human pancreatic cancer cells. J Gastrointest Surg 2001;5:603–612; discussion 12–13.

101. Khoshnan A, Tindell C, Laux I, Bae D, Bennett B, Nel AE: The NF-kappa B cascade is important in Bcl-xL expression and for the anti-apoptotic effects of the CD28 receptor in primary human CD4 + lymphocytes. J Immunol 2000;165:1743–1754.

102. Khanbolooki S, Nawrocki ST, Arumugam T, et al.: Nuclear factor-kappaB maintains TRAIL resistance in human pancreatic cancer cells. Mol Cancer Ther 2006;5:2251–2260.

103. Braeuer SJ, Buneker C, Mohr A, Zwacka RM: Constitutively activated nuclear factor-kappaB, but not induced NF-kappaB, leads to TRAIL resistance by up-regulation of X-linked inhibitor of apoptosis protein in human cancer cells. Mol Cancer Res 2006;4:715–728.

104. Nawrocki ST, Bruns CJ, Harbison MT, et al.: Effects of the proteasome inhibitor PS-341 on apoptosis and angiogenesis in orthotopic human pancreatic tumor xenografts. Mol Cancer Ther 2002;1:1243–1253.

105. Nawrocki ST, Carew JS, Pino MS, et al.: Bortezomib sensitizes pancreatic cancer cells to endoplasmic reticulum stress-mediated apoptosis. Cancer Res 2005;65:11658–11666.

106. Nawrocki ST, Sweeney-Gotsch B, Takamori R, McConkey DJ: The proteasome inhibitor bortezomib enhances the activity of docetaxel in orthotopic human pancreatic tumor xenografts. Mol Cancer Ther 2004;3:59–70.

107. Shah SA, Potter MW, McDade TP, et al.: 26S proteasome inhibition induces apoptosis and limits growth of human pancreatic cancer. J Cell Biochem 2001;82:110–122.

108. Marten A, Zeiss N, Serba S, Mehrle S, von Lilienfeld-Toal M, Schmidt J: Bortezomib is ineffective in an orthotopic mouse model of pancreatic adenocarcinoma. Mol Cancer Ther 2008;7:3624–3631.

109. Alberts SR, Foster NR, Morton RF, et al.: PS-341 and gemcitabine in patients with metastatic pancreatic adenocarcinoma: a North Central Cancer Treatment Group (NCCTG) randomized phase II study. Ann Oncol 2005;16:1654–1661.

110. Davies AM, Ruel C, Lara PN, et al.: The proteasome inhibitor bortezomib in combination with gemcitabine and carboplatin in advanced non-small cell lung cancer: a California Cancer Consortium Phase I study. J Thorac Oncol 2008;3:68–74.

111. Ryan DP, Appleman LJ, Lynch T, et al.: Phase I clinical trial of bortezomib in combination with gemcitabine in patients with advanced solid tumors. Cancer 2006;107:2482–2489.

112. McConkey DJ, Zhu K: Mechanisms of proteasome inhibitor action and resistance in cancer. Drug Resist Updat 2008;11:164–179.

113. Li L, Braiteh FS, Kurzrock R: Liposome-encapsulated curcumin: in vitro and in vivo effects on proliferation, apoptosis, signaling, and angiogenesis. Cancer 2005;104:1322–1331.

114. Lev-Ari S, Vexler A, Starr A, et al.: Curcumin augments gemcitabine cytotoxic effect on pancreatic adenocarcinoma cell lines. Cancer Invest 2007;25:411–418.

115. Dhillon N, Aggarwal BB, Newman RA, et al.: Phase II trial of curcumin in patients with advanced pancreatic cancer. Clin Cancer Res 2008;14:4491–4499.

116. Pan X, Arumugam T, Yamamoto T, et al.: Nuclear factor-kappaB p65/relA silencing induces apoptosis and increases gemcitabine effectiveness in a subset of pancreatic cancer cells. Clin Cancer Res 2008;14:8143–8151.

117. Ashkenazi A, Herbst RS: To kill a tumor cell: the potential of proapoptotic receptor agonists. J Clin Invest 2008;118:1979–1990.

118. Kang Y, Massague J: Epithelial-mesenchymal transitions: twist in development and metastasis. Cell 2004;118:277–279.

119. Peinado H, Olmeda D, Cano A: Snail, Zeb and bHLH factors in tumour progression: an alliance against the epithelial phenotype? Nat Rev Cancer 2007;7:415–428.

120. Mani SA, Yang J, Brooks M, et al.: Mesenchyme Forkhead 1 (FOXC2) plays a key role in metastasis and is associated with aggressive basal-like breast cancers. Proc Natl Acad Sci USA 2007;104: 10069–10074.

121. Onder TT, Gupta PB, Mani SA, Yang J, Lander ES, Weinberg RA: Loss of E-cadherin promotes metastasis via multiple downstream transcriptional pathways. Cancer Res 2008;68:3645–3654.

122. Yang J, Mani SA, Donaher JL, et al.: Twist, a master regulator of morphogenesis, plays an essential role in tumor metastasis. Cell 2004;117:927–939.

123. Yang J, Mani SA, Weinberg RA: Exploring a new twist on tumor metastasis. Cancer Res 2006; 66:4549–4552.

124. Burk U, Schubert J, Wellner U, et al.: A reciprocal repression between ZEB1 and members of the miR-200 family promotes EMT and invasion in cancer cells. EMBO Rep 2008;9:582–589.

125. Gregory PA, Bert AG, Paterson EL, et al.: The miR-200 family and miR-205 regulate epithelial to mesenchymal transition by targeting ZEB1 and SIP1. Nat Cell Biol 2008;10:593–601.

126. Gregory PA, Bracken CP, Bert AG, Goodall GJ: MicroRNAs as regulators of epithelial-mesenchymal transition. Cell Cycle 2008;7:3112–3118.

127. Korpal M, Lee ES, Hu G, Kang Y: The miR-200 family inhibits epithelial-mesenchymal transition and cancer cell migration by direct targeting of E-cadherin transcriptional repressors ZEB1 and ZEB2. J Biol Chem 2008;283:14910–14914.

128. Park SM, Gaur AB, Lengyel E, Peter ME: The miR-200 family determines the epithelial phenotype of cancer cells by targeting the E-cadherin repressors ZEB1 and ZEB2. Genes Dev 2008;22:894–907.

129. Dumont N, Wilson MB, Crawford YG, Reynolds PA, Sigaroudinia M, Tlsty TD: Sustained induction of epithelial to mesenchymal transition activates DNA methylation of genes silenced in basal-like breast cancers. Proc Natl Acad Sci USA 2008;105: 14867–14872.

130. Mani SA, Guo W, Liao MJ, et al.: The epithelial-mesenchymal transition generates cells with properties of stem cells. Cell 2008;133:704–715.

131. Radisky DC, LaBarge MA: Epithelial-mesenchymal transition and the stem cell phenotype. Cell Stem Cell 2008;2:511–512.

132. Haddad Y, Choi W, McConkey DJ: Delta-crystallin enhancer binding factor 1 controls the epithelial to mesenchymal transition phenotype and resistance to the epidermal growth factor receptor inhibitor erlotinib in human head and neck squamous cell carcinoma lines. Clin Cancer Res 2009;15:532–542.

133. Rho JK, Choi YJ, Lee JK, et al.: Epithelial to mesenchymal transition derived from repeated exposure

to gefitinib determines the sensitivity to EGFR inhibitors in A549, a non-small cell lung cancer cell line. Lung Cancer 2009;63:219–226.

134. Thomson S, Buck E, Petti F, et al.: Epithelial to mesenchymal transition is a determinant of sensitivity of non-small-cell lung carcinoma cell lines and xenografts to epidermal growth factor receptor inhibition. Cancer Res 2005;65:9455–9462.

135. Yauch RL, Januario T, Eberhard DA, et al.: Epithelial versus mesenchymal phenotype determines in vitro sensitivity and predicts clinical activity of erlotinib in lung cancer patients. Clin Cancer Res 2005;11:8686–8698.

136. Marks PA, Breslow R: Dimethyl sulfoxide to vorinostat: development of this histone deacetylase inhibitor as an anticancer drug. Nat Biotechnol 2007;25:84–90.

137. Hess-Stumpp H, Bracker TU, Henderson D, Politz O: MS-275, a potent orally available inhibitor of histone deacetylases–the development of an anticancer agent. Int J Biochem Cell Biol 2007; 39:1388–1405.

138. Witta SE, Gemmill RM, Hirsch FR, et al.: Restoring E-cadherin expression increases sensitivity to epidermal growth factor receptor inhibitors in lung cancer cell lines. Cancer Res 2006;66: 944–950.

139. Richon VM, Sandhoff TW, Rifkind RA, Marks PA: Histone deacetylase inhibitor selectively induces p21WAF1 expression and gene-associated histone acetylation. Proc Natl Acad Sci USA 2000;97: 10014–10019.

140. Farrow B, Sugiyama Y, Chen A, Uffort E, Nealon W, Mark Evers B: Inflammatory mechanisms contributing to pancreatic cancer development. Ann Surg 2004;239:763–769; discussion 9–71.

141. Albazaz R, Verbeke CS, Rahman SH, McMahon MJ: Cyclooxygenase-2 expression associated with severity of PanIN lesions: a possible link between chronic pancreatitis and pancreatic cancer. Pancreatology 2005;5:361–369.

142. Vonlaufen A, Phillips PA, Xu Z, et al.: Pancreatic stellate cells and pancreatic cancer cells: an unholy alliance. Cancer Res 2008;68:7707–7710.

143. Apte MV, Haber PS, Applegate TL, et al.: Periacinar stellate shaped cells in rat pancreas: identification, isolation, and culture. Gut 1998;43:128–133.

144. Kruse ML, Hildebrand PB, Timke C, Folsch UR, Schafer H, Schmidt WE: Isolation, long-term culture, and characterization of rat pancreatic fibroblastoid/stellate cells. Pancreas 2001;23:49–54.

145. Sparmann G, Hohenadl C, Tornoe J, et al.: Generation and characterization of immortalized rat pancreatic stellate cells. Am J Physiol Gastrointest Liver Physiol 2004;287:G211–G219.

146. Hwang RF, Moore T, Arumugam T, et al.: Cancer-associated stromal fibroblasts promote pancreatic tumor progression. Cancer Res 2008; 68:918–926.

147. Hebrok M, Kim SK, Melton DA: Notochord repression of endodermal Sonic hedgehog permits pancreas development. Genes Dev 1998;12: 1705–1713.

148. Kim SK, Hebrok M: Intercellular signals regulating pancreas development and function. Genes Dev 2001;15:111–127.

149. Ischenko I, Seeliger H, Schaffer M, Jauch KW, Bruns CJ: Cancer Stem Cells: How can we Target them? Curr Med Chem 2008;15:3171–3184.

150. Pasca di Magliano M, Biankin AV, Heiser PW, et al.: Common activation of canonical Wnt signaling in pancreatic adenocarcinoma. PLoS ONE 2007;2: e1155.

151. Xie K, Abbruzzese JL: Developmental biology informs cancer: the emerging role of the hedgehog signaling pathway in upper gastrointestinal cancers. Cancer Cell 2003;4:245–247.

152. Berman DM, Karhadkar SS, Maitra A, et al.: Widespread requirement for Hedgehog ligand stimulation in growth of digestive tract tumours. Nature 2003;425:846–851.

153. Morton JP, Mongeau ME, Klimstra DS, et al.: Sonic hedgehog acts at multiple stages during pancreatic tumorigenesis. Proc Natl Acad Sci USA 2007;104: 5103–5108.

154. Yauch RL, Gould SE, Scales SJ, et al.: A paracrine requirement for hedgehog signalling in cancer. Nature 2008;455:406–410.

155. Ruiz i Altaba A: Therapeutic inhibition of Hedgehog-GLI signaling in cancer: epithelial, stromal, or stem cell targets? Cancer Cell 2008; 14:281–283.

156. Mimeault M, Brand RE, Sasson AA, Batra SK: Recent advances on the molecular mechanisms involved in pancreatic cancer progression and therapies. Pancreas 2005;31:301–316.

157. Wang Z, Zhang Y, Banerjee S, Li Y, Sarkar FH: Inhibition of nuclear factor kappab activity by genistein is mediated via Notch-1 signaling pathway in pancreatic cancer cells. Int J Cancer 2006;118: 1930–1936.

158. Wang Z, Zhang Y, Banerjee S, Li Y, Sarkar FH: Notch-1 down-regulation by curcumin is associated with the inhibition of cell growth and the induction of apoptosis in pancreatic cancer cells. Cancer 2006;106:2503–2513.

15 EGFR Signaling Pathways in Pancreatic Cancer Pathogenesis

Caroline R. Sussman · Gwen Lomberk · Raul Urrutia

1 Introduction 388

2 EGF Ligands 388

3 EGF Receptors 390

4 Post-receptor EGF Signaling 390

5 Signaling Via the Canonical EGF-RAS-ERK Pathway 393

6 EGF Signaling Via Other Important, Non-canonical Intracellular Pathways 394

7 Anti-Erb-Mediated Therapy for Pancreatic Cancer 397

8 Erb-Mediated Molecular Imaging Modalities 398

9 Concluding Remarks 399

J. P. Neoptolemos, R. Urrutia, J. L. Abbruzzese, M. W. Büchler (eds.), *Pancreatic Cancer*,
DOI 10.1007/978-0-387-77498-5_15, © Springer Science+Business Media, LLC 2010

Abstract: The Epidermal Growth Factor Receptor (EGFR/ErbB) signaling axis influences the development, maintenance, and disease of tissues throughout the body. Effects have been demonstrated on normal cell proliferation, migration, differentiation, adhesion, and apoptosis in the pancreas as well as the heart, muscle, nervous system and a wide variety of organ epithelia. In addition, alterations in the EGF pathway, including overexpression of ErbBs, mutations in downstream mediators (e.g., Ras), as well as aberrant signaling, are present in the vast majority of pancreatic and other solid tissue tumors. The importance of the ErbB signaling axis to cancer is illustrated by the number of articles and reviews published on this topic to date (>20,000 and >3,000, respectively). In line with the importance of ErbB signaling to cancer, several anti-cancer therapies have been developed targeting various parts of the ErbB signaling axis. Three are currently in use, and more are undergoing intense development and investigation. Presently, the NIH lists 165 clinical studies of ErbB signaling in cancer.

1   Introduction

Studies of EGF date back to the 1950s when its roles in gastrointestinal ulcers, and subsequently in cancer, were discovered [1,2]. We now know EGF as the founding member of the EGF family of ligands. EGF ligands signal through the ErbB family of receptors to alter intracellular protein activity, gene transcription, and cell biological status with respect to proliferation, migration, differentiation and more.

ErbB signaling has roles in numerous diseases, most notably cancer, but also psoriasis, Alzheimer's disease, and schizophrenia [3,4]. ErbB1 is overexpressed in colorectal, gastric, ovarian, renal, prostate, cervical, brain (including glioblastoma multiforme, GBM), NSCLC, and squamous cell head and neck cancer. ErbB2 is a potent inducer of neuroblastoma and metastatic mammary tumors in rats, and is overexpressed or mutated in many human cancers including breast, brain (including GBM), and non-small cell lung cancer. In mouse, an increase in ErbB signaling causes cancers of the pancreas, breast, lung, colon, stomach, ovary, brain, prostate, and kidney.

In the pancreas, ErbB signaling affects development and growth of both the endocrine and exocrine pancreas [5–7], and its receptors influence the development and progression of pancreatic cancer. In fact, ErbB1 is overexpressed in 30–90% of pancreatic cancer [8] where neoplastic cells appear to enter the lymph node and establish metastasis to other organs [9]. EGFR has become a model of translational research that raises the stature of basic science. Many of us have seen how a molecule discovered in the laboratory can transcend the bench and become a therapeutic proof-of-principle. Moreover, studies on EGFR have inspired the birth of other molecular-targeted areas, such as anti-VEGF, anti-TGFβ, anti-c-KIT and others. A more detailed description of the role and impact of studying ErbB signaling in pancreatic cancer follows in subsequent paragraphs.

2   EGF Ligands

EGF ligands have different affinities for the different ErbB receptors [4,10,11]. Seven ligands have high affinity for ErbB1 (Amphiregulin (AREG), Betacellulin (BTC), EGF, Epigen, Epiregulin (EREG), Heparin-Binding EGF-like Growth Factor (HBEGF), and TGFα). Of these, BTC, Epigen, and EREG also bind ErbB4, as does Neuregulin (NRG)-1, NRG-2,

NRG-3, NRG-4, and Tomoregulin. NRG-1 and NRG-2 also bind ErbB3, as does Neuroglycan C (❯ *Fig. 15-1*).

All of the EGF ligands are single transmembrane glycoproteins with an N-terminal extracellular region and C-terminal cytoplasmic tail [10,11]. A juxtamembrane extracellular EGF domain is common to all ligands. This EGF domain contains six conserved cysteines, which form three disulfide bonds providing a common secondary structure, and allowing interaction with ErbB receptors. EGF is unique in that it has nine repeats of the EGF domain. The presence of AR, BTC, and EPR in syntenic regions of human chromosome 4 and mouse chromosome 5 suggests these ligands arose by a gene duplication event that preceded the divergence of human and mouse [10].

Ligands may signal while membrane bound or as a proteolytically cleaved, soluble, extracellular portion [12]. The cleaved form is generated in a process called ectodomain shedding by the activity of a sheddase (a protease of the matrix metalloprotease (MMP) or a disintegrin and metalloprotease (ADAM) family). The efficiency of cleavage is determined by the sequence at the site of cleavage, the length of the juxtamembrane domain [13], and availability of particular sheddases, which have preferential activity for specific ligands [14]. Following cleavage, signaling may be autocrine (on the same cell), juxtacrine (on an adjacent cell), paracrine (on a nearby cell), or endocrine (on a distant cell).

⬛ Fig. 15-1

ErbB receptors and their ligands: The four ErbB receptors with their corresponding high affinity activating ligands are shown. All four receptors have an extracellular amino terminus with two cysteine rich (CR) domains (green) containing the dimerization domain (DD) and two leucine rich ligand binding domains (L) (purple). Receptors all have a single transmembrane domain (blue), an intracellular kinase domain (pink), and carboxy terminal tail with tyrosine phosphorylation sites (open circle). Receptors are shown here as inactivated monomers (no ligand bound). In the inactivated state of ErbB1, ErbB3, and ErbB4, the two CR domains are tethered by disulfide bonds (shaded green) sequestering the DD so that it is unavailable for dimerization. In contrast, ErbB2 does not bind ligand and has a constitutively exposed DD. ErbB3 is unique in that its kinase domain is inactive. Abbreviations for ligands are defined in the text.

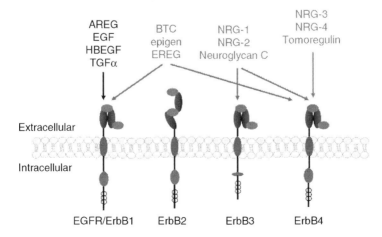

3   EGF Receptors

The receptor family consists of four single-transmembrane glycoproteins, ErbB1 (EGFR, HER1), ErbB2 (HER2, *neu* in rodents), ErbB3 (HER3), and ErbB4 (HER4). The four ErbB receptors share several common functional domains (◉ *Fig. 15-1*). The extracellular domain includes the N-terminus, leucine rich domain (LD) 1, cysteine-rich domain (CD) 1, LD2, and CD2. There is a dimerization domain (DD) in CD1, which is hidden in ErbB1, ErbB3, and ErbB4, but not ErbB2, due to disulfide bonds tethering CD1 and CD2 [4]. These bonds are absent in ErbB2, leaving the DD constitutively available. Intracellular domains include the juxtamembrane domain, tyrosine kinase domain, and C-terminal tail containing tyrosine phosphorylation sites. ErbB3 differs from the other ErbB receptors in that it has an inactive tyrosine kinase domain [4].

Classical activation of ErbB1, ErbB3, and ErbB4 results from binding of a single ligand to a single receptor monomer, inducing a conformational change exposing the dimerization domain within CD1 (◉ *Fig. 15-1*) [4]. ErbB2 has no known ligand, but does not need one for dimerization since its DD is constitutively exposed. Homo- and heterodimerization follows exposure of the dimerization domain (◉ *Fig. 15-2*). Most ErbBs have the highest affinity for ErbB2 as a dimerization partner; however, dimer composition is ultimately a function of both affinity and levels of expression of receptor monomers [15,16]. Following dimerization, the tyrosine kinase domain of ErbB1, ErbB2, and ErbB4 phosphorylates the C-terminal tail of its dimerization partner [4]. Due to its inactive kinase domain, ErbB3 cannot phosphorylate another ErbB receptor, although another ErbB receptor can phosphorylate ErbB3. Together, these events, initiated by the dimerization of different ErbB family members, can be referred to as the ErbB canonical pathway.

Non-canonical pathways can also activate ErbB receptors. Anything that can activate ADAM family metalloproteinases, such as activation of G protein coupled receptors by non-EGF ligands, such as endothelin-1, bombesin, thrombin, lysophosphatidic acid, Wnt1, Wnt5, and angiotensin-II, can induce cleavage of EGF ligands, and activation of ErbB receptors [4]. Integrins can increase the translation of ErbB2 and ErbB3, and form a complex with ErbB2 and Src resulting in ErbB2 phosphorylation and activation. In addition, ECM proteins [17], cell adhesion proteins, proteins related to the immune response, and several poxviruses [18] utilize the ErbB signaling pathway. Understandably, the identification of non-canonical pathways has elicited significant excitement since several of them help explain processes that were obscure before their discovery.

4   Post-receptor EGF Signaling

Phosphotyrosines on activated ErbB receptors create binding sites for Grb2 and Src homology 2 (SH2) proteins, activating signaling of the RAS/RAF/MAPK, PLCγ1/PKC, PI3kinase/AKT, and STAT pathways (◉ *Fig. 15-3*) [19]. An analysis of the affinity and specificity of ErbB receptors for signaling proteins showed that ErbB1 and ErbB2 are the most promiscuous, with ErbB3 following, and ErbB4 showing the most specificity [20]. Downstream signaling varies depending on the specific ligand bound and the monomer composition of the ErbB dimer [21,22].

Following signaling, receptors may be dephosphorylated, cleaved, or endocytosed [4]. Dephosphorylation stops signaling by removing sites for adaptor proteins to bind, and results from the activity of phosphatases such as density enhanced phosphatase-1 (DEP1) and protein

⬛ Fig. 15-2

ErbB dimers: There are nine possible signaling ErbB dimer combinations. Monomers of ErbB1 (purple), ErbB3 (pink), and ErbB4 (blue) change conformation with ligand binding (light blue) such that the DD becomes available and the monomer forms a dimer. Upon dimerization with all ErbB monomers except ErbB3, tyrosines in the C-terminal tail become phosphorylated (yellow) by the dimerization partner. ErbB2 (green) does not bind ligand and has a constitutively available DD. The kinase domain of ErbB3 is inactive, thus ErbB3 cannot phosphorylate its dimerization partner; however, ErbB3 can be phosphorylated. The phosphorylated tyrosines bind and activate intracellular proteins with SH2 and PTB domains. Shown on top are the possible activated ErbB homodimers (ErbB1, ErbB2, and ErbB4), and on bottom the activated heterodimers.

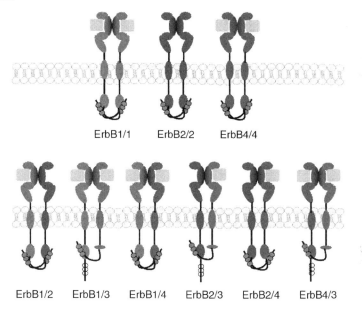

tyrosine phosphatase (PTP) 1B. Endocytosis may stop or promote signaling by promoting ligand dissociation, lysosomal degradation, and possibly nuclear targeting. Once in lysosomes, receptors remaining bound to ligand are more often degraded, while those dissociated from ligand are more often recycled to the membrane. This may provide a regulatory step to stop signaling preferentially of high-affinity ligand-receptor combinations. One notable exception is the ErbB1/ErbB2 dimer, which preferentially escapes degradation and is recycled, thus tends to signal longer. ErbB1 signaling induces several proteins with a negative feedback effect, promoting its own degradation, such as Sprouty-2, LRIG-1, MIG-6/RALT and suppressor of cytokine signaling-5 (SOC-5).

All ErbB receptors have been found in the nucleus where they may function as transcription factors or co-factors [4]. ErbB receptors contain three clusters of basic amino acids in the juxtamembrane domain with homology to known nuclear localization sequences. Nuclear localization of ErbB1 causes the upregulation of several cancer-related genes, such as cyclinD1, B-myb, cyclooxygenase-2, and members of the iNOS/NO pathway [23]. ErbB4 undergoes a ligand-dependent proteolytic cleavage of the intracellular domain [24]. However, investigation on the

☑ Fig. 15-3

ERB signaling pathways: EGF receptor activation initiates a diverse array of cellular pathways via dimerization (represented by the light blue cylinders in the cell membrane). Each receptor dimer recruits different SH2-containing effector proteins triggering distinct signaling pathways, culminating in cellular responses such as cell proliferation or apoptosis. The activated receptor complexes with the adaptor protein, Grb2, which is coupled to the guanine nucleotide releasing factor, SOS1. This Grb2-SOS1 complex can either directly bind to receptor phosphotyrosine sites or indirectly through SHC. As a result of these interactions, SOS is localized in close proximity to RAS, allowing for Ras activation. Subsequently, the ERK and JNK signaling pathways are activated, which ultimately lead to the activation of transcription factors, such as c-fos, AP-1, and Elk-1, that promote gene expression and contribute to cell proliferation. In addition, in response to EGFR activation, JAK kinases activate STAT-1 and STAT-3 transcription factors, contributing to further proliferative signaling. Protein kinase C (PKC) is also activated via phosphatidylinositol signaling (PIP2 to PIP3) and calcium release, which serves as another node of EGF signaling. See text for further details.

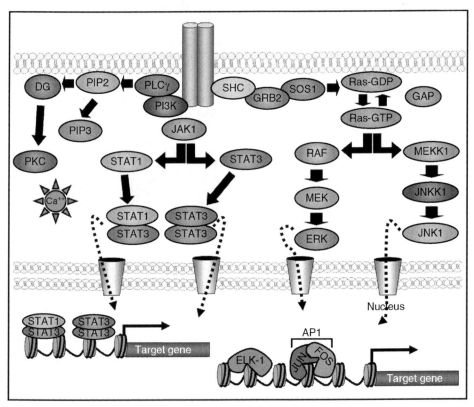

nuclear role of ErbBs is still in its infancy in many organs and certainly underrepresented in the field of pancreatic cancer research. Therefore, this area of research offers a unique opportunity for potential fruitful discoveries that can advance our knowledge on this painful disease.

5   Signaling Via the Canonical EGF-RAS-ERK Pathway

This pathway is of paramount importance for the pathobiology of pancreatic cancer since its alteration, at many levels, associates frequently with this disease [25–27]. Upon dimerization, the ErbB receptor becomes autophosphorylated at multiple tyrosines within its cytoplasmic domain (reviewed in [19,28]). The generation of a phosphorylated tyrosine acts as a docking site on this receptor for proteins containing domains similar to a portion of the Src oncogene, and thus termed Src homology 2 domains (SH2 domains). The SH2 domain-containing protein, Grb2, binds to the receptor and subsequently recruits the guanine nucleotide exchange factor, SOS (❍ Fig. 15-3). Another Src-homology domain in Grb2, called an SH3 domain, is a proline-binding motif that interacts with many proteins. SOS acts as the guanine nucleotide exchange factor (GEF) for RAS which unloads GDP and binds GTP to become activated (❍ Fig. 15-4). Inactivation of RAS requires the exchange of GTP for GDP again. This GTP hydrolysis can be accelerated by GTPase-activating proteins (GAPs). Noteworthy, the human genome encodes three *RAS* genes that give rise to four ubiquitously expressed gene products, though only one of them, *K-RAS*, is mutated in more than 90% of pancreatic

◘ Fig. 15-4

Downstream RAS signaling: After receptor activation (represented by the light blue cylinders in the cell membrane), RAS activation is regulated by the cycle of hydrolysis of bound GTP. The activated receptor signals to a guanine nucleotide exchange factor, such as SOS1 (see ❍ Fig. 15-3), which then ejects GDP from RAS to allow RAS to bind free GTP to become active. Opposing this activation are the GTPase-activating proteins (GAPs), which stimulate the endogenous GTPase of RAS, thereby creating inactive RAS-GDP. Although PI3K can be activated via its recruitment to ErbB receptors, PI3K can also be activated by RAS directly. Activation of PI3K results in not only activation of AKT and its downstream effectors (see ❍ Fig. 15-6) to mediate cell survival, but an increase in PtdIns(3,4,5)P3 at the plasma membrane as well. This leads to the activation of the Rho family of small GTPases, Rho, Rac1, and Cdc42 via recruitment of GEFs to the plasma membrane.

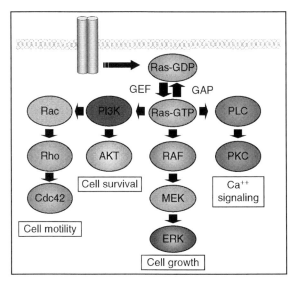

tumors [25,29]. This family of proteins is composed of H-RAS, N-RAS, K-RAS A and K-RAS B (K-RAS A and K-RAS B are splice variants of single gene). The *H-RAS* gene was named such due to its homology to the oncogene of the Harvey murine sarcoma virus, while the *K-RAS* acquired its name from homology to the oncogene of the Kirsten murine sarcoma virus. The *N-RAS* gene does not have a retroviral homolog, but it is identified this way because it was originally isolated from neuroblastoma cells.

The process of Ras activation involves the migration of GTP-bound RAS to the membrane where it recruits RAFs, a group of three serine/threonine kinases (A-RAF, B-RAF, C-RAF) whose regulation is complex and not completely understood. Membrane-localized RAF is activated by multiple phosphorylations and de-phosphorylations. Subsequently, RAF phosphorylates two serine residues in the activation loop of MEK1/2 (❯ *Fig. 15-4*). MEK is a dual specificity kinase that phosphorylates ERK on both the threonine and tyrosine within a conserved TEY motif in the activation loop. Two isoforms of this enzyme exist, ERK1 and ERK2, which share many functions, though independent knock-outs of these proteins in mice suggest that sometimes they may have non-redundant functions in vivo. Activated ERK can phosphorylate more than 100 substrates at various locations in the cell, creating a multidimensional network. Specifically within the nucleus alone, the dimerized form of ERK actively translocates into the nucleus where it phosphorylates many substrates. These substrates include transcription factors that are regulated by MAP kinase phosphorylation, including Elk-1, c-Myc, c-Jun, c-Fos, and C/EBP β among others. For instance, the phosphorylation of the ETS family of transcription factors, such as ELK-1, which modulate *c-fos* and *c-jun* expression, leads to activation of the AP-1 transcription factor, which is made up of a Fos-Jun heterodimer (❯ *Fig. 15-3*). These regulators are able, among others, to regulate the expression of proteins, such as D-type cyclins, which instruct the cell to enter into the G1 phase of the cell cycle. Thus, the MAP kinase pathway represents signals originating from receptors at the cell surface to the nucleus that result in the regulation of gene expression.

Due to the diverse nature of the downstream substrates this pathway acts upon, normally, the process of activation must be tightly regulated. Thus, evidence for negative feedback loops is found at several levels. For example, ERK-mediated phosphorylation of MEK inactivates the pathway. ERK also activates the kinase RSK2, which can inhibit the ERK pathway by phosphorylating SOS. In contrast, ERK phosphorylation of RAF appears to enhance activation of the ERK pathway. Finally, there are several phosphatases, including the dual specificity phosphatases (DUSPs), that can inactivate ERK either in the cytoplasm or the nucleus. Therefore, due to their incredible regulatory potential, this pathway relies on maintaining tight checks and balances, which, unsurprisingly, when altered, can easily contribute to the development and maintenance of the cancer phenotype.

6   EGF Signaling Via Other Important, Non-canonical Intracellular Pathways

In addition to the MAPK pathway, ErbB can regulate many cancer associated cell functions by activating other intracellular kinases and their signaling cascades. Although the detailed description of these cascades are beyond the scope of this article, we will briefly provide a description of pathways that are among the most important in cancer-associated processes, such PI3Ks, PDK, AKT, GSK3β, and mTOR. PI3Ks (Phosphoinositide 3-kinases) were originally discovered as enzymatic activity which transduce signals downstream of several oncoproteins and growth factor receptors thereby signaling to induce cell proliferation, survival, and migration. These proteins comprise a family of lipid kinases which are classified into three subfamilies according to structure and substrate specificity (reviewed in [30–32]). The class IA PI3Ks are of the most relevance to this article due to their clear involvement in cancer [31,32]. This class is divided into two subgroups. The PI3K that acts downstream of ErbB receptors is composed of both, a regulatory (85 kDa) and a catalytic subunit (110 kDa). There are three catalytic isoforms (p110α, p110β, and p110δ) and five regulatory isoforms (p85α, p85β and p55γ encoded by separate genes and p55α and p50α that are produced via alternate splicing of the p85α gene).

Recruitment and activation of PI3K to Tyr-phosphorylated ErbB receptors occurs via an SH2 domain within the regulatory subunit [28,33,34] (◉ Fig. 15-5). Noteworthy, however, PI3K can also be activated by Ras directly (◉ Fig. 15-4) [35,36]. ErbB-mediated activation of PI3K within the plasma membrane microenvironment phosphorylates phosphoinositides (PtdIns) at the 3'-OH position of the inositol ring. The most studied product of PI3K activity is PtdIns(3,4,5)P3 from the phosphorylation of PtdIns(4,5)P2. The PtdIns(3,4,5)P3 molecules

◘ Fig. 15-5

PTEN regulation of phosphoinositide 3-kinase (pi3k) signaling: Upon activation via receptor signaling (represented by the light blue cylinders in the cell membrane), the main substrate of PI3K is phosphoinositide (4,5) bisphosphate (PIP2). Phosphorylation of PIP2 by PI3K generates PtdIns(3,4,5)P3 (PIP3). PIP3 and its 5'-dephosphorylation product, PIP2, are important second messengers that promote cell survival, cell growth, protein synthesis, mitosis, and motility. Cell survival, mitosis, and protein synthesis are all promoted via PI3K-dependent activation of the PDK-1/AKTpathway. Importantly, PTEN is a tumor suppressor gene that is able to dephosphorylate PIP3 in order to regulate this process. Since the activation of AKT is regulated via its phosphorylation by PDK-1, along with integrin-linked kinase (ILK), inactivation of PTEN permits constitutive and unregulated activation of the AKT pathway. In addition to regulating the AKT signaling pathway, PTEN also inhibits EGF-induced SHC phosphorylation to suppress the MAP kinase signaling cascade. Thus, inactivation of PTEN also facilitates the constitutive and unregulated signaling of MAP kinase, lending to an increase in cell growth.

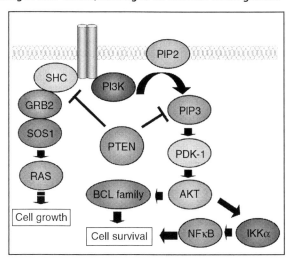

bind to pleckstrin homology (PH) domains with one of the relevant PH domains in this context is that of AKT, also known as protein kinase B (PKB). Through this mechanism, AKT localizes to the membrane, where it is activated by phosphorylation on Thr-308 by PDK1 (3-phosphoinositide-dependent protein kinase 1).

Interestingly, PDK1 contains a PH domain with higher affinity for PtdIns(3,4,5)P3 than AKT [37]. This PDK1 PH domain can, in addition, complex to PtdIns(3,4)P2 which is produced by hydrolysis of PtdIns(3,4,5)P3 in the membrane. This mechanism allows the existence of basal levels of activated PDK1, however phosphorylation of AKT at S473 is required for its full activation. This important step is mediated by mTOR (mammalian target of rapamycin) signaling complex 2, or mTORC2. After full activation, AKT phosphorylates several proteins that mediate the crosstalk to other pathways (❯ Fig. 15-6), such as glycogen synthase kinase 3 (GS3K) and mTOR, regulates the activity of p70 ribosomal S6 kinase-1, and activates eukaryotic translation initiation factor 4E-binding protein-1. These steps are critical to mediate protein synthesis. Thus, together, these cascades of phosphorylations promote growth and survival in many different cell populations. For instance, the activation of PI3K and AKT, as well as the subsequent downstream signaling, promote survival via a RAS/PIK3/AKT1/IKBKA(IκB kinase-α)/NFKB1 pathway that induces anti-apoptotic gene transcription [31,35].

AKT is negatively regulated by the tumor suppressor PTEN (phosphatase and tensin homolog deleted on chromosome 10). PTEN is a lipid phosphatase that catalyzes the reverse reaction of PI3K, by dephosphorylating the D3 position of its lipid products and thereby

◘ Fig. 15-6

AKT and its downstream effectors: As shown in ❯ Fig. 15-3, EGFR activation results in direct or indirect activation of PI3K. AKT is located downstream of PI3K and, therefore, functions as a key effector of ERB signaling. Activated AKT promotes cell survival through via inhibition of apoptosis by phosphorylating the Bad component of the Bad/Bcl-XL complex. This phosphorylation causes Bad to dissociate from the Bad/Bcl-XL complex through binding to 14-3-3. In addition, AKT triggers activation of IKK-α that ultimately leads to NFκB activation and cell survival. AKT also regulates cell growth through its effects on the mTOR pathway, as well as cell cycle and cell proliferation through its actions on GSK3β, resulting in inhibition of cyclin D1, and MDM2, thus indirectly inhibiting p53.

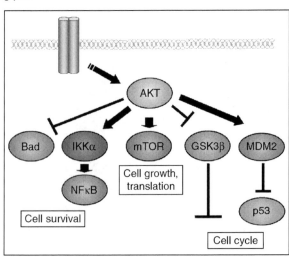

inhibiting the activation of AKT [35]. Aberrant AKT/PTEN signaling, often found in different human cancers, plays an important role in cancer development, progression and therapeutic resistance [31,35].

ErbB can also signal via members of the Rho family of small GTPases, namely Rho, Rac1, and Cdc42 (◉ Fig. 15-4). Like Ras, these proteins are activated when bound to GTP and inactive in the GDP-bound state, steps that are mediated by specific GEFs and GAPs respectively. As mentioned above, receptor activation stimulates PI3K, resulting in an increase in PtdIns(3,4,5)P3 at the plasma membrane. This increased in PtdIns(3,4,5)P3 recruits, via the PH domain members of the Vav family of proteins (Vav1, 2, and 3), which by acting as a GEFs, lead to the activation of Rho, Rac1, and more discriminately, Cdc42 [38, 39]. Vav is not the exclusive GEF for this protein since, for example, several others GEFs, including Sos1, Sos2, and Tiam1, have been shown to transduce the growth signal from the EGF receptor to Rac1 [40, 41]. Small GTPases of the Rho family are involved in a variety of functions in different cells, though they are notorious for their role in cytoskeletal reorganization and cell migration. For instance, Cdc42 controls the assembly of filopodia [42], Rac1 stimulates the formation of lamellipodia and membrane ruffles, and RhoA regulates the assembly of stress fibers [43].

The proteins Diaphanous 1 (Dia1) and ROCK signal the activation of some Rho GTPases to their action on the actin cytoskeleton [44]. Dia1 stimulates actin polymerization and actin bundle formation. ROCK activates myosin to cross-link actin bundles and as a result, the formation of actomyosin bridges to induce contractility. Besides their role in motility, Rho GTPases are also emerging as important regulators of the Wnt-APC-beta-catenin signaling, which is of paramount importance for the regulation of cytoskeletal dynamics, cell adhesion, gene expression, and cell growth (reviewed in [45]). Interestingly, at least some part of this pathway appears to be necessary for pancreatic cancer since, it has been demonstrated that aberrant expression of Vav1 acts as a dominant oncogenic factor in these tumors and its levels correlate with patient survival [46]. Therefore, future studies this area may uncover additional pathobiological mechanisms as well as therapeutic targets for pancreatic cancer.

7 Anti-Erb-Mediated Therapy for Pancreatic Cancer

There are two categories of ErbB targeted therapies for cancer, monoclonal antibodies and tyrosine kinase inhibitors [47]. Monoclonal antibodies bind to the extracellular domain of the receptor, preventing ligand-induced activation. Tyrosine kinase inhibitors bind to the intracellular kinase domain, inhibiting phosphorylation and subsequent signaling. In general, the monoclonal antibodies developed to date are more specific than the tyrosine kinase inhibitors, yet they also may be immunogenic themselves.

Trastuzumab (Herceptin) was the first anti Erb (ErbB2)- targeted therapy used clinically [3]. Additional Erb-targeted inhibitors include erlotinib (Tarceva), a kinase inhibitor, and two anti-ErbB1 monoclonal antibodies, cetuximab (Erbitux), and panitumumab (Vectibix) [3,47–51]. These are approved in NSCLC, colorectal cancer, squamous-cell carcinoma of the head and neck. Additionally, Erlotinib is approved for use in advanced pancreatic cancer [47]. Another tyrosine kinase inhibitor, gefitinib (Iressa), is no longer used in the United States or the European Union due to low efficacy, but is still used in eastern Asia. Overall, more Erb-targeted therapeutics is under development and investigation due to these initial proof-of-concepts. In fact, this is a difficult, but potentially fruitful area where hard-core basic science research can generate a conceptual framework for novel drugs via interactions with other academicians in the fields of molecular modeling, crystallography, and synthetic chemistry, as well as pancreatic cancer diagnosis and management teams. Thus, this pipeline of investigations to take drugs from the bench to the bedside, as demonstrated for EGF inhibitors, is the paradigm that we may need to follow in order to defeat this dismal disease.

Studies investigating anti-Erb therapies in pancreatic cancer are beginning to show modest improvements. Cetuximab in combination with gemcitabine in advanced pancreatic cancer yields mixed results [52,53]. Erlotinib in combination with gemcitabine modestly, but significantly, improves response and survival rates, hence its approval in the US and EU as a first line treatment for pancreatic cancer [54].

Several putative predictors of the efficacy of ErbB-targeted therapy have emerged [47]. The presence of skin toxicity (rash) is positively correlated with efficacy, and may be indicative of blood or tissue anti-ErbB concentration. Interestingly, immunohistochemical labeling showing increased ErbB expression is not a good predictor of response, and good responses have been observed in tumors that stain negative for Erbs [55,56]. The presence of mutations in Erbs seems to be a good indicator of efficacy, as well as an increase in *ErbB* copy number. Tumors with an activated K-RAS do not appear to respond well to anti-Erb therapy [47,57]. This may explain the modest effects of anti-Erb therapy in pancreatic cancer, as activated K-RAS in pancreatic cancer is almost universal. However, this type of therapy, for which development and testing is still at the early stages, can potentially be further improved by combining the anti-ERB compounds with inhibitors of RAS, RAF, MEK, PI3K, PDK, AKT, mTOR and some downstream targets, against which several drugs have been developed and many are currently in clinical trials.

8   Erb-Mediated Molecular Imaging Modalities

Erb targeting with the goal of generating molecular imaging modalities for tumors is another new area of investigation, however a detailed description is beyond the scope of this chapter [58]. Briefly, radiopharmaceutical, in particular, labeled humanized monoclonal antibodies, that can specifically target cell surface proteins, including receptors, have been used with the goal of either neoplastic cell ablation (molecular-targeted chemotherapy) or for imaging (molecular imaging) in many tissues. Molecular medicine offers many modalities, including Single Photon Computed Tomography (SPCT) or Positron Emission Tomography (PET), which, in combination with MRI and CT, have the potential to give a good definition, anatomical-functional map of a tumor. Several types of antibodies, either whole or as a fragment, are being currently tested against ErbB1 [47]. Some molecules of particular interest due to their potential higher biodistribution and more rapid clearance are the so called anti-ErbB1 "affibodies". Affibodies are made from three bundle molecules based on 58 amino acids from IgG, and they bind can bind to their targets at low nanomolar concentration. For example, some of these molecules have been shown to bind to specific tumors in vivo. This is important if the therapy is dependent upon the expression of a distinct cell surface protein. Molecular imaging techniques to image other ErbB members, which can also contribute to the cancer phenotype, need to be derived. Furthermore, this proof-of-principle predicts that it could be possible to use a similar approach to other cell surface markers which start to be expressed at the stage of carcinoma in situ (PanIN3). Therefore, molecular imaging offers another wide-open field of study in pancreatic cancer research, and we are optimistic that future development in this area has the potential to profoundly impact the diagnosis and therapy of this disease.

Therefore, it is important to reflect on all of the theoretical frameworks underlying how these signaling cascades work and can be targeted. However, their expected results are "epithelium-centric" and do not integrate the potential modulation of ErbB signaling that can occur by other molecules present in the tumor microenvironment. Pancreatic cancer is characterized by a robust desmoplastic reaction, which influences pancreatic cell growth. However, whether other pathways, which are active in the tumor microenvironment, modulate the outcome of ERB signaling is an area of current investigation. For instance, the existence of cross-talk between ErbB1 and integrin signaling has recently been demonstrated to be involved in carcinoma cell invasion and metastasis, which may explain, in part, how inhibitors of EGFR affect malignant disease [59]. However, studies on the role of the desmoplastic reaction in the tumor biology of pancreatic cancer is another nascent and very promising area of pancreatic cancer research, where we predict that most of the discoveries possessing the highest translational potential may occur in the very near future.

9   Concluding Remarks

Given the central role of ErbB signaling in the regulation of proliferation, migration, and differentiation, it seems likely that therapeutically tapping into this high-level control mechanism can prove useful for pancreatic cancer treatment. It is interesting to note that ErbB-targeted therapies developed thus far target an ErbB monomer and, as a result all dimers containing that monomer, thus potentially affecting ErbB signaling in complex ways. A more refined strategy with more specific targeting may prove to be significantly more effective. This may be at the level of targeting specific receptor dimers or specific downstream signaling events activated by tumorigenic dimers, but not by dimers promoting healthy tissue differentiation. While anti-EGF inhibitors have elicited modest success in the treatment of pancreatic cancer, additional combinations of these agents with small drugs targeting Ras, Raf, MEK, PI3K, PDK, AKT, mTOR, small GTPases, or Wnt signaling may have synergistic effects and thus offer better therapeutic options. Several important areas of investigation on factors that affect ErbB-mediated signaling, such as non-canonical pathways, the likely modulatory role of factors from the tumor microenvironment, how other cellular pathways are altered under the almost universal presence of oncogenic K-ras mutations, and the effects of nuclear ErbBs, remain among the less understood areas of basic research in pancreatic cancer with highly promising translational potential.

Key Research Points

- Four ErbB isoforms are differentially expressed in human tissues. They form different types of dimers which then complex with distinct ligands, some found overexpressed in pancreatic cancer (ErbB2-EGF).
- A good understanding of the biochemistry and cell biological processes associated to these receptors is important, not only for the biology, but also the pathobiology of pancreatic cancer. Unfortunately, besides ErbB1/EGFR, little detailed information is available to reconstruct pathways that can be specific to the other isoforms.
- The knowledge of some of these ERB-mediated pathways such as EGFR are among the best-understood signaling cascades in many organs. However the role of ERB proteins in pancreatic development and cell homeostasis remains an underrepresented area of biomedical research.

Future Scientific Directions

- EGFR/ErbB1 is the best-studied ERB receptor isoform and its contribution to pancreatic cancer, though still far from complete, is better understood. However, pancreatic cancer cells express other combinations of ERB isoforms, which biology and signaling is less known but may be of significant biomedical relevance in this disease.

- More knowledge must be gained on how to modulate the response of anti-EGFR therapy in a manner that can be more beneficial to pancreatic cancer patients. Fortunately, there are numerous signaling nodes that have been identified during the last two decades, which can serve as targets for combined therapeutic modalities designed to achieve this goal. Many of these targeted therapies being developed are entering into preclinical trials and the more advanced of these efforts are already in clinical trials. Thus, combination therapies that target different nodes in this pathway are close to hard-core testing.

- The interaction of pancreatic cancer cells with the tumor microenvironment, which is full of growth factors that bind to ERB receptors and extracellular matrix proteins that crosstalk with these pathways, may provide the basis for future application of this important basic science knowledge to the design of therapy. Therefore, more basic science is needed in this area to inform the development of novel molecularly targeted drugs by focusing on several members of the EGF pathway.

Clinical Implications

- Anti-EGFR therapy has shown a limited benefit in treating pancreatic cancer patients. Interestingly, mutations in K-ras are a predictor of non-responsiveness to EGFR therapy. Therefore, investigations on molecular mechanisms that can help to design new drugs that can increase the sensitivity to established anti-EGFR by targeting other molecules within this pathway are of paramount medical importance.

- The role of EGFR and, in particular other members of the ERB family of tyrosine kinase receptors, in normal pancreatic molecular cell biology warrant further investigations. Their translational potential to human disease is unknown. However, this has been already an area of fruitful research, which because of its translational potential, deserves to be further expanded.

- The area of molecular targeted-imaging has extensively benefited on investments on EGFR as a probe. Some of these techniques remain to be refined, but represent promising areas of translational research as well as evidence-based medical care.

Acknowledgments

Work in the authors' laboratories is supported by AHA SDG 06-30137N (to CRS), NIH DK-52913 (to RU) and Mayo Clinic Pancreatic SPORE P50 CA102701 (to RU).

References

1. Reynolds VH, Boehm FH, Cohen S Enhancement of chemical carcinogenesis by an epidermal growth factor. Surg Forum 1965;16:108–109.

2. Debray C, Reversat R [Antiulcer extracts taken from the gastrointestinal mucosa and the urine.]. Sem Hop 1950;26(50):2419–2429.

3. Rivera F, Vega-Villegas ME, Lopez-Brea MF Cetuximab, its clinical use and future perspectives. Anticancer Drugs 2008;19(2):99–113.

4. Wieduwilt MJ, Moasser MM The epidermal growth factor receptor family: biology driving targeted therapeutics. Cell Mol Life Sci 2008;65(10):1566–1584.

5. Kritzik MR, et al.: Expression of ErbB receptors during pancreatic islet development and regrowth. J Endocrinol 2000;165(1):67–77.

6. Huotari MA, et al.: ErbB signaling regulates lineage determination of developing pancreatic islet cells in embryonic organ culture. Endocrinology;2002:143 (11):4437–4446.

7. Means A, et al.: Overexpression of heparin-binding EGF-like growth factor in mouse pancreas results in fibrosis and epithelial metaplasia. Gastroenterology 2003;124(4):1020–1036.

8. Burtness B Her signaling in pancreatic cancer. Expert Opin Biol Ther 2007;7(6):823–829.

9. Pryczynicz A, et al.: Expression of EGF and EGFR strongly correlates with metastasis of pancreatic ductal carcinoma. Anticancer Res 2008;28(2B): 1399–1404.

10. Harris RC, Chung E, Coffey RJ EGF receptor ligands. Exp Cell Res 2003;284(1):2–13.

11. Schneider MR, Wolf E The epidermal growth factor receptor ligands at a glance. J Cell Physiol 2009;218 (3):460–466.

12. Sanderson MP, Dempsey PJ, Dunbar AJ Control of ErbB signaling through metalloprotease mediated ectodomain shedding of EGF-like factors. Growth Factors 2006;24(2):121–36.

13. Hinkle CL, et al.: Selective roles for tumor necrosis factor alpha-converting enzyme/ADAM17 in the shedding of the epidermal growth factor receptor ligand family: the juxtamembrane stalk determines cleavage efficiency. J Biol Chem 2004;279(23): 24179–24188.

14. Sahin U, et al.: Distinct roles for ADAM10 and ADAM17 in ectodomain shedding of six EGFR ligands. J Cell Biol 2004;164(5):769–779.

15. Graus-Porta D, et al.: ErbB-2, the preferred heterodimerization partner of all ErbB receptors, is a mediator of lateral signaling. Embo J 1997;16(7): 1647–1655.

16. Tzahar E, et al.: A hierarchical network of interreceptor interactions determines signal transduction by Neu differentiation factor/neuregulin and epidermal growth factor. Mol Cell Biol 1996;16(10): 5276–5287.

17. Swindle CS, et al.: Epidermal growth factor (EGF)-like repeats of human tenascin-C as ligands for EGF receptor. J Cell Biol 2001;154(2):459–468.

18. Tzahar E, et al.: Pathogenic poxviruses reveal viral strategies to exploit the ErbB signaling network. Embo J 1998;17(20):5948–5963.

19. Scaltriti M, Baselga J The epidermal growth factor receptor pathway: a model for targeted therapy. Clin Cancer Res, 2006;12(18):5268–5272.

20. Jones RB, et al.: A quantitative protein interaction network for the ErbB receptors using protein microarrays. Nature 2006;439(7073):168–174.

21. Carpenter G ErbB-4: mechanism of action and biology. Exp Cell Res 2003;284(1):66–77.

22. Citri A, Skaria KB, Yarden Y The deaf and the dumb: the biology of ErbB-2 and ErbB-3. Exp Cell Res 2003;284(1):54–65.

23. Massie C, Mills IG The developing role of receptors and adaptors. Nat Rev Cancer 2006;6(5):403–409.

24. Schlessinger J, Lemmon MA Nuclear signaling by receptor tyrosine kinases: the first robin of spring. Cell 2006;127(1):45–48.

25. Bardeesy N, DePinho RA Pancreatic cancer biology and genetics. Nat Rev Cancer 2002;2(12): 897–909.

26. Hruban RH, Wilentz RE, Kern SE Genetic progression in the pancreatic ducts. Am J Pathol 2000; 156(6):1821–1825.

27. Hruban RH, et al.: Pathology of genetically engineered mouse models of pancreatic exocrine cancer: consensus report and recommendations. Cancer Res 2006;66(1):95–106.

28. Yarden Y, Sliwkowski MX Untangling the ErbB signalling network. Nat Rev Mol Cell Biol 2001; 2(2):127–37.

29. Hruban RH, et al.: Pancreatic intraepithelial neoplasia: a new nomenclature and classification system for pancreatic duct lesions. Am J Surg Pathol 2001;25(5):579–586.

30. Skwarek LC, Boulianne GL Great expectations for PIP: phosphoinositides as regulators of signaling during development and disease. Dev Cell 2009; 16(1):12–20.

31. Garcia-Echeverria C, Sellers WR Drug discovery approaches targeting the PI3K/Akt pathway in cancer. Oncogene 2008;27(41):5511–5526.

32. Wymann MP, Schneiter R Lipid signalling in disease. Nat Rev Mol Cell Biol 2008;9(2):162–176.

33. Carpenter CL, et al.: Phosphoinositide 3-kinase is activated by phosphopeptides that bind to the SH2

domains of the 85-kDa subunit. J Biol Chem 1993;268(13):9478–9483.

34. Mattoon DR, et al.: The docking protein Gab1 is the primary mediator of EGF-stimulated activation of the PI-3K/Akt cell survival pathway. BMC Biol 2004;2:24.

35. Cantley LC The phosphoinositide 3-kinase pathway. Science 2002;296(5573):1655–1657.

36. Sjolander A, et al.: Association of p21ras with phosphatidylinositol 3-kinase. Proc Natl Acad Sci USA 1991;88(18):7908–7912.

37. Currie RA, et al.: Role of phosphatidylinositol 3,4,5-trisphosphate in regulating the activity and localization of 3-phosphoinositide-dependent protein kinase-1. Biochem J 1999;337(Pt 3):575–583.

38. Abe K, et al.: Vav2 Is an Activator of Cdc42, Rac1, and RhoA. J Biol Chem. 2000;275(14):10141–10149.

39. Movilla N, et al.: How Vav proteins discriminate the GTPases Rac1 and RhoA from Cdc42. Oncogene 2001;20(56):8057–8065.

40. Scita G, et al.: EPS8 and E3B1 transduce signals from Ras to Rac. Nature 1999;401(6750):290–293.

41. Ray R, Vaidya R, Johnson L: MEK/ERK regulates adherens junctions and migration through Rac1. Cell Motility Cytoskeleton 2007;64(3):143–156.

42. Nobes CD, Hall A Rho, Rac, and Cdc42 GTPases regulate the assembly of multimolecular focal complexes associated with actin stress fibers, lamellipodia, and filopodia. Cell 1995;81(1):53–62.

43. Hall A Rho GTPases and the Actin Cytoskeleton. Science 1998;279(5350):509–514.

44. Watanabe N, et al.: Cooperation between mDia1 and ROCK in Rho-induced actin reorganization. Nat Cell Biol 1999;1(3):136–143.

45. Schlessinger K., Hall A, Tolwinski N Wnt signaling pathways meet Rho GTPases. Genes Dev 2009; 23(3):265–277.

46. Fernandez-Zapico ME, et al.: Ectopic expression of VAV1 reveals an unexpected role in pancreatic cancer tumorigenesis. Cancer Cell 2005;7(1): 39–49.

47. Ciardiello F, Tortora G EGFR antagonists in cancer treatment. N Engl J Med 2008;358(11): 1160–1174.

48. Harari PM, Wheeler DL, Grandis JR Molecular target approaches in head and neck cancer: epidermal

growth factor receptor and beyond. Semin Radiat Oncol 2009;19(1):63–68.

49. Zhang X, Chang A Molecular predictors of EGFR-TKI sensitivity in advanced non-small cell lung cancer. Int J Med Sci 2008;5(4):209–217.

50. Yang CH EGFR tyrosine kinase inhibitors for the treatment of NSCLC in East Asia: present and future. Lung Cancer 2008;60(Suppl 2):S23–30.

51. Wong KK Searching for a magic bullet in NSCLC: the role of epidermal growth factor receptor mutations and tyrosine kinase inhibitors. Lung Cancer 2008;60(Suppl 2):S10–18.

52. Xiong HQ, et al.: Cetuximab, a monoclonal antibody targeting the epidermal growth factor receptor, in combination with gemcitabine for advanced pancreatic cancer: a multicenter phase II Trial. J Clin Oncol 2004;22(13):2610–2616.

53. Philip PA Improving treatment of pancreatic cancer. Lancet Oncol 2008;9(1):7–8.

54. Moore MJ, et al.: Erlotinib plus gemcitabine compared with gemcitabine alone in patients with advanced pancreatic cancer: a phase III trial of the National Cancer Institute of Canada Clinical Trials Group. J Clin Oncol 2007;25(15):1960–1966.

55. Galizia G, et al.: Cetuximab, a chimeric human mouse anti-epidermal growth factor receptor monoclonal antibody, in the treatment of human colorectal cancer. Oncogene 2007;26(25):3654–3660.

56. Chung KY, et al.: Cetuximab shows activity in colorectal cancer patients with tumors that do not express the epidermal growth factor receptor by immunohistochemistry. J Clin Oncol 2005; 23(9):1803–1810.

57. Massarelli E, et al.: KRAS mutation is an important predictor of resistance to therapy with epidermal growth factor receptor tyrosine kinase inhibitors in non-small-cell lung cancer. Clin Cancer Res 2007; 13(10):2890–2896.

58. Mishani E, et al.: Imaging of EGFR and EGFR tyrosine kinase overexpression in tumors by nuclear medicine modalities. Curr Pharm Des 2008; 14(28):2983–2998.

59. Ricono JM, et al.: Specific cross-talk between epidermal growth factor receptor and integrin alphavbeta5 promotes carcinoma cell invasion and metastasis. Cancer Res 2009;69(4):1383–1391.

16 Hedgehog Signaling Pathways in Pancreatic Cancer Pathogenesis

Marina Pasca di Magliano · Matthias Hebrok

1	*Key Research Points*	*404*
1.1	The Hedgehog Signaling Pathway	404
1.2	The Hedgehog Signaling Pathway in Cancer	405
1.3	Different Modalities of Hedgehog Signaling Activation	406
1.4	Pancreatic Adenocarcinoma	408
1.5	Hedgehog Signaling in Pancreatic Adenocarcinoma	409
1.6	Hedgehog Signaling in Tumor Stroma	411
1.7	Hedgehog Signaling and Pancreatic Regeneration	412
1.8	Hedgehog Signaling in Invasive Tumors and Metastasis	413
1.9	Hedgehog Signaling in Other Pancreatic Lesions and Tumors	413
2	*Future Scientific Directions*	*414*
3	*Clinical Implications*	*414*

J. P. Neoptolemos, R. Urrutia, J. L. Abbruzzese, M. W. Büchler (eds.), *Pancreatic Cancer*,
DOI 10.1007/978-0-387-77498-5_16, © Springer Science+Business Media, LLC 2010

Abstract: Recent research has identified the Hedgehog signaling pathway as a key player in pancreatic cancer. The pathway is normally silent in the adult pancreas, but it gets activated in precursor lesions of pancreatic cancer as well as in invasive and metastatic pancreatic adenocarcinoma. Interestingly, mutations in the components of Hedgehog signaling have not been identified in pancreatic cancer; instead, the mechanism of activation relies on overexpression of one of the pathway ligands, Sonic Hedgehog, by the tumor cells. It is under investigation whether the secreted Hedgehog ligand mediates interactions among different cell types within the tumor. Our current knowledge indicates that the Hedgehog signaling pathway gets activated downstream of Kras (which is activated through a mutation in the vast majority of pancreatic cancers) and it synergizes with the Kras activity to promote tumor progression. Interestingly, the activity of the Hedgehog pathway appears to regulate processes such as tumor metastasis, one of the factors that preclude treatment in human patients. Current research is aimed at fully understanding the role of the pathway in pancreas cancer formation and progression and at establishing whether inhibition of this pathway might represent a valid approach to treat pancreatic cancer in the clinic.

1   Key Research Points

1.1   The Hedgehog Signaling Pathway

The study of the mammalian Hedgehog signaling pathway ◉ *Fig. 16-1* is a constantly evolving field fueled by continuous discoveries of novel signaling and cellular components that modulate the activity of the pathway in a cell type specific manner. In the context of this chapter,

◘ Fig. 16-1

The Hedgehog signaling pathway. a. In absence of ligands the Hedgehog pathway is inactive. Patched (Ptch) is localized at the cell membrane while Smoothened (Smo) is retained in the cytoplasm. The Gli transcription factors are processed to their repressor form (GliR) which prevents transcription of the Hedgehog target genes. The processing of Gli occurs in the cilia, a cellular organelle that is essential to regulate the activity of the Hedgehog pathway. b. When one of the Hedgehog ligands binds Patched, Smoothened enters the cilium and blocks the formation of GliR while initiating the accumulation of the activator form of Gli (GliA) which translocates to the nucleus and activates transcription of Hedgehog target genes.

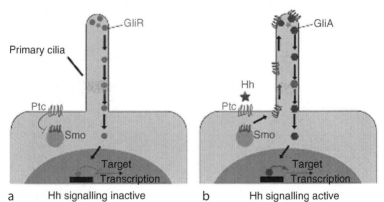

we will discuss only the basic components of the pathway. More detailed information can be found in excellent recent reviews [1,2].

We currently know of three distinct Hedgehog ligands in mammals, Sonic Hedgehog (Shh), Indian Hedgehog (Ihh) and Desert Hedgehog (Dhh), all of which bind to the same transmembrane receptor, Patched (Ptch). In the absence of ligands, Patched serves as an inhibitor of the pathway by blocking the downstream signaling component, Smoothened (Smo). Binding of a Hedgehog ligand to Ptch represses its ability to inhibit Smo function and, as a consequence, members of the Gli family of transcription factors translocate to the nucleus where they activate expression of Hedgehog target genes. Three members of this family are known in mammals: Gli1, Gli2 and Gli3. While Gli1 and Gli2 mostly act as activators of target transcription (Gli-A), Gli3 has been shown to mainly repress gene transcription in absence of Hedgehog ligands (Gli-R).

More recently, the primary cilium, a cellular appendage present on many vertebrate cells, has been identified as a node of Hedgehog regulation (expertly reviewed in [3]). Present evidence suggests that all cell types responsive to Hedgehog signaling possess a primary cilium and that pathway components localize within this structure and undergo posttranslational modifications. For example, in the absence of ligands, Gli3 is localized at the tip of the cilia and undergoes modifications that result in the formation of the repressor form of the protein [4,5]. Activator versions of Gli2 and Gli3 are not generated under these conditions. Upon ligand induction, Smo protein enters the cilia and appears to interact with Suppressor of Fused (SuFu), a negative regulator of the pathway, to block the formation of Gli3-R while initiating the generation of Gli2-A. Experimental evidence for cilia function in Hedgehog signal transduction has been obtained from studies in mutant mice lacking essential components for cilia formation. Assembly and function of primary cilia depends on interflagellar transport (IFT) proteins and elimination of genes coding for these proteins causes phenotypes similar to those observed in the absence of Hedgehog and Gli activity [3]. Thus, primary cilia do not only function as nodes in which Hedgehog signaling components aggregate, but they also mediate both the activator and repressor functions of the Gli proteins.

1.2 The Hedgehog Signaling Pathway in Cancer

Numerous studies have demonstrated a key role for the Hedgehog signaling pathway during embryonic organ formation. However, pathway activity is reduced significantly in cells of adult tissues. A notable exception to this rule are cells with progenitor properties in organs characterized by frequent turnover such as the skin. Increasing evidence points at adult progenitor cells as the potential cell of origin for certain cancers. Therefore, it is intriguing that inappropriate activation of the Hedgehog signaling pathway in adult cells has been linked to tumor formation in several organs, including the skin, the cerebellum, the lung, the pancreas and the prostate. Here, we will provide a brief, general overview of the distinct roles Hedgehog signaling plays in diverse cancers.

The earliest studies on the connection between Hedgehog pathway activation and carcinogenesis focused on basal cell carcinoma of the skin and on medulloblastoma (reviewed in [6]). Individuals with an inherited inactivating mutation in the **PTCH** gene (Gorlin's syndrome or basal cell nevus syndrome) develop numerous basal cell carcinomas. In addition, these individuals are at high risk for the development of medulloblastoma, a childhood cerebellar tumor with dismal prognosis. Often the second copy of the **PTCH** gene is lost in these patients, further promoting the hypothesis that PTCH acts like a classic tumor suppressor in this context. Studies of sporadic cases of basal cell carcinoma and medulloblastoma have demonstrated a reduction in PTCH function, either through deletion or loss of function mutation. Thus, studies from both familiar and sporadic cases of basal cell carcinoma point to activation of the Hedgehog pathway as a key event in the onset of these tumors.

It should further be noted that mutations in other Hedgehog pathway components have also been identified in certain cases of basal cell carcinoma and medulloblastoma. These include mutant forms of **SMO** that are not inhibited by PTCH and, less frequently, mutations in other pathway components such as **SUPPRESSOR OF FUSED (SUFU)** [7–9]. More recently, a series of surprising findings has linked inappropriate inactivation of the Hedgehog signaling pathway to other tumor types normally not observed in patients with Gorlin's syndrome. While these different tumors have distinct characteristics, one common feature is the lack of activating mutations in components of the Hedgehog pathway. As discussed in detail below, this suggests the existence of distinct mechanisms for Hedgehog activation during tumorigenesis in different tissues.

1.3   Different Modalities of Hedgehog Signaling Activation

A key difference exists in the modality of Hedgehog signaling activation in different tumor types ● *Fig. 16-2*. In general terms, the tumors can be divided in two categories: in the first category the Hedgehog signaling pathway is deregulated due to a mutation of one of the pathway components. As an example, loss-of-function PTCH mutations are common in basal cell carcinoma as well as in medulloblastoma. Activating mutations of SMO are also found in

◘ Fig. 16-2

Cell autonomous and non-cell autonomous activation of Hedgehog signaling. a. Mutations in *Ptch* or *Smo* cause constitutive, cell autonomous activation of the Hedgehog pathway. b, c. Overexpression of the Shh ligand in non-cell autonomous activation of the Hedgehog pathway. b. Shh activates the Hedgehog pathway in the same tumor cells that secrete it through an autocrine loop. c. Shh is secreted by the tumor cells and it works in a paracrine fashion to activate the pathway in surrounding components of the stroma. Autocrine and paracrine signaling can occur simultaneously.

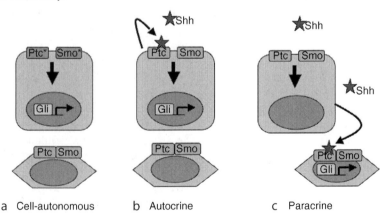

a Cell-autonomous   b Autocrine   c Paracrine

basal cell carcinomas [7]. Therefore, mutation-driven, cell-autonomous activation of the pathway at the level of PTCH/SMO is sufficient to increase the activity above a threshold required to initiate tumorigenesis.

A second category includes those tumors in which activation of the Hedgehog pathway is induced by ligand overexpression within the epithelial tumor cells. This category includes solid tumors such as small cell lung cancer, prostate cancer, and several gastrointestinal tumors. Since ligands are secreted molecules they could either act on the cells that produce them through an autocrine loop, or on the surrounding, non-tumor cells types through a juxtacrine/paracrine loop. It should be noted that autocrine and juxtacrine/paracrine action are not mutually exclusive and both could occur in the setting of a given tumor. A good example for a tumor driven in this non-cell-autonomous, ligand-driven manner is prostate cancer. During embryogenesis the Hedgehog pathway provides essential cues required for proper patterning of the prostate. In the adult prostate, progenitor cells are required for organ homeostasis, a process controlled by the interplay of different pathways including Hedgehog signaling. Components of the Hedgehog pathway are expressed in human prostate cancer cell lines [10] as well as human tumors [11,12] with the highest expression levels being found in metastatic tumors. Moreover, Hedgehog signaling appears to be required for tumor growth as demonstrated in experiments using the Hedgehog inhibitor cyclopamine both in vitro and in mouse xenograft experiments. Most prostate tumors overexpress the ligand SHH, however, a controversy exists on whether SHH secreted by the epithelial tumor cells activates Hedgehog function through an autocrine loop or whether it mainly controls pathway activity in surrounding stromal cells. The controversy stems in part from the absence of a set of reliable methods to determine Hedgehog pathway activation in a given tissue. Expression of GLI1 and PTCH are commonly accepted markers for Hedgehog activation, however; disparate results have been obtained with regard to their expression profile in the epithelial and stromal compartments of prostrate cancer. An answer to these questions awaits the generation of better immunohistochemical tools as well as reliable mouse models for prostrate cancer that could be combined with transgenic reporter mice to define the cells marked by Hedgehog activation.

Finally, there is an interesting subset of tumors with non-cell autonomous Hedgehog signaling represented by B-cell lymphomas and plasmacytoma. Neither activating mutations in Hedgehog pathway components nor excessive expression of ligands has been noted in these tumor cells. Instead, proliferation of tumor cells only occurs in lymphoid organs, such as spleen, bone marrow and lymph nodes, where the tissue stroma provides a source of SHH. Thus, the lack of ligand expression in the tumor cells themselves precludes autocrine signaling [13] and restricts tumor growth to niches that provide ample Hedgehog ligands. Interestingly, when tumor cells are experimentally engineered to ectopically activate Hedgehog signaling, they acquire the ability to leave the niche and grow in other locations, such as the skin.

Summarily, these observations indicate that Hedgehog signaling regulates tumor formation in at least two distinct manners. In tumors with cell-autonomous signaling, the activity of the pathway, marked by increased expression of *PTCH* and *GLI1*, is found within the epithelial compartment of the tumors. Given the fact that Hedgehog signaling often promotes cell proliferation and survival, this suggests that specific inhibition of the pathway needs to be considered as a possible treatment option for patients suffering from these types of tumors. Tumors marked by non-cell autonomous Hedgehog signaling could not be directly targeted via pathway inhibition. However, it is likely that Hedgehog signaling has beneficial effects on the stromal tissue surrounding the epithelial cancer cells, either by promoting proliferation of these cells or by eliciting secondary effects through increased vascularization or positive feedback signals that promote expansion of the epithelial compartment. Thus, while Hedgehog inhibition would not directly block epithelial cell survival and growth, abrogation of these secondary effects could also result in tumor shrinkage. Future studies are required to determine the exact responses Hedgehog signaling has on the diverse cell types of the stromal compartment

1.4   Pancreatic Adenocarcinoma

One of the tumors with ligand-driven activation of Hedgehog signaling is pancreatic adenocarcinoma. Pancreatic adenocarcinoma is the most common pancreatic malignancy, and it is a devastating disease with limited treatment options. Currently, the only chance for cure requires resecting the primary tumor. However, the majority of patients are diagnosed only after the cancer has become locally invasive or metastasized, thus precluding surgical intervention.

Considerable effort has been put into defining new treatment options and identifying novel biomarkers for early diagnosis. Both these aspects depend on an accurate knowledge of the biology of pancreatic cancer. Here, we describe the role of Hedgehog signaling as a marker of early stages of neoplastic lesions and tumor progression. We also describe ongoing studies to define the requirement of the pathway in tumor progression and metastasis.

A progression model for pancreatic cancer has been described based on pathological findings and molecular analysis of mutations in oncogenes and tumor suppressors in human pancreas specimens [14]. According to this model, pre-cancerous lesions known as Pancreatic Intra-epithelial Neoplasia (PanINs) precede the onset of the invasive phase of the disease in most cases. In addition, pancreatic adenocarcinoma can be linked to different types of pre-malignant lesions known as intraductal papillary mucinous neoplasms (IPMNs) and mucinous cystic neoplasms (MCNs) [15].

The PanIN lesions are classified based on histological criteria and on the appearance of signature mutations in oncogenes and tumor suppressors. Genetic changes accumulate in a remarkably conserved pattern during the progression from the early PanIN lesions (PanIN1A) to the advanced lesions (PanIN3 or carcinoma in situ). The most characteristic genetic alteration almost invariably present in pancreatic ductal adenocarcinoma is a single amino acid change in position 12 of the KRAS protein [16,17]. The amino acid substitution results in a constitutively active form of KRAS that is thought to initiate the tumorigenesis process. Studies in mice confirm the importance of Kras activation in pancreatic cancer. The most accurate mouse models of pancreatic cancer are based on conditionally activating a mutated allele of Kras within its endogenous genomic locus in epithelial cells of the mouse pancreas [18]. After a long period of latency, these transgenic mice develop PanIn that occasionally develop into invasive disease.

While ectopic expression of activated Kras is sufficient for PanIN induction in transgenic mice, pancreatic adenocarcinoma occurs only late in life, suggesting that other genetic or signaling changes need to occur for efficient transformation of pancreatic cells. Similarly, KRAS activation in humans does not appear to promote rapid pancreatic cancer formation. For instance, activating mutations in *KRAS* are often present in PanIN 1As found in cadaveric specimen of adult human pancreata [19] at an incidence significantly higher than the rate of pancreatic cancer diagnosis, suggesting that most PanIN will never progress to pancreatic adenocarcinoma. Mutations in tumor suppressor genes, including INK4A/ARF and p53, are believed to be required for tumorigenesis. In support of this notion, functional losses of tumor suppressor genes, such as of p53 [20] or of Arf/Ink4A [21], accelerate the onset of PanIN lesions and the progression to invasive cancer in transgenic Kras models of the disease.

Substantial effort has been placed on the identification of mutations in oncogenes and tumor suppressors during this process (expertly reviewed in [22]). However, more recent studies have provided evidence that embryonic signaling pathways, including the Hedgehog, Wnt, and Notch pathways, also play critical roles in pancreas tumor formation. This chapter will focus on our current knowledge about how Hedgehog signaling affects pancreas tumorigenesis.

1.5   Hedgehog Signaling in Pancreatic Adenocarcinoma

The role of Hedgehog signaling in pancreatic tissue is complex and changes throughout the life of an organism. At the earliest stages of pancreas organogenesis, Hedgehog signaling is excluded from the pancreas proper and ectopic activation of Shh in the pancreas anlage blocks organ formation. In later embryogenesis, expression of Hedgehog components is upregulated but remains relatively low when compared to pathway activity in adjacent tissues. In the adult pancreas, the Hedgehog signaling pathway is active only in a restricted subset of cells, including the endocrine cells located within the islets of Langerhans and the duct cells. However, similar to results obtained from studies performed in other organs, the Hedgehog pathway is upregulated during exocrine regeneration [23]. Thus, pancreatic injury leads to transient reactivation of Hedgehog signaling to promote acinar cell regeneration.

The first evidence for the importance of Hedgehog signaling in pancreatic cancer was the observation that PanIN lesions as well as invasive pancreatic adenocarcinomas express the SHH ligand [24,25] ◉ *Fig. 16-3*. This finding was somewhat surprising as SHH expression has not been found in normal embryonic or adult pancreatic tissue, suggesting that the transcriptional profile of pancreatic cells is aberrant during tumor formation. Mouse models have been used extensively to determine how activation of the Hedgehog pathway contributes to pancreatic cancer onset and progression. The first attempt at upregulating the Hedgehog pathway in the pancreas was based on overexpressing **Shh** under control of the **pancreatic and duodenal homeobox 1 promoter 1** (**Pdx1**) which is active in endodermal cells at the earliest stage of pancreas formation. As previously mentioned, Shh is normally excluded from the developing pancreatic epithelium and its forced activation leads to pancreatic agenesis [26]. Due to the severely impaired pancreas function, **Pdx1-Shh** transgenic animals survive only a few weeks after birth and are therefore not suitable as a cancer model. However, the pancreatic remnants that are found in some of the transgenic animals have enlarged ducts and lesions resembling human PanINs. Thus, activation of Hedgehog signaling via ectopic ligand expression might be able to drive the early stages of PanIN formation [24].

In a different model, an active form of the transcription factor **GLI2**, a mediator of Hedgehog signaling, was expressed in the pancreatic epithelium [27]. Interestingly, cell-autonomous Hedgehog activation within the pancreatic epithelium does not recapitulate the phenotypes observed upon overexpression of the Hedgehog ligand Shh. Neither loss of pancreatic tissue nor evidence of PanIN or PanIN-like lesions was observed in the pancreata of these animals. However, some of the transgenic mice develop pancreatic tumors that appear highly undifferentiated and do not resemble the normal pathology found in samples of human pancreatic ductal adenocarcinoma. Therefore, cell-autonomous activation of

⬛ Fig. 16-3

Genetic changes in pancreatic cancer progression. The cell of origin of PDA is controversial. The current data point to the acinar cell as the most likely candidate that can de-differentiated to assume duct-like cell characteristics, although the possibility that pancreatic cancer arises from pancreatic duct cells cannot be excluded. The most common precursor lesions for pancreatic cancer are known as Pancreatic Intraepithelial Neoplasia (PanIN). The lesions progress from PanIN1A to PanIN3 and the classification of individual lesions is based on histological and molecular criteria. Several genetic alterations that mark pancreatic ductal adenocarcinoma are already found in PanIN lesions: mutations in the Kras gene are present in the vast majority of PanIN1As, while tumor suppressor genes like Her2/Neu, p16, p53, DPC4 and BRCA2 are often inactivated in PanIN lesions of higher grade. Sonic Hedgehog (Shh) is not expressed in normal adult pancreatic acini or ducts. However, its expression is detectable in most PanIN1As, and it increases with PanIN progression with the highest levels being observed in invasive pancreatic adenocarcinoma. (modified from Hruban et al. 2001 #14).

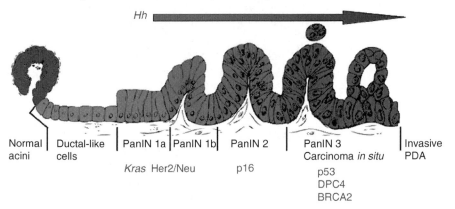

Hedgehog signaling in pancreatic epithelial cells is insufficient to initiate PanIN or pancreatic cancer formation.

In humans, KRAS mutation is the first step during PanIN formation followed by an increase in Hedgehog signaling. Transgenic mice with both activated Kras and Hh mutations (Kras/GLI2) were generated to address the question of whether cell-autonomous Hedgehog activation can accelerate PanIN formation. Pancreata isolated from these compound transgenic mice display early onset of multiple PanIN lesions that progress rapidly towards carcinoma in situ. However, the end stage tumors that form in *Kras/GLI2* mice are also of an undifferentiated type that does not resemble human pancreatic adenocarcinoma. At least two alternative explanations for the presence of undifferentiated tumors should be considered. It is possible that uncontrolled activation of Hedgehog signaling via ectopic expression of GLI2 might be incompatible with the differentiation state of the cells that form the basis of pancreatic adenocarcinoma. Alternatively, increased Hedgehog activation in an as of yet undefined cell type might lead to significant expansion of these cells, eventually resulting in the displacement of forming PanIN and pancreatic adenocarcinoma. Future studies using more defined Cre alleles allowing expression in specific subsets of pancreatic epithelial cells, e.g., specifically in duct or acinar cells should help to distinguish between these two alternatives [28–30].

In summary, these data show that: (1) cell-autonomous activation of Hedgehog signaling does not result in pancreatic adenocarcinoma or its precursor lesions; (2) Hedgehog and Kras activation synergize in promoting and accelerating the onset of pancreatic cancer precursor lesions. As a side note, further support for the notion that upregulation of Shh expression in PanIN lesions and pancreatic cancer is a general phenomenon comes from the recent observations that describe similar lesions in transgenic zebrafish marked by deregulated Kras signaling in pancreatic epithelium [31]. These data are exciting as they point to substantial conservation in pancreatic ductal adenocarcinoma not only between mammalian but along vertebrate species. Considering the suitability of the zebrafish both for genetic and small chemical screens, it should be possible to exploit this system to identify novel therapeutic targets for treatment of human patients.

1.6   Hedgehog Signaling in Tumor Stroma

Detailed analysis of mouse models of pancreatic adenocarcinoma have also implicated Hedgehog signaling in the desmoplastic component of the cancer. An important difference between pancreatic adenocarcinoma and the undifferentiated tumors present in the Kras/GLI2 animals is the absence of stromal desmoplasia in the latter. Detailed investigation of the molecular mechanisms underlying tumor formation suggest an important role for Hedgehog signaling in the recruitment and possible expansion of the mesenchymal component of the tumor. Progressively increasing levels of Hedgehog ligands are observed in the epithelial compartment of developing PanIN lesions. Increasing evidence suggests that epithelial-produced Hedgehog ligands, including SHH and IHH, act on surrounding mesenchymal cells and are instrumental in the desmoplastic reaction that supports tumor growth and is known to contribute to tumor malignancy. The importance of Hedgehog ligands in this process is supported by the fact that these proteins are absent in undifferentiated Kras/GLI2 tumors composed of a solid mass of tumor cells, with no evidence of a mesenchymal population. Thus, albeit circumstantial, these data support the notion that non cell-autonomous Hedgehog signaling participates in the expansion and function of the tumor stroma.

While intriguing, the current data do not provide conclusive evidence for a requirement for Hedgehog signaling in shaping the desmoplastic response and thus deciphering the exact relationships between the tumor cells and the stroma is the focus of ongoing investigation. However, additional support for Hedgehog-mediated epithelial to mesenchyme interactions comes from embryonic studies in which ectopic expression of Shh in epithelial cells leads to profound changes in the nature and differentiation state of the surrounding mesenchyme [26]. Pancreatic mesenchyme in these transgenic mice assumes properties of gut mesenchyme, a finding that is in line with the expression pattern of Hedgehog ligands that is minimal in the pancreatic area but high in gut tissue. Interestingly, a gene profiling study has identified a cluster of extrapancreatic foregut markers expressed in PanIN lesion that possibly reflects the effect of activated Hedgehog signaling in the lesions [32]. Future studies will have to determine whether increased Hedgehog activity in tumor mesenchyme also impacts the differentiation state. Efforts to define which cell types within the pancreatic tumors respond to Hedgehog ligands will be important to fully understand the role of the pathway in pancreas cancer formation and progression.

1.7   Hedgehog Signaling and Pancreatic Regeneration

A number of open key questions in pancreatic cancer are still unanswered. For example, which cell types give rise to the tumor? What causes pancreatic cells to initiate lesion formation and ultimately cancer? A partial answer to both these questions has been provided by a remarkable study recently published by Guerra and colleagues [33]. In order to understand their work, it is necessary to point out the most obvious differences between human pancreatic cancer and its counterpart in transgenic mice. In humans, mutations in Kras occur sporadically and presumably in adult cells. On the other hand, most mouse models of pancreatic cancer are based on activating the active form of Kras in the entire pancreatic epithelial compartment beginning at the early stages of pancreatic development. Hence, the transgene is activated in precursor cells prior to their differentiation along the different pancreatic lineages.

Guerra and colleagues developed an inducible model in which the activated Kras can be activated at will at different time points. It is important to note that they used the elastase promoter, so that the mutant Kras is expressed only in the acinar lineage (and possibly in some centroacinar cells) within the adult pancreas but does induce recombination in other cell types when activated during embryogenesis. Using this model, activating Kras during development leads to extensive PanIN lesions that eventually progress to invasive pancreatic cancer, recapitulating what has been observed with other models of Kras activation in the pancreas. However, if the transgene is kept silent during development and only activated in adult animals, there is evidence of neither PanIN development nor cancer. One interpretation is that undifferentiated pancreatic cells provide a permissive environment for Kras activation and tumor onset, while adult cells, possibly because they are mostly removed from the cell cycle, might not become transformed even in presence of an active form of Kras. In humans, however, the Kras mutations arise presumably in the adult pancreas, so some additional event must occur to drive their progression to cancer. The additional event could be another mutation occurring in the same cells, or it could be an environmental cause, such as inflammation. Consistent with the last possibility, one of the known risk factors for pancreatic cancer is chronic pancreatitis. Chronic pancreatitis can be induced in mouse by treating the animals with caerulein. Interestingly, wild-type mice treated with caerulein develop pancreatitis, characterized at the histological level by loss of acinar cells and their replacement by duct-like cells, a phenomenon known as acinar-ductal metaplasia. However, once the treatment is suspended, the tissue recovers completely, revealing a seldom appreciated regenerative capacity of the pancreatic acinar cells. In contrast, mice carrying an activated form of Kras in their acinar cells [33] develop PanIN lesions following pancreatitis. Therefore, it appears that in the presence of the activated form of Kras the acinar-ductal metaplasia progresses to PanIN lesions. It is intriguing to speculate that a similar mechanism might exist in human patients, whereby following injury the pancreas initiates a regeneration response, aimed at re-establishing its normal architecture and function, but where cells harbor mutations in Kras the regeneration process gets sidetracked and causes the onset of cancer. Pancreatitis, especially the chronic form of it, is an extreme form of injury to the pancreas, and not all the pancreatic cancer patients have experienced it. However, is possible that much milder, even subclinical forms of inflammation are sufficient to trigger Kras mutated cells to induce cancer. There are two main conclusions that can be drawn from this study: the *first* one is that adult pancreatic acinar cells can give rise to pancreatic cancer, challenging the belief that the disease originates from pancreatic ducts (although the study does not allow to exclude duct cells as another possible cell of origin of pancreatic cancer). The **second** finding is that the effect of Kras activation is context-dependent, being profoundly different in embryonic pancreatic cells, in healthy adult cells and in adult cells in the context of tissue injury.

Recent results have implicated Hedgehog signaling during exocrine pancreas regeneration. One of the important inflammatory pathways that is activated in pancreatitis is the NFκ-B pathway [33,34]. Interestingly, Shh expression in pancreatic cancer has been shown to be activated downstream of the NFκ-B pathway [35]. In cancer, NFκ-B is downstream of Kras activation, and therefore a cascade of events can be identified with Kras, NFκ-B and Shh as key players during tumor initiation. Given that NFκ-B is activated in pancreatitis as well as cancer, an interesting question to ask was whether the Hedgehog pathway is activated in the context of pancreatitis. Recent data [23] shows that the Hedgehog pathway is activated in a transient manner when acinar cells undergo acinar-ductal metaplasia induced by acute pancreatitis. However, the pathway is immediately downregulated as soon as the metaplastic ducts re-differentiate into acinar cells. Based on the data described above, one can speculate that in the presence of mutated Kras the Hedgehog pathway becomes chronically activated. The failure to downregulate Hedgehog signaling could in turn promote PanIN lesion formation and progression, possibly by modifying the reciprocal signaling between the tumor epithelial cells and the surrounding cells of mesenchymal origin. This hypothesis could easily be tested using the available mouse model of pancreatic cancer.

1.8 Hedgehog Signaling in Invasive Tumors and Metastasis

Pancreatic cancer patients often present with metastatic disease at the time of diagnosis, a finding that prevents them from undergoing surgical resection and significantly worsens their prognosis. A deeper understanding of the metastatic process is required in order to generate drugs that can specifically target this aspect of the disease. Hedgehog signaling has been shown to affect two key processes during tumor invasiveness, namely angiogenesis and metastasis [10,36,37]. Currently, there is evidence that SHH secreted by the tumor cells can stimulate the angiogenic function of tumor endothelial cells [38]. Moreover, the Hedgehog pathway's possible implication in pancreatic cancer metastasis has been recently addressed [39]. As observed in other contexts [40], Hedgehog signaling appears to positively regulate Snail expression in a highly metastatic pancreatic cancer cell line. Activation of the Hedgehog pathway results in downregulation of E-cadherin in the same cells. Snail is a mediator of epithelial-mesenchymal transition, a process that is believed to play an important role in tumor metastasis, whereas E-cadherin is essential for cell-cell adhesion while preventing cell movement. Taken together, these findings indicate that Hedgehog signaling might play a role in promoting pancreatic cancer cell migration. Strikingly, inhibition of the Hedgehog pathway was able to almost completely abolish formation of metastasis in an orthotopic xenograft model of pancreatic cancer. This finding has potential clinical implications, and, if confirmed in human patients, would indicate the possibility to use Hedgehog inhibition to prevent spreading of the tumor. It remains to be addressed whether Hedgehog inhibition has any effect on metastases that are already established before diagnosis.

1.9 Hedgehog Signaling in Other Pancreatic Lesions and Tumors

Little information about the role of Hedgehog signaling in other pancreatic cancers is currently available. Intraductal papillary mucinous neoplasms (IPMNs) and mucinous cystic neoplasms

(MCNs) are less common progenitor lesions to pancreatic adenocarcinoma than PanIN. Both these neoplasms have significantly improved outcomes if they are resected in the premalignant stage. Interestingly, Hedgehog signaling components have been shown to be expressed both in IPMNs [41–43] and in MCNs [44]. Mouse models of MCNs [45] and of IPMNs [46] have recently become available, opening the possibility to perform functional studies to test whether manipulation of Hedgehog signaling affects the formation or progression of these tumors.

2   Future Scientific Directions

While significant progress has been made in the understanding of the role of Hedgehog signaling in pancreatic cancer, several important questions remain and are the focus of ongoing research.

One of the key issues is how the pathway acts in pancreatic cancer, namely which cell types respond to the ligand secreted by the tumor cells. Fortunately, this question can be addressed using mouse models currently available. An in vivo readout of cells with active signaling within the tumor will provide an indication of which cells would be affected by Hedgehog inhibition. Moreover, it would allow to study the downstream effectors of Hedgehog signaling, which are so far poorly understood.

At this moment, it is not clear how epithelial and stromal Hedgehog signaling contribute to tumor progression. It is important to note that the tumor stroma is composed by a heterogeneous mix of different cell types, and that the interactions between these different cell types are not well defined. It is likely that future studies will elucidate whether Hedgehog signaling mediates some of the interactions between different cell types within the tumor.

Another area of research that has recently emerged is the role of cilia regarding regulation of the Hedgehog signaling pathway. While strong progress has been made in the understanding of the basic mechanisms by which cilia and hedgehog signaling interact during the development of different organs, little is know on whether the cilia play a role in mediating the activity of this pathway in cancer. However, a recent study conducted on pancreatic cancer cell lines [47] has provided data indicating that cilia are indeed present at least in a percentage of tumor cells and that components of the Hedgehog pathway accumulate within the cilia in this context. It is likely that future studies on Hedgehog signaling and cilia in pancreatic cancer will be performed using the currently available mouse models of this disease, and possibly taking advantage of the several available cilia mutant mouse strains.

Finally, an extremely active area of research is represented by the study of tumor stem cells. A stem cell population has been identified in human pancreatic cancer [48] and interestingly these cells express the components of the Hedgehog pathway. What is the role of Hedgehog signaling in these cells? Does it control cell renewal or proliferation? Does it have an effect on their niche? All these questions are still open and will likely be addressed by the scientific community in the near future.

3   Clinical Implications

There are two main potential clinical implications of studying Hedgehog signaling in pancreatic cancer. The first possibility, is that components of the Hedgehog pathway could be used as diagnostic markers of the disease. Shh has been detected in the pancreatic juice of pancreatic cancer patients [41] at levels significantly different than those found in chronic pancreatitis.

Moreover, studies on Hedgehog signaling in the tumor stroma components might lead to the identifycation of secreted molecules that are downstream of the Hedgehog pathway, and that might potentially accumulate in the patients serum or pancreatic juice. A panel of biomarkers that provides a clear indication to distinguish pancreatic cancer patients from pancreatitis patients and healthy individuals would be paramount for early detection.

The second potential clinical implication is whether hedgehog inhibition might prove a viable clinical option to aide the treatment of pancreatic cancer. Early findings using cyclopamine as a hedgehog inhibitor showed marked tumor size reduction [24,25] for a percentage of the tumor cell lines used in those experiments. However, there studies were based on subcutaneous xenograft of human cancer cell lines in mice. This model is not a reliable prediction of clinical efficacy. Interestingly, a recent study has addressed the question of whether cyclopamine treatment would prolong the survival in a mouse model of pancreatic cancer [49]. The results indicated a modest but significant effect on the life span of the treated animals compared to controls. Since the specificity of cyclopamine as a Hedgehog inhibitor has recently been questioned, it would be important to confirm the findings using different inhibitors of the pathway. Recently, new and more potent inhibitors of the Hedgehog signaling pathway have been described [50,51], including one that acts downstream of SMO [51]. In conclusion, further research is needed to validate the possibility of using anti-Hedgehog therapy in the treatment of pancreatic cancer.

Key Research Points

- Hedgehog signaling is inactive in normal adult pancreas. The pathway is ectopically activated in PanIN lesions and pancreatic cancer.
- The Sonic Hedgehog ligand is overexpressed by the epithelial cells of PanIN lesions and pancreatic cancer. It is still unknown whether it operates through an autocrine loop on epithelial cancer cells and/or in a paracrine manner by regulating survival and proliferaion of components of the tumor stroma.
- Hedgehog signaling is transiently activated in the pancreas following tissue injury such as pancreatitis. It is possible that the activation might become chronic in the context of cells marked by genetic damage, including activating mutations in the K-ras gene.
- Epithelial activation of Hedgehog signaling accelerates PanIN and tumor formation in the context of Kras mutation.

Future Scientific Directions

- What is the relative contribution of epithelial and stromal Hedgehog signaling to tumor progression?
- Given their importance in regulating the pathway during embryogenesis of different organs, are cilia an important regulator of Hedgehog signaling in cancer,?
- Is Hedgehog signaling important for the maintenance of pancreatic cancer stem cells and their interaction with their niche?

Clinical Implications

- Components of the Hedgehog pathway or target genes of the pathway could be explored as biomarkers for pancreatic cancer.
- Hedgehog signaling inhibition might provide a new treatment option for pancreatic cancer.

References

1. Jacob L, Lum L: Hedgehog signaling pathway. Sci STKE 2007;2007(407):cm6.
2. Wang Y, McMahon AP, Allen BL: Shifting paradigms in Hedgehog signaling. Curr Opin Cell Biol 2007;19 (2):159–165.
3. Eggenschwiler JT, Anderson KV: Cilia and developmental signaling. Annu Rev Cell Dev Biol 2007;23:345–373.
4. Haycraft CJ, Banizs B, Aydin-Son Y, Zhang Q, Michaud EJ, Yoder BK: Gli2 and Gli3 localize to cilia and require the intraflagellar transport protein polaris for processing and function. PLoS Genet 2005;1(4):e53.
5. Huangfu D, Anderson KV: Cilia and Hedgehog responsiveness in the mouse. Proc Natl Acad Sci USA 2005;102(32):11325–11330.
6. Ingham PW: The patched gene in development and cancer. Curr Opin Genet Dev 1998;8(1):88–94.
7. Xie J, Murone M, Luoh SM, Ryan A, Gu Q, Zhang C, Bonifas JM, Lam CW, Hynes M, Goddard A, Rosenthal A, Epstein EH, Jr, de Sauvage FJ. Activating Smoothened mutations in sporadic basal-cell carcinoma. Nature 1998;391 (6662):90–92.
8. Taylor MD, Liu L, Raffel C, Hui CC, Mainprize TG, Zhang X, Agatep R, Chiappa S, Gao L, Lowrance A, Hao A, Goldstein AM, Stavrou T, Scherer SW, Dura WT, Wainwright B, Squire JA, Rutka JT, Hogg D: Mutations in SUFU predispose to medulloblastoma. Nat Genet 2002;31(3):306–310.
9. Reifenberger J, Wolter M, Knobbe CB, Köhler B, Schönicke A, Scharwächter C, Kumar K, Blaschke B, Ruzicka T, Reifenberger G: Somatic mutations in the PTCH, SMOH, SUFUH and TP53 genes in sporadic basal cell carcinomas. Br J Dermatol 2005;152 (1):43–51.
10. Sanchez P, Hernández AM, Stecca B, Kahler AJ, DeGueme AM, Barrett A, Beyna M, Datta MW, Datta S, Ruiz i Altaba A: Inhibition of prostate cancer proliferation by interference with SONIC HEDGEHOG-GLI1 signaling. Proc Natl Acad Sci USA 2004;101(34):12561–12566.
11. Karhadkar SS, Bova GS, Abdallah N, Dhara S, Gardner D, Maitra A, Isaacs JT, Berman DM, Beachy PA: Hedgehog signalling in prostate regeneration, neoplasia and metastasis. Nature 2004;431(7009):707–712.
12. Sheng T, Li C, Zhang X, Chi S, He N, Chen K, McCormick F, Gatalica Z, Xie J: Activation of the hedgehog pathway in advanced prostate cancer. Mol Cancer 2004;3:29.
13. Dierks C, Grbic J, Zirlik K, Beigi R, Englund NP, Guo GR, Veelken H, Engelhardt M, Mertelsmann R, Kelleher JF, Schultz P, Warmuth M: Essential role of stromally induced hedgehog signaling in B-cell malignancies. Nat Med 2007;13(8):944–951.
14. Hruban RH, Adsay NV, Albores-Saavedra J, Compton C, Garrett ES, Goodman SN, Kern SE, Klimstra DS, Klöppel G, Longnecker DS, Lüttges J, Offerhaus GJ: Pancreatic intraepithelial neoplasia: a new nomenclature and classification system for pancreatic duct lesions. Am J Surg Pathol 2001;25 (5):579–586.
15. Hingorani SR: Location, location, location: precursors and prognoses for pancreatic cancer. Gastroenterology 2007;133(1):345–350.
16. Hruban RH, van Mansfeld AD, Offerhaus GJ, van Weering DH, Allison DC, Goodman SN, Kensler TW, Bose KK, Cameron JL, Bos JL: K-ras oncogene activation in adenocarcinoma of the human pancreas. A study of 82 carcinomas using a combination of mutant-enriched polymerase chain reaction analysis and allele-specific oligonucleotide hybridization. Am J Pathol 1993;143(2):545–554.
17. Hruban RH, Wilentz RE, Kern SE: Genetic progression in the pancreatic ducts. Am J Pathol 2000;156 (6):1821–1825.
18. Hingorani SR, Petricoin EF, Maitra A, Rajapakse V, King C, Jacobetz MA, Ross S, Conrads TP, Veenstra TD, Hitt BA, Kawaguchi Y, Johann D, Liotta LA, Crawford HC, Putt ME, Jacks T, Wright CV, Hruban RH, Lowy AM, Tuveson DA: Preinvasive and invasive ductal pancreatic cancer and its early detection in the mouse. Cancer Cell 2003;4(6):437–450.
19. Tada M, Ohashi M, Shiratori Y, Okudaira T, Komatsu Y, Kawabe T, Yoshida H, Machinami R, Kishi K, Omata M: Analysis of K-ras gene mutation in hyperplastic duct cells of the pancreas without

pancreatic disease. Gastroenterology 1996;110 (1):227–231.

20. Hingorani SR, Wang L, Multani AS, Combs C, Deramaudt TB, Hruban RH, Rustgi AK, Chang S, Tuveson DA: Trp53R172H and KrasG12D cooperate to promote chromosomal instability and widely metastatic pancreatic ductal adenocarcinoma in mice. Cancer Cell 2005;7(5):469–483.

21. Aguirre AJ, Bardeesy N, Sinha M, Lopez L, Tuveson DA, Horner J, Redston MS, DePinho RA: Activated Kras and Ink4a/Arf deficiency cooperate to produce metastatic pancreatic ductal adeno-carcinoma. Genes Dev 2003;17(24):3112–3126.

22. Hezel AF, Kimmelman AC, Stanger BZ, Bardeesy N, Depinho RA: Genetics and biology of pancreatic ductal adenocarcinoma. Genes Dev 2006;20 (10):1218–1249.

23. Fendrich V, Esni F, Garay MV, Feldmann G, Habbe N, Jensen JN, Dor Y, Stoffers D, Jensen J, Leach SD, Maitra A: Hedgehog signaling is required for effective regeneration of exocrine pancreas. Gastroenterology 2008;135(2):621–631.

24. Thayer SP, Pasca di Magliano M, Heiser PW, Nielsen CM, Roberts DJ, Lauwers GY, Qi YP, Gysin S, Fernández-del Castillo C, Yajnik V, Antoniu B, McMahon M, Warshaw AL, Hebrok M: Hedgehog is an early and late mediator of pancreatic cancer tumorigenesis. Nature 2003;425(6960): 851–856.

25. Berman DM, Karhadkar SS, Maitra A, Montes De Oca R, Gerstenblith MR, Briggs K, Parker AR, Shimada Y, Eshleman JR, Watkins DN, Beachy PA: Widespread requirement for Hedgehog ligand stim-ulation in growth of digestive tract tumours. Nature 2003;425(6960):846–851.

26. Apelqvist A, Ahlgren U, Edlund H: Sonic hedge-hog directs specialised mesoderm differentiation in the intestine and pancreas. Curr Biol 1997;7 (10):801–814.

27. Pasca di Magliano M, Sekine S, Ermilov A, Ferris J, Dlugosz AA, Hebrok M: Hedgehog/Ras interactions regulate early stages of pancreatic cancer. Genes Dev 2006;20(22):3161–3173.

28. Desai BM, Oliver-Krasinski J, De Leon DD, Farzad C, Hong N, Leach SD, Stoffers DA: Preexisting pancre-atic acinar cells contribute to acinar cell, but not islet beta cell, regeneration. J Clin Invest 2007;117(4): 971–977.

29. Means AL, Xu Y, Zhao A, Ray KC, Gu G: A CK19 (CreERT) knockin mouse line allows for conditional DNA recombination in epithelial cells in multiple endodermal organs. Genesis 2008;46(6):318–323.

30. Murtaugh LC, Law AC, Dor Y, Melton DA: Beta-catenin is essential for pancreatic acinar but not islet development. Development 2005;132 (21):4663–4674.

31. Park SW, Davison JM, Rhee J, Hruban RH, Maitra A, Leach SD: Oncogenic KRAS induces progenitor cell expansion and malignant transformation in zebra-fish exocrine pancreas. Gastroenterology 2008;134 (7):2080–2090.

32. Prasad NB, Biankin AV, Fukushima N, Maitra A, Dhara S, Elkahloun AG, Hruban RH, Goggins M, Leach SD: Gene expression profiles in pancreatic intraepithelial neoplasia reflect the effects of Hedge-hog signaling on pancreatic ductal epithelial cells. Cancer Res 2005;65(5):1619–1626.

33. Guerra C, Schuhmacher AJ, Cañamero M, Grippo PJ, Verdaguer L, Pérez-Gallego L, Dubus P, Sandgren EP, Barbacid M: Chronic pancreatitis is essential for induction of pancreatic ductal adenocarcinoma by K-Ras oncogenes in adult mice. Cancer Cell 2007;11(3):291–302.

34. Steinle AU, Weidenbach H, Wagner M, Adler G, Schmid RM: NF-kappaB/Rel activation in cerulein pancreatitis. Gastroenterology 1999;116(2):420–430.

35. Nakashima H, Nakamura M, Yamaguchi H, Yamanaka N, Akiyoshi T, Koga K, Yamaguchi K, Tsuneyoshi M, Tanaka M, Katano M: Nuclear factor-kappaB contributes to hedgehog signaling pathway activation through sonic hedgehog induc-tion in pancreatic cancer. Cancer Res 2006;66 (14):7041–7049.

36. Pola R, Ling LE, Silver M, Corbley MJ, Kearney M, Blake Pepinsky R, Shapiro R, Taylor FR, Baker DP, Asahara T, Isner JM: The morphogen Sonic hedge-hog is an indirect angiogenic agent upregulating two families of angiogenic growth factors. Nat Med 2001;7(6):706–711.

37. Kanda S, Mochizuki Y, Suematsu T, Miyata Y, Nomata K, Kanetake H: Sonic hedgehog induces capillary morphogenesis by endothelial cells through phosphoinositide 3-kinase. J Biol Chem. 2003;278 (10):8244–8249.

38. Yamazaki M, Nakamura K, Mizukami Y, Ii M, Sasa-jima J, Sugiyama Y, Nishikawa T, Nakano Y, Yana-gawa N, Sato K, Maemoto A, Tanno S, Okumura T, Karasaki H, Kono T, Fujiya M, Ashida T, Chung DC, Kohgo Y: Sonic hedgehog derived from human pan-creatic cancer cells augments angiogenic function of endothelial progenitor cells. Cancer Sci 2008;99 (6):1131–1138.

39. Feldmann G, Dhara S, Fendrich V, Bedja D, Beaty R, Mullendore M, Karikari C, Alvarez H, Iacobuzio-Donahue C, Jimeno A, Gabrielson KL, Matsui W, Maitra A: Blockade of hedgehog signaling inhibits pancreatic cancer invasion and metastases: a new paradigm for combination therapy in solid cancers. Cancer Res 2007;67(5):2187–2196.

40. Li X, Deng W, Nail CD, Bailey SK, Kraus MH, Ruppert JM, Lobo-Ruppert SM: Snail induction is an early response to Gli1 that determines the

efficiency of epithelial transformation. Oncogene 2006;25(4):609–621.

41. Ohuchida K, Mizumoto K, Fujita H, Yamaguchi H, Konomi H, Nagai E, Yamaguchi K, Tsuneyoshi M, Tanaka M: Sonic hedgehog is an early developmental marker of intraductal papillary mucinous neoplasms: clinical implications of mRNA levels in pancreatic juice. J Pathol 2006;210(1):42–48.

42. Satoh K, Kanno A, Hamada S, Hirota M, Umino J, Masamune A, Egawa S, Motoi F, Unno M, Shimosegawa T: Expression of Sonic hedgehog signaling pathway correlates with the tumorigenesis of intraductal papillary mucinous neoplasm of the pancreas. Oncol Rep 2008;19(5):1185–1190.

43. Jang KT, Lee KT, Lee JG, Choi SH, Heo JS, Choi DW, Ahn G: Immunohistochemical expression of Sonic hedgehog in intraductal papillary mucinous tumor of the pancreas. Appl Immunohistochem Mol Morphol 2007;15(3):294–298.

44. Liu MS, Yang PY, Yeh TS: Sonic hedgehog signaling pathway in pancreatic cystic neoplasms and ductal adenocarcinoma. Pancreas 2007;34(3):340–346.

45. Izeradjene K, Combs C, Best M, Gopinathan A, Wagner A, Grady WM, Deng CX, Hruban RH, Adsay NV, Tuveson DA, Hingorani SR: Kras (G12D) and Smad4/Dpc4 haploinsufficiency cooperate to induce mucinous cystic neoplasms and invasive adenocarcinoma of the pancreas. Cancer Cell 2007;11(3):229–243.

46. Siveke JT, Einwächter H, Sipos B, Lubeseder-Martellato C, Klöppel G, Schmid RM: Concomitant pancreatic activation of Kras(G12D) and Tgfa results in cystic papillary neoplasms reminiscent of human IPMN. Cancer Cell 2007;12(3):266–279.

47. Nielsen SK, Møllgård K, Clement CA, Veland IR, Awan A, Yoder BK, Novak I, Christensen ST: Characterization of primary cilia and Hedgehog signaling during development of the human pancreas and in human pancreatic duct cancer cell lines. Dev Dyn 2008;237(8):2039–2052.

48. Li C, Heidt DG, Dalerba P, Burant CF, Zhang L, Adsay V, Wicha M, Clarke MF, Simeone DM: Identification of pancreatic cancer stem cells. Cancer Res 2007;67(3):1030–1037.

49. Feldmann G, Habbe N, Dhara S, Bisht S, Alvarez H, Fendrich V, Beaty R, Mullendore M, Karikari C, Bardeesy N, Oullette MM, Yu W, Maitra A: Hedgehog inhibition prolongs survival in a genetically engineered mouse model of pancreatic cancer. Gut 2008;57(10):1420–1430.

50. Brunton SA, Stibbard JH, Rubin LL, Kruse LI, Guicherit OM, Boyd EA, Price S: Potent inhibitors of the hedgehog signaling pathway. J Med Chem 2008;51(5):1108–1110.

51. Lee J, Wu X, Pasca di Magliano M, Peters EC, Wang Y, Hong J, Hebrok M, Ding S, Cho CY, Schultz PG: A small-molecule antagonist of the hedgehog signaling pathway. Chembiochem 2007;8(16):1916–1919.

17 Smad4/TGF-β Signaling Pathways in Pancreatic Cancer Pathogenesis

Alixanna Norris · Murray Korc

1	*Pancreatic Ductal Adenocarcinoma*	*420*
1.2	Disease Description	420
1.3	Overview of Molecular Alterations in PDAC	420
2	*TGF-β Background*	*421*
2.1	TGF-β	421
2.2	TGF-β Receptors	421
2.3	Smad Proteins	422
2.4	Smad4	424
2.5	Consequences of Normal TGF-β Signaling	424
2.6	TGF-β in Normal Development	425
2.7	TGF-Beta Signaling in the Adult Pancreas	426
2.8	Smad-Independent Pathways of TGF-β	426
3	*TGF-β and Pancreatic Cancer*	*427*
3.1	Noted Alterations	427
3.2	Smad4 and Pancreatic Cancer	428
3.3	TGF-β and Acute Pancreatitis	429
3.4	TGF-β and Chronic Pancreatitis	430
4	*Translational Implications*	*430*
4.1	Overview	430
4.2	Blocking TGF-β Actions in Models of PDAC	431
4.3	TGF-β in the Clinic?	431
4.4	The Future of TGF-β	432

J. P. Neoptolemos, R. Urrutia, J. L. Abbruzzese, M. W. Büchler (eds.), *Pancreatic Cancer*,
DOI 10.1007/978-0-387-77498-5_17, © Springer Science+Business Media, LLC 2010

Abstract: Pancreatic ductal adenocarcinoma (PDAC) is an extremely aggressive disease with dismal survival statistics. Extensive research efforts have focused on the elucidation of the specific molecular alterations behind pancreatic cancer, with the goals of understanding PDAC pathobiology and devising new and effective targeted therapies. These studies have yielded surprisingly consistent results, indicating that key genetic alterations include a high frequency of mutations in the K-*ras*, p53, p16 and Smad4 genes. In addition, there is excessive activation of mitogenic pathways, overexpression of TGF-β isoforms, and an intense desmoplastic reaction that is driven, in part, by the proliferation of pancreatic stellate cells, and marked apoptosis resistance. This chapter focuses on the potential role of the TGF-β signaling pathway in PDAC progression and metastasis while highlighting the importance of Smad4 in TGF-β signal transduction.

1 Pancreatic Ductal Adenocarcinoma

1.2 Disease Description

Pancreatic ductal adenocarcinoma (PDAC) is the deadliest form of pancreatic cancer and is presently the fourth leading cause of cancer-related mortality in the United States. Patients have an extremely poor prognosis, with a 5-year survival less than 5% [1] and a median survival of 6 months [2]. These dismal statistics are due to a combination of a low rate of resectability at presentation [3,4] and inherently aggressive tumor behavior. The poor survival of this malignancy has initiated an impetus of research efforts to understand the molecular mechanisms driving pancreatic cancer.

1.3 Overview of Molecular Alterations in PDAC

A number of common pathways are known to be frequently altered in PDAC. Often, it is the somatic mutation of only one or a few key regulatory genes within a pathway that leads to its signaling dysfunction. As shown in ⊙ *Table 17-1*, the most common alterations include mutations of the K-*ras* oncogene (∼90%), the p53 (∼85%) and SMAD4 (∼50%) tumor suppressor genes and the p16 cell cycle inhibitory gene (∼85% mutated and ∼15% epigenetically silenced) [5,6]. Conversely, elevated expression of multiple tyrosine kinase receptors and/or their ligands is documented in PDAC as well as over-activation of the src, NFκB and Stat3 signaling pathways [7,8]. The somatic alterations outlined here have the potential to increase cell proliferation while reducing normal apoptotic mechanisms that protect against tumor development, thereby laying the groundwork for cancer initiation.

Molecular alterations have also been documented in PDAC which are likely contributors to the inherently aggressive cancer phenotype. For instance, the KAI1 tetraspan receptor and NK4 are often lost [9], leading to increased cancer cell motility. Additional contributing factors may include increased activation of proangiogenic factors, altered epithelial-mesenchymal interactions and the alteration of transforming growth factor-β (TGF-β) signaling [10–12]. While a combination of these molecular alterations is likely to contribute to cancer cell invasion and metastatic potential, the remainder of this chapter will focus on the specific role of the TGF-β signaling pathway in pancreatic cancer.

⊙ Table 17-1

Genetic alterations in PDAC

Gene	Alteration	Frequency	Function
K-ras	Activation mutation	90%	Mitogenic signaler
p16	Inactivation mutation or silencing	85–95%	Cell cycle arrest
p53	Inactivation mutation	70%	Apoptosis & cell cycle arrest
DPC4 (Smad4)	Homozygous deletion or missense mutations	50%	Mediator of TGF-β signaling
AKT2	Amplification or overexpression	10–20%	Mediator of PI3K signaling
MYB	Amplification or overexpression	10%	Transcription factor
BRCA2	Mutation	5%	Mitotic maintenance and DNA repair
ALK5	Mutation	1–4%	Receptor for TGF-β
MKK4	Mutation or deletion	<4%	Mediator of JNK signaling

2   TGF-β Background

2.1   TGF-β

TGF-β is a cytokine that has been implicated in a diverse range of biological processes. After its initial discovery in 1983, it was shown to have transforming ability in rat fibroblasts [13] and was initially named "sarcoma growth factor." Following further study, it became clear that TGF-β is one of the most potent biological regulators of proliferation in normal cells. In addition to proliferation, the TGF-β signaling pathway has been implicated in numerous cellular and biological processes including embryogenesis, differentiation, apoptosis, angiogenesis, immunosuppression and wound healing.

TGF-β is a member of a large family of structurally related polypeptide growth factors. The TGF-β superfamily comprises nearly thirty members in human, mouse, *Xenopus* and other vertebrates [14,15]. Seven members are known to exist in *Drosophila* [16] and four in *C. elegans* [17]. The proteins within this family are divided into two main branches as defined by sequence similarity: the BMP/GDF/MIS branch and the TGF-β/activin/nodal branch [18,19]. There are three mammalian TGF-β isoforms (TGF-β1, TGF-β2, and TGF-β3 that are encoded by different genes with different expression patterns [20]. All three isoforms are highly conserved and all are expressed in epithelial, endothelial, mesenchymal and hematopoetic cells, with TGF-β1 being the most abundantly expressed isoform. The TGF-β1 protein is made and secreted into the extracellular matrix where it forms a complex comprised of a TGF-β1 dimer and one of many latent TGF-β1 binding proteins. Upon release from this complex, the TGF-β1 ligand is activated and is free to propagate signaling by binding to defined receptors.

2.2   TGF-β Receptors

As depicted in ⊚ *Fig. 17-1*, TGF-β ligands initiate signaling by acting through specific cell surface receptors that belong to a family of transmembrane serine/threonine kinase receptors.

◘ Fig. 17-1

The TGF-β/Smad signaling pathway. TGF-β actions are initiated following binding by a TGF-β dimeric ligand to the TβRII homodimer at the cell's membrane. This leads to the recruitment, binding and phosphorylation of the TβRI homodimer at its GS site (GSGS). Activated TβRI then, with the help of the Smad anchor for receptor activation (SARA) protein, activates the R-Smads (Smad2/3) by phosphorylation. This step is inhibited by the I-Smads (Smad6/7). Following binding with the Co-Smad (Smad4), the activated R-Smads are translocated to the nucleus. Here, they interact with nuclear transcription factors (TF) and co-activators/co-repressors to mediate the transcription of target genes. This pathway is reviewed to greater detail in the text.

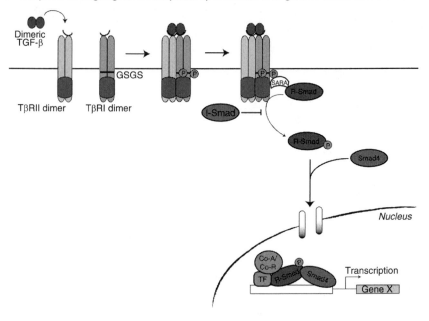

Thus, TGF-βs act through two receptors, designated as type I (TβRI) and type II TGF-β (TβRII) [19,21,22]. In addition, there is a type III TGF-β receptor (TβRIII) which differs from the other two receptors in that it has no intrinsic signaling function and instead serves to present activated TGF-β1 to the other two receptors [15]. Both TβRI and TβRII exist as homodimers and consist of an extracellular ligand binding domain, a transmembrane domain, and an intracellular serine/threonine kinase domain. In the presence of TGF-β ligand and following binding to the TβRII homodimer, TβRII complexes with and phosphorylates TβRI within a conserved 30 amino acid segment known as the GS region (GSGS) [23]. Phosphorylation at this GS site results in the activation of TβRI kinase activity and subsequent phosphorylation of TGF-β signal transducers: the Smad family proteins [19,24–27].

2.3   Smad Proteins

Smad proteins are a family of transcription factors that are divided into three structure/function subcategories: the receptor-regulated Smads (R-Smads), the common-partner

Smad (Co-Smad) and the inhibitory Smads (I-Smads). In total, there are eight Smad family members: Smad1–8 [28]. Smads1, 5 and 8 mediate bone morphogenic protein (BMP) signals, however, and are generally not relevant to TGF-β signaling. Smad proteins have a highly conserved MH1 domain at the N-terminus and a highly conserved MH2 domain at the C-terminus. The MH1 domain facilitates Smad binding to DNA, namely the promoters of target genes (○ Fig. 17-2). The MH2 domain has been shown to mediate Smad transcriptional activity, oligomerization and protein-protein interactions with receptors and nuclear co-factors [19,23,26,27]. Smads2 and 3 have been shown to have intrinsic nuclear import activity in the MH2 domain [29]. In a dormant state, the Smads are primarily localized to the cytoplasm, which ensures their active response to activated receptors. The cytoplasmic retention of Smads2 and 3 is facilitated by the binding of the protein to the Smad anchor for receptor activation (SARA) protein [30]. In addition to tethering the Smads in the cytoplasm, bound SARA prevents exposure of the nuclear import signal in the Smad MH2 domain [29] and aids in the presentation of Smads to activated receptors [30].

Following binding with and activation by TβRII, TβRI directly phosphorylates the R-Smads, Smad2 and Smad3, at their C-terminal SSXS motif [10,12,31–34]. The phosphory-lated R-Smads then heterodimerize with the Co-Smad, Smad4, and the resulting complex is translocated to the nucleus. The exact mechanisms behind Smad nuclear translocation are still unknown, however one report by Xu et al. (2002) suggests the shuttling is dependent on nucleoporins [35]. Once in the nucleus, the complex is free to modulate gene transcription in conjunction with co-activators and co-repressors such as AP-1, FAST, TFE3, p300/CBP and Ski [19,22,24,25,27,36]. It is the specific interactions of the Smad complex with these nuclear factors that facilitates the specificity and complexity of TGF-β signaling (○ Fig. 17-1). These

■ Fig. 17-2

Smad protein domain structures. (a) Shown are schematic representations of the R-Smads (Smad2/3) and Co-Smad (Smad4) structural domains. Domain structures are labeled and include the MH1 domain (DNA binding), the MH2 domain (oligomerization and protein-protein interactions) and the proline tyrosine (PY, PPXY) motif (ubiquitination site). (b) In an unphosphorylated state, the MH1 and MH2 domains of the R-Smads are folded such that their activity is inhibited. Following phosphorylation of the SSXS motif by activated TβRI, the protein is unfolded and free to interact with the Co-Smad.

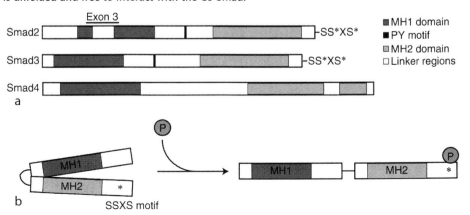

nuclear factors are required for Smad genetic regulation because, although Smads are able to bind to DNA on their own, their affinity for the Smad cognate sequence is too low to achieve unassisted binding to DNA [37].

The I-Smads (Smad6 and Smad7) act to inhibit activation of Smad2 and Smad3 phosphorylation [38]. This inhibition is enhanced by Smad7 associating proteins such as STRAP, p300, the Yes-Associated Protein 65 (YAP65), Smurf1/2 and GADD34/PP1c [39–43]. I-Smads have been shown to be transcriptional targets of the TGF-β pathway, suggesting they also function in a negative-feedback loop to modulate TGF-β signaling.

2.4 Smad4

The Co-Smads associate with the R-Smads after TGF-β receptor activation and prior to Smad complex nuclear accumulation. Smad4 is the only known member of the Co-Smad family in humans and mice. Despite being structurally similar to the R-Smads, Smad4 is unable to become phosphorylated by the TβRI receptor and contains a nuclear export signal that prevents nuclear localization in the absence of agonist stimulation [44]. Smad4 is not required for the nuclear accumulation of Smad complexes, but it is required for the formation of active transcriptional complexes [45]. Gene activation is mediated by the presence of a Smad binding motif (CAGAC) and nuclear Smad-interacting DNA binding proteins mentioned above. Ultimately, Smad4 is essential for the specific binding of these nuclear proteins to their consensus DNA binding sites and subsequent TGF-β-induced gene regulation.

2.5 Consequences of Normal TGF-β Signaling

TGF-β has been shown to affect cell growth and differentiation by enhancing the proliferation of mesenchymal cells while inhibiting the proliferation of epithelial cells [34,46]. The TGF-β-mediated growth inhibition is due to suppression of the G1 phase of the cell cycle via several mechanisms [47–49]. One mechanism is by the TGF-β-dependent up-regulation of cyclin-dependent kinase (CDK) inhibitors (● Fig. 17-3). The CDK inhibitors known to be affected by TGF-β include p16, p21Cip1, p27Kip1 and p15Ink4b [18,19,23]. p15Ink4b directly binds to CDK4/6 and interferes with cyclin D-CDK4/6 complex formation, while simultaneously inducing the redistribution of p27Kip1 from the cyclin D-CDK4 complex to the cyclin E-CDK2 complex, leading also to CDK2 inhibition. p21Cip1 directly inhibits the activity of cyclin E-CDK2. Induction of these CDK inhibitors by TGF-β contributes to the accumulation of a hypophosphorylated (active) form of the retinoblastoma protein (pRb), a key regulator of the G1-S transition [50,51].

A second mechanism of TGF-β-dependent cell cycle arrest is by the suppression of the cell cycle machinery. The list of suppressed cell cycle players includes c-Myc, Cdc25A [52,53], cyclin E [54,55], cyclin A [56–58], Cdc2 [59,60] CDK2 and CDK4 [47–49,54,61–63]. Also, in one report by Kornmann et al. (1999), TGF-β1-dependent growth inhibition was shown to be associated with an increase in cyclin D1 levels [64] but this observation may be a peculiarity of that particular cell line. Some of these effects on the cell cycle machinery are likely cell-type specific and/or secondary events to global G1 inhibition [18].

◘ Fig. 17-3

Direct cell cycle effects of TGF-β signaling. (a) During normal cellular proliferation, CDK/cyclin complexes are upregulated following induction by mitogenic growth factors. The ensuing activation of CDKs facilitates the hyperphosphorylation and inactivation of pRb. This leads to the release and subsequent binding of E2F to E2F consensus sites in the genome. In cooperation with basal transcriptional machinery, this binding by E2F promotes the transcription of genes associated with S-phase progression including cyclin E, E2F-1, cdc-25 (controls entry and progression through cell cycle), cyclin A, dihydrofolate reductase and thymidine kinase. (b) Smad4 is activated in response to TGF-β signaling and subsequently upregulates cyclin-dependent kinase inhibitors p16, p15, p27 and p21. These proteins inhibit the activity of the cdk/cyclin complexes, allowing for the accumulation of hypophosphorylated (active) Rb. Active Rb sequesters E2F, thereby inhibiting E2F-mediated transcriptional activity and promoting G1 cell cycle arrest.

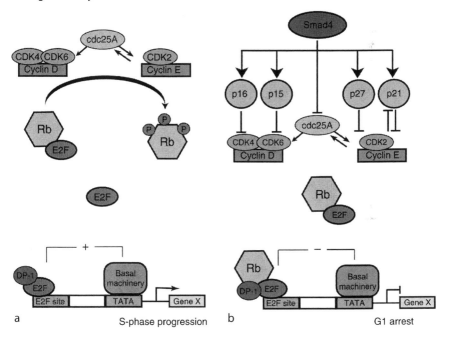

2.6   TGF-β in Normal Development

TGF-β1 is thought to be an important regulator of pancreatic organogenesis, due to the effects on both exocrine and endocrine pancreas when it is altered during development [65]. At embryonic day 12.5, TGF-β1 is expressed solely in the embryonic pancreatic epithelium and is devoid of expression in the mesenchyme. Approaching embryonic day 15.5, TGF-β1 mRNA begins to localize to the developing acini at modest levels. Towards the end of gestation, TGF-β1 is upregulated and then becomes essential for terminal acinar differentiation. This upregulation may also be important for islet formation and inhibition of proliferation of pluripotent cell growth [66].

To determine the specific roles for TGF-β in pancreatic development, transgenic mice were developed which expressed a dominant-negative form of TβRII, thereby inactivating TGF-β signaling [67]. The mice developed increased proliferation in the acinar cells combined with reduced acinar differentiation. The mice also developed fibrosis, inflammatory infiltration into the pancreas and acute neo-angiogenesis. These results indicate that TGF-β negatively controls the growth of acinar cells and is essential for acinar differentiation in the developing exocrine pancreas.

Another important role for TGF-β is in the regulation of epithelial-mesenchymal interactions. Treatment of cells with follistatin, a TGF-β and activin antagonist, was shown to decrease the differentiation of endocrine cells and promote embryonic exocrine cell differentiation [68]. Conversely, the induction of TGF-β signaling in embryonic mouse pancreas led to the formation of endocrine cells [69], the disruption of epithelial branching and the reduced formation of acinar cells [68]. Thus, TGF-β is a key player in the developing pancreas due to its ability to regulate cross-talk between the epithelium and mesenchyme. This function becomes important in tumorigenesis, as well.

2.7   TGF-Beta Signaling in the Adult Pancreas

TGF-βs are known to be expressed at low levels in both the exocrine and endocrine compartments of the normal pancreas [22]. TGF-β1 is specifically expressed in both the developing and adult pancreas. The endocrine islets show expression of both TGF-β2 and TGF-β3. The ductal cells are equally positive for all three TGF-β isoforms, while the acinar cells also stain for all three isoforms but show predominance towards TGF-β1 [70]. Additionally, TGF-β signaling is known to elicit an immunosuppressive response. Thus, TGF-βs may also act to inhibit harmful immune-mediated attacks against the endocrine or exocrine pancreas.

2.8   Smad-Independent Pathways of TGF-β

In addition to its canonical roles, TGF-β can signal independently of Smad-mediated transcription (❯ *Fig. 17-4*). Some of the pathways affected include the ERK, JNK and p38 MAPK kinase pathways. Cells that are deficient in Smad4 or express mutated TβRII (that are deficient in Smad signaling) were able to activate p38 signaling in response to TGF-β [71,72]. Kinetics studies suggest that the activation of pathways with slow kinetics may depend on Smad-dependent transcription while rapid activation may occur independently of transcription [73].

The specific mechanisms guiding Smad-independent pathway signaling by TGF-β are not well understood. *In vitro* studies suggest that Ras, MAPK kinase kinases, TGF-β-activated kinase 1 (TAK1), X-linked inhibitor of apoptosis (XIAP), MEKK1, and NF-κB may all be players in TGF-β-mediated Smad-independent signaling [74].

These signals may also be important feedback loops for the canonical TGF-β pathway. Activation of the ERK and JNK pathways by TGF-β results in the regulation of the Smad family proteins [71,75]. Smad4 is activated in response to TGF-β-dependent signaling through the MAPK pathway [76]. MAPK effectors were also shown to interact with Smad-interacting nuclear transcription factors (e.g., c-Jun and ATF-2) following TGF-β [73,77].

Smad4-independent signaling is an important factor in the overall cellular response to TGF-β. Signaling through the p38/MAPK pathway allows TGF-β to regulate epithelial-to-mesenchymal differentiation and enhances its pro-invasion effects. The associations

⬛ Fig. 17-4

Smad dependent and independent pathways of TGF-β signaling. The activated TGF-β receptor complex signals both through Smad-dependent (right side of figure) and Smad-independent (left side of figure) pathways, resulting in the activation of multiple signaling pathways and the regulation of important cellular functions. Details and references are cited in the text.

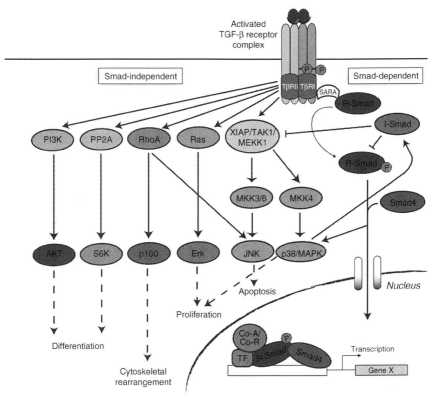

between the TGF-β and the mitogenic pathways can also be counteractive. Smad6 can down-regulate the activity of TAK1 [78] while Smad7 can promote the activation of JNK [79]. Conversely, c-Jun is known to inhibit Smad2 signaling (through interaction with Smad co-repressors) in a JNK-dependent manner [80]. Therefore, it is ultimately the balance between the Smad and MAPK signaling pathways that ultimately defines the outcome of TGF-β signaling in a cell.

3   TGF-β and Pancreatic Cancer

3.1   Noted Alterations

Both precursor and malignant lesions of the pancreas express TGF-β1, suggesting a role for it in pancreatic tumorigenesis. Similarly to normal epithelium, TGF-βs act as tumor suppressors in the early stages of pancreatic tumorigenesis [18]. Cultured pancreatic cancer cells, on the other hand, demonstrate an attenuated response towards TGF-β-mediated growth inhibition [49,81–84] and the expression of TGF-β at later stages of cancer progression fosters a more aggressive phenotype. This apparent dichotomy is the subject of much debate and the detailed mechanisms contributing to this functional "switch" remain to be elucidated. A number of alterations in the TGF-β signaling pathway are suggested to contribute to the resistance to TGF-β-mediated growth inhibition by cancer cells.

The overexpression of TGF-β correlates with pancreatic cancer progression and other malignancies [85,86]. TGF-β1 was shown to be differentially expressed in increasing grades of PanIN lesions and in PDAC, all three mammalian TGF-β isoforms have been shown to be expressed at high levels in the cancer cells by both protein and RNA. That elevated expression also associated with advanced stage and poor survival of PDAC patients [87]. The expression of these isoforms is capable of exerting paracrine growth-promoting properties that enhance tumor angiogenesis, growth and metastasis. Additionally, cancer cells have been shown to secrete higher amounts of TGF-β than their normal cell counterparts resulting in high levels of the TGF-β ligand in the tumor-associated microenvironment and tumor stroma. The reduced levels of circulating TGF-β isoforms in patient serum was also shown to be associated with prolonged survival [88]. These data suggest a possible role for altered epitheli-al-mesenchymal interactions by TGF-β signaling in pancreatic tumorigenesis. TβRII is also known to be overexpressed in PDAC and correlate with advanced tumor stage [89], decreased patient survival [90] and increased expression of genes known to promote angiogenesis and invasion (e.g., plasminogen activator 1 and matrix-metalloproteinase-9) [91]. Additionally, high levels of Smad2 have been documented in PDAC [91], leading to a more potent response to TGF-β signals.

In addition to overexpression of TGF-β components, loss-of-function or deletion altera-tions in the TGF-β signaling pathway have been documented. Smad4 mutations are the most frequent TGF-β alteration in PDAC [92], followed by decreased TβRI expression [84,93], increased TβRII expression, overexpression of I-Smads [94,95] and rarely mutations in TβRI/TβRII [96]. The net result of these alterations is a loss of the negative growth constraints imposed by TGF-β signaling at later stages in PDAC progression and may prove to be the basis for the dichotomy behind TGF-β.

3.2   Smad4 and Pancreatic Cancer

The mutation or deletion of Smad4 is one of the best characterized disruptions of TGF-β signaling in pancreatic cancers [92,97,98]. It has been estimated that 50–60% of all pancreatic cancer patients have alterations in Smad4, leading to aberrant cell cycle regulation by TGF-β [99,100]. As one of the first novel candidate tumor suppressors identified in pancreatic cancer, the original name for *Smad4* was *DPC4* (*deleted in pancreatic carcinoma locus 4*) [97]. Homozygous deletion of *Smad4* has been estimated for approximately 30% of cases while allelic loss of the *Smad4* chromosome (18q) is found in about 90% of all pancreatic cancers [101]. Inactivating mutations of Smad4 occurs in approximately 20% of all pancreatic cancer and are typically within either the MH1 (DNA binding) or MH2 (transcriptional activation) domains of the protein. Documented mutations include deletion of the entire chromosome and a combination of point, frame-shift, nonsense and missense mutations. Missense mutations found within the MH2 domain typically result in the loss of stability and disruption of the dimerization ability of the Smads [102]. Further, a study by Xu et al. (2000) found that mutated

Smad4 proteins with an arginine mutation in the MH1 domain are translated at similar rates as wild type proteins, but are degraded more rapidly by a ubiquitin-mediated pathway [102].

A juvenile polyposis syndrome (JPS) co-segregates with the transmission of germline defects in *Smad4*. JPS is an autosomal dominant disorder in which patients have an increased risk of gastrointestinal cancers and have widespread intestinal polyps [103]. Occasionally, *Smad4* mutations have been found in conjunction with *TβRI* and *TβRII* mutations in biliary [96] and colon cancer [104], respectively. Deletion of Smad4 in pancreatic cancer cell lines leads to the alteration of genes that modulate multiple biological functions, including ECM remodeling, cell adhesion, membrane transport, signaling transduction, intracellular transport, metabolism and transcriptional regulation [105]. These observations suggest that Smad4 may have nonoverlapping tumor suppressive functions with the TGF-β receptors.

Murine knockout studies have been performed for Smad4. Homozygous deletion of *Smad4* was embryonic lethal, with mutants dying before day 7.5 of embryogenesis [106]. Mutant embryos were shown to be smaller, to not express a mesodermal marker and to have abnormal visceral endoderm development. Further, it was concluded that the *Smad4* knockout embryos had reduced cellular proliferation (not increased apoptosis). These results suggested that Smad4 is specifically required for the differentiation of the visceral endoderm. Additionally, it was determined that Smad4 has an important role in anterior patterning during embryogenesis, as rescue experiments resulted in embryos with severe anterior truncations. In contrast, *Smad4* heterozygotes are viable and developed gastric polyps that progress into full tumors later in life [107].

Despite its prevalence in pancreatic cancer, Smad4 re-expression may not be a viable therapeutic option. The presence of Smad4 *in vitro* was associated with a prolonged doubling time and an enhanced sensitivity to TGF-β-mediated growth inhibition [108]. Smad4 re-expression *in vitro* was also shown to induce a TGF-β-independent angiogenic response which correlated with a decrease in vascular endothelial growth factor (VEGF) and increase in thrombospondin-1, leading to reduced tumor formation and vascular density [109]. Also, experiments in human cervical cancer cell lines showed that Smad4 re-expression led to transcriptional induction of ECM-associated genes in response to TGF-β, without alteration of classical TGF-β cell cycle targets (e.g., p21, p15 and c-myc) [110]. Similarly, in a nude mouse model of PDAC, the initial re-expression of *Smad4* in Smad4 deficient tumor cells was found to be associated with an immediate elongation of the lag phase of *in vivo* tumor growth [108]. The prolonged lag phase was attributed to restoration of the TGF-β signaling pathway and reduced proliferative capacity in Smad4 expressing cells. Following the initial delay, however, the Smad4-expressing tumors exhibited renewed growth and proliferation, indicating that cells are able to escape the growth suppressive effects of a reactivated TGF-β pathway. Taken together, these observations suggest that Smad4 re-expression may not necessarily be sufficient to inhibit tumor growth in the pancreatic setting and that Smad4 growth inhibitory actions are circumvented in later stages of pancreatic tumorigenesis.

3.3 TGF-β and Acute Pancreatitis

There is enhanced expression of TGF-βs in acute pancreatitis in humans [111] as well as in rodent models [112]. Interestingly, the administration of the pancreatic secretagogue caerulein, which binds and activates the cholecystokinin (CCK) receptor, to transgenic mice that are heterozygous for a dominant negative TβRII (called FVB) results in a markedly attenuated inflammatory response in comparison to that observed in wild type mice [113]. Caerulein injection in wild type mice resulted in 6- and 36-fold increases in serum amylase and lipase levels, respectively, as well as increased serum trypsinogen activation peptide (TAP) levels, gross edema and a marked inflammatory response in the pancreas that consisted mainly of neutrophils and macrophages. There was an associated increase in TGF-β1 mRNA levels in pancreas of these mice [113]. By contrast, FVB heterozygous mice exhibited minimal alterations in response to caerulein, with attenuated neutrophil-macrophage infiltrates and a blunted increase in TGF-β1 mRNA levels [113]. Moreover, pancreatic acini from FVB heterozygotes did not exhibit restricted stimulation at high caerulein concentrations, even though CCK receptor mRNA levels were not decreased. Thus, a functional TGF-β signaling pathway may be required for caerulein to induce acute pancreatitis, for the CCK receptor to induce acinar cell damage at high ligand concentrations and for the injury response to lead to TGF-β1 up-regulation.

3.4   TGF-β and Chronic Pancreatitis

Several studies have emphasized the potential role of chronic pancreatitis, which may occur in the context of repeated episodes of acute pancreatitis, in the pathobiology of PDAC in humans [114–116], as well as in mouse models of this malignancy [117]. Given the abundance of TGF-β in chronic pancreatitis and PDAC, its marked up-regulation in acute pancreatitis, and the important role of TGF-β in stem and progenitor self renewal, it is not surprising that aberrant TGF-β signaling pathways could be viewed as contributing to the genesis of PDAC. In addition, activated pancreatic stellate cells (PSCs) are known to be key contributors to stroma formation and fibrosis in both chronic pancreatitis and PDAC. In the normal pancreas, PSCs consist of approximately 4% of the total cell population and are located in the inter-acinar spaces. Recent studies have drawn correlations between PSCs and progenitor cells. For instance, stellate cells were shown to express the stem cell markers nestin and CD133 [118] and rat pancreatic stellate cells were able to differentiate *in vitro* into lineages from all three germ layers [119]. PSCs require a progenitor phenotype because their normal role is as part of a healing process after pancreatic injury. Activated PSCs also inhibit matrix metallioproteases-3 and -9, thereby enhancing fibrogenesis by reducing collagen degradation [120]. It is the perpetuation of these activated PSCs in response to CP and PDAC that are thought to promote tumor pathobiology.

The TGF-β pathway is thought to be a key activator of PSC activation. Thus, the elevated TGF-β levels in the pancreas of patients with CP lead to PSC activation and proliferation, functioning in both autocrine and paracrine pathways to activate Smads2 and 3 in these cells [121]. Additionally, a potential mediator of PSC activation and well-established target gene of TGF-β is connective tissue growth factor (CTGF). CTGF is upregulated in PDAC [122] and binds to α5β1 integrin and heparan sulphate proteoglycan receptors [123], thereby stimulating PSC adhesion and migration.

4   Translational Implications

4.1   Overview

The use of new and emerging therapies is crucial in the battle against PDAC. The Food and Drug Administration recently approved the use of erlontinib, an inhibitor of the tyrosine kinase activity of the epidermal growth factor (EGF) receptor, in combination with gemcitabine, a nucleoside analogue. Gemcitabine is converted intracellularly to active metabolites difluor-odeoxycytidine di- and triphosphate (dFdCDP, dFdCTP), which both inhibit ribonucleotide reductase and decrease the amount of deoxynucleotide that is available for DNA synthesis. In addition, dFdCTP is incorporated into DNA, resulting in DNA strand termination and apopto-sis. It is currently used as a first-line therapy and radiosensitizer in the treatment of pancreatic cancer [124]. The combined use of gemcitabine and elontinib improved the median survival by 0.5 month (5.9 mo. of gemcitabine alone vs. 6.4 mo. of combination) [125]. Due to the prevalence of TGF-β alterations in pancreatic cancer, similar targeting of TGF-β pathways at the receptor and ligand level, or at the level of their downstream gene targets, may yield more promising results.

4.2   Blocking TGF-β Actions in Models of PDAC

Several approaches have been used to suppress the paracrine actions of TGF-βs. These approaches include the use of antisense strategies to inhibit TGF-β synthesis [126,127] and anti-TGF-β neutralizing antibodies to block the action of TGF-β [128]. Efforts have also been made to express a mutated form of the TGF-β1 precursor, thereby inhibiting the mature processing of all three TGF-β isoforms [129]. In addition, small molecule inhibitors that target the kinase activity of TβRI have been tested [130]. In all cases, the blockade of TGF-β actions was sufficient to reduce cellular proliferation *in vitro*, and attenuate tumor growth and metastasis *in vivo*.

Investigators have also used the expression of soluble TβRII or TβRIII to sequester free TGF-β ligand [131,132]. When use of a soluble TβRII was explored, tumor growth and metastasis was found to be attenuated in both a subcutaneous or orthotopic model of pancreatic cancer [133,134]. The treated tumors were also found to have less angiogenesis and impaired expression of genes associated with growth and metastasis (e.g., plasminogen activator inhibitor 1 and urokinase plasminogen activator) [133,134]. These results suggest that the observed TGF-β overexpression in pancreatic cancer has both proliferative and angiogenic paracrine effects *in vivo*. Due to the far-spanning biology of the TGF-β pathway, it has been suggested that additional paracrine effects might include the modification of the composition of the extracellular matrix (ECM), stimulation of fibroblast and stellate cell proliferation and the suppression of cancer-directed immune mechanisms.

Another mechanism by which TGF-β signaling can be implemented to attack PDAC would be the manipulation of known TGF-β gene targets. One such attempt was made by blocking the action of connective tissue growth factor (CTGF). As mentioned above, CTGF is up-regulated by TGF-β and is known to be overexpressed in PDAC [122]. *In vitro*, CTGF increases pancreatic cell proliferation and invasion [135]. *In vivo*, blocking CTGF by an antibody (e.g., FG-3019) reduces tumor growth, metastasis and angiogenesis in an orthotopic mouse model of pancreatic cancer [136]. These results indicate that the blockage of TGF-β molecular targets may prove to be therapeutic in the treatment of PDAC.

4.3   TGF-β in the Clinic?

Due to its complexity, the TGF-β signaling pathway contains multiple options for intervention by targeted therapies in patients [37,137–139]. For instance, interference with the physical binding of active TGF-β ligand to its receptor could be achieved by preventing the formation of processed and active TGF-β ligand, by scavenging circulating TGF-β with excess binding proteins (e.g., latency-associated protein), or by blocking receptor binding using an inhibitory antibody. Small molecule inhibitors might be targeted to the intracellular portions of TGF-β receptors, thus inhibiting signal transduction, or degradation of TGF-β isoforms using antisense technology could be employed. Pharmacologic and/or biological inhibitors (e.g., FKBP12 and TRAP-1) could be used to inhibit the kinase activity of activated TGF-β receptors. Alternatively, elevated expression of the I-Smads would prevent phosphorylation of Smads2 and 3, thereby eliminating TGF-β signaling. As all of these options are viable approaches to the inhibition of the pro-cancer effects of TGF-β, continued investigation is needed to evaluate clinical relevance.

Currently, several efforts are underway to define the potential for TGF-β inhibition in PDAC patients to improve survival. New TGF-β inhibitors are already being tested pre-clinically and, in a few instances, in human clinical trials. These new therapies are designed to block activity of or interrupt signaling by TGF-β in tumor cells or activated immune cell populations [128,140,141]. While early results are encouraging, the dichotomous role of TGF-β in tumorigenesis complicates the facile implementation of TGF-β inhibitors into clinical practice. The global suppression of TGF-β, while beneficial in terms of tumor reduction, has the potential to also affect TGF-β signaling in normal (or close-to-normal) tissue and thereby contribute to the formation of new tumors or hyperplasia. To circumvent this outcome, novel strategies should seek to target specific members of the TGF-β pathway which are known to play a role in tumor progression, while avoiding members that are involved in growth inhibition and cell cycle arrest. Continued research into the intricacies of TGF-β associated proteins will help to elucidate specific mechanisms for future targeted therapies. The possibility of devising therapies that target specific pathways that are known to be altered in pancreatic cancer may also lead to individualized therapies that are based on the specific alterations in the cancer of PDAC patients, thereby presenting new hope for efficient therapeutic modalities that minimize potential side effects.

4.4   The Future of TGF-β

As regulators of global cellular biology in virtually every cell type, maintenance of the TGF-β pathway is crucial to maintaining healthy growth. Therefore, it is not surprising that altered expression or regulation of TGF-β family members is a predisposition for aberrant physiological behavior and pathology [18]. New and exciting research is exploring the epigenetic aspects of TGF-β expression and signaling. Epigenetic modifications are emerging as important modulators of cellular biology and include a diverse set of regulators and mechanisms. The variability in epigenetics can be used to partly explain the discrete differences between cells that otherwise have identical genomes. The epigenetic regulation of the TGF-β signaling pathway and its downstream targets is currently poorly described and future studies in this area will surely reveal potential therapeutic targets in PDAC.

The complexity of TGF-β signaling is also the target of ongoing research. In addition to the canonical TGF-β/Smad pathways presented in this review, there is intricate and undefined cross-talk between TGF-β and other signaling pathways within the cell and surrounding microenvironment [74]. The mechanisms of regulation and downstream biological consequences of these signaling networks underscores the complex influences of the TGF-β superfamily in both normal development and tumorigenesis. Additionally, evidence has suggested that there are TGF-β-independent functions for the Smad proteins. The delineation of these functions is lacking and is likely an area of future research. All of these network and TGF-β-independent interactions are likely the reason for the acute toxicity witnessed after TGF-β targeted therapy and will need to be better understood before more efficacious and specific therapies can be designed.

Key Research Points

- The TGF-β pathway is responsible for a diverse range of physiological and cellular processes.
- TGF-β is a key regulator of normal pancreatic development and organogenesis.
- TGF-β signaling is aberrant in pancreatic cancer and associates with a more aggressive phenotype.
- Smad4 mutations are one of the most common and well-documented alterations of the TGF-β pathway in pancreatic cancer.

Future Scientific Directions

- The use of animal models of pancreatic cancer to delineate the specific roles of all members of the canonical TGF-β/Smad family in cancer initiation and development
- The characterization of epigenetic modifications regulating TGF-β signaling
- The continued elucidation of the intricate interactions between the TGF-β pathway and a multitude of other cellular signaling networks
- The investigation into TGF-β-independent functions of the Smad proteins

Clinical Implications

- Continued research into the biology governing TGF-β regulation will unveil new and more specific avenues for TGF-β targeted therapy in pancreatic cancer.
- Compounds and molecular therapeutics will need to be chosen based on their specificity for targeting the pro-tumorigenic properties of TGF-β signaling while sparing the "good" tumor suppressive outcomes.
- Knowledge of the spectrum of TGF-β alterations in an individualized setting may be used to help predict patient response to current anti-cancer therapy and/or the stage of their disease progression.

References

1. Gudjonsson B: Cancer of the pancreas. 50 years of surgery. Cancer 1987;60(9):2284–2303.
2. DiMagno EP, Reber HA, Tempero MA: AGA technical review on the epidemiology, diagnosis, and treatment of pancreatic ductal adenocarcinoma. American Gastroenterological Association. Gastroenterology 1999;117(6):1464–1484.
3. Ho CK, Kleeff J, Friess H, Buchler MW: Complications of pancreatic surgery. HPB (Oxford) 2005;7(2):99–108.

4. Buchler MW, Kleeff J, Friess H: Surgical treatment of pancreatic cancer. J Am Coll Surg 2007;205(4 Suppl): S81–86.

5. Hansel DE, Kern SE, Hruban RH: Molecular pathogenesis of pancreatic cancer. Annu Rev Genomics Hum Genet 2003;4:237–256.

6. Jiao L, Zhu J, Hassan MM, Evans DB, Abbruzzese JL, Li D: K-ras mutation and p16 and preproenkephalin promoter hypermethylation in plasma DNA of pancreatic cancer patients: in relation to cigarette smoking. Pancreas 2007;34(1):55–62.

7. Summy JM, Trevino JG, Baker CH, Gallick GE: c-Src regulates constitutive and EGF-mediated VEGF expression in pancreatic tumor cells through activation of phosphatidyl inositol-3 kinase and p38 MAPK. Pancreas 2005;31(3):263–274.

8. Greten FR, Weber CK, Greten TF, Schneider G, Wagner M, Adler G, et al.: Stat3 and NF-kappab activation prevents apoptosis in pancreatic carcinogenesis. Gastroenterology 2002;123(6):2052–2063.

9. Guo X, Friess H, Graber HU, Kashiwagi M, Zimmermann A, Korc M, et al.: KAI1 expression is up-regulated in early pancreatic cancer and decreased in the presence of metastases. Cancer Res 1996;56(21):4876–4880.

10. Korc M: Pathways for aberrant angiogenesis in pancreatic cancer. Mol Cancer 2003;2:8.

11. Truty MJ, Urrutia R: Basics of TGF-beta and pancreatic cancer. Pancreatology 2007;7(5–6):423–435.

12. Korc M: Role of growth factors in pancreatic cancer. Surg Oncol Clin N Am 1998;7(1):25–41.

13. Anzano MA, Roberts AB, Smith JM, Sporn MB, De Larco JE: Sarcoma growth factor from conditioned medium of virally transformed cells is composed of both type alpha and type beta transforming growth factors. Proc Natl Acad Sci USA 1983;80(20): 6264–6268.

14. Hogan BL: Bone morphogenetic proteins: multifunctional regulators of vertebrate development. Genes Dev 1996;10(13):1580–1594.

15. Massague J: TGF-beta signal transduction. Annu Rev Biochem 1998;67:753–791.

16. Raftery LA, Sutherland DJ: TGF-beta family signal transduction in Drosophila development: from Mad to Smads. Dev Biol 1999;210(2):251–268.

17. Padgett RW, Das P, Krishna S: TGF-beta signaling, Smads, and tumor suppressors. Bioessays 1998;20 (5):382–390.

18. Massague J, Blain SW, Lo RS: tgfbeta signaling in growth control, cancer, and heritable disorders. Cell 2000;103(2):295–309.

19. Shi Y, Massague J: Mechanisms of TGF-beta signaling from cell membrane to the nucleus. Cell 2003;113(6):685–700.

20. Derynck R, Akhurst RJ, Balmain A: TGF-beta signaling in tumor suppression and cancer progression. Nat Genet 2001;29(2):117–129.

21. Kingsley DM: The TGF-beta superfamily: new members, new receptors, and new genetic tests of function in different organisms. Genes Dev 1994;8(2):133–146.

22. Siegel PM, Massague J: Cytostatic and apoptotic actions of TGF-beta in homeostasis and cancer. Nat Rev Cancer 2003;3(11):807–821.

23. Derynck R, Feng XH: TGF-beta receptor signaling. Biochim Biophys Acta 1997;1333(2):F105–150.

24. Attisano L, Wrana JL: Signal transduction by the TGF-beta superfamily. Science 2002;296(5573): 1646–1647.

25. Massague J, Seoane J, Wotton D: Smad transcription factors. Genes Dev 2005;19(23):2783–2810.

26. Heldin CH, Miyazono K, ten Dijke P: TGF-beta signalling from cell membrane to nucleus through SMAD proteins. Nature 1997;390(6659):465–471.

27. Derynck R, Zhang Y, Feng XH: Smads: transcriptional activators of TGF-beta responses. Cell 1998;95 (6):737–740.

28. Derynck R, Gelbart WM, Harland RM, Heldin CH, Kern SE, Massague J, et al.: Nomenclature: vertebrate mediators of tgfbeta family signals. Cell 1996;87(2):173.

29. Xu L, Chen YG, Massague J: The nuclear import function of Smad2 is masked by SARA and unmasked by tgfbeta-dependent phosphorylation. Nat Cell Biol 2000;2(8):559–562.

30. Tsukazaki T, Chiang TA, Davison AF, Attisano L, Wrana JL: SARA, a FYVE domain protein that recruits Smad2 to the tgfbeta receptor. Cell 1998; 95(6):779–791.

31. Shi Y, Wang YF, Jayaraman L, Yang H, Massague J, Pavletich NP: Crystal structure of a Smad MH1 domain bound to DNA: insights on DNA binding in TGF-beta signaling. Cell 1998; 94(5):585–594.

32. Massague J, Wotton D: Transcriptional control by the TGF-beta/Smad signaling system. EMBO J 2000;19(8):1745–1754.

33. Murakami M, Nagai E, Mizumoto K, Saimura M, Ohuchida K, Inadome N, et al.: Suppression of metastasis of human pancreatic cancer to the liver by transportal injection of recombinant adenoviral NK4 in nude mice. Int J Cancer 2005;117 (1):160–165.

34. Gold LI: The role for transforming growth factor-beta (TGF-beta) in human cancer. Crit Rev Oncog 1999;10(4):303–360.

35. Xu L, Kang Y, Col S, Massague J: Smad2 nucleocytoplasmic shuttling by nucleoporins CAN/Nup214 and Nup153 feeds tgfbeta signaling complexes in the cytoplasm and nucleus. Mol Cell 2002;10(2): 271–282.

36. Feng XH, Derynck R: Specificity and versatility in tgf-beta signaling through Smads. Annu Rev Cell Dev Biol 2005;21:659–693.

37. Roberts AB, Wakefield LM: The two faces of transforming growth factor beta in carcinogenesis. Proc Natl Acad Sci U S A 2003;100(15):8621–8623.

38. ten Dijke P, Miyazono K, Heldin CH: Signaling inputs converge on nuclear effectors in TGF-beta signaling. Trends Biochem Sci 2000;25(2):64–70.

39. Datta PK, Moses HL: STRAP and Smad7 synergize in the inhibition of transforming growth factor beta signaling. Mol Cell Biol 2000;20(9):3157–3167.

40. Ferrigno O, Lallemand F, Verrecchia F, L'Hoste S, Camonis J, Atfi A, et al.: Yes-associated protein (YAP65) interacts with Smad7 and potentiates its inhibitory activity against TGF-beta/Smad signaling. Oncogene 2002;21(32):4879–4884.

41. Monteleone G, Del Vecchio Blanco G, Monteleone I, Fina D, Caruso R, Gioia V, et al.: Post-transcriptional regulation of Smad7 in the gut of patients with inflammatory bowel disease. Gastroenterology 2005;129(5):1420–1429.

42. Ogunjimi AA, Briant DJ, Pece-Barbara N, Le Roy C, Di Guglielmo GM, Kavsak P, et al.: Regulation of Smurf2 ubiquitin ligase activity by anchoring the E2 to the HECT domain. Mol Cell 2005;19(3):297–308.

43. Shi W, Sun C, He B, Xiong W, Shi X, Yao D, et al.: GADD34-PP1c recruited by Smad7 dephosphorylates tgfbeta type I receptor. J Cell Biol 2004;164(2):291–300.

44. Watanabe M, Masuyama N, Fukuda M, Nishida E: Regulation of intracellular dynamics of Smad4 by its leucine-rich nuclear export signal. EMBO Rep 2000;1(2):176–182.

45. Shi Y, Hata A, Lo RS, Massague J, Pavletich NP: A structural basis for mutational inactivation of the tumour suppressor Smad4. Nature 1997;388(6637):87–93.

46. Roberts AB: Molecular and cell biology of TGF-beta. Miner Electrolyte Metab 1998;24(2–3):111–119.

47. Boyer Arnold N, Korc M: Smad7 abrogates transforming growth factor-beta1-mediated growth inhibition in COLO-357 cells through functional inactivation of the retinoblastoma protein. J Biol Chem 2005;280(23):21858–21866.

48. Ravitz MJ, Wenner CE: Cyclin-dependent kinase regulation during G1 phase and cell cycle regulation by TGF-beta. Adv Cancer Res 1997;71:165–207.

49. Kleeff J, Korc M: Up-regulation of transforming growth factor (TGF)-beta receptors by TGF-beta1 in COLO-357 cells. J Biol Chem 1998;273(13):7495–7500.

50. Laiho M, DeCaprio JA, Ludlow JW, Livingston DM, Massague J: Growth inhibition by TGF-beta linked to suppression of retinoblastoma protein phosphorylation. Cell 1990;62(1):175–185.

51. Herrera RE, Makela TP, Weinberg RA: TGF beta-induced growth inhibition in primary fibroblasts requires the retinoblastoma protein. Mol Biol Cell 1996;7(9):1335–1342.

52. Iavarone A, Massague J: Repression of the CDK activator Cdc25A and cell-cycle arrest by cytokine TGF-beta in cells lacking the CDK inhibitor p15. Nature 1997;387(6631):417–422.

53. Iavarone A, Massague J: E2F and histone deacetylase mediate transforming growth factor beta repression of cdc25a during keratinocyte cell cycle arrest. Mol Cell Biol 1999;19(1):916–922.

54. Geng Y, Weinberg RA: Transforming growth factor beta effects on expression of G1 cyclins and cyclin-dependent protein kinases. Proc Natl Acad Sci U S A 1993;90(21):10315–10319.

55. Reddy KB, Hocevar BA, Howe PH: Inhibition of G1 phase cyclin dependent kinases by transforming growth factor beta 1. J Cell Biochem 1994;56(3):418–425.

56. Ralph D, McClelland M, Welsh J: RNA fingerprinting using arbitrarily primed PCR identifies differentially regulated rnas in mink lung (Mv1Lu) cells growth arrested by transforming growth factor beta 1. Proc Natl Acad Sci USA 1993;90(22):10710–10714.

57. Satterwhite DJ, Aakre ME, Gorska AE, Moses HL: Inhibition of cell growth by TGF beta 1 is associated with inhibition of B-myb and cyclin A in both BALB/MK and Mv1Lu cells. Cell Growth Differ 1994;5(8):789–799.

58. Feng XH, Filvaroff EH, Derynck R: Transforming growth factor-beta (TGF-beta)-induced down-regulation of cyclin A expression requires a functional TGF-beta receptor complex. Characterization of chimeric and truncated type I and type II receptors. J Biol Chem 1995;270(41):24237–24245.

59. Landesman Y, Pagano M, Draetta G, Rotter V, Fusenig NE, Kimchi A: Modifications of cell cycle controlling nuclear proteins by transforming growth factor beta in the hacat keratinocyte cell line. Oncogene 1992;7(8):1661–1665.

60. Eblen ST, Fautsch MP, Burnette RJ, Joshi P, Leof EB: Cell cycle-dependent inhibition of p34cdc2 synthesis by transforming growth factor beta 1 in cycling epithelial cells. Cell Growth Differ 1994;5(2):109–16.

61. Ewen ME, Sluss HK, Whitehouse LL, Livingston DM: TGF beta inhibition of Cdk4 synthesis is linked to cell cycle arrest. Cell 1993;74(6):1009–1020.

62. Koff A, Ohtsuki M, Polyak K, Roberts JM, Massague J: Negative regulation of G1 in mammalian cells: inhibition of cyclin E-dependent kinase by TGF-beta. Science 1993;260(5107):536–539.

63. Senderowicz AM: Inhibitors of cyclin-dependent kinase modulators for cancer therapy. Prog Drug Res 2005;63:183–206.

64. Kornmann M, Tangvoranuntakul P, Korc M: TGF-beta-1 up-regulates cyclin D1 expression in

COLO-357 cells, whereas suppression of cyclin D1 levels is associated with down-regulation of the type I TGF-beta receptor. Int J Cancer 1999;83(2): 247–254.

65. Ellenrieder V, Fernandez Zapico ME, Urrutia R: tgfbeta-mediated signaling and transcriptional regulation in pancreatic development and cancer. Curr Opin Gastroenterol 2001;17(5):434–440.

66. Crisera CA, Maldonado TS, Kadison AS, Li M, Alkasab SL, Longaker MT, et al.: Transforming growth factor-beta 1 in the developing mouse pancreas: a potential regulator of exocrine differentiation. Differentiation 2000;65(5):255–259.

67. Bottinger EP, Jakubczak JL, Roberts IS, Mumy M, Hemmati P, Bagnall K, et al.: Expression of a dominant-negative mutant TGF-beta type II receptor in transgenic mice reveals essential roles for TGF-beta in regulation of growth and differentiation in the exocrine pancreas. EMBO J 1997;16 (10):2621–2633.

68. Ritvos O, Tuuri T, Eramaa M, Sainio K, Hilden K, Saxen L, et al.: Activin disrupts epithelial branching morphogenesis in developing glandular organs of the mouse. Mech Dev 1995;50(2–3):229–245.

69. Sanvito F, Herrera PL, Huarte J, Nichols A, Montesano R, Orci L, et al.: TGF-beta 1 influences the relative development of the exocrine and endocrine pancreas in vitro. Development 1994;120(12): 3451–3462.

70. Yamanaka Y, Friess H, Buchler M, Beger HG, Gold LI, Korc M: Synthesis and expression of transforming growth factor beta-1, beta-2, and beta-3 in the endocrine and exocrine pancreas. Diabetes 1993;42 (5):746–756.

71. Engel ME, McDonnell MA, Law BK, Moses HL: Interdependent SMAD and JNK Signaling in Transforming Growth Factor-beta -mediated Transcription. J. Biol. Chem 1999;274(52):37413–37420.

72. Yu L, Hebert MC, Zhang YE: TGF-beta receptor-activated p38 MAP kinase mediates Smad-independent TGF-beta responses. EMBO J 2002;21 (14):3749–3759.

73. Massague J: How cells read TGF-[beta] signals. Nat Rev Mol Cell Biol 2000;1(3):169–178.

74. Derynck R, Zhang YE: Smad-dependent and Smad-independent pathways in TGF-beta family signalling. Nature 2003;425(6958):577–584.

75. Kretzschmar M, Doody J, Timokhina I, Massague J: A mechanism of repression of tgfbeta/Smad signaling by oncogenic Ras. Genes Dev 1999;13(7):804–816.

76. Yue J, Mulder KM: *Activation of the Mitogen-Activated Protein Kinase Pathway by Transforming Growth Factor-β*, in *Transforming Growth Factor-Beta Protocols*. 2000. p. 125–131.

77. Itoh S, Itoh F, Goumans MJ, Ten Dijke P: Signaling of transforming growth factor-beta family members through Smad proteins. Eur J Biochem 2000;267 (24):6954–6967.

78. Kimura N, Matsuo R, Shibuya H, Nakashima K, Taga T: BMP2-induced Apoptosis Is Mediated by Activation of the TAK1-p38 Kinase Pathway That Is Negatively Regulated by Smad6. J. Biol. Chem 2000;275(23):17647–17652.

79. Mazars A, Lallemand F, Prunier C, Marais J, Ferrand N, Pessah M, et al.: Evidence for a Role of the JNK Cascade in Smad7-mediated Apoptosis. J. Biol. Chem 2001;276(39):36797–36803.

80. Pessah M, Marais J, Prunier C, Ferrand N, Lallemand F, Mauviel A, et al.: c-Jun Associates with the Oncoprotein Ski and Suppresses Smad2 Transcriptional Activity. J. Biol. Chem 2002;277(32): 29094–29100.

81. Beauchamp RD, Lyons RM, Yang EY, Coffey RJ, Jr., Moses HL: Expression of and response to growth regulatory peptides by two human pancreatic carcinoma cell lines. Pancreas 1990;5(4): 369–380.

82. Baldwin RL, Korc M: Growth inhibition of human pancreatic carcinoma cells by transforming growth factor beta-1. Growth Factors 1993;8(1):23–34.

83. Friess H, Kleeff J, Korc M, Buchler MW: Molecular aspects of pancreatic cancer and future perspectives. Dig Surg 1999;16(4):281–290.

84. Wagner M, Kleeff J, Lopez ME, Bockman I, Massaque J, Korc M: Transfection of the type I TGF-beta receptor restores TGF-beta responsiveness in pancreatic cancer. Int J Cancer 1998;78(2): 255–260.

85. Derynck R, Jarrett JA, Chen EY, Eaton DH, Bell JR, Assoian RK, et al.: Human transforming growth factor-beta complementary DNA sequence and expression in normal and transformed cells. Nature 1985;316(6030):701–705.

86. Glynne-Jones E, Harper ME, Goddard L, Eaton CL, Matthews PN, Griffiths K: Transforming growth factor beta 1 expression in benign and malignant prostatic tumors. Prostate 1994;25(4):210–218.

87. Friess H, Yamanaka Y, Buchler M, Ebert M, Beger HG, Gold LI, et al.: Enhanced expression of transforming growth factor beta isoforms in pancreatic cancer correlates with decreased survival. Gastroenterology 1993;105(6):1846–1856.

88. Bellone G, Smirne C, Mauri FA, Tonel E, Carbone A, Buffolino A, et al.: Cytokine expression profile in human pancreatic carcinoma cells and in surgical specimens: implications for survival. Cancer Immunol Immunother 2006;55(6):684–698.

89. Lu Z, Friess H, Graber HU, Guo X, Schilling M, Zimmermann A, et al.: Presence of two signaling TGF-beta receptors in human pancreatic cancer correlates with advanced tumor stage. Dig Dis Sci 1997;42(10):2054–2063.

90. Wagner M, Kleeff J, Friess H, Buchler MW, Korc M: Enhanced expression of the type II transforming growth factor-beta receptor is associated with decreased survival in human pancreatic cancer. Pancreas 1999;19(4):370–376.

91. Kleeff J, Friess H, Simon P, Susmallian S, Buchler P, Zimmermann A, et al.: Overexpression of Smad2 and colocalization with TGF-beta1 in human pancreatic cancer. Dig Dis Sci 1999;44(9):1793–1802.

92. Hahn SA, Schutte M, Hoque AT, Moskaluk CA, da Costa LT, Rozenblum E, et al.: DPC4, a candidate tumor suppressor gene at human chromosome 18q21.1. Science 1996;271(5247):350–353.

93. Baldwin RL, Friess H, Yokoyama M, Lopez ME, Kobrin MS, Buchler MW, et al.: Attenuated ALK5 receptor expression in human pancreatic cancer: correlation with resistance to growth inhibition. Int J Cancer 1996;67(2):283–288.

94. Kleeff J, Maruyama H, Friess H, Buchler MW, Falb D, Korc M: Smad6 suppresses TGF-beta-induced growth inhibition in COLO-357 pancreatic cancer cells and is overexpressed in pancreatic cancer. Biochem Biophys Res Commun 1999;255(2):268–273.

95. Arnold NB, Ketterer K, Kleeff J, Friess H, Buchler MW, Korc M: Thioredoxin is downstream of Smad7 in a pathway that promotes growth and suppresses cisplatin-induced apoptosis in pancreatic cancer. Cancer Res 2004;64(10):3599–3606.

96. Goggins M, Shekher M, Turnacioglu K, Yeo CJ, Hruban RH, Kern SE: Genetic alterations of the transforming growth factor beta receptor genes in pancreatic and biliary adenocarcinomas. Cancer Res 1998;58(23):5329–5332.

97. Hahn SA, Hoque AT, Moskaluk CA, da Costa LT, Schutte M, Rozenblum E, et al.: Homozygous deletion map at 18q21.1 in pancreatic cancer. Cancer Res 1996;56(3):490–494.

98. Riggins GJ, Thiagalingam S, Rozenblum E, Weinstein CL, Kern SE, Hamilton SR, et al.: Mad-related genes in the human. Nat Genet 1996;13(3):347–349.

99. Jaffee EM, Hruban RH, Canto M, Kern SE: Focus on pancreas cancer. Cancer Cell 2002;2(1):25–28.

100. Wilentz RE, Hruban RH: Pathology of cancer of the pancreas. Surg Oncol Clin N Am 1998;7(1):43–65.

101. Furukawa T, Sunamura M, Horii A: Molecular mechanisms of pancreatic carcinogenesis. Cancer Sci 2006;97(1):1–7.

102. Xu J, Attisano L: Mutations in the tumor suppressors Smad2 and Smad4 inactivate transforming growth factor beta signaling by targeting Smads to the ubiquitin-proteasome pathway. Proc Natl Acad Sci USA 2000;97(9):4820–4825.

103. Howe JR, Roth S, Ringold JC, Summers RW, Jarvinen HJ, Sistonen P, et al.: Mutations in the SMAD4/DPC4 gene in juvenile polyposis. Science 1998;280(5366):1086–1088.

104. Grady WM, Myeroff LL, Swinler SE, Rajput A, Thiagalingam S, Lutterbaugh JD, et al.: Mutational inactivation of transforming growth factor beta receptor type II in microsatellite stable colon cancers. Cancer Res 1999;59(2):320–324.

105. Cao D, Ashfaq R, Goggins M, Hruban RH, Kern SE, Iacobuzio-Donahue CA: Differential Expression of Multiple Genes in Association with MADH4/DPC4/SMAD4 Inactivation in Pancreatic Cancer. Int J Clin Exp Pathol 2008;1(6):510–517.

106. Sirard C, de la Pompa JL, Elia A, Itie A, Mirtsos C, Cheung A, et al.: The tumor suppressor gene Smad4/Dpc4 is required for gastrulation and later for anterior development of the mouse embryo. Genes Dev 1998;12(1):107–119.

107. Xu X, Brodie SG, Yang X, Im YH, Parks WT, Chen L, et al.: Haploid loss of the tumor suppressor Smad4/Dpc4 initiates gastric polyposis and cancer in mice. Oncogene 2000;19(15):1868–1874.

108. Yasutome M, Gunn J, Korc M: Restoration of Smad4 in bxpc3 pancreatic cancer cells attenuates proliferation without altering angiogenesis. Clin Exp Metastasis 2005;22(6):461–473.

109. Schwarte-Waldhoff I, Volpert OV, Bouck NP, Sipos B, Hahn SA, Klein-Scory S, et al.: Smad4/DPC4-mediated tumor suppression through suppression of angiogenesis. Proc Natl Acad Sci USA 2000;97(17):9624–9629.

110. Klein-Scory S, Zapatka M, Eilert-Micus C, Hoppe S, Schwarz E, Schmiegel W, et al.: High-level inducible Smad4-reexpression in the cervical cancer cell line C4-II is associated with a gene expression profile that predicts a preferential role of Smad4 in extracellular matrix composition. BMC Cancer 2007;7:209.

111. Friess H, Lu Z, Riesle E, Uhl W, Brundler AM, Horvath L, et al.: Enhanced expression of TGF-betas and their receptors in human acute pancreatitis. Ann Surg 1998;227(1):95–104.

112. Riesle E, Friess H, Zhao L, Wagner M, Uhl W, Baczako K, et al.: Increased expression of transforming growth factor beta s after acute oedematous pancreatitis in rats suggests a role in pancreatic repair. Gut 1997;40(1):73–79.

113. Wildi S, Kleeff J, Mayerle J, Zimmermann A, Bottinger EP, Wakefield L, et al.: Suppression of transforming growth factor beta signalling aborts caerulein induced pancreatitis and eliminates restricted stimulation at high caerulein concentrations. Gut 2007;56(5):685–692.

114. Lowenfels AB, Maisonneuve P, Cavallini G, Ammann RW, Lankisch PG, Andersen JR, et al.:

Pancreatitis and the risk of pancreatic cancer. International Pancreatitis Study Group. N Engl J Med 1993;328(20):1433–1437.

115. Farrow B, Sugiyama Y, Chen A, Uffort E, Nealon W, Mark Evers B: Inflammatory mechanisms contributing to pancreatic cancer development. Ann Surg 2004;239(6):763–769; discussion 9–71.

116. Whitcomb DC: Inflammation and Cancer V. Chronic pancreatitis and pancreatic cancer. Am J Physiol Gastrointest Liver Physiol 2004;287(2): G315–319.

117. Guerra C, Schuhmacher AJ, Canamero M, Grippo PJ, Verdaguer L, Perez-Gallego L, et al.: Chronic pancreatitis is essential for induction of pancreatic ductal adenocarcinoma by K-Ras oncogenes in adult mice. Cancer Cell 2007;11(3):291–302.

118. Lardon J, Rooman I, Bouwens L: Nestin expression in pancreatic stellate cells and angiogenic endothelial cells. Histochemistry and Cell Biology 2002;117 (6):535–540.

119. Kruse C, Kajahn J, Petschnik AE, Maaß A, Klink E, Rapoport DH, et al.: Adult pancreatic stem/progenitor cells spontaneously differentiate in vitro into multiple cell lineages and form teratoma-like structures. Annals of Anatomy - Anatomischer Anzeiger 2006;188(6):503–517.

120. Shek FW, Benyon RC, Walker FM, McCrudden PR, Pender SL, Williams EJ, et al.: Expression of transforming growth factor-beta 1 by pancreatic stellate cells and its implications for matrix secretion and turnover in chronic pancreatitis. Am J Pathol 2002;160(5):1787–1798.

121. Ohnishi H, Miyata T, Yasuda H, Satoh Y, Hanatsuka K, Kita H, et al.: Distinct roles of Smad2-, Smad3-, and ERK-dependent pathways in transforming growth factor-beta1 regulation of pancreatic stellate cellular functions. J Biol Chem 2004;279(10):8873–8878.

122. Wenger C, Ellenrieder V, Alber B, Lacher U, Menke A, Hameister H, et al.: Expression and differential regulation of connective tissue growth factor in pancreatic cancer cells. Oncogene 1999;18(4): 1073–1080.

123. Gao R, Brigstock DR: Connective Tissue Growth Factor (CCN2) in Rat Pancreatic Stellate Cell Function: Integrin [alpha]5[beta]1 as a Novel CCN2 Receptor. Gastroenterology 2005;129(3): 1019–1030.

124. Crane C, Janjan N, Evans D, Wolff R, Ballo M, Milas L, et al.: Toxicity and Efficacy of Concurrent Gemcitabine and Radiotherapy for Locally Advanced Pancreatic Cancer. Int J Gastrointest Cancer 2001;29(1):9–18.

125. Moore MJ: Brief communication: a new combination in the treatment of advanced pancreatic cancer. Semin Oncol 2005;32(6 Suppl 8):5–6.

126. Fitzpatrick DR, Bielefeldt-Ohmann H, Himbeck RP, Jarnicki AG, Marzo AL, Robinson BW: Transforming growth factor-beta: antisense RNA-mediated inhibition affects anchorage-independent growth, tumorigenicity and tumor-infiltrating T-cells in malignant mesothelioma. Growth Factors 1994;11 (1):29–44.

127. Marzo AL, Fitzpatrick DR, Robinson BW, Scott B: Antisense oligonucleotides specific for transforming growth factor beta2 inhibit the growth of malignant mesothelioma both in vitro and in vivo. Cancer Res 1997;57(15):3200–3207.

128. Hoefer M, Anderer FA: Anti-(transforming growth factor beta) antibodies with predefined specificity inhibit metastasis of highly tumorigenic human xenotransplants in nu/nu mice. Cancer Immunol Immunother 1995;41(5):302–308.

129. Lopez AR, Cook J, Deininger PL, Derynck R: Dominant negative mutants of transforming growth factor-beta 1 inhibit the secretion of different transforming growth factor-beta isoforms. Mol Cell Biol 1992;12(4):1674–1679.

130. Halder SK, Beauchamp RD, Datta PK: A specific inhibitor of TGF-beta receptor kinase, SB-431542, as a potent antitumor agent for human cancers. Neoplasia 2005;7(5):509–521.

131. Won J, Kim H, Park EJ, Hong Y, Kim SJ, Yun Y: Tumorigenicity of mouse thymoma is suppressed by soluble type II transforming growth factor beta receptor therapy. Cancer Res 1999;59(6): 1273–1277.

132. Bandyopadhyay A, Zhu Y, Cibull ML, Bao L, Chen C, Sun L: A soluble transforming growth factor beta type III receptor suppresses tumorigenicity and metastasis of human breast cancer MDA-MB-231 cells. Cancer Res 1999;59(19): 5041–5046.

133. Rowland-Goldsmith MA, Maruyama H, Kusama T, Ralli S, Korc M: Soluble type II transforming growth factor-beta (TGF-beta) receptor inhibits TGF-beta signaling in COLO-357 pancreatic cancer cells in vitro and attenuates tumor formation. Clin Cancer Res 2001;7(9):2931–2940.

134. Rowland-Goldsmith MA, Maruyama H, Matsuda K, Idezawa T, Ralli M, Ralli S, et al.: Soluble type II transforming growth factor-beta receptor attenuates expression of metastasis-associated genes and suppresses pancreatic cancer cell metastasis. Mol Cancer Ther 2002;1(3):161–167.

135. Hartel M, Di Mola FF, Gardini A, Zimmermann A, Di Sebastiano P, Guweidhi A, et al.: Desmoplastic reaction influences pancreatic cancer growth behavior. World J Surg 2004;28(8):818–825.

136. Aikawa T, Gunn J, Spong SM, Klaus SJ, Korc M: Connective tissue growth factor-specific antibody attenuates tumor growth, metastasis, and

angiogenesis in an orthotopic mouse model of pancreatic cancer. Mol Cancer Ther 2006;5(5): 1108–1116.

137. Akhurst RJ, Derynck R: TGF-beta signaling in cancer–a double-edged sword. Trends Cell Biol 2001;11(11):S44–51.

138. Marten A, Buchler MW: Immunotherapy of pancreatic carcinoma. Curr Opin Investig Drugs 2008;9(6):565–569.

139. Yingling JM, Blanchard KL, Sawyer JS: Development of TGF-beta signalling inhibitors for cancer therapy. Nat Rev Drug Discov 2004;3 (12):1011–1022.

140. Wojtowicz-Praga S, Verma UN, Wakefield L, Esteban JM, Hartmann D, Mazumder A: Modulation of B16 melanoma growth and metastasis by anti-transforming growth factor beta antibody and interleukin-2. J Immunother Emphasis Tumor Immunol 1996;19(3):169–175.

141. Arteaga CL, Hurd SD, Winnier AR, Johnson MD, Fendly BM, Forbes JT: Anti-transforming growth factor (TGF)-beta antibodies inhibit breast cancer cell tumorigenicity and increase mouse spleen natural killer cell activity. Implications for a possible role of tumor cell/host TGF-beta interactions in human breast cancer progression. J Clin Invest 1993;92(6):2569–2576.

18 Notch Signaling in Pancreatic Morphogenesis and Pancreatic Cancer Pathogenesis

Gwen Lomberk · Raul Urrutia

1   Introduction 442

2   Notch Receptor 443

3   Notch Ligand 445

4   Crosstalk with Other Signaling Cascades 446

5   Notch-TGFβ Interactions 447

6   Notch-VEGF Interactions 447

7   The Notch-Hes Pathway in Pancreatic Morphogenesis 448

8   Notch and Pancreatic Cancer 449

9   Pharmacological and Genetic Manipulation of the Notch Pathway 450

10 Concluding Remarks 451

J. P. Neoptolemos, R. Urrutia, J. L. Abbruzzese, M. W. Büchler (eds.), *Pancreatic Cancer*,
DOI 10.1007/978-0-387-77498-5_18, © Springer Science+Business Media, LLC 2010

Abstract: Notch signaling is becoming the focus of investigation in a large number of laboratories around the world due to its pleiotropic effect in regulating normal development and alterations in cancer. During the last decade, the scientific community studying this pathway has made significant contributions to our understanding of the cellular role of Notch signaling in regulating proliferation, differentiation, apoptosis, migration, branching morphogenesis, and angiogenesis. Similar to observations with other signaling cascades, such as TGBβ, besides its role in morphogenesis, Notch signaling becomes dysregulated in adult tissue and contributes to the development and maintenance of the cancer phenotype. Elegant studies in this field of research have lead to not only the better understanding of the molecules within the pathway, but as a consequence, rational design of drugs that can inhibit Notch signaling with promising results. The study of Notch signaling in the pancreas has dawned on solid ground and thus, we predict that in the next few years, a better understanding of the pathway at the mechanistic level, along with a strict testing of pharmacological antagonists, will advance the field of pancreatic cancer research in a significant manner.

1   Introduction

Notch signaling has elicited significant attention from the basic science community because of its ability to regulate normal morphogenesis in a conserved manner from flies to human. This remarkable conservation throughout the animal kingdom suggests that evolution has exercised a strong pressure for maintaining this morphogenetic cascade for millions of years, thus underscoring its importance for life. Developmentally, Notch signaling became first known as a robust mediator of lateral inhibition, a key patterning process that organizes the regular spacing of different cell types within tissues, including branching morphogenesis of a similar type as that observed in the pancreas [1–7]. In fact, several molecules from the Notch signaling pathway are potent regulator of normal pancreas organogenesis and/or neoplastic transformation in this organ [2–7]. Initially, the interest of Notch signaling as a modulator of disease states developed from studies of its role in hereditary diseases that result from abnormal morphogenesis, such as Alagille syndrome, spondylocostal dysostosis, and several cancers, all of which display aberrant ligand expression [8–14]. However, in the adult pancreas, Notch has also been shown to recapitulate some of its developmental functions, thus aiding in both regeneration [15] and the acquisition of the neoplastic phenotype [3–5,7,16]. As a result, the current concept is that Notch signaling is associated not only with pancreatic morphogenesis but also with the development and/or maintenance of the pancreatic cancer cell phenotype.

The attractiveness of studying this pathway for pancreatic cancer investigators is due to an increased need to better understand the pathobiological role of this type of signaling in pancreatic cancer along with the relative ease that exists for pharmacologically targeting this pathway. We believe that this increased understanding on how Notch signaling regulates an aggressive cancer phenotype in this organ, at the fine cellular and molecular level, is very promising to derive potential "biomolecular-based therapeutic modalities" that can be combined with the currently existing therapies to fight this disease. Thus, in the current chapter, we update the current knowledge that exists in the field of Notch signaling research, as well as develop a theoretical framework that covers the molecular to the pathobiological role of this biochemical cascade in pancreatic cells.

2   Notch Receptor

Receptors of the Notch family are cell-surface type I transmembrane proteins. Upon ligand binding, Notch receptors undergo successive proteolytic cleavages that lead to the release of the Notch Intra-Cellular Domain (NICD) (❯ Fig. 18-1) [4,14,17–19]. This cleaved notch intracellular domain is the active form of the receptor. In fact, several studies have shown that this pathway can be activated, in a ligand-independent manner, by simply overexpressing the NICD.

In order to better understand the mechanism of Notch signaling, it is important to remember the domain composition of this receptor since its interaction with other proteins,

⬛ Fig. 18-1

The Notch signaling pathway. The figure illustrates the key events in the Notch signaling pathway. Ligands of the delta and jagged families expressed on an adjacent signal-sending cell initiate the signal through Notch receptor recognition on the signal-receiving cell (a). This interaction between receptor and ligand leads to a cascade of proteolytic cleavages of the Notch receptor, beginning with metalloprotease cleavage just outside the membrane (b). This proteolytic step facilitates the subsequent intramembrane cleavage of Notch by the γ-secretase complex (c) to release the Notch intracellular domain (NICD) from the membrane. The NICD then translocates to the nucleus (d) and enters into a transcriptional activation complex with the transcription factor CSL along with co-activators, including Mastermind-like proteins (Maml) and CBP/p300, thereby activating transcription of target genes (e).

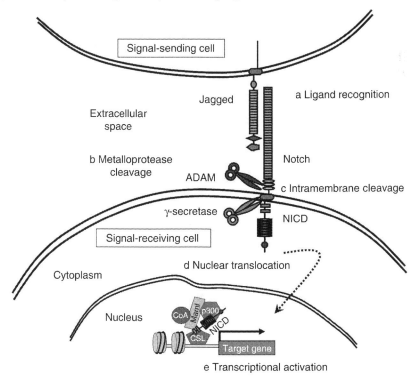

including ligands, depends upon this structural composition and domain organization [17]. Most notably, the extracellular domain of Notch is composed of 36 EGF repeats in vertebrates, though their number varies according to the organism being considered (⊙ *Fig. 18-2*). Another important motif includes three Lin12/Notch repeats. Careful biochemical analysis has demonstrated that the repeats 11 and 12 EGF function as binding sites for Delta and Serrate [20]. The Notch intracellular domain includes six ankyrin repeats and two classically basic residue-charged nuclear localization signals. The positions of the S1–S4 cleavage sites are crucial, since cleavage at these sites, which is achieved by the γ-secretase enzyme, releases the intracellular domain [21]. In turn, the intracellular domain subsequently migrates to the nucleus to function as a transcriptional regulator. Thus, this system appears to have evolved to mediate the characteristic long term transcriptional response that is necessary to trigger a hierarchical cascade of gene expression that is responsible of regulating cell differentiation, tissue remodeling, and morphogenesis.

⬛ Fig. 18-2

The human Notch receptors. Schematic diagram of the structural domain features of the human Notch receptors 1–4. The arrows mark the approximate locations of the cleavage sites for the ADAM metalloprotease and γ-secretase for release of the NICD. The double line represents the cellular membrane. The legend box identifies the graphic representation of each structural feature.

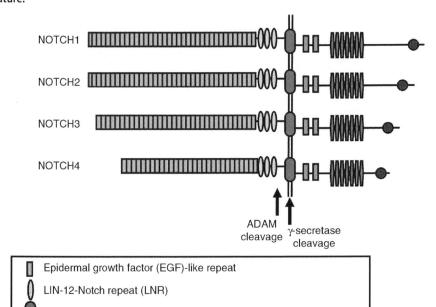

3   Notch Ligand

Initially, most of the mechanistic information gained about the Notch signaling pathway was gathered from experiments in *Drosophila melanogaster* [11,22]. The two ligands found as results of these experiments, Delta and Serrate, and Lag2, another molecule with similar domains, are known today as the canonical DSL (Delta, Serrate, Lag2) ligands, which are believed to be responsible for most Notch functions [20]. Noteworthy, however, nonca-nonical ligands have also been shown to activate Notch, though little is known about these pathways [23].

Similar to the Notch receptor, the canonical ligands are also type 1 cell-surface proteins containing tandem epidermal growth factor (EGF) repeats in their extracellular domains (◉ *Fig. 18-3*). The DSL domain, the N-terminal (NT) domain as well as the first two EGF repeats are required for binding of these ligands to Notch [24,25]. The mammalian canonical ligands are identified by their homology to the two *Drosophila* ligands, Delta and Serrate, and are designated as either Delta-like (Dll1, Dll3 and Dll4) or Serrate-like (Jagged1 and Jagged2)

◘ Fig. 18-3

The human DSL ligands. Schematic diagram of the structural domain features of the human DSL ligands for Notch with the double line representing the cellular membrane. The legend box identifies the graphic representation of each structural feature.

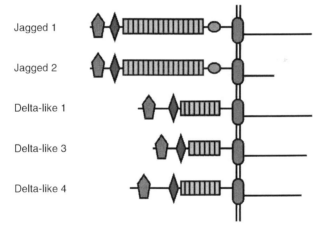

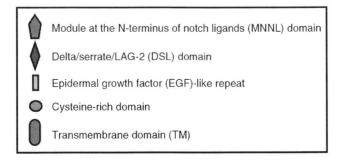

[20,26]. The intracellular domain of DSL ligands contain a C-terminal PDZ motif [27], which is required for signaling and interactions with the cytoskeleton. The currently accepted model for Notch signaling activation is initiated at the cell membrane by the DSL ligand expressed in one cell (signal-sending cell) and a Notch receptor (Notch1–4) expressed on another cell in close proximity (signal-receiving cell). Consequently, since cell-to-cell contact is necessary to activate this pathway, one can envision a Notch-bearing cell would be regulated by its neighboring cells expressing the Delta and Serrate ligands to achieve lateral inhibition. Lateral inhibition, as it has been classically described for early neuroblast differentiation, is a process in which Notch mediates reciprocal inhibitory signaling between neuroblasts that otherwise have a similar potential for cell phenotype determination [28]. In order to present Notch to its ligand, these molecules form heterodimers produced as a result of processing by a furin-like protease during transit to the plasma membrane [29,30]. Ligand binding initiates additional cleavages of Notch, first by a disintegrin and metalloprotease (ADAM) within the juxtamembrane region, followed by γ-secretase within the transmembrane domain, thereby resulting in the release of the Notch intracellular domain (❯ Fig. 18-1) [4,18]. γ-Secretase is made of four subunits, namely presenilin (PS), APH-1, nicastrin, and PEN-2. PS is the catalytic peptide, which provides the aspartyl protease activity to the entire complex [31]. Therefore, pharmacologically inhibiting this process, as is commonly done using γ-secretase via pharmacological inhibitors [32], can disrupt Notch signaling, raising the possibilities that tools of this type can be used to manipulate this pathway for therapeutic purposes, though its disruption is not necessarily cell specific and may have unwanted consequences.

Intracellular Signaling Molecules for the Notch Pathway: The first intracellular signaling peptide that must be considered the beginning of the Notch signaling pathway is, as mentioned above, the NICD which is produced by proteolytic cleavages of the receptors. This peptide translocates to the nucleus and associates with the CSL (CBF1/Su(H)/Lag-1) family of transcription factor complexes (❯ Fig. 18-1), resulting in subsequent activation of Notch target genes, such as *Myc*, *p21* and HES and Hey family members, via the mastermind-like transcriptional coactivators [33,34]. *Hes* and *Hey* genes are the mammalian counterparts of the Hairy and Enhancer-of-split type of genes in *Drosophila,* and they represent the primary targets of the Delta-Notch signaling pathway [18,35]. In this review, we primarily focus on describing the role of Hes proteins as Notch signaling molecules because of their role in pancreatic morphogenesis [3,36,37]. In mammals, there are seven members in the Hes family (Hes1–7), although Hes4 is absent in the mouse genome.

4 Crosstalk with Other Signaling Cascades

Continuous tissue remodeling during embryogenesis requires coordinated regulation among many signaling pathways to maintain the balance between proliferation and differentiation, stem cells and immature progenitor cells. Canonical Notch signaling has long been regarded as a signaling cascade that is sufficient for morphogenesis. However, recent studies have shown that Notch signaling can establish a crosstalk with other cascades in order to achieve its pleiotrophic effects [38–41]. Some of these pathways include Hedgehog, TGFβ, BMP, VEGF, and Wnt signaling. Following, we describe the crosstalk between Notch with TGFβ and VEGF signaling for two very important reasons; namely, these pathways are the best known Notch interactors, and they both play an important role in cancer-related functions, such as angiogenesis.

Interestingly, most of the data regarding the role of Notch in angiogenesis has been derived from experiments in animal models. For instance, mice in which *Notch1* has been disrupted, in the whole animal, by homologous recombination, are lethal at E10.5 because the primary vascular plexi in the yolk sac and brain undergo aberrant remodeling [42]. In addition, this phenotype also includes alterations in large vessels. Supporting the validity of this data, experiments performed using a vascular-specific knockout of *Notch1* displays remarkably similar defects [42]. Alterations in vascular biology have also been observed in genetically engineered animals expressing genes encoding proteins from the Notch signaling pathway [43–46]. For instance, knockout of a single allele of *dll4* leads to lethality at E9.5 due also to a failure in remodeling the primary vascular plexus. This phenotype is also recapitulated in jagged1-deficient mice and RBP-J–deficient mice. Additional experiments using a gain-of-function paradigm based on expressing the NICD have shown alterations in angiogenesis [47]. Thus, the role of Notch signaling in endothelial cell biology and angiogenesis is well-established.

5   Notch-TGFβ Interactions

As mentioned above, under defined circumstances, Notch signaling has been found to interact with TGFβ signaling. Members of the TGFβ family of cytokines form distinct signaling subfamilies, including TGFβ, BMPs, Activin, and Inhibin, among others. Signaling via these cytokines begins at the cell surface by activating distinct serine/threonine kinases, which in turn, transduce the intracellular signal to the nucleus through either Smad-dependent or independent mechanisms [48]. In endothelial cells, TGFβ induces cell migration while arresting proliferation [1]. In addition, many members of the TGFβ family of cytokines not only have the ability to display similar effects on endothelial cells, but also stimulate pericytes, which are critical for vessel formation [49]. Therefore, the role of these cytokines in angiogenesis is well-established.

In the past several years, emerging evidence supports a role for an interaction among these pathways in angiogenesis. For instance, TGFβ induces endothelial cell migration in a manner dependent upon a pathway that involves Jagged-1-Notch-Hey-1-Smad3 [50]. TGFβ-mediated arrest of cell proliferation has been found to require Notch signaling [39]. Many TGFβ-inducible genes require an additional stimulation with Notch to achieve full expression. Knock-out of the Notch ligand, Jagged-1, leads to a reduction of TGFβ-mediated induction of p21 and rescues the cell cycle arrest that is so characteristic of this pathway [51]. Lastly, signaling via the intracellular domain of certain Notch receptors has been found to interact with Smads from the BMP pathway and appear to participate in signaling by this cytokine [50,52].

6   Notch-VEGF Interactions

Basic evidence for an interaction between angiogenic factors and Notch signaling has been gathered by the observation that VEGF induces both Notch receptor and ligand [53,54]. For instance, Notch1 and dll4 are upregulated by VEGF, via both, VEGFR1 and VEGFR2, in human arterial cells [55]. This upregulation in Notch requires signaling through phosphatidylinositol

3-kinase/Akt, but not MAPK/ERK or src kinases. Interestingly, similar results have been found in the mouse retina, where VEGF induction of dll4 was demonstrated [56]. Administration of VEGF in mouse retinas increases expression of dll4, whereas injection of the VEGF antagonist, VEGF-Trap, downregulates the expression of this molecule. Noteworthy, however, dll4 in this situation forms part of a negative feedback loop where notch signaling upregulates HESR1 (HEY1), which then functionally interacts with SP1 sites to silence *VEGFR2* gene expression. At the cellular level, the dll4+/− phenotype increases filopodia and branching angiogenesis, which can be antagonized, at least partially, by reducing VEGF levels with sFlt1 (soluble VEGFR1 extracellular domain) or by blocking VEGFR2 using specific antibodies. These studies on dll4 in developing retina indicate that, in the presence of Notch signaling, cells may migrate toward a VEGF gradient in order to facilitate the initial steps of angiogenesis. Remarkably, subsequent downregulation of these signals correlate with subsequent steps in angiogenesis, such as anastomoses, tube formation, and vessel maturation. Lastly, the VEGF-Notch signaling interaction has been validated using zebrafish, *Danio rerio*, as an in vivo animal model [54]. In zebrafish, this pathway appears to underlie arteriovenous specification. In VEGF morphants, the dorsal aorta loses arterial markers, such as ephrin B2, and ectopically expresses the vein marker, Flt4. The aberrant arterial phenotype is rescued by activated Notch in VEGF morphants, but not conversely, by VEGF in Notch mutants. These experiments are extremely informative because, together, they locate Notch downstream of VEGF in zebrafish arterial specification.

7   The Notch-Hes Pathway in Pancreatic Morphogenesis

Through the analyses of many experiments performed in various organisms ranging from *Drosophila melanogaster* to human, Notch has been found to play several functions that are important for development, normal physiology and diseases. These functions include but are not limited to cell proliferation, cell differentiation, apoptosis, cell migration, angiogenesis, and branching morphogenesis. Having this concept in mind, in fact, allows us to understand how Notch is of significant importance for both, pancreatic development and carcinogenesis [4].

During development, the pancreas originates from the endodermal foregut epithelium as two primordial parts of the organ, namely the dorsal and ventral pancreatic buds, which fuse to form the entire gland. In both pancreatic buds, the epithelium gives rise to both exocrine and endocrine cells: exocrine progenitors become acinar cells, which secrete digestive enzymes, whereas endocrine cells emigrate from the epithelium to form islets. The liver and biliary systems also originate from the endodermal epithelium of the foregut. Together, this data indicate that both systems share a pattern of branch morphogenesis which is not only needed under physiological conditions but during cancer development both the biliary and pancreatic ducts give rise to similar type of cancers, both with an extremely aggressive behavior. Therefore, we can predict that both malignancies may, at least in part, overlap in the molecular mechanisms that give rise to and maintain their cancer phenotype.

At the molecular level, in the developing pancreas, the Ptf1a transcription factor promotes exocrine cell differentiation [57], whereas the bHLH gene, *Ngn3*, mediates the differentiation of all types of endocrine cells [58], including α (glucagon-producing), β (insulin-producing), δ (somatostatin-producing) and PP (pancreatic polypeptide-producing) cells. The role of the Notch pathway in this phenomenon can be better understood via its relationship with Ngn3.

The inactivation of the murine *Hes1* by homologous recombination triggers an upregulation of *Ngn3*, creating a bias toward endocrine cell differentiation and severe hypoplasia of the gland [59]. Further supporting a critical role of Notch in pancreatic development is the fact that similar phenotypes are observed after either knocking out the delta-like 1 (*Dll1*) ligand or the transcription factor that is an effector of Notch, namely RBP-J (Recombination Signal Sequence-Binding Protein) [5,7] showing accelerated differentiation of pancreatic endocrine cells, as well as by the overexpression of either *Ngn3* or the intracellular form of Notch3 (repressor of Notch signaling) [60]. Together, this data strongly suggests that the Dll1-Notch-RBP-J-Hes1 pathway inhibits premature endocrine differentiation.

Hes1 also antagonizes the function of Ptf1a, the master regulator of exocrine cell differentiation, by directly targeting the Ptf1a promoter and silencing its expression [2]. Moreover, expression of the intracellular domain of Notch inhibits acinar cell differentiation by antagonizing the function of Ptf1a [6,36]. Thus, in summary, Notch-Hes1 signaling promotes the maintenance of pancreatic progenitor cells by antagonizing Ptf1a and Ngn3. However, in Hes1-null mice, Ptf1a and Ngn3 are ectopically expressed in the common bile duct, leading to the formation of an ectopic pancreas [59]. Thus, this observation emphasizes that the biliary tree has similarity with the pancreatic buds at the molecular level, at least enough as to adopt a pancreas phenotype when key pancreas-specific regulators are expressed in these cells. This is not a trivial finding since this type of transdifferentiation is not a common event in every tissue type. Thus, both the biliary and the pancreas epithelium appear to go through a phase of "capacitation," in which the expression of key Notch-induced transcription factors is able to push their phenotype either way. The potential contribution of this concept to better understanding normal bile and pancreatic duct morphogenesis and their cancers is potentially very insightful, though it remains an underrepresented area of research.

Elegant studies in zebrafish have also been very useful for learning the role of Notch in pancreatic morphogenesis. For instance, activated Notch and Notch target genes impair zebrafish acinar cell differentiation [36]. In fact, strong evidence supporting a role for Notch in regulating exocrine pancreatic differentiation has been derived from this work on zebrafish embryos, in which Notch signaling is disrupted (homozygous *mindbomb* mutations) [36]. Mutant embryos appear to have accelerated exocrine pancreatic differentiation as compared with wild-type controls. Similar alterations were also observed after expressing a dominant negative *Suppressor of Hairless* [*Su(H)*]. Mechanistic studies, using transient transfection assays in COS7 cells involving a Ptf1-responsive reporter gene, demonstrated that Notch and Notch/Su(H) target genes directly inhibit Ptf1 activity. Thus, since Ptf1 is a critical regulator of acinar cell differentiation and zymogen gene expression, this work in zebrafish has not only defined a role for Notch in acinar cell differentiation, but also provides at least one mechanism by which this pathway functions.

8   Notch and Pancreatic Cancer

Many of the functions that Notch performs during embryonic development is found to be, to some extent, recapitulated during cancer. Consequently, after organogenesis, it is critical that this signaling pathway undergoes tight regulation in order to prevent aberrant signaling, which has the potential to lead to neoplastic transformation, as described in other organs. Notch either promotes or suppresses tumor growth depending upon the tumor type via its role in differentiation, proliferation, angiogenesis, and immune regulation [4]. This is one of the manners in which Notch behaves as potential tumor promotor. Another manner by which Notch signaling can mediate tumorigenesis is by acquiring activating mutations in members of this signaling pathway, such as the ones found in the Notch1 receptor in a high fraction of T-cell acute lymphoblastic leukemias and lymphomas [61].

Notch is also emerging as a mediator of cell transdifferentiation, also known as metaplasia [16,59]. This function is important for the pancreatic cancer field since frank ductal pancreatic adenocarcinoma is thought to originate in a multistep fashion where ductular-like preneoplastic lesions with metaplastic components, known as Pancreatic Intraepithelial Neoplasia (PanIN), progress by the accumulation of distinct mutations in oncogenes and tumor suppressor genes. Initial evidence for the re-expression of Notch signaling components in metaplasia of the pancreas was obtained through the use of genetically engineered mice (GEM). Mice overexpressing TGFα, as driven by the Elastase I promoter/enhancer in acininar cells, undergo a massive metaplasia where the pancreas can be often replaced by ductular-like structures, which have lost most of the acinar phenotype and are surrounded by a robust desmoplastic reaction [62]. These lesions undergo neoplastic transformation, a process that can be significantly speed up by crossing the mice with p53 null animals [63]. Interestingly, the expression of Notch receptors, ligands, and target genes is higher in metaplastic ducts than in adjacent normal appearing tissue in vivo and in organ explants exposed to TGFα. More importantly, however, is recent data, which demonstrates that a two- to threefold increase in Notch receptors, ligands, and downstream Notch target genes, in primary human pancreatic carcinoma samples [64,65]. Thus, together, the available evidence derived from work in both mice and human suggest a model in which the postnatal expression of Notch signaling molecules occurs in the metaplastic pancreatic epithelium, a phenomenon that correlates with cancer development.

Evidence of an upregulation of Notch signaling during pancreatic carcinogenesis has elicited interest in finding molecules, which by downregulating this pathway to normal levels may be useful in the therapy of pancreatic cancer. Several useful molecules already exist from previous studies on the biology of Notch signaling, such as γ-secretase inhibitors, though new agents are being investigated, as discussed further in the following section. For instance, recent reports using cultured pancreatic cancer cells have shown that in BxPC-3, HPAC, and PANC-1 pancreatic cancer cells, Notch-1 downregulation causes the upregulation of NF-κB, a potential downstream target of this pathway and induces apoptosis [66]. In this work, the authors found that naturally occurring molecules, such as genistein and curcumin (substances of great interest to the field of chemoprevention), are efficient in downregulating Notch signaling, thus adding to the arsenal of compounds that may serve as the foundation for developing several generations of new drugs, which can be tested for either the chemoprevention of pancreatic cancer at the PanIN stage or even later when a frank tumor develops.

9   Pharmacological and Genetic Manipulation of the Notch Pathway

Different types of small drugs, such as ADAM inhibitors, Notch antisense, anti-Notch monoclonal antibodies, RNA interference, and natural products, such as genistein and curcumin, as mentioned above, have been proposed for inhibiting Notch. Unfortunately, however, these agents have not reached clinical trials yet. The most promising and most widely tested manner of inhibiting Notch signaling is by using γ-Secretase Inhibitors (GSI); many of them at least being tested in preclinical trials for several cancers [10]. Again, before Notch becomes competent for signaling, it is processed by two important enzymes, furin-like activity and γ-secretase [18]. Thus, in theory, any manipulation that interferes with Notch processing in adult tissue should impair signaling by this pathway. Thus far, blocking the final cleavage of Notch mediated by the γ-secretase complex has been the most successful strategy for development of small drugs for therapeutic purposes [41]. A new line of drugs, collectively known as γ-secretase inhibitors (GSI), is being developed and is under intense testing. The idea of generating GSI was derived from the Alzheimer's field [67]. Interestingly, most γ-secretase inhibitors (GSI), tested to date, interfere with Notch receptor processing, thus supporting the hypothesis that these agents may be useful for the treatment of malignancies where Notch signaling is altered.

Relative specificity and high anti-Notch activity make GSIs promising as drugs that have the potential to soon pass the preclinical trial phase. The clinical use of GSIs, however, will develop from whether their benefits are out-shadowed by their side-effects. For instance, gastrointestinal toxicity has been recently reported [68]. Moreover, although chronic treatment with the GSI, LY-411,575, inhibits beta-amyloid peptide production, it produces complex side-effects, such as alterations in lymphopoiesis and intestinal cell differentiation. It remains to be determined whether the side-effects are related to disrupting the physiological effect of Notch signaling in normal adult tissues or to a lack of selectivity of GSIs, since the γ-secretase complex can process numerous different substrates in addition to Notch [31]. Therefore, an aggressive testing of these drugs, not only for their beneficial effects but also for their potential side-effects, is necessary before more conclusions can be reached about their potential usefulness in the therapy of any cancer.

10   Concluding Remarks

During the last decade a significant amount of information has been gained about Notch signaling. Studies initiated in model organisms such as the fruit fly provided a detailed understanding on how this pathway works at the biochemical level. Notch signaling has been associated with both normal morphogenesis and neoplastic transformation. Complementary studies in both zebrafish and mice have revealed the significant relevance of this pathway in normal pancreatic morphogenesis, as well as pancreatic cancer. Moreover, alterations in this pathway have been detected in human tissue. Thus, together, these studies put Notch signaling at the center of the signaling cascades which are important to study in the pancreas. Initial therapeutic promises to target this pathway come from studies on γ-secretase inhibitors. Unfortunately, these compounds have significant gastrointestinal side effects, which may limit their use until newer generations of these agents without this shortcoming are developed. Therefore, we still have to wait to see whether this strategy to manipulate Notch signaling will be beneficial for either chemoprevention or therapy of pancreatic cancer. In summary, the area of Notch signaling is an attractive, poorly understood, and promising area of investigation. Thus far, the data obtained in pancreas demonstrate that investigation of Notch signaling is of significant biomedical relevance and may help to better understand pancreatic cell homeostasis along with the development and maintenance of the pancreatic cancer phenotype.

Key Research Points

- Notch signaling is a master regulator of embryonic development in many cells and organisms. It is involved in the process of lateral inhibition where cell-to-cell contact between a signaling and a receiving cell determine fate outcome. In the exocrine pancreas, Notch is involved in acinar cell differentiation.
- Notch signaling interacts with key exocrine pancreatic transcription factors, like PTF-1, thus providing at least one mechanism by which this pathway specifies cell fate in this organ.
- Alterations in Notch signaling are a cause of several diseases, including certain malignancies. Notch is altered during the metaplastic progression that leads to pancreatic cancer and in ductal adenocarcinoma. These findings make Notch a potential therapeutic target for therapeutic interventions.

Future Scientific Directions

- Notch is involved in both pancreatic morphogenesis and pancreatic cancer. Fortunately, different types of animal models and model organisms exist to better understand the mechanism by which this pathway instructs these processes.
- Studies on crosstalk between Notch signaling with other cascades in pancreatic cells is very well-established for a few pathways. Therefore, expanding this area of research will provide a better understanding of pancreatic physiology and pathobiology.
- Historically, some of the knowledge on the Notch pathway that has been derived from studies in non-pancreatic cell systems has been directly applied to normal and neoplastic pancreatic cell biology. However, recent studies, which indicate that well-known mediators of the Notch pathway regulate pancreatic morphogenesis in a Notch independent manner, require a careful extrapolation of data from the literature and in depth molecular experimentation in the pancreas itself.

Clinical Implications

- Fortunately, prototype drugs have been derived from the knowledge gained on the biochemistry of Notch signaling. These include several protease inhibitors, in particular, the γ-secretase inhibitors (GSIs). The hope is that these research directions will ultimately lead to another molecularly targeted therapy for pancreatic cancer, such as the one developed for VEGF or EGF.
- GSIs, which are the major tool for manipulating Notch signaling in Alzheimer, are among the most advanced drugs in preclinical trials and early human trials. However, these drugs are not very specific, as γ-secretase cleaves numerous substrates besides Notch. Therefore, side effects are common. An improvement of these drugs using structural data, molecular modeling, and screening of combinatorial libraries derived from GSI-related compounds are necessary in order to achieve a higher therapeutic index.
- Since Notch deregulation appears to already occur at the preneoplastic stage (PanINs) and these lesions are very frequent in normal and pancreatitis patients, it remains to be explored if GSI or other small drugs that target this pathway are beneficial in the chemoprevention of pancreatic cancer.

Acknowledgments

Work in the author's laboratory (R.U.) is supported by funding from the National Institutes of Health DK 52913 and Mayo Clinic Pancreatic SPORE (P50 CA102701).

References

1. Horowitz A, Simons M: Branching morphogenesis. Circ Res 2008;103:784–795.

2. Ghosh B, Leach SD: Interactions between hairy/enhancer of split-related proteins and the pancreatic transcription factor Ptf1-p48 modulate function of the PTF1 transcriptional complex. Biochem J 2006;393:679–685.

3. Leach S: Epithelial differentiation in pancreatic development and neoplasia: new niches for nestin and Notch. J Clin Gastroenterol 2005;39:S78–S82.

4. Lomberk G, Fernandez-Zapico M, Urrutia R: When developmental signaling pathways go wrong and their impact on pancreatic cancer development. Curr Opin Gastroenterol 2005;21:555–560.

5. Masui T, Long Q, Beres T, Magnuson M, MacDonald R: Early pancreatic development requires the vertebrate suppressor of hairless (RBPJ) in the PTF1 bHLH complex. Genes Dev 2007;21:2629–2643.

6. Murtaugh LC, Stanger BZ, Kwan KM, Melton DA: Notch signaling controls multiple steps of pancreatic differentiation. Proc Natl Acad Sci USA 2003;100:14920–14925.

7. Nakhai H, Siveke J, Klein B, Mendoza-Torres L, Mazur P, Algul H, Radtke F, Strobl L, Zimber-Strobl U, Schmid R: Conditional ablation of Notch signaling in pancreatic development. Development 2008;135:2757–2765.

8. McDaniell R, Warthen DM, Sanchez-Lara PA, Pai A, Krantz ID, Piccoli DA, Spinner NB: NOTCH2 mutations cause Alagille syndrome, a heterogeneous disorder of the Notch signaling pathway. Am J Hum Gen 2006;79:169–173.

9. Miele L, Golde T, Osborne B: Notch signaling in cancer. Curr Mol Med 2006;6:905–918.

10. Miele L, Miao H, Nickoloff BJ: NOTCH signaling as a novel cancer therapeutic target. Curr Cancer Drug Targets 2006;6:313–323.

11. Talora C, Campese AF, Bellavia D, Felli MP, Vacca A, Gulino A, Screpanti I: Notch signaling and diseases: an evolutionary journey from a simple beginning to complex outcomes. Biochim Biophys Acta 2008;1782:489–497.

12. Turnpenny P, Alman B, Cornier A, Giampietro P, Offiah A, Tassy O, Pourquié O, Kusumi K, Dunwoodie S: Abnormal vertebral segmentation and the notch signaling pathway in man. Dev Dyn 2007;236:1456–1474.

13. Warthen D, Moore E, Kamath B, Morrissette J, Sanchez P, Piccoli D, Krantz I, Spinner N: Jagged1 (JAG1) mutations in Alagille syndrome: increasing the mutation detection rate. Hum Mutat 2006;27:436–443.

14. Watt FM, Estrach S, Ambler CA: Epidermal Notch signalling: differentiation, cancer and adhesion. Curr Opin Cell Biol 2008;20:171–179.

15. Siveke T, ÄìMartellato CL, Lee M, Mazur P, Nakhai H, Radtke F, Schmid R: Notch signaling is required for exocrine regeneration after acute pancreatitis. Gastroenterology 2008;134:544–555.

16. De La O J-P, Emerson LL, Goodman JL, Froebe SC, Illum BE, Curtis AB, Murtaugh LC: Notch and Kras reprogram pancreatic acinar cells to ductal intraepithelial neoplasia. Proc Natl Acad Sci USA 2008;105:18907–18912.

17. Fleming RJ: Structural conservation of Notch receptors and ligands. Semin Cell Dev Biol 1998;9:599–607.

18. Lomberk G, Urrutia R: Primers on molecular pathways – notch. Pancreatology 2008;8:103–104.

19. Wilson A, Radtke F: Multiple functions of Notch signaling in self-renewing organs and cancer. FEBS Lett 2006;580:2860–2868.

20. D'Souza B, Miyamoto A, Weinmaster G: The many facets of Notch ligands. Oncogene 2008;27:5148–5167.

21. LaVoie MJ, Selkoe DJ: The Notch ligands, jagged and delta, are sequentially processed by {alpha}-secretase and presenilin/{gamma}-secretase and release signaling fragments. J Biol Chem 2003;278:34427–34437.

22. Gonczy P: Mechanisms of asymmetric cell division: flies and worms pave the way. Nat Rev Mol Cell Biol 2008;9:355–366.

23. Gordon WR, Arnett KL, Blacklow SC: The molecular logic of Notch signaling – a structural and biochemical perspective. J Cell Sci 2008;121:3109–3119.

24. Parks AL, Stout JR, Shepard SB, Klueg KM, Dos Santos AA, Parody TR, Vaskova M, Muskavitch MAT: Structure-function analysis of delta trafficking, receptor binding and signaling in drosophila. Genetics 2006;174:1947–1961.

25. Shimizu K, Chiba S, Kumano K, Hosoya N, Takahashi T, Kanda Y, Hamada Y, Yazaki Y, Hirai H: Mouse jagged1 physically interacts with

Notch2 and other Notch receptors. Assessment by quantitative methods. J Biol Chem 1999;274: 32961–32969.

26. Fiuza U-M, Arias AM: Cell and molecular biology of Notch. J Endocrinol 2007;194:459–474.

27. Pintar A, De Biasio A, Popovic M, Ivanova N, Pongor S: The intracellular region of Notch ligands: does the tail make the difference? Biol Direct 2007;2:19.

28. Wheeler SR, Stagg SB, Crews ST: Multiple Notch signaling events control drosophila CNS midline neurogenesis, gliogenesis and neuronal identity. Development 2008;135:3071–3079.

29. Nichols J, Miyamoto A, Weinmaster G: Notch signaling: constantly on the move. Traffic 2007;8: 959–969.

30. Nichols JT, Miyamoto A, Olsen SL, D'Souza B, Yao C, Weinmaster G: DSL ligand endocytosis physically dissociates Notch1 heterodimers before activating proteolysis can occur. J Cell Biol 2007;176:445–458.

31. Steiner H, Fluhrer R, Haass C: Intramembrane proteolysis by {gamma}-secretase. J Biol Chem 2008;283:29627–29631.

32. Six E, Ndiaye D, Laabi Y, Brou C, Gupta-Rossi N, Israel A, Logeat F: The Notch ligand Delta1 is sequentially cleaved by an ADAM protease and gamma-secretase. Proc Natl Acad Sci USA 2003; 100:7638–7643.

33. Borggrefe T, Oswald F: The Notch signaling pathway: transcriptional regulation at Notch target genes. Cell Mol Life Sci 2009. Epub ahead of print.

34. McElhinny AS, Li JL, Wu L: Mastermind-like transcriptional co-activators: emerging roles in regulating cross talk among multiple signaling pathways. Oncogene 2008;27:5138–5147.

35. Fischer A, Gessler M: Delta Notch and then? Protein interactions and proposed modes of repression by Hes and Hey bHLH factors. Nucl Acids Res 2007;35:4583–4596.

36. Esni F, Ghosh B, Biankin AV, Lin JW, Albert MA, Yu X, MacDonald RJ, Civin CI, Real FX, Pack MA, Ball DW, Leach SD: Notch inhibits Ptf1 function and acinar cell differentiation in developing mouse and zebrafish pancreas. Development 2004;131: 4213–4224.

37. Kimura K, Satoh K, Kanno A, Hamada S, Hirota M, Endoh M, Masamune A, Shimosegawa T: Activation of Notch signaling in tumorigenesis of experimental pancreatic cancer induced by dimethylbenzanthracene in mice. Cancer Sci 2007;98:155–162.

38. Guo X, Wang X-F: Signaling cross-talk between TGF-[beta]/BMP and other pathways. Cell Res 2009;19:71–88.

39. Holderfield MT, Hughes CCW: Crosstalk between vascular endothelial growth factor, Notch, and transforming growth factor-{beta} in vascular morphogenesis. Circ Res 2008;102:637–652.

40. Krejcí A, Bernard F, Housden B, Collins S, Bray S: Direct response to Notch activation: signaling crosstalk and incoherent logic. Sci Signal 2009;2:ra1.

41. Shih I-M, Wang T-L: Notch signaling, {gamma}-secretase inhibitors, and cancer therapy. Cancer Res 2007;67:1879–1882.

42. Limbourg FP, Takeshita K, Radtke F, Bronson RT, Chin MT, Liao JK: Essential role of endothelial Notch1 in angiogenesis. Circulation 2005;111: 1826–1832.

43. Doi H, Iso T, Sato H, Yamazaki M, Matsui H, Tanaka T, Manabe I, Arai M, Nagai R, Kurabayashi M: Jagged1-selective Notch signaling induces smooth muscle differentiation via a rbp-j{kappa}-dependent pathway. J Biol Chem 2006;281:28555–28564.

44. Dufraine J, Funahashi Y, Kitajewski J: Notch signaling regulates tumor angiogenesis by diverse mechanisms. Oncogene 2008;27:5132–5137.

45. Gridley T: Notch signaling in vascular development and physiology. Development 2007;134:2709–2718.

46. Trindade A, Ram Kumar S, Scehnet JS, Lopes-da-Costa L, Becker J, Jiang W, Liu R, Gill PS, Duarte A: Overexpression of delta-like 4 induces arterialization and attenuates vessel formation in developing mouse embryos. Blood 2008;112:1720–1729.

47. MacKenzie F, Duriez P, Larrivee B, Chang L, Pollet I, Wong F, Yip C, Karsan A: Notch4-induced inhibition of endothelial sprouting requires the ankyrin repeats and involves signaling through RBP-J {kappa}. Blood 2004;104:1760–1768.

48. Truty M, Urrutia R: Basics of TGF-beta and pancreatic cancer. Pancreatology 2007;7:423–435.

49. Armulik A, Abramsson A, Betsholtz C: Endothelial/pericyte interactions. Circ Res 2005;97:512–523.

50. Blokzijl A, Dahlqvist C, Reissmann E, Falk A, Moliner A, Lendahl U, Ibanez CF: Cross-talk between the Notch and TGF-{beta} signaling pathways mediated by interaction of the Notch intracellular domain with Smad3. J Cell Biol 2003;163:723–728.

51. Niimi H, Pardali K, Vanlandewijck M, Heldin C-H, Moustakas A: Notch signaling is necessary for epithelial growth arrest by TGF-{beta}. J Cell Biol 2007;176:695–707.

52. Itoh F, Itoh S, Goumans M, Valdimarsdottir G, Iso T, Dotto G, Hamamori Y, Kedes L, Kato M, ten Dijke P: Synergy and antagonism between Notch and BMP receptor signaling pathways in endothelial cells. EMBO J 2004;23:541–551.

53. Thurston G, Kitajewski J: VEGF and delta-Notch: interacting signalling pathways in tumour angiogenesis. Br J Cancer 2008;99:1204–1209.

54. Siekmann AF, Lawson ND: Notch signalling limits angiogenic cell behaviour in developing zebrafish arteries. Nature 2007;445:781–784.

55. Banerjee S, Mehta S, Haque I, Sengupta K, Dhar K, Kambhampati S, Van Veldhuizen PJ, Banerjee SK: VEGF-A165 induces human aortic smooth muscle cell migration by activating Neuropilin-1-VEGFR1-PI3K Axis†. Biochemistry 2008;47: 3345–3351.

56. Lobov IB, Renard RA, Papadopoulos N, Gale NW, Thurston G, Yancopoulos GD,.Wiegand SJ: Delta-like ligand 4 (Dll4) is induced by VEGF as a negative regulator of angiogenic sprouting. Proc Natl Acad Sci USA 2007;104:3219–3224.

57. Jiang Z, Song J, Qi F, Xiao A, An X, Liu N-a, Zhu Z, Zhang B, Lin S: exdpf is a key regulator of exocrine pancreas development controlled by retinoic acid and ptf1a in Zebrafish. PLoS Biol 2008;6:e293.

58. Bernardo AS, Hay CW, Docherty K: Pancreatic transcription factors and their role in the birth, life and survival of the pancreatic [beta] cell. Mol Cell Endocrinol 2008;294:1–9.

59. Fukuda A, Kawaguchi Y, Furuyama K, Kodama S, Horiguchi M, Kuhara T, Kawaguchi M, Terao M, Doi R, Wright CVE, Hoshino M, Chiba T, Uemoto S: Reduction of Ptf1a gene dosage causes pancreatic hypoplasia and diabetes in mice. Diabetes 2008; 57:2421–2431.

60. Apelqvist A, Li H, Sommer L, Beatus P, Anderson DJ, Honjo T, de Angelis MH, Lendahl U, Edlund H: Notch signalling controls pancreatic cell differentiation. Nature 1999;400:877–881.

61. Pear W, Aster J: T cell acute lymphoblastic leukemia/lymphoma: a human cancer commonly associated with aberrant NOTCH1 signaling. Curr Opin Hematol 2004;11:426–433.

62. Miyamoto Y, Maitra A, Ghosh B, Zechner U, Argani P, Iacobuzio-Donahue CA, Sriuranpong V, Iso T, Meszoely IM, Wolfe MS, Hruban RH, Ball DW, Schmid RM, Leach SD: Notch mediates TGF [alpha]-induced changes in epithelial differentiation during pancreatic tumorigenesis. Cancer Cell 2003;3:565–576.

63. Wagner M, Greten F, Weber C, Koschnick S, 1 Torsten Mattfeldt T, Deppert W, Kern H, Adler G, Roland M, Schmid R: A murine tumor progression model for pancreatic cancer recapitulating the genetic alterations of the human disease. Genes Dev 2001;15(3):286–293.

64. Büchler P, Gazdhar A, Schubert M, Giese N, Reber H, Hines O, Giese T, Ceyhan G, Müller M, Büchler M, Friess H: The Notch signaling pathway is related to neurovascular progression of pancreatic cancer. Ann Surg 2005;242:791–800.

65. Doucas H, Mann C, Sutton C, Garcea G, Neal C, Berry D, Manson M: Expression of nuclear notch3 in pancreatic adenocarcinomas is associated with adverse clinical features, and correlates with the expression of STAT3 and phosphorylated Akt. J Surg Oncol 2008;97:63–68.

66. Wang Z, Zhang Y, Li Y, Banerjee S, Liao J, Sarkar FH: Down-regulation of Notch-1 contributes to cell growth inhibition and apoptosis in pancreatic cancer cells. Mol Cancer Ther 2006;5:483–493.

67. Wolfe M: Gamma-secretase modulators. Curr Alzheimer Res 2007;4:571–573.

68. Imbimbo B: Therapeutic potential of γ-secretase inhibitors and modulators. Curr Top Med Chem 2008;8:54–61.

19 Molecular Characterization of Pancreatic Cancer Cell Lines

David J. McConkey · Woonyoung Choi · Keith Fournier · Lauren Marquis · Vijaya Ramachandran · Thiruvengadam Arumugam

1	Introduction: Preclinical Models of Pancreatic Cancer	458
2	Common Assumptions About Established Cell Lines	459
2.1	"Cell Lines Are Genetically Scrambled"	459
2.2	"The Effects of Drugs on Cancer Cells in Tissue Culture Cannot Predict their Activities in Patients"	460
2.3	"Effects of Drugs in Two Dimensional Growth Conditions Have No Relationship to Their Effects in 3D and/or In Vivo"	461
3	Heterogeneity in Human Pancreatic Cancer Cell Lines	462
4	Characteristics of Orthotopic Xenografts Derived from Established Cell Lines	464
5	Summary and Concluding Remarks	466

J. P. Neoptolemos, R. Urrutia, J. L. Abbruzzese, M. W. Büchler (eds.), *Pancreatic Cancer*,
DOI 10.1007/978-0-387-77498-5_19, © Springer Science+Business Media, LLC 2010

Abstract: A Relatively large number of very well characterized human pancreatic cancer cell lines is available for preclinical investigation. However, there is a perception that continuous passage in tissue culture coupled with genomic instability has made them poor models of human disease and that preclinical attempts to identify active therapeutic regimens that employed them as models have uniformly failed when they were translated into clinical trials. Here we will review the current status of some high profile studies employing cell lines to model human cancer biology and identify the potential strengths and weaknesses associated with the approach. We will also discuss results that challenge the notion that cell lines are poor models of human cancer biology.

1   Introduction: Preclinical Models of Pancreatic Cancer

Pancreatic cancer is a uniformly lethal disease, and identifying new approaches for early detection and therapeutic intervention are exceptionally high priorities in cancer research. Fortunately, even though less funding has been allocated to the study of pancreatic cancer than to other types of cancer, a relative wealth of preclinical models are available to researchers in the field. They can be grouped broadly into three categories: established human cell lines (and xenografts derived from them), transgenic mice, and "tumorgrafts" (also known as "primary human xenografts"). All are being used to better understand the biology of human disease and to develop biology-based therapies that will be more effective than the current standard of care, which is gemcitabine-based chemo- and radiotherapy. Preclinical models are important tools for establishing the cause–effect mechanisms that control pancreatic cancer biology since they all can be genetically manipulated (and primary tumors in patients still cannot be). In addition, they can be used to rapidly and efficiently screen candidate therapeutics to prioritize those that should be evaluated in clinical trials.

There is currently a very active dialog among pancreatic cancer researchers concerning which model(s) best capture sentinel aspects of neoplastic transformation and cancer progression. Among proponents of transgenic mouse models, Tuveson's group has been most influential in terms of defending their relative merits as compared to the other models [1,2]. The transgenic models are all based on pancreas-specific expression of mutant active K-ras, either driven to high levels on its own or expressed in conjunction with loss of various tumor suppressors (p16, p53, and/or SMAD4). Investigators largely agree that they recapitulate the pathologic phenotypes of disease progression through PanINs to overt cancer, and where directly studied they display drug resistance that is similar to that observed in patients [1,2]. Furthermore, the genetic makeup of transgenic mouse tumors can be cleanly modified by breeding, and gains and losses of particular genes can now be done with precise timing using Cre-Lox and other approaches. However, tumor latency can be quite long, and perhaps as a result distant metastases are rare. Furthermore, although it has not yet been comprehensively quantified, the genetic complexity (mutations and gene copy number gains and losses) is probably not as great as is present in human disease. Whether this is a strength or a weakness depends on perspective (i.e., it is possible that a large fraction of the mutations observed in human cancers are unnecessary), but these factors do raise questions that need to be addressed concerning how completely transgenics capture the inter-tumoral heterogeneity that is most likely present in primary tumors.

Tumorgrafts (primary tumor xenografts) are a second class of preclinical models that are gaining many enthusiastic proponents [3,4]. Unlike transgenic mouse models, there is no concern about whether or not tumorgrafts possess the spectrum of genetic alterations that are present in these models since they are directly derived from human cancers. However, unlike the tumors that develop in transgenics, tumorgrafts tend to closely resemble primary human tumors, particularly with respect to their abilities to recapitulate ductal architecture and recruit an extensive tumor-associated stroma, and many of them can produce spontaneous metastases [3]. Because of this, there is a growing sense that tumorgrafts are better models for studying the biology of tumor–stromal interactions, particularly the roles of developmental pathways like Hedgehog, Notch, and Wnt [5]. Recently, tumorgrafts were used as an important tool to obtain a comprehensive picture of the panoply of genetic alterations that are found in human pancreatic cancers because they allow for clean separation of tumor epithelial cells from contaminating stromal cells while presumably not having drifted too far from the original tumors they were derived from. (Murine cells rapidly replace the human stromal cells that were present in the original primary tumors.)

Finally, a very large collection of human pancreatic cancer cell lines is readily available (through ATCC and other sources). Again, one major strength associated with using human cancer cell lines is that no assumptions have to be made about which genetic and epigenetic defects gave rise to the disease, since in each case disease arose in a patient. Furthermore, genetic manipulation of cell lines is now very straightforward (through the use of transient or stable RNAi), and functional studies can be performed on cells in tissue culture or in tumor xenografts in vivo even more rapidly than can be done in tumorgrafts. However, the reason that cell lines and conventional xenografts have started to fall out of favor is that many investigators feel that they have lost key features of the original tumor biology due to extended passage in tissue culture. Furthermore, much has been made recently about how cell lines and xenografts have failed to predict drug efficacy in patients, and they are often used as the comparator to defend the superiority of transgenics or tumorgrafts. The purpose of this chapter is to provide what will hopefully be a balanced appraisal of the strengths and weaknesses of established cell lines, in part by challenging some of the assumptions that are currently held about them.

2   Common Assumptions About Established Cell Lines

2.1   "Cell Lines Are Genetically Scrambled"

Some cell lines have literally been maintained in continuous culture since the 1950s (HeLa) [6], and some of the pancreatic cancer cell lines that are in routine use are over 30 years old [7,8]. Given that cancers display genomic instability, there is valid concern that cell lines could acquire new genetic changes when they are propagated in tissue culture. The development of reproducible, genome-wide approaches to study genetic and epigenetic changes now makes it possible to quantify genetic "scrambling" and render solid conclusions based on data.

Our multidisciplinary research team is currently actively involved in thoroughly characterizing large sets of established human pancreatic cancer cell lines, subcutaneous and orthotopic tumor xenografts derived from them, transgenic mice, and tumorgrafts (produced here at MD Anderson) by gene expression profiling using the Illumina platform. Although these studies are incomplete and it would be premature to generate conclusions from them, it is already clear that the transgenics and tumorgrafts are "different" from the established cell lines and they will therefore be better models for certain studies than the cell lines are. Nonetheless, our results also partially dispel the notion that the cell lines are poor models of human tumors, because they do retain gene expression patterns that are similar to those found in primary tumors, and these patterns are highly reproducible across time (years) and between institutions (in our case, MD Anderson and USCF). The conclusion that the gene expression signatures in cell lines are more stable than might be anticipated is consistent with earlier results obtained by one member of our group [9].

Other groups have more mature results using panels of human cell lines derived from different solid tumors. While these examples do not prove that pancreatic cancer cell lines will also accurately model human disease, they do serve to challenge long-held ideas about how the biology of cell lines may "drift" excessively from the original biology of the human tumors they are derived from. They also demonstrate the power of using large panels of human cell lines to capture the molecular heterogeneity that is present in primary tumors and to link this heterogeneity to sensitivity or resistance to particular therapeutic modalities.

Work performed by Gray's group provides some of the strongest evidence against the assumption that genetic instability in cancer cell lines causes them to drift far from the genetic phenotypes of the original tumors they were derived from. They assembled a relatively large panel (n = 51) of human breast cancer cell lines and used comparative genomic hybridization (CGH) to evaluate the high copy number gains and losses that were present at the whole genome level [10]. They then compared the results to those obtained in a set of 145 primary human tumors. The results demonstrated that very similar patterns of gains and losses were observed in both sets of material, and they went on to show that these similarities extended to transcriptome patterns and Herceptin sensitivity [10]. As introduced above, we have had very similar experience in pancreatic cancer cell lines and have also performed analogous studies with human bladder cancer cell lines (W. Choi, J. Shah, manuscript in preparation). One problem we have identified in the existing pancreatic cancer patient datasets is that in general bulk tumors have been profiled without concern for isolating the epithelial compartment away from the extensive tumor-associated stroma (and complicating the situation, in many cases pancreatic neoplasms of varying histologies have been grouped together). However, by using chronic pancreatitis as a filter to "subtract" the inflammatory stromal signature from the bulk tumor profile, Logsdon's group found good concordance between cell lines and primary pancreatic tumors as well [9].

2.2   "The Effects of Drugs on Cancer Cells in Tissue Culture Cannot Predict their Activities in Patients"

There are clearly important examples of tumor–stromal interactions are critical determinants of therapeutic activity in preclinical models. One of the more obvious ones can be found in studies of angiogenesis inhibitors, where the drug target is not the tumor cell itself. Recent studies have demonstrated that interactions with other types of stromal cells (including pancreatic stellate cells) impart drug resistance [11], and as noted above, interactions between tumor and stromal cells are thought to be important determinants of activation of developmental pathways like Hedgehog [5]. Nonetheless, autocrine pathways are probably also important features of tumor biology, and these pathways probably can be identified in tissue culture. Furthermore, intrinsic mechanisms probably also contribute to cell proliferation and apoptosis resistance, and these too can be detected relatively easily in cell lines.

One recent example that demonstrates that in vitro studies with cell lines can be used to predict therapeutic efficacy in patients comes from a project from Genentech, Inc.

(San Francisco, CA) that was designed to identify molecular markers associated with sensitivity or resistance to the small molecule epidermal growth factor receptor (EGFR) inhibitor, erlotininb (Tarceva, which is also approved in combination with gemcitabine for the treatment of pancreatic cancer). They screened a panel of 42 human non-small cell lung cancer (NSCLC) cell lines for sensitivity to transforming growth factor-alpha (TGFα)-induced proliferation and erlotinib-mediated inhibition of proliferation and compared the patterns observed to the basal gene expression profiles obtained from the cells using microarrays [12]. They discovered that a multi-gene signature of epithelial-to-mesenchymal transition (EMT) was a strong predictor of therapeutic resistance in the cell lines, and they went on to show that markers of EMT were also predictive of therapeutic benefit in a NSCLC clinical trial that compared the effects of erlotinib plus chemotherapy to chemotherapy alone [12]. Since then, several other groups have shown that EMT is associated with resistance to EGFR inhibitors in many other solid tumor cell lines, including bladder, head and neck squamous cell carcinoma (HNSCC), colon cancer, and pancreatic cancer [13–20]. We have designed a neoadjuvant clinical trial to directly examine whether EMT is associated with biological resistance to erlotinib in primary bladder tumors (A. Siefker-Radtke, Principal Investigator).

There are other examples of how cell line-based screens have been used to create hypotheses about how tumor heterogeneity affects drug sensitivity or resistance. Theodorescu's group used in vitro drug sensitivity information from the NCI-60 panel of cell lines coupled with their own experience with a panel of 40 human bladder cancer cell lines to develop an algorithm (termed "COXEN") that they subsequently used to predict therapeutic efficacy in patients [21]. The predictive value of COXEN is now being evaluated prospectively in a cooperative group clinical trial led by the Southwest Oncology Group (SWOG), and the group has developed similar strategies to predict the outcome of combination chemotherapy [22]. Furthermore, recent work by investigators associated with the Harvard Melanoma SPORE demonstrated that cells with activating mutations in B-raf are hypersensitive to small molecule inhibitors of MEK [23], a finding that has since been confirmed by other groups in other tumor models and preliminarily in patients [24] (personal communication). Finally, two other recent screens performed by Genentech have identified candidate markers of sensitivity to TRAIL [25] and hedgehog pathway inhibitors [5], and it will be of interest to see how these preclinical predictions fare within the contexts of clinical trials.

2.3 "Effects of Drugs in Two Dimensional Growth Conditions Have No Relationship to Their Effects in 3D and/or In Vivo"

Several years ago investigators at the National Cancer Insitute's Cancer Therapeutics Evaluation Program (CTEP) assembled a large collection of human cancer cell lines and then extensively characterized them in terms of their sensitivities to a large number of conventional and investigational anti-cancer therapies [26]. Known as the "NCI-60," this panel of lines and the data derived from them have been enormously valuable for subsequent studies of the heterogeneity of drug action in cancer [26]. Unfortunately, the power of the NCI-60 to predict drug activity in patients is imperfect [27], in that a variety of different agents show promising activity in the screen but then fail to display much clinical activity in patients. An excellent example of one such compound is the proteasome inhibitor bortezomib (Velcade, formerly known as PS-341), which displayed unprecedented activity in the NCI-60 [28] but did not produce much single-agent activity in solid tumors in patients [29].

At the root of this concern is the same unresolved question that applies to all preclinical models – do they accurately and completely reflect the biology of human disease? Unfortunately, an answer to this question is not yet available but should be soon. A more approachable question is whether the biology of drug sensitivity or resistance is qualitatively different when cells are grown in two-dimensional culture in vitro compared to three-dimensional growth in an appropriate local microenvironment in vivo. We will discuss our own (relatively extensive) experience with this issue in the sections that follow.

Three other key points need to be considered when using cell lines (or any other preclinical models) to attempt to predict clinical activity in patients. First, it is important that experiments be designed to mimic the pharmacokinetic properties of the drug in patients. These include maximal serum and tumor concentrations (if the latter can be estimated) and the length of time tumor cells are likely to be exposed to these concentrations before they are cleared from the system. Most investigators expose cells in tissue culture to drugs continuously (for up to 96 h in some cases), whereas most conventional and investigational agents have in vivo half lives that can be measured in hours or minutes. MTD levels of drugs in rodents can be higher or lower than corresponding MTD levels in patients.

It is also important to have good information about how the pathway being targeted regulates cancer cell biology. Conventional cytotoxic therapy most likely "works" because it causes cancer cell death. However, the type of cell death being induced (apoptosis, necrosis, autophagy, etc.) is usually drug- and often cell type-dependent, so applying a "one size fits all" method to measure cell death might misrepresent response. Even more importantly, in our experience most biologicals (growth factor receptor inhibitors, anti-angiogenic agent, or signal transduction inhibitors) exert cytostatic rather than cytotoxic responses. (This is especially true at concentrations of the drugs that can actually be reached in patients.) These cytostatic effects can occur by inducing various checkpoints that act at different points in the cell cycle, so once again using an assay that measures "proliferation" might miss the most relevant effects of such agents.

Finally, and related to the two points highlighted above, it is critical that assays are chosen that are highly quantitative and specifically measure what is thought to be the most important biological effect(s) of the agent in question. For example, the typical assays that are used in high throughput settings (MTT, SRB, Cell Glo Titer, etc.) measure a mixture of growth arrest and cell death, and depending on the duration of the assay, the growth arrest component often dominates (in a manner that is related to cell doubling time). While many investigators (especially radiation biologists) consider clonogenic assays to be the "gold standard" methods for measuring cell kill, once again these assays measure many different cell fates, including apoptosis, "terminal" autophagy, "mitotic catastrophe," necrosis, and senescence. In addition, it is possible that the most rapid forms of cell death (i.e., apoptosis) might in many cases be more preferable than delayed cell death and correlate better with clinical outcome [30]. In any case, setting the bar higher seems to be important to increase the value of our preclinical models.

3 Heterogeneity in Human Pancreatic Cancer Cell Lines

Work performed over the last 2 decades has shown that mutations in the genes encoding K-ras, p16INK4, DPC4/SMAD4, and p53 accumulate in a majority of primary human pancreatic cancers [31]. The importance of these mutations has recently been confirmed by large-scale sequencing of 24 human pancreatic cancer cell lines and tumorgrafts [32]. In total, the mean number of genetic alterations observed in pancreatic cancers is actually lower than corresponding rates in human colon or breast cancer for reasons that are not immediately clear [32]. Nonetheless, the genetic complexity is impressive (mean number of mutations = 63), resulting in alterations in at least 12 core biological pathways [32]. How these mutations arise is also not clear – it is conceivable that the four sentinel events drive the rest of the genetic complexity that is present in primary tumors. If not, then it is unlikely that transgenic mouse models will encompass a significant portion of this heterogeneity, and their predictive power in informing personalized approaches to pancreatic cancer therapy may be limited.

On the other hand, comparisons made between the 24 cell lines and tumorgrafts and 94 primary tumor specimens revealed relatively good concordance between the two sources of human cancer cells [32]. If anything, it appeared that genetic defects were more common in the primary tumors than they were in the preclinical models, supporting the idea that in vitro and in vivo passage of the cells does not lead to substantial genomic "scrambling."

As introduced above, a relatively large number of established human pancreatic cancer cell lines are available for preclinical study. Our own group has assembled a panel of 47 different cell lines and is in the process of performing DNA fingerprinting, gene expression profiling, array CGH, and drug sensitivity studies on the panel through a collaboration with a group at UCSF/Lawrence Livermore. These cell lines display heterogeneity in terms of the presence of the four major mutations observed in primary tumors (⊘ Table 19-1) (also see http://pathology2.jhu.edu/pancreas/geneticsweb/Profiles.htm), and preliminary analyses of a subset of the lines has revealed remarkable heterogeneity in gene expression (⊘ Fig. 19-1) and sensitivity to various conventional and investigational agents (⊘ Table 19-1).

Our group has already arrived at several general conclusions based on our experience with these cell lines to date. First, there appears to be a subset of the lines (including COLO357, its derivative L3.6pl, BxPC-3, SU8686, and CFPac) that is sensitive to apoptosis induced by a variety of different conventional and investigational agents (gemcitabine, 5-FU, cisplatin, TRAIL, and proteasome inhibitors), and another subset that is generally resistant (including mPANC96, Panc-1, MiaPaCa2, and HS766T) (⊘ Table 19-1). Interestingly, the drug-sensitive and drug-resistant lines co-cluster together when their gene expression patterns are analyzed by unsupervised clustering (⊘ Fig. 19-1), and further analysis of the pathways that are different between the subsets indicates that the drug-resistant cells display features of epithelial-to-mesenchymal transition (EMT)(T. Arumugam et al. Cancer Research, in press). Furthermore, erlotinib sensitivity is limited to a subset of these gemcitabine-sensitive, "epithelial" cell lines [16,33]. This EMT appears to be driven (at least in part) by the transcriptional repressor Zeb-1 [34], because knockdown of Zeb-1 restores expression of epithelial markers and sensitivity to gemcitabine and erlotinib (T. Arumugam et al. Cancer Research, in press; K. Fournier et al. manuscript in preparation). Importantly, Zeb-1 functions as an adaptor protein to recruit histone deacetylases (HDACs) to chromatin, and recent studies demonstrate that they can also restore expression of epithelial markers and sensitivity to EGFR inhibitors in other solid tumor models [35]. We have found that the HDAC inhibitors vorinostat (SAHA) and SNDX-275 [35] can also restore sensitivity to gemcitabine and erlotinib in pancreatic cancer cells (K. Fournier et al. manuscript in preparation), raising the possibility that they could also be used to increase drug sensitivity in patients.

Co-culture of established cell lines with isolated stromal cells affords an opportunity to enhance the predictive power of in vitro drug efficacy experiments. Rosa Hwang in our research program has developed immortalized human pancreatic cancer stellate cells and has used them to show that relevant tumor–stromal interactions can be recapitulated in vitro [11]. (We are currently involved in collaborative studies aimed at determining whether the

□ Table 19-1

Molecular properties of representative gemcitabine-sensitive and –resistant human pancreatic cancer cell lines. Molecular genotypes were obtained from ATCC, the Johns Hopkins website (see text), or references in the literature. DNA fingerprinting was performed using the PowerPlex 16 kit (Promega, Inc. Madison, WI). Gemcitabine sensitivity was determined by exposing cells to 10 μM drug for 48-72 h and measuring growth inhibition by MTT reduction and apoptosis by propidium iodide staining and FACS analysis (Arumugam et al. *Cancer Research*, in press.) Invasion was measured at 48 h using modified Boyden chambers. "Epithelial" and "mesenchymal" phenotypes were determined by expression of molecular markers using gene expression profiling (Illumina platform)(Arumugam et al. *Cancer Research*, in press).

Cell line*	K-ras	P16	SMAD4	P53	Gem sensitivity	Invasion	Epithelial or mesenchymal
HPDE	Wt	Wt	Wt	Wt	S	N.D.	E
BxPC3	Wt	Wt	Mut	Mut	S	++	E
L3.6pl	Mut	N.D.	Mut	Wt	S	+	E
SU.86.86	Mut	Mut	Mut	Mut	S	+	E
CFPac-1	Mut	Mut	Mut	Mut	S	+	E
MiaPaCa-2	Mut	Mut	Wt	Mut	R	+	M
AsPC-1	Mut	Mut	Mut	Mut	R	+	M
mPanc-96	Mut	Mut	Mut	Mut	R	+++	M
Panc-1	Mut	Mut (del)	Wt	Mut	R	+++	M
HS766T	Mut	Wt	Mut	Mut	R	++++	M

*HPDE is a normal ductal epithelial cell that has been immortalized with SV40 large T antigen. Therefore, the p53 and Rb pathways are not fully operational in the cells. DNA fingerprinting indicates that ASPC-1 and mPanc-96 are clonally related; the apparent differences in tumorigenicity may therefore be due to epigenetic mechanisms. "N.D.," not determined, either because the gene has not been sequenced for the presence of mutations or because conflicting data are present in the published literature

stellate cells can interact with established cell lines to restore the paracrine hedgehog pathway activation that can be observed in tumor xenografts in vivo.) Importantly, co-culture with stellate cells increases tumor cell drug resistance [11], suggesting that co-culture models might be useful for defining the molecular mechanisms involved and testing candidate therapeutic approaches to circumvent them.

4 Characteristics of Orthotopic Xenografts Derived from Established Cell Lines

As noted above, the utility of using in vitro drug sensitivities to predict in vivo efficacy is now being questioned. The same is true for xenografts derived from established human cancer cell lines [36]. It seems likely that part of the problem is due in part to poor model selection and in part to problems with data interpretation. First most investigators use ectopic (subcutaneous) rather than orthotopic (intra-pancreatic) implantation of tumor cell lines to generate their xenografts, and previous studies have demonstrated that the orthotopic microenvironment

■ Fig. 19-1

Gene expression profiles of gemcitabine-sensitive and –resistant pancreatic cancer cell lines.
Global gene expression profiles were obtained from two independent RNA isolates using the
Illumina platform. Unsupervised clustering of the data segregated the cell lines according to
drug sensitivity (blue = drug-sensitive, red = drug-resistant). Pathway analysis revealed that EMT
is one prominent feature of the drug-resistant cells (Arumugam et al. *Cancer Research*, in press).

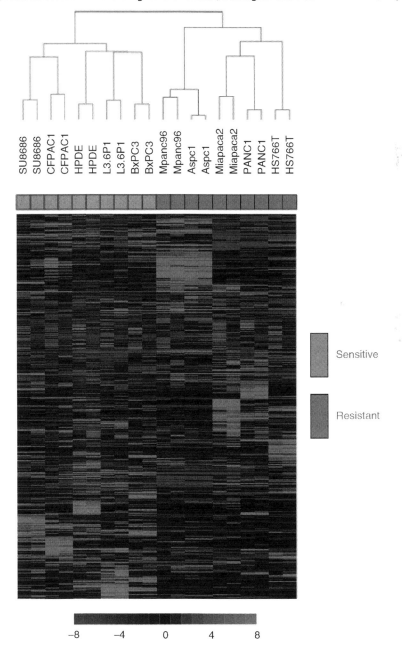

can have a significant influence on tumor biology [37] and gene expression [38]. Second, a large fraction of previous studies have employed drug-sensitive cells (like L3.6pl or BxPC-1), which we think has biased experiments in favor of response. Finally, the effects of therapy on tumor growth have often been overstated, and cytostatic responses that would by analogy merely produce temporary disease stabilization or partially inhibit progression in patients have been interpreted as successes. All three of these points can be easily addressed by employing drug-resistant lines (like HPAC or mPANC96) in orthotopic models with imaging strategies that can distinguish tumor growth inhibition from regression [39,40].

Another, essentially opposite concern is that the tumor microenvironment can provide important survival signals, and therefore drugs that are active in vitro may be completely inactive in vivo. Our own experience suggests that this problem is more quantitative rather than qualitative. We have found remarkable concordance in tumor cell sensitivities to gemcitabine, cisplatin, docetaxel, EGFR inhibitors, TRAIL, and proteasome inhibitors in comparisons of drug efficacy in vitro and in orthotopic tumor xenografts in vivo [33,39,41–43].

Finally, there is also a concern that conventional cancer cell lines become independent of tumor–stromal interactions for their growth. Our own indirect evidence tends to support this view. Compared to our tumorgrafts or primary patient specimens, our conventional xenografts (ectopic or orthotopic) tend to grow as relatively homogeneous masses of tumor cells. This does not seem to be caused by the immunosuppressed state of the host, since tumorgrafts growing in the same strain of animals display extensive stromal involvement. There are conventional models (i.e., Capan-2) that do display a relatively organized tumor-associated stroma (T. Arumugam, unpublished observations), and it is possible that other conventional models could be "encouraged" to do so by using lower tumor innocula and/or isolated progenitor ("stem") cells rather than bulk cell cultures to establish the tumors. Even though the extent of stromal involvement may be less impressive, the biology of the tumor–stromal interactions that do exist may well be appropriate, as demonstrated in a recent study of the effects of hedgehog pathway inhibitors in some of them [5]. Comparative gene expression profiling (using human and mouse chips) will enable us to more precisely define the differences in the nature of the tumor–stromal interactions that form in tumorgrafts versus conventional orthotopic xenografts.

5   Summary and Concluding Remarks

Human pancreatic cancer cell lines offer several advantages over transgenic mice and tumorgrafts. They probably do retain many (if not most) of the genetic properties that were present in the primary tumors they were derived from, and when large enough panels of cell lines are employed they are currently the best option if one wants to capture the biological heterogeneity present in human pancreatic cancers. Furthermore, they can be used to rapidly screen for biomarkers of drug sensitivity and resistance, and they can be genetically modified to establish whether such markers play a causal role in the phenotypes observed. Finally, when implanted orthotopically in nude mice, they do appear to recapitulate some of the important tumor–stromal interactions that are now considered important determinants of overall tumor biology, including angiogenesis and paracrine developmental pathway signaling [5].

It is also clear that transgenic mice and tumorgrafts possess some features that make them better models of certain processes than cell lines. Transgenic mice are available that reproduce the whole spectrum of pancreatic progression, from inflammation through PanINs to overt adenocarcinoma, and if their similarities to primary human tumors can be confirmed at the whole genome/molecular level, then they will be essential tools for studying early stages of disease progression and identifying biomarkers that can be used for early detection. Likewise, tumorgrafts appear to capture more of the phenotypic features of primary tumors than do conventional xenografts, and it is likely that they will ultimately prove to be better models for predicting drug efficacy in patients. The major weaknesses with both are that experiments take much longer and are much more expensive than tissue culture studies, and they are not amenable to high throughput approaches. Overall, we conclude that all three types of model possess crucial strengths and weaknesses. Given that there are too many attractive candidate therapies for pancreatic cancer to evaluate them all in patients, the research community should continue to make them all better tools for understanding human disease biology and the way heterogeneous biological properties dictate tumor response to conventional and novel agents.

Key Research Points

- Human pancreatic cancer cell lines are not genetically "scrambled"
- Cell lines display marked heterogeneity in sensitivity to gemcitabine and other anti-cancer agents, and one limitation with previous studies is that they have often employed the most drug-sensitive models
- In our experience, in vitro drug sensitivity or resistance correlates relatively well with sensitivity or resistance in orthotopic xenografts
- Epithelial-to-mesenchymal transition (EMT) is a major underlying pattern in human pancreatic cancer cell lines and is linked to drug resistance
- Cell lines and xenografts derived from them probably are probably inferior models of tumor–stromal interactions as compared to transgenics and tumorgrafts ("primary xenografts")

Future Scientific Directions

- Gene expression profiling and other global analytic strategies should be employed to more precisely determine whether cell lines and other preclinical models capture the biological heterogeneity present in primary human tumors
- This work will require comparisons of tumor biological properties in cells maintained in two-dimensional and three-dimensional culture in vitro and in subcutaneous and orthotopic xenografts derived from them
- It seems likely that these studies will reveal that each of the three major preclinical models (cell lines, transgenics, and tumorgrafts) possesses important strengths and weaknesses

Clinical Implications

- Given the increasingly large number of candidate therapies coupled with the limited number of pancreatic cancer patients available for enrollment in clinical trials, preclinical models must be used to "rank" candidate therapies prior to clinical evaluation

- It is essential that all of our preclinical models become better predictors of clinical activity in patients and that drug efficacy be linked to tumor biology
- Where studied, large scale studies of investigational agents in cell lines have produced valuable information for clinical development

References

1. Frese KK, Tuveson DA: Maximizing mouse cancer models. Nat Rev Cancer 2007;7(9):645–658.

2. Olive KP, Tuveson DA: The use of targeted mouse models for preclinical testing of novel cancer therapeutics. Clin Cancer Res 2006;12(18):5277–5287.

3. Embuscado EE, Laheru D, Ricci F, et al.: Immortalizing the complexity of cancer metastasis: genetic features of lethal metastatic pancreatic cancer obtained from rapid autopsy. Cancer Biol Ther 2005;4(5):548–554.

4. Li C, Heidt DG, Dalerba P, et al.: Identification of pancreatic cancer stem cells. Cancer Res 2007;67 (3):1030–1037.

5. Yauch RL, Gould SE, Scales SJ, et al.: A paracrine requirement for hedgehog signalling in cancer. Nature 2008;455(7211):406–410.

6. Scherer WF, Syverton JT, Gey GO: Studies on the propagation in vitro of poliomyelitis viruses. IV. Viral multiplication in a stable strain of human malignant epithelial cells (strain HeLa) derived from an epidermoid carcinoma of the cervix. J Exp Med 1953;97(5):695–710.

7. Lieber M, Mazzetta J, Nelson-Rees W, Kaplan M, Todaro G: Establishment of a continuous tumor-cell line (panc-1) from a human carcinoma of the exocrine pancreas. Int J Cancer 1975;15(5):741–747.

8. Yunis AA, Arimura GK, Russin DJ: Human pancreatic carcinoma (MIA PaCa-2) in continuous culture: sensitivity to asparaginase. Int J Cancer 1977;19 (1):128–135.

9. Logsdon CD, Simeone DM, Binkley C, et al.: Molecular profiling of pancreatic adenocarcinoma and chronic pancreatitis identifies multiple genes differentially regulated in pancreatic cancer. Cancer Res 2003;63(10):2649–2657.

10. Neve RM, Chin K, Fridlyand J, et al.: A collection of breast cancer cell lines for the study of functionally distinct cancer subtypes. Cancer Cell 2006;10 (6):515–527.

11. Hwang RF, Moore T, Arumugam T, et al.: Cancer-associated stromal fibroblasts promote pancreatic tumor progression. Cancer Res 2008;68(3):918–926.

12. Yauch RL, Januario T, Eberhard DA, et al.: Epithelial versus mesenchymal phenotype determines in vitro sensitivity and predicts clinical activity of erlotinib in lung cancer patients. Clin Cancer Res 2005;11(24 Pt 1):8686–8698.

13. Barr S, Thomson S, Buck E, et al.: Bypassing cellular EGF receptor dependence through epithelial-to-mesenchymal-like transitions. Clin Exp Metastasis 2008;25(6):685–693.

14. Fuchs BC, Fujii T, Dorfman JD, et al.: Epithelial-to-mesenchymal transition and integrin-linked kinase mediate sensitivity to epidermal growth factor receptor inhibition in human hepatoma cells. Cancer Res 2008;68(7):2391–2399.

15. Haddad Y, Choi W, McConkey DJ: Delta-crystallin enhancer binding factor 1 controls the epithelial to mesenchymal transition phenotype and resistance to the epidermal growth factor receptor inhibitor erlotinib in human head and neck squamous cell carcinoma lines. Clin Cancer Res 2009;15(2):532–542.

16. Pino MS, Balsamo M, Di Modugno F, et al.: Human Mena+11a isoform serves as a marker of epithelial phenotype and sensitivity to epidermal growth factor receptor inhibition in human pancreatic cancer cell lines. Clin Cancer Res 2008;14(15): 4943–4950.

17. Thomson S, Buck E, Petti F, et al.: Epithelial to mesenchymal transition is a determinant of sensitivity of non-small-cell lung carcinoma cell lines and xenografts to epidermal growth factor receptor inhibition. Cancer Res 2005;65(20):9455–9462.

18. Frederick BA, Helfrich BA, Coldren CD, et al.: Epithelial to mesenchymal transition predicts gefitinib resistance in cell lines of head and neck squamous cell carcinoma and non-small cell lung carcinoma. Mol Cancer Ther 2007;6(6):1683–1691.

19. Black PC, Brown GA, Inamoto T, et al.: Sensitivity to epidermal growth factor receptor inhibitor requires E-cadherin expression in urothelial carcinoma cells. Clin Cancer Res 2008;14(5):1478–1486.

20. Shrader M, Pino MS, Brown G, et al.: Molecular correlates of gefitinib responsiveness in human bladder cancer cells. Mol Cancer Ther 2007;6(1): 277–285.

21. Lee JK, Havaleshko DM, Cho H, et al.: A strategy for predicting the chemosensitivity of human cancers and its application to drug discovery. Proc Natl Acad Sci USA 2007;104(32):13086–13091.

22. Havaleshko DM, Cho H, Conaway M, et al.: Prediction of drug combination chemosensitivity in human bladder cancer. Mol Cancer Ther 2007;6 (2):578–586.

23. Lin WM, Baker AC, Beroukhim R, et al.: Modeling genomic diversity and tumor dependency in malignant melanoma. Cancer Res 2008;68(3):664–673.

24. Adjei AA, Cohen RB, Franklin W, et al.: Phase I pharmacokinetic and pharmacodynamic study of the oral, small-molecule mitogen-activated protein kinase kinase 1/2 inhibitor AZD6244 (ARRY-142886) in patients with advanced cancers. J Clin Oncol 2008;26(13):2139–2146.

25. Wagner KW, Punnoose EA, Januario T, et al.: Death-receptor O-glycosylation controls tumor-cell sensitivity to the proapoptotic ligand Apo2L/TRAIL. Nat Med 2007;13(9):1070–1077.

26. Shoemaker RH: The NCI60 human tumour cell line anticancer drug screen. Nat Rev Cancer 2006;6 (10):813–823.

27. Johnson JI, Decker S, Zaharevitz D, et al.: Relationships between drug activity in NCI preclinical in vitro and in vivo models and early clinical trials. Br J Cancer 2001;84(10):1424–1431.

28. Adams J, Palombella VJ, Sausville EA, et al.: Proteasome inhibitors: a novel class of potent and effective antitumor agents. Cancer Res 1999;59 (11):2615–2622.

29. McConkey DJ, Zhu K: Mechanisms of proteasome inhibitor action and resistance in cancer. Drug Resist Updat 2008;11(4–5):164–179.

30. Davis DW, Buchholz TA, Hess KR, Sahin AA, Valero V, McConkey DJ: Automated quantification of apoptosis after neoadjuvant chemotherapy for breast cancer: early assessment predicts clinical response. Clin Cancer Res 2003;9(3):955–960.

31. Hruban RH, Goggins M, Parsons J, Kern SE: Progression model for pancreatic cancer. Clin Cancer Res 2000;6(8):2969–2972.

32. Jones S, Zhang X, Parsons DW, et al.: Core signaling pathways in human pancreatic cancers revealed by global genomic analyses. Science 2008;321(5897): 1801–1806.

33. Pino MS, Shrader M, Baker CH, et al.: Transforming growth factor alpha expression drives constitutive epidermal growth factor receptor pathway activation and sensitivity to gefitinib (Iressa) in human pancreatic cancer cell lines. Cancer Res 2006;66 (7):3802–3812.

34. Peinado H, Olmeda D, Cano A: Snail, Zeb and bHLH factors in tumour progression: an alliance against the epithelial phenotype? Nat Rev Cancer 2007;7(6):415–428.

35. Witta SE, Gemmill RM, Hirsch FR, et al.: Restoring E-cadherin expression increases sensitivity to epidermal growth factor receptor inhibitors in lung cancer cell lines. Cancer Res 2006;66(2): 944–950.

36. Sausville EA, Burger AM: Contributions of human tumor xenografts to anticancer drug development. Cancer Res 2006;66(7):3351–3354, discussion 4.

37. Bruns CJ, Harbison MT, Kuniyasu H, Eue I, Fidler IJ: In vivo selection and characterization of metastatic variants from human pancreatic adenocarcinoma by using orthotopic implantation in nude mice. Neoplasia 1999;1(1):50–62.

38. Nakamura T, Fidler IJ, Coombes KR: Gene expression profile of metastatic human pancreatic cancer cells depends on the organ microenvironment. Cancer Res 2007;67(1):139–148.

39. Khanbolooki S, Nawrocki ST, Arumugam T, et al.: Nuclear factor-kappaB maintains TRAIL resistance in human pancreatic cancer cells. Mol Cancer Ther 2006;5(9):2251–2260.

40. Pan X, Arumugam T, Yamamoto T, et al.: Nuclear factor-kappaB p65/relA silencing induces apoptosis and increases gemcitabine effectiveness in a subset of pancreatic cancer cells. Clin Cancer Res 2008;14 (24):8143–8151.

41. Nawrocki ST, Bruns CJ, Harbison MT, et al.: Effects of the proteasome inhibitor PS-341 on apoptosis and angiogenesis in orthotopic human pancreatic tumor xenografts. Mol Cancer Ther 2002;1 (14):1243–1253.

42. Nawrocki ST, Carew JS, Pino MS, et al.: Bortezomib sensitizes pancreatic cancer cells to endoplasmic reticulum stress-mediated apoptosis. Cancer Res 2005;65(24):11658–11666.

43. Nawrocki ST, Sweeney-Gotsch B, Takamori R, McConkey DJ: The proteasome inhibitor bortezomib enhances the activity of docetaxel in orthotopic human pancreatic tumor xenografts. Mol Cancer Ther 2004;3(1):59–70.

20 Mouse Models of Pancreatic Exocrine Cancer

Michelle Lockley · David Tuveson

1	Introduction	472
2	The Origins of Human PDA	472
3	Chemically-Induced Pancreatic Cancer	473
3.1	Hamsters	473
3.2	Rats	476
3.3	Mice	476
4	Transplanted, Chemically-Induced Tumors	477
5	Immunodeficient Models	478
6	Genetically Engineered Mouse Models	479
6.1	Early Transgenic Models	479
6.2	Mutant *KRAS* Transgenic Models	481
7	Pancreatic Development	481
8	Endogenous Murine Models of PDA	482
8.1	The Cre-Lox System	482
8.2	Endogenous Mutant *KRAS* Mice	483
8.3	Activated *KRAS* and *Ink4a/Arf* Deficiency	483
8.4	Activated *KRAS* and the *p53* Pathway	484
8.5	The Role of Inflammation	486
8.6	Cystic Neoplasms: Activated *KRAS* and *Smad4/TGF-β* Signaling	487
9	Limitations of Current Models	489
10	The Future	489
10.1	Uncovering the Cell of Origin	490
10.2	Improving Disease Detection and Treatment	490

J. P. Neoptolemos, R. Urrutia, J. L. Abbruzzese, M. W. Büchler (eds.), *Pancreatic Cancer*,
DOI 10.1007/978-0-387-77498-5_20, © Springer Science+Business Media, LLC 2010

Abstract: Pancreatic ductal adenocarcinoma (PDA) is a common and lethal disease. Despite the prevalence of PDA, our understanding of the critical events underlying disease pathogenesis and therapeutic resistance is woefully inadequate. To accelerate progress, much effort has been directed at recapitulating PDA in suitable animal models. Early efforts to model PDA in rodents utilized chemical carcinogenesis, and although useful for certain applications, crucial limitations prevented their widespread utility. Traditional transgenic approaches also failed to produce accurate models of pancreatic cancer in mice, potentially due to the non-physiological control of gene expression. The advent of gene targeting in embryonic stem cells and a deeper understanding of the molecular and cellular events that occur during pancreatic neoplasia enabled the development of accurate models of pre-invasive and invasive PDA. Such models are now yielding fruitful information of direct relevance to patients with pancreatic cancer.

1 Introduction

Pancreatic ductal adenocarcinoma (PDA) is a lethal disease that typically presents at an advanced stage, metastasizes early and is resistant to conventional treatments such as radiation and chemotherapy. In the UK in 2003 there were 7,000 deaths from pancreatic cancer, making it the sixth most common cause of cancer death. In the same year, 7,156 people were diagnosed with pancreatic cancer, emphasizing the bleak prognosis for patients with this disease [1]. In recent years, immense efforts have been made to understand the molecular mechanisms of pancreatic carcinogenesis in an attempt to devise novel methods of disease detection and treatment. The ultimate platform on which to evaluate this is human tissue but late presentation and the inaccessibility of the human organ necessitate the use of surrogates. Examination of cells in tissue culture is limited by the absence of stromal tissues and a functioning immune system, which are thought to be important in the initiation and progression of this disease [2]. Other features of pancreatic cancer such as angiogenesis and metastasis are also difficult to evaluate in this setting. It is hoped that the development of accurate animal models of pancreatic cancer will circumvent many of these limitations and thus improve our understanding of this devastating disease. Owing to their physiological and genetic similarity to humans, mammals are preferred for animal modeling. The short life span and size of rodents, as well as their ability to breed readily in captivity, makes small rodents particularly suitable [3].

2 The Origins of Human PDA

The generation of accurate animal models of PDA required a thorough understanding of the molecular and cellular events underlying the cognate human disease, and as these topics are extensively highlighted elsewhere in this monograph they will be only briefly summarized here. PDA can be distinguished from other pancreatic and non-pancreatic malignancies by a characteristic set of somatic and inherited mutations. The most consistent genetic abnormality found in pre-invasive and invasive PDA is activating mutation of the *KRAS* oncogene [4]. Indeed, 90–95% of all PDA cases contain missense mutations in *KRAS* that attenuate the GTPase enzymatic activity of *Kras* and thereby cause constitutive signaling through multiple effector pathways to influence cellular proliferation, survival, differentiation and motility

[4–6]. The tumor suppressor gene and cell cycle inhibitor *p16/Ink4a* is also usually mutated in PDA, due to allelic deletion, point mutation and promoter methylation [7]. *p16/Ink4a* alterations occur subsequent to *KRAS* mutations and are observed in approximately 90% of PDA cases [8]. Inactivation of the tumor suppressor gene *p53* occurs in approximately 75% of PDA cases, usually through missense mutation together with loss of the remaining wild-type allele [9,10]. *p53* mutation confers multiple transforming effects upon cells including dysfunction of apoptotic regulation and loss of genome integrity mechanisms, and accordingly, *p53* mutation is associated with a more advanced stage of PDA such as early metastasis [11,12]. Additionally, the TGF-β pathway is frequently inactivated in PDA due predominantly to mutations in the "deleted in pancreatic carcinoma 4" gene, *Dpc4* (also known as *Smad4*). *Smad4/Dpc4* is mutated in approximately 50% of PDA [13]. A recent extensive analysis of tissue obtained from 114 human pancreatic cancers has confirmed the prime importance of the four genes described above [14]. In this study, additional mutant genes were noted at lower frequencies. These can be grouped into 12 core pathways that are altered in PDA tumorigenesis. Importantly, *Kras*, *p16/Ink4a*, *p53* and *Dpc* interact with many of these core pathways and thus their mutation provides a framework for the rational design of murine models of PDA.

PDA is hypothesized to develop from pre-invasive neoplasms that include pancreatic intra-epithelial neoplasms (PanIN), intraductal papillary mucinous neoplasms (IPMN) and mucinous cycstic neoplasms (MCN). PanINs are located in small pancreatic ducts and are composed of columnar and cuboidal cells that frequently contain intracytoplasmic mucin. They are classified as PanIN-1, -2 or -3 depending on the extent of cytological and architectural atypia. Telomere shortening and several genetic abnormalities characteristic of PDA are observed with increasing frequency in progressively advanced PanINs. These features, together with the observation that *KRAS* is mutated in 36% of PanIN-1A and 87% of PanIN-2/3, support the hypothesis that PanIN is a primary precursor to PDA and implies a role for mutant *KRAS* in tumor initiation [15]. In contrast to PanINs, IPMNs are mucin-producing cystic neoplasms that grow in papillary clusters in large pancreatic ducts. MCNs are also cystic, tend not to communicate with pancreatic ducts, are more common in women and have an "ovarian-type" stroma that is often positive for the oestrogen receptor. IPMNs and MCNs can both progress to PDA but have a dramatically more favorable prognosis than PanINs. As all three precursor neoplasms can progress to PDA, their detection and treatment is an important area of intensive clinical investigation. Therefore, animal models that include evidence of progression from a pre-invasive stage to frank PDA are highly desired (⊙ *Fig. 20-1*).

3 Chemically-Induced Pancreatic Cancer

3.1 Hamsters

The first animal models of pancreatic cancer were generated in the 1970's by administering chemical carcinogens to small rodents (⊙ *Table 20-1*). Following the discovery of the carcinogenic properties of nitrosamines, Pour and co-workers evaluated a variety of these compounds in Syrian golden hamsters. Initially, they found that weekly injections of 2, 2-dihydroxy-di-n-propylnitrosamine (DHPN) gave rise to tumors of the respiratory tract, pancreas, liver, and kidneys, with most pancreatic tumors being ductal adenomas and adenocarcinomas [16]. A related compound, 2,2'-dioxopropyl-n-propylnitrosamine

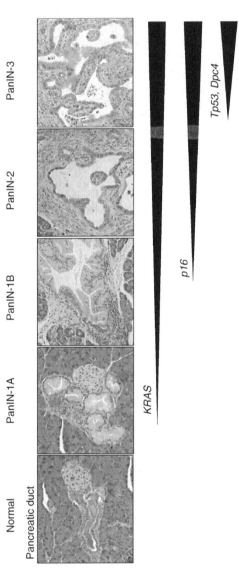

Fig. 20-1

Histological and molecular sequence of events in the evolution of PanIN to PDA.

Normal   PanIN-1A   PanIN-1B   PanIN-2   PanIN-3

Pancreatic duct

KRAS

p16

Tp53, Dpc4

⬛ Table 20-1

Tumors induced by chemical carcinogens in rodents

Species	Carcinogen	Pancreatic pathology	Extra-pancreatic tumors	Reference
Hamsters	DHPN	PDA	liver, lung kidney,	[16]
	DOPN	PDA	liver, lung	[17]
	DIPN	PDA	liver, lung kidney,	[18]; [19]
	BOP (s/c weekly)	PDA, cystic mucinous neoplasms, intraductal papillary neoplasms	liver, lung, kidney, gallbladder	[20]
Rats	DMBA (intrapancreatic injection)	Acinar tumors	NR	[21]
	Azaserine	Acinar tumors, PDA	kidney, skin, breast	[22]
Mice	DMBA (intrapancreatic implantation)	PDA	NR	[23]

DHPN = 2, 2-dihydroxy-di-n-propylnitrosamine, DOPN = 2,2'-dioxopropyl-n-propylnitrosamine, DIPN = N-Nitroso-bis(2-hydroxypropyl)amine, BOP = N-Nitrosobis(2-oxopropyl)amine, DMBA = 7,12-dimethylbenz-α-anthracene. s/c = subcutaneously, NR = none reported

(DOPN), conferred carcinogenesis that was more restricted to the pancreas, although a few tumors were reported in the lungs and liver [17]. N-Nitroso-bis(2-acetoxyproply)amine and the related compound N-Nitroso-bis(2-hydroxypropyl)amine (DIPN) were also shown to be carcinogenic in the hamster pancreas, liver, respiratory tract and kidneys [18,19]. Using high resolution light and transmission electron microscopy, Levitt et al. demonstrated that DIPN caused progressive proliferation of ductal cells, followed by the development of multicentric foci of cystic adenomas, intraductal carcinomas and eventually invasive ductal neoplasms, implying a sequential histological evolution of PDA [24].

Further work identified N-Nitrosobis(2-oxopropyl)amine (BOP) as the most potent and selective pancreatic carcinogen in Syrian hamsters, however tumors could also occur in additional sites depending upon the route of administration [20]. Indeed, when administered orally to Syrian hamsters for 90 days, BOP resulted in a high incidence of intra- and extra-hepatic bile duct, but not pancreatic, neoplasms [25]. In contrast, a single subcutaneous dose of BOP caused a few pancreatic adenomas after a latency of at least 28 weeks but a high incidence of pancreatic tumors was only achieved by administering BOP weekly for life [20]. These were predominantly ductal in origin, although cystic mucinous neoplasms and intraductal papillary neoplasms were also reported [26]. Pathologically, the neoplasms observed in hamsters following BOP administration had striking similarities to those found in humans, with a pronounced desmoplastic reaction and perineural invasion. At the molecular level, *KRAS* was frequently mutated at codon 12, although *p53* mutations were not a feature of these tumors [27]. Pathologically, neoplasms invaded locally and metastasized to lymph nodes, liver and lungs [28] and a clinical syndrome of weight loss, jaundice, ascites and vascular thrombosis was observed that closely mimicked that of the human disease [29]. The BOP-induced hamster model of pancreatic cancer therefore achieved remarkable molecular, pathological and clinical approximation to the human disease. Unfortunately, nitrosamines do not seem to induce PDAs in other more commonly used laboratory animals such as mice and rats [30], limiting the widespread use of this approach.

3.2   Rats

Several chemical carcinogens have been investigated as inducers of PDA in rats, with the most success achieved using 7,12-dimethylbenz-α-anthracene (DMBA) and azaserine. Dissin et al. induced adenocarcinomas by implanting the polycyclic hydrocarbon, DMBA, into the pancreatic head of rats. These tumors exhibited invasive and metastatic behavior but the tumor prevalence was only 8% [21], and their appearance on electron microscopy suggested an acinar rather than ductal cell of origin [31]. Longnecker and co-workers identified azaserine as a potential pancreatic carcinogen after investigating mutagenic chemicals that localize to the pancreas following systemic administration [22]. They observed that azaserine delivered intraperitoneally every week for 6 months caused more than 25% of the rats to develop pancreatic carcinomas by the age of one year, with metastasis noted to lymph nodes, liver and lung [22]. Malignant tumors of the kidney, skin and breast were also observed but were not as frequent as pancreatic tumors. In common with DMBA, the administration of azaserine to rats also induced acinar tumors dramatically more frequently than ductal tumors. Despite the long latency for overt azaserine-induced carcinogenesis, focal abnormalities of acinar cell differentiation were seen as early as two months after azaserine treatment [22], which were described as atypical acinar cell nodules (AACN). A small percentage of these AACN progressed by 9 months to carcinomas *in situ*. Moreover, pancreatic carcinomas were only seen in rats with multiple pancreatic AACNs, implicating them as a putative precursor neoplasm in this model [32]. Azaserine-induced pancreatic carcinomas in rats are considered a good model for acinar cell cancers but, in contrast to the human disease, they exhibit *KRAS* mutations [33]. Although foci of dysplastic acinar cells are commonly observed in the human adult pancreas, the low incidence of acinar cell tumors in man has restricted the usefulness of this model.

3.3   Mice

More recently, DMBA has been administered to mice by surgical implantation in the head of the pancreas [23]. When left *in situ* for 30 days, 16 mice (67%) developed PanINs and 4 (17%) developed adenocarcinomas. A longer exposure to DMBA of 60 days increased the prevalence of PDA to 38%. Although molecular changes were not assessed in this study, two independent pathologists considered these DMBA-induced neoplasms to resemble human PanIN/PDA histology closely. The increased frequency of PDA induction by DMBA in mice, compared to the low frequency observed in rats, suggested that this was a feasible model for further evaluation. Further investigations revealed a co-operative induction of PDA by DMBA and carcinogens known to promote pancreatic carcinogenesis in humans, including alcohol [34] and nicotine [35]. These findings demonstrate that chemical carcinogens can induce PanIN and PDA in laboratory mice however the requirement for surgical implantation of DMBA is technically encumbering and limits the utility of this model.

4   Transplanted, Chemically-Induced Tumors

A major limitation of chemically-induced pancreatic cancers is the development of a species-specific phenotype that does not recapitulate critical aspects of human PDA. For example, carcinogens induce acinar rather than ductal carcinomas in rats, reflecting the histology of the rare pancreatic carcinomas that develop spontaneously in this species [28]. Additionally, although ductal carcinomas can develop in azaserine-treated hamsters, they differ from the human disease by the absence of *p53* mutations. These limitations have been addressed by the generation of cancer cell lines from chemically-induced tumors (❯ *Fig. 20-2*). For example, pancreatic ductal cancer cell lines prepared from azaserine-treated hamsters spontaneously acquired *p53* mutations in vitro [36]. These cell lines have been successfully transplanted orthotopically into the pancreata of wild-type hamsters to generate invasive and metastatic PDA [37]. Additionally, a cell line derived from an acinar cell carcinoma arising in an azaserine-treated rat was observed to acquire ductal features during cell culture and subsequent regrafting into the rat pancreas. Orthotopic injection of these DSL-6A/C1 cells into the pancreas of recipient rats that had not been treated with azaserine resulted in the development of small, clinically innocuous tumors. By prior growth of DSL-6A/C1 cells as subcutaneous tumors in "donor" rats followed by orthotopic implantation of excised tumor

☐ Fig. 20-2

Diagramatic representation of pancreatic tumor induction in rodents following azaserine treatment. Subsequent harvest of pancreatic ductal (hamster) and acinar (rat) tumor cells and growth *in vitro* promotes the *p53* mutation in hamster PDA and differentiation of rat acinar cell cancers to metastatic PDA.

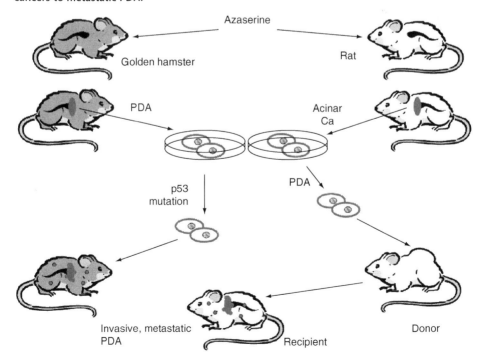

fragments into the pancreata of "recipient" rats, larger, locally invasive and metastatic tumors developed. These tumors demonstrated a ductal phenotype, were surrounded by dense stroma and caused a clinical syndrome similar to that seen in humans [38]. These rat orthotopic models therefore mimicked many aspects of human PDA in an immunocompetent host. However, serious limitations have prevented the widespread use of these models, including the laborious and artificial manner of model generation, and the concern that additional uncharacterized molecular events that occurred in cell culture may not reflect attributes of the cognate human disease.

5   Immunodeficient Models

The advent of immunocompromised mice enabled the generation of PDA xenografts in which human tumor tissue and cell lines were expanded in vivo. Early efforts chiefly involved subcutaneous engraftment models, and these facilitated molecular studies such as the identification of *Smad4/Dpc4* mutation in PDA [13]. To mimic the anatomic environment of PDA better, Tan et al. orthotopically inoculated the human pancreatic adenocarcinoma cell line, AsPC-1, into the pancreas of nude mice resulting in the rapid formation of moderately- to poorly-differentiated pancreatic tumors [39]. In contrast to subcutaneous grafts, which did not display metastatic behavior, these tumors invaded locally and metastasized to intraperitoneal structures and the lungs. Other groups have also observed aggressive, more poorly differentiated tumors when the human PDA cell line HPAC was injected into the pancreas of severe combined immunodeficient (SCID) mice, compared to subcutaneous grafts of the same cell line. This was suggested to be due to the effects of local tropic factors on tumor growth [40]. Whilst it is possible that the anatomical location of engrafted human cells alters their behavior, the increased metastasis seen in the orthotopic AsPC-1 and other models [41] could simply represent seeding of cells at the time of injection. Nonetheless, the availability of these early PDA xenograft models greatly facilitated molecular and therapeutic studies.

A potential shortcoming of PDA xenograft models is the inability of the rapidly expanding tumor to recapitulate the heterogeneous neoplastic cellularity and tumor microenvironment present in native tumors. Indeed, prior cell culturing is associated with the outgrowth of clonal populations of tumor cells (reviewed in [3]). Additionally, xenografts poorly recapitulate the tumor microenvironment architecture present in resected PDA tumors, as reflected by abnormalities in stromal cells, the vasculature and lymphatic channels, and the immune system. Therefore, in efforts to improve the accuracy of human pancreatic cancer xenografts, fresh human tumor tissue fragments have been implanted orthotopically in immunodeficient mice. In one such study, Fu et al. sutured 1 mm^3 pieces of PDA tumors into the pancreata of nude mice and observed that the majority grew locally with extension into surrounding tissues [42]. Additionally, distant metastases developed in mice and expression of tumor-associated antigens was similar before and after implantation, suggesting a resemblance between the original human tumor and the xenograft mouse model. A criticism of this approach has been the necessary trauma caused by the implantation procedure and the inflammatory response associated with the use of sutures, both of which might be expected to alter tumor behavior in these models compared to the human disease [28].

Xenograft models have frequently been used to investigate the efficacy of anti-cancer agents however they are typically more sensitive to systemic therapies than the corresponding human disease. The considerable short-comings of these models have led some to describe them as "animal culture" and to advise their use only as an intermediate step between cell culture and more appropriate animal cancer models [3].

6 Genetically Engineered Mouse Models

Genetically engineered animal models have been created to express mutant versions of genes that have been implicated in human carcinogenesis. Since the genome of the laboratory mouse, *mus muscularis*, has been sequenced in its entirety, almost all efforts in genetically engineered animal models have been focused on this species. The most common genes to be manipulated in this way are oncogenes and tumor suppressor genes. When oncogenes and dominant negative tumor-suppressor genes are expressed non-physiologically in mice by ectopic promoter and enhancer regions, mutant animals are described as transgenic mice. These models have the disadvantage that random incorporation of transgenes and the use of heterologous promoters lead to unpredictable effects on gene expression. In contrast, endogenous animal models are mice in which tumor-suppressor genes have been lost or oncogenes expressed from their physiological promoters [3].

6.1 Early Transgenic Models

The pancreas was one of the first organs in which tissue-specific transgene expression was achieved over twenty years ago. In 1984, Swift et al. published a report describing the expression of the rat serine protease *elastase I* in the murine pancreas [43]. This was achieved by micro-injection of a cDNA construct containing the rat *elastase I* gene, together with flanking sequences, into the pro-nucleus of fertilized murine oocytes. These oocytes were subsequently transferred to foster mothers whose transgenic offspring showed germline expression of one or more copies of the rat *elastase I* gene (⊙ *Fig. 20-3*). High pancreatic expression of rat *elastase I* was observed in the adult transgenic mice, mirroring the high physiological expression of this gene in the rat pancreas. In contrast, *elastase I* gene expression in non-pancreatic murine tissues was minimal. In order to identify which DNA elements were required for pancreas-specific expression of the rat *elastase I* gene, Ornitz et al. introduced a fusion gene comprising the human growth hormone structural gene joined to the 5' flanking region of the rat *elastase I* gene. They found that only 213 base pairs of the *elastase I* gene sequence was sufficient to direct exclusive expression of human growth hormone in pancreatic acinar tissue, thereby identifying a pancreatic acinar cell-specific promoter [44].

Subsequent efforts produced a genetic model of pancreatic cancer by creating transgenic mice in which the transforming gene from the simian virus 40 (SV40) T-antigen was placed under the control of the regulatory element from the rat *elastase I* promoter [45]. All four mutant mouse strains created in this way died of pancreatic cancer by 6.5 months. Breeding of founder mice prior to tumor formation led to the creation of three transgenic lines which developed pancreatic cancer. Although these early experiments established transgenic mice as a means of modeling human pancreatic cancer, the use of the acinar-specific *elastase* promoter resulted in the generation of acinar cell as opposed to ductal malignancies.

The ability of cellular oncogenes to induce pancreatic carcinogenesis was been investigated by using the rat *elastase I* promoter to drive expression of activated human *HRAS* and *c-MYC* in transgenic mice. Mutant *HRAS* induced massive acinar cell cancers in mice during fetal

☐ Fig. 20-3

Micro-injection of cDNA constructs, such as the rat *elastase I* gene, into the pro-nucleus of fertilized murine oocytes and subsequent injection into pseudo-pregnant females, creates transgenic offspring with germline expression of the exogenous gene.

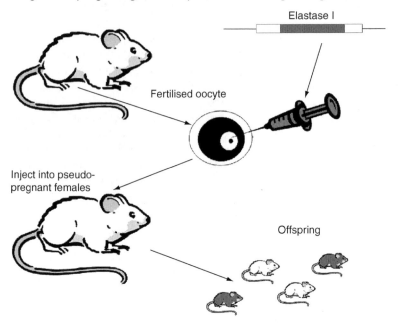

development, resulting in death in utero or shortly after birth [46]. In contrast, when *c-MYC* expression was driven by the rat *elastase I* promoter, transgenic mice developed mixed acinar and ductal pancreatic cancers between two and seven months of age [47]. Since *elastase I* was expected to be an acinar cell-specific promoter, it is interesting to note that in younger mice, transformed acinar-derived cells were seen in pancreatic islets. By later stages in the disease process, neoplastic ductal cells appeared within acinar cell tumors giving rise to mixed or ductal adenocarcinomas and implying that acinar cells contribute to pancreatic ductal carcinogenesis in this model.

The hypothesis that acinar cells transdifferentiate to ductal pancreatic cancers was further pursued by Sandgren and colleagues, who generated transgenic elastase-TGF-α mutant mice following the identification of TGF-α over-expression in human pancreatic cancers, [48]. Elastase-TGF-α mice developed pancreatic fibrosis with massive expansion of the pancreatic micro-fibroblast population and accumulation of extracellular matrix. Pancreata demonstrated acinar cell abnormalities which resembled some features of early stage PanINs. In mice older than one year, occasional papillary and cystic pancreatic cancers were observed in close association with dysplastic foci [49]. Despite their acinar origin, these tumors expressed the duct specific antigen, Duct-1, suggesting an acinar to ductal evolution of pancreatic cancer and supporting the observations made by Sandgren et al. in their *c-MYC* transgenic mouse [47]. However, the overall distortion of the pancreatic acinar architecture, the absence of clear evolution of PanINs to PDA, and the lack of mutant *Kras* as the dominant oncogene restricted the usefulness of this model.

6.2   Mutant *KRAS* Transgenic Models

To directly address whether oncogenic *Kras* might yield improved transgenic mouse models of pancreatic cancer, Grippo et al. [50] generated multiple lines of elastase-*KRAS*^{G12D} transgenic mice. The majority of these mice were born underweight but with distended abdomens. At *post mortem* examination, pancreatic tissue was largely replaced by stroma and normal ducts were sparse. Two founder mice appeared normal at birth and, when mated, their offspring had normal appearing pancreata with occasional hyperplastic acini. As they aged, the pancreatic tissue became progressively more abnormal with prominent acinar hyperplasia that was frequently associated with dysplasia, lymphocyte infiltration and fibrosis. Between 6 and 18 months of age, acinar to ductal metaplasia was observed although ductal lesions did not follow a typical PanIN progression pattern to yield PDA. These observations imply a role for *KRAS* in the initiation of malignant pancreatic pathology and, when targeted to acinar cells by the elastase I promoter, it appears that *KRAS* is capable of inducing acinar to ductal differentiation.

In an attempt to target mutant *KRAS* expression to the pancreatic ductal lineage, Brembeck et al. [51] created transgenic mice in which oncogenic *KRAS*^{G12V}, was expressed ectopically from the cytokeratin 19 promoter that is expressed in many simple cuboidal cells including mature pancreatic ductal cells. They observed dramatic periductal infiltration of predominantly CD4 positive lymphocytes but morphological changes in ductal cells were rare. Since targeting mutant *KRAS* expression to mature ductal cells caused predominantly inflammation in this model, it is possible that additional genetic events are required in addition to activating mutations of *KRAS* to initiate PanIN, or conversely that differentiated ductal cells are not the cell of origin for PDA. The failure of mutant *KRAS* expression, in both acinar and mature ductal compartments, to produce ductal neoplasia gave support to the hypothesis that pancreatic cancer arises from undifferentiated ductal progenitor cells.

Since pancreatic ductal adenocarcinoma presents late clinically, it has been difficult to study the pathological evolution of the human disease. These early transgenic experiments provided a unique platform on which to investigate the ability of oncogenes either to drive carcinogenesis within a specific cell type or to promote transdifferentiation of pre-malignant cells. They generated hypotheses relating to the cell of origin of pancreatic cancer but did not enable the creation of a murine model of classical PanIN or invasive PDA. The generation of mouse models that accurately replicated human PDA was facilitated by the advent of gene targeting approaches in embryonic stem cells, the delineation of molecules and cellular features controlling pancreatic development, the recognition and acceptance of pre-invasive pancreatic neoplasms and the unraveling of the genetic events that characterize human pancreatic cancer.

7   Pancreatic Development

Advances in the understanding of pancreatic developmental biology identified the homeodomain protein, *Pdx-1*, and the helix-loop-helix protein, *Ptf1α/p48*, as critical regulators of early pancreatic development [52]. Targeted deletion of either of these genes severely impairs pancreatic morphogenesis and cell differentiation [53–55]. In early development, common pancreatic precursor cells expressing both *Pdx-1* and *Ptf1α/p48* give rise to all differentiated endocrine and exocrine cells of the mature organ. *Pdx-1* is expressed from embryonic day 8.5 and, at maturity, is expressed at the highest levels in islet β cells. *Ptf1α/p48* expression initiates at embryonic day 9.5 and only persists in the acinar compartment postnatally [56]. These tissue-specific promoters have been exploited to enable pancreas-specific, physiological expression of mutant genes to create endogenous murine models of PDA.

8   Endogenous Murine Models of PDA

8.1   The Cre-Lox System

Endogenous models of human PDA have utilized site-specific recombinase enzymes (SSRs) to generate conditional murine cancer models. Most commonly, the bacteriophage Cre-Lox system has been employed (❯ *Fig. 20-4*). In this system, the *Cre* SSR recognizes a pair of DNA sequences known as Lox-P sites and enzyme activity catalyses their recombination such that the intervening DNA sequence is excised or inverted [57]. Endogenous murine cancer models can therefore be generated by flanking tumor suppressor genes with Lox-P sites and exposing the mouse to *Cre* recombinase. Alternatively, a transcriptional and translational

☐ Fig. 20-4

Genetic recombination at Lox-P sites (denoted by triangles) following the action of Cre recombinase results in excision of the intervening sequence. (a.) In conditional knock-in alleles, excision of a "stop" cassette enables expression of an oncogene. (b) In conditional knock-out alleles, *Cre* expression excises exons to disrupt tumor-suppressor genes (TSGs).

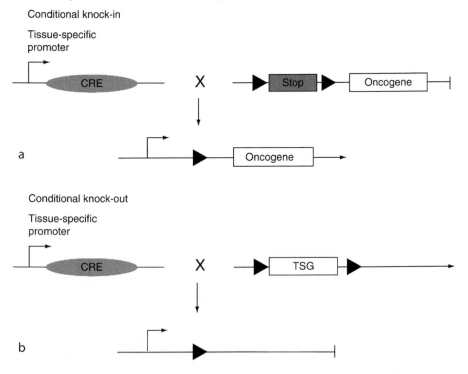

"stop" cassette can be flanked by Lox-P sites and inserted immediately upstream of an oncogenic sequence such that excision of the "stop" cassette enables expression of the oncogene. By using tissue-specific promoters to direct *Cre* expression, genetic manipulations can be limited to the organ of interest.

8.2   Endogenous Mutant *KRAS* Mice

The first description of the use of this technology to generate endogenous murine models of pancreatic cancer was published in 2003. Jacks and co-workers had previously produced mice in which the endogenous *KRAS* locus was replaced by a mutant $KRAS^{G12D}$ allele, preceded by a Lox-stop-Lox cassette [58]. These mice were crossed with mice expressing *Cre* recombinase in pancreatic tissue either through a *Pdx-1* promoter-driven transgene or by knocking in *Cre* at the *Ptf1α/p48* locus [59]. *Pdx1-Cre* transgenic animals showed stochastic pancreatic *Cre* expression whilst *Ptf1α/p48* knock-in strains had uniform *Cre* expression throughout the pancreas. Mutant *KRAS* activation in both mice resulted in increased levels of GTP-bound Ras that was associated with progressive ductal pathology. From two weeks of age, focal cuboidal to columnar epithelial transition was observed in pancreatic ducts, representing early PanIN-1a neoplasms. Over the following year, these early changes were succeeded by more pronounced architectural and cytological abnormality, including the development of papillary lesions with increasing nuclear atypia, resembling the progression of human PanINs from grade 1 to 3. In addition to these pre-invasive ductal neoplasms, pancreatic parenchyma underwent marked inflammatory and fibrotic changes, similar to that seen in human pancreatic cancer. Despite this, progression to overt pancreatic ductal adenocarcinoma associated with invasion and widespread metastasis was only observed in approximately 10% of mice over the first year, implying the need for additional genetic events during malignant progression.

8.3   Activated *KRAS* and *Ink4a/Arf* Deficiency

In human PDA, loss of the cyclin-dependant kinase inhibitor $p16^{Ink4a}$ is an almost universal event that follows *KRAS* mutation. In addition, the $p14^{ARF}$ tumor-suppressor gene (known as $p19^{ARF}$ in mice) that is also encoded by the *Ink4a* gene locus (◉ *Fig. 20-5*) is likely to be inactivated in PDA. To investigate the contribution of *Ink4a/ARF* deficiency to PDA, Aguirre et al. generated conditional *Ink4a/ARF* mice with exons 2 and 3 of the *Ink4a* gene (encoding $p16^{Ink4a}$ and $p19^{ARF}$ respectively) flanked by Lox-P sites [60]. Pancreas-specific *Cre*-mediated excision of $p16^{Ink4a}$ and $p19^{ARF}$ together with heterozygous expression of $KRAS^{G12D}$ (as previously described by Hingorani et al. [59]) was achieved by crossing with *Pdx1-Cre* transgenic mice (*Pdx1-Cre;LSL-KRAS ^{G12D};Ink4a/Arf $^{lox/lox}$*). Low grade PanIN lesions were observed in these mice as early as three weeks of age, which increased in number and grade over the following month. Most mice succumbed to pancreatic cancer between weeks seven and eleven, after presenting with weight loss, jaundice, ascites and palpable abdominal masses. At *post mortem* examination, the pancreatic tumors were solid and frequently invaded adjacent organs. Although metastasis occurred to lymph nodes, hepatic metastases were rare and pulmonary metastases were not reported. Microscopically, the primary tumors had a predominantly sarcomatoid differentiation pattern, with well- to moderately-differentiated

□ Fig. 20-5

Ink4a encodes *p14^ARF* and *p16^Ink4a*. *p14^ARF* inhibits *mdm2*-mediated *p53* degradation, whilst *p16^Ink4a* inhibits cyclin-dependant kinase (CDK) activity.

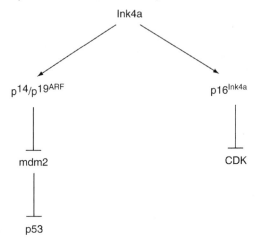

PDA and anaplastic morphology reported less frequently. This contrasted with mice expressing mutant *KRAS^{G12D}* without inactivation of the *Ink4A/ARF* locus (*Pdx1-Cre;LSL-KRAS^{G12D}*) that, in agreement with the findings of Hingorani et al. [59], developed PanIN lesions and progressive fibrosis but not invasive pancreatic cancer. *Pdx1-Cre;Ink4a/Arf^{lox/lox}* mice that lacked activated *KRAS^{G12D}* did not develop pancreatic tumors, supporting a model in which activating *KRAS* mutation initiates the formation of PanINs, which progress to invasive malignancy upon loss of *Ink4a/ARF.*

8.4 Activated *KRAS* and the *p53* Pathway

Following the findings of Aguirre et al., it was hypothesized that *p16^Ink4a* and *p19^ARF* initially restrain the oncogenic activity of mutant *KRAS*, although their relative contribution to pancreatic oncogenesis remained unknown. *p14^ARF* and *p16^Ink4a* deletions co-exist in approximately 40% of human PDA [61]. Since *p14^ARF* inhibits *mdm2*-mediated *p53* degradation, some of its biological function might be expected to mirror that of *p53*. Nonetheless, co-existent mutations of *p53* and loss of *p14^ARF* are found in 38% of human PDA [10], implying non-overlapping tumor suppressor roles for these two proteins. In humans, *p53* is mutated in up to 75% of PDA [10], typically in tumors that have already undergone *KRAS* mutation and *p16^Ink4a* loss [11]. Interestingly, the *Pdx1-Cre;LSL-KRAS^{G12D};Ink4a/Arf^{lox/lox}* mice described by Aguirre et al. did not acquire mutations of *p53* or any other tumor suppressor implicated in pancreatic cancer [60], perhaps implying that *p53* is not rate-limiting for the generation of pancreatic cancer in mice when its upstream regulators are absent. In order to understand the relative contribution of these factors, Bardeesy et al. [62] investigated the impact of loss of *p16^Ink4a*, *p19^ARF* and *p53* in the previously described *Pdx1-Cre; LSL-KRAS^{G12D}* model [59]. When *Pdx1-Cre;LSL-Kras^{G12D}* mice were interbred with mice bearing null mutations in $p53$ and $p16^{Ink4a}$ or in $p16^{Ink4a}$ and $p19^{ARF}$, all tumor suppressor mutations, either alone or in combination, were found to give rise to invasive pancreatic cancer. Homozygous loss of $p53$ resulted in the generation of lethal tumors by eight weeks of age, a comparable time course to that seen with combined loss of $p16^{Ink4a}$ and $p19^{ARF}$. The addition of homozygous deletion of $p16^{Ink4a}$ to homozygous $p53$ loss did not alter the latency of PDA formation, suggesting that developmental inactivation of $p53$ diminishes the need for $p16^{Ink4a}$ loss. Interestingly, $p16^{Ink4a}$ deletion in the context of wild-type $p53$ and $p19^{ARF}$ significantly accelerated the development of lethal PDA to a mean of 18.3 weeks, demonstrating that mutation of the $p53$ pathway *per se* was not required for the development of PDA. In $KRAS^{G12D}$ mutant mice heterozygous for $p53$ (*Pdx1-Cre; LSL-KRAS^{G12D}; p53$^{lox/+}$*) the addition of a heterozygous mutation of $p16^{Ink4a}$ (*Pdx1-Cre; LSL-KRAS^{G12D}; p53$^{lox/+}$; p16$^{lox/+}$*), significantly shortened the time to development of lethal PDA from 21.8 to 14.7 weeks. Heterozygous deletion of $p16^{Ink4a}/p19^{ARF}$ (*Pdx1-Cre; LSL-KRAS^{G12D}; p16/p19$^{lox/+}$*) also gave rise to lethal PDA but with a much greater latency of 34.2 weeks. Histologically, nearly all tumors generated were ductal adenocarcinomas with a dense stromal reaction. In homozygous mice, the highest proportion of PDA was found in the setting of $p53$ loss. The additional loss of $p16^{Ink4a}$ tended to increase the number of tumors with anaplastic features, whereas $p16^{Ink4a}$ deletion in the presence of wild-type $p53$, gave rise to pancreatic cancers with areas of sarcomatoid differentiation. In compound heterozygous mice, PDA was most common in *Pdx1-Cre;LSL-KRAS^{G12D};p53$^{lox/+}$;p16$^{lox/+}$* mice, whereas *Pdx1-Cre; LSL-KRAS^{G12D};p16/p19$^{lox/+}$* frequently showed a sarcomatoid histology. Invasion and metastasis were more frequently observed in heterozygous mice of all genotypes, perhaps because of their enhanced survival compared to homozygotes. This work provided insight into the unique and redundant roles of the tumor suppressors $p53$, $p16^{Ink4a}$ and $p19^{ARF}$ on pancreatic tumor histology and behavior.

In human PDA, inactivation of $p53$ usually occurs through missense mutation combined with loss of the second allele [9,10]. One of the most common $p53$ mutations in human PDA is $p53^{R175H}$ [63] and therefore Hingorani et al. investigated the influence of the orthologous $p53^{R172H}$ mutation together with $KRAS^{G12D}$ expressed endogenously in the developing mouse pancreas [64]. This was achieved by generating conditional $LSL-p53^{R172H}$ mice and interbreeding with conditional *Pdx1-Cre;KRAS^{G12D}* transgenic mice such that offspring were triply heterozygous (*Pdx1-Cre;LSL-KRAS^{G12D};LSL-p53$^{R172H/+}$*). The authors postulated that this genotype was likely to be an accurate approximation of that found in humans following spontaneous acquisition of heterozygous mutations. Compared to control littermates and $KRAS$ mutant mice (*Pdx1-Cre;LSL-KRAS^{G12D}*), double mutants had a significantly reduced median survival of five months. In agreement with their previous work, *Pdx1-Cre;LSL-KRAS^{G12D}* mice developed predominantly pre-invasive disease. All *Pdx1-Cre;LSL-KRAS^{G12D};LSL-p53$^{R172H/+}$* mice developed a clinical syndrome reminiscent of human PDA consisting of cachexia and abdominal distension. At *post mortem*, large volumes of haemorrhagic ascites together with large, firm tumors of the pancreas were invariably found. There was also macroscopic evidence of local invasion and metastasis to the liver, lung and peritoneum. Microscopically, the pancreatic tumors of compound mutant mice were moderately- or well-differentiated ductal carcinomas and were associated with all grades of PanIN. Notably, the pancreata of very young mice were overall of normal histology except for the occurrence of PanIN-1a, suggesting that genetic mutations acquired during adulthood are necessary for disease progression. Analysis of cell lines derived from pancreatic tissue and PDAs revealed that the wild-type $p53$ allele was uniformly lost over time, thereby mirroring the situation in human PDA. Additionally, aneuploidy and chromosomal instability were observed in most of the PDA cell lines, similar to these features in human PDA cells. Interestingly, expression of the *Ink4a* locus and *Smad4/Dpc4* was retained in all PDA cell lines evaluated. This study provided further evidence of the importance of the *p53* pathway in suppressing invasive pancreatic cancer initiated by activating *KRAS* mutations. These models are summarized in ● *Table 20-2*.

8.5 The Role of Inflammation

Previously described models utilized mutant gene expression that initiated during embryonic development. Guerra et al. used an inducible Cre-Lox system to investigate the influence of oncogenic *KRAS* expression at various stages in development and adult life [65]. They interbred mice harboring a conditional *KRAS*^{G12V} mutant allele to mouse strains harboring an acinar cell doxycycline responsive Cre transgene. This system enabled *Cre* to be "switched off" by exposing mice to doxycycline and "switched on" when this drug was removed. In contrast to previous work [50], they observed the full range of PanINs and PDA when

◘ Table 20-2

Summary Table of studies into endogenous murine models of pancreatic ductal carcinogenesis

Genetics	Predominant histology	Clinical	Metastasis	Survival	Reference
LSL-Kras^{G12D}	PDA (10%)	–	50%	–	[64]
Ink4a/Arf$^{lox/lox}$	Sarcomatoid (Minimal PDA with anaplastic regions)	Weight loss, jaundice, ascites	Lymph nodes and rarely liver	7–11 weeks	[60]
p53$^{lox/lox}$	PDA (100%)		0%	6.2 weeks	[62]
p16/p19$^{lox/lox}$	PDA (48%)		11%	8.5 weeks	
	Sarc. (26%)				
	Ana. (26%)				
p53$^{lox/lox}$; p16$^{lox/lox}$	Ana. (60%)		20%	7.2 weeks	
	PDA (40%)				
p16$^{lox/lox}$	Sarc. (100%)		33%	18.3 weeks	
p53$^{lox/+}$	PDA (100%)		33%	21.8 weeks	
p16/p19$^{lox/+}$	PDA (57%)		69%	34.2 weeks	
	Sarc. (43%)				
p53$^{lox/+}$; p16$^{lox/+}$	PDA (81%)		25%	14.7 weeks	
	Sarc. (19%)				
LSL-p53^{R172H}	PDA (96%)	Weight loss, ascites	74%	20 weeks	[64]

All mice had *Pdx-Cre* directed expression of a conditional *LSL-Kras*^{G12D} allele Sarc. = sarcomatoid differentiation, Ana. = anaplastic histology

$KRAS^{G12V}$ was "switched on" in murine embryonic acinar cells. This implies that mutant $KRAS$ is capable of promoting acinar to ductal metaplasia and of stimulating oncogenesis in this background. Activating $KRAS^{G12V}$ in the adult pancreas did not result in pancreatic neoplasia. However, if chronic pancreatitis was induced by first exposing adult mice to caerulein, animals developed the full spectrum of PanINs and invasive PDA. Acinar cell injury in the adult organ therefore appears to render these cells, or a sub-population within them, receptive to the transforming effect of mutant $KRAS$. This work provided a possible mechanism for the well known association between chronic pancreatitis and PDA in humans [66]. It upheld the importance of mutant $KRAS$ in initiating pancreatic oncogenesis as well as suggesting that PDA can originate from adult pancreatic acinar cells in the context of pancreatic inflammation.

8.6   Cystic Neoplasms: Activated *KRAS* and *Smad4/TGF-β* Signaling

Another important genetic event in human PDA is the inactivation of *Smad4/Dpc4* that occurs in approximately 50% of cases [67]. This tumor suppressor gene, which is lost in the hereditary juvenile polyposis cancer syndrome [68], encodes a signal mediator downstream of the receptors for transforming growth factor β (TGF-β). Physiological functions of TGF-β include apoptosis induction, cell-cycle modulation and growth inhibition in epithelial cells [69]. In human epithelial cancers, TGF-β is frequently inactivated, allowing cellular escape from growth inhibition such that tumor cell growth is enhanced and a metastatic phenotype promoted. TGF-β is also thought to have a role in pancreatic development. In mice, germline deletion of *Smad4/Dpc4* is lethal during early embryogenesis, while heterozygous deletion gives rise to upper gastrointestinal polyps but not pancreatic pathology [70]. Data acquired *in vitro* and in xenograft models of pancreatic cancer gave conflicting conclusions regarding the role of *Smad4/Dpc4*. Very recently, efforts have been made to understand the significance of this pathway in human pancreatic cancer through the use of genetic mouse models.

Bardeesy et al. [71] investigated the role of *Smad4/Dpc4* in pancreatic development and pathology by flanking exons 8 and 9 in the mouse germline with Lox-P sites and crossing with *Pdx1-Cre* or *Ptf1α/p48-Cre* transgenic mice. They found that mice with homozygous deletion of *Smad4/Dpc4* were born at the expected frequency with normal pancreata although many mice had duodenal polyps. Deletion of this tumor suppressor in isolation therefore seems to be insufficient to induce PDA. When mice were generated with conditional deletion of *Smad4/Dpc4* and conditional expression of $KRAS^{G12D}$ using either *Pdx1-Cre* or *Ptf1α/p48-Cre* (collectively known as *Cre;LSL-KRAS^{G12D};Smad4$^{lox/lox}$*), abdominal masses were observed between the ages of seven and twelve weeks and survival was dramatically reduced compared to *Pdx1-Cre;LSL-KRAS^{G12D}* controls. Interestingly, histological examination of *post mortem* specimens from *Cre;LSL-KRAS^{G12D};Smad4$^{lox/lox}$* mice revealed predominantly cystic pancreatic neoplasms resembling IPMNs in 17 out of 20 animals. PanINs were also seen although PDA was only found in 2 out of 20 mice. *Smad4/Dpc4* therefore seems to accelerate disease progression and to divert *KRAS*-induced carcinogenesis to a more cystic histology. More detailed analysis of *Cre;LSL-KRAS^{G12D};Smad4$^{lox/lox}$* and control *Cre;LSL-KRAS^{G12D}* mice sacrificed at sequential time points demonstrated that additional deletion of *Smad4/Dpc4* was influential early in the disease course with an increase in the number and size of PanIN lesions being observed in *Cre;LSL-KRAS^{G12D};Smad4$^{lox/lox}$* mice from 4 weeks of age. Further mice were created incorporating deletions of the *Ink4a* locus. Combined mutation of *Smad4/Dpc4* and

Ink4a in the absence of *KRAS* activation gave rise to only one IPMN-like tumor in 23 mice, confirming the importance of mutant *KRAS* for tumor initiation. Mice with combined deletions of *Smad4/Dpc4* and heterozygous loss of *Ink4a* on a *KRAS* mutant background (*Cre;LSL-KRAS^{G12D};Ink4a/Arf$^{lox/+}$;Smad4$^{lox/lox}$*) had a significantly reduced median survival of 12.6–14 weeks (depending on the promoter used to direct *Cre* expression) compared to 38 weeks in *Cre;LSL-Kras^{G12D};Ink4a/Arf$^{lox/+}$* controls. 12 out of 13 *Ptf1α/p48-Cre; LSL-KRAS^{G12D};Ink4a/Arf$^{lox/+}$,Smad4$^{lox/lox}$* died of PDA whereas gastric cancer was noted in similar mice directed from the *Pdx1-Cre* transgene. Compared to the PDA tumors observed in control mice (*Cre;LSL-KRAS^{G12D};Ink4a/Arf$^{lox/+}$*), *Smad4* loss promoted a more differentiated tumor morphology with cystic lesions resembling IPMN. This work provided a histologically accurate murine model of human IPMN although surprisingly, corresponding mutations of *Smad4/Dpc4* are rare in IPMN and are instead more common in MCN [72]. Nonetheless, a role for *Smad4/Dpc4* is implicated in suppressing *KRAS*-induced oncogensis and regulating cellular differentiation. It also confirmed previous findings that, in the context of *KRAS^{G12D}*, additional mutations in tumor suppressor genes are necessary for reliable pancreatic tumorigenesis.

The induction of cystic neoplasms by abnormalities of *Smad4/Dpc4* was explored further by Izeradjene et al. [73]. They generated mice with deletions of *Smad4/Dpc4* alone or in combination with *KRAS^{G12D}* using the Cre-lox system. Again, hetero- and homozygous pancreatic deletion of *Smad4/Dpc4* alone did not result in any phenotypic abnormalities. When combined with mutant *KRAS* expression, heterozygous animals (*Pdx1-Cre;LSL-KRAS$_{G12D}$;Smad4$_{lox/+}$*) had a significantly reduced survival of eight months. At *post mortem*, the double mutant animals were found to have PanIN lesions as well as cystic lesions in the pancreas and stomach. Gastric lesions were primarily squamous cell carcinomas with evidence of local invasion and distant metastatic spread. They were again interpreted as being due to the extra-pancreatic expression of *Pdx-1* and were thought to be the primary cause of premature death in these mice. When similar mice were generated using the more pancreas-specific *Ptf1α/p48* promoter no gastric lesions were seen. Heterozygous *Ptf1α/p48-Cre; KRAS^{G12D};Smad$^{lox/+}$*, mice had a comparable survival to *Ptf1α/p48-Cre;KRAS^{G12D}* animals, with the former developing palpable abdominal masses due to large mucin-containing cystic neoplasms affecting the body and tail of the pancreas. PanINs were also seen, although they tended to be of a lower grade than those found in age-matched *Ptf1α/p48-Cre; KRAS^{G12D}* littermates. Homozygous deletion of *Smad4/Dpc4* together with mutant *KRAS* expression once again reduced survival compared to heterozygous counterparts. There was also an increase in the extent of mucin-containing pancreatic cysts, implicating loss of heterozygosity at *Smad4/Dpc4* as a major contributor to disease progression. Indeed, immunohistochemical analysis of pancreatic tissue obtained from heterozygous mice demonstrated that *Smad4/Dpc4* expression was retained in cystic pre-malignant lesions but lost in adjacent areas of invasive PDA. Microscopically, the pancreatic cystic lesions in *Ptf1α/p48-Cre;KRAS^{G12D};Smad$^{lox/+}$* mice resembled human MCN, being lined by columnar, mucin-filled epithelial cells with a lower proliferative index than PanIN cells. The surrounding stroma was cellular with typical "ovarian" features including positivity for progesterone and oestrogen receptors. Local invasion and metastasis was much lower than that previously described for *Pdx1-Cre; LSL-KRAS^{G12D};LSL-p53^{R172H}* mice [64], correlating with the less aggressive phenotype seen with cystic pancreatic neoplasms compared to PDA in humans. It is unclear why similar genetic models have produced different cystic neoplasms. Possibilities include the different strains of mice used or a discrepancy in the pathological interpretation of tumor specimens between the two groups. Despite this, the development of endogenous murine models of pre-invasive, pancreatic cystic neoplasia by these two groups has provided an important biological resource. Intuitively, detection and treatment of the three known PDA precursor lesions: PanIN, IPMN and MCN is predicted to influence patient outcomes and interrogation of the models described here is therefore imperative. The slower progression of IPMN and MCNs make them particularly attractive as a target for novel screening methods and therapies.

9 Limitations of Current Models

The progressive sophistication of genetic engineering and the consequent development of murine models of pancreatic cancer have generated considerable enthusiasm that such models will be useful for pre-clinical investigation. It is important to remember however that differences exist between mice and humans and attempts must always be made to minimize or account for them.

At the genetic level, one possible limitation when using the Cre-Lox system is that the placement of a "stop" cassette between a promoter and the gene of interest will necessarily render the mouse heterozygous for that gene prior to *Cre* expression. The *KRAS* mice described here, could therefore be exposed to the reported tumor-suppressor role of wild-type *KRAS* [74] prior to *Cre*-mediated activation of mutant *KRAS*. In addition, the mutant genes activated in genetically engineered models will be induced in many cells of a tissue simultaneously and, when compound mutant mice are created, all mutant alleles are likely to be expressed together. This differs from the accepted mechanism by which human tumors are thought to develop from a single mutated cell that subsequently acquires additional mutations in a step-wise manner (*Fig. 20-1*). These limitations can be addressed to some extent by the use of different site-specific recombinases in addition to *Cre*, as well as by utilizing drug-inducible recombinase enzymes [3]. A fundamental species difference with relevance to pancreatic cancer is the increased length of murine telomeres in comparison to human telomeres. Telomere shortening has been shown to be one of the earliest genetic events in pancreatic cancer [75] but as yet shortening murine telomeres to increase their approximation to the human equivalent has proved difficult [3]. A current challenge is therefore to minimize many of these limitations in future models.

10 The Future

Successive advances in the field of animal modeling have resulted in the creation of a variety of genetically engineered mice that accurately represent pre-invasive and invasive pancreatic neoplasms at the genetic, biochemical, histological and clinical level. Despite these impressive advances, human pancreatic cancer remains difficult to detect in its early stages, treatments are unchanged and the outlook for patients with pancreatic cancer is bleak. Although the models described here have attempted to uncover the cell of origin of PDA, the answer to this important question remains elusive. Whilst existing models could be improved by incorporating additional genetic and environmental abnormalities common to human PDA, it is predicted that interrogation of existing models should lead to earlier disease detection and improved therapeutic options.

10.1 Uncovering the Cell of Origin

The cellular niche that gives rise to PanIN and PDA is still unclear. The use of *Pdx1-Cre* to express mutant $KRAS^{G12D}$ in the developing mouse embryo produced only PanINs and PDA, suggesting that *KRAS* is capable of initiating oncogenesis in the immature ductal compartment or other cellular lineages [59]. In efforts to further define the cell type responsible, the expression of $KRAS^{G12V}$ in the embryonic pancreatic acinar compartment and adult acinar compartment provided evidence that this cell type could transdifferentiate to PanIN and PDA under certain conditions [65]. In support of this hypothesis, the intermediate filament protein nestin, a marker of progenitor cells in the pancreas and other organs, has been identified in populations of differentiated acinar cells [76]. In contrast, no direct evidence currently supports ductal cells as the cell of origin for PanIN or PDA, although no studies with ductal specific Cre transgenes and conditionally mutant *KRAS* mice have been reported. Current efforts should soon determine the plasticity of the various pancreatic lineages in the initiation of PanIN and PDA.

Evidence is accumulating in support of the concept of tumor-initiating stem cells in solid cancers and a stem cell population has recently been isolated in human pancreatic cancer [77]. These cancer-initiating cells, which are thought to account for less than 1% of cells within the tumor and are particularly resistant to therapeutic agents, were characterized by cell surface marker expression including CD24 and CD44 [78,79]. Cancer stem cells expressing CD133 have also recently been reported in human pancreatic cancer tissue [80]. Only 500 of these cells were necessary to induce oncogenesis when injected orthotopically in nude mice, whereas injection of a million CD133 negative cells did not result in tumorigenesis. Cells co-expressing CD133 and the chemokine receptor, CXCR4, were critical to the development of a metastatic phenotype in these mice. Although it is unclear whether these tumor-initiating cells are also the cell of origin for PDA, the existence of analogous populations of cells in endogenous animal models of PDA should be pursued for biological and therapeutic insights.

10.2 Improving Disease Detection and Treatment

The ultimate reason for devising intricate murine models of human cancer is to improve the outlook for people with cancer. It is imperative that these models are exploited to provide novel biomarkers, imaging strategies and therapies for use in patients. Resection of even very early stage human pancreatic cancer is rarely curative, implying that significant advances in patient survival will only be achieved through detection and treatment at the pre-invasive stage. Since PanINs are rarely clinically apparent in humans prior to the development of PDA, the availability of murine models of pre-invasive cancer, should expedite the discovery of biomarkers to detect preinvasive neoplasms in patients. The only routinely available serum biomarker of pancreatic cancer currently in clinical use is Ca19.9. Although this marker at presentation correlates with disease prognosis [81], it is rarely raised in PanINs, precluding its use for screening. In a small pilot study, Hingorani et al. [59] were able to identify a serum proteomic signature in *KRAS* mutant mice with histologically confirmed PanIN, but not PDA, using surfaced enhanced laser desorption ionisation time-of-flight (SELDI-TOF). The proteomic signature generated was able to distinguish PanIN mice from littermate controls with a sensitivity of 90.5% and specificity of 97.7%. Further investigation of the serum of murine cancer models could identify the secreted products of genes with differential expression in tumor-prone mice, supporting the feasibility of such an approach. In a recently published landmark study using *Pdx-Cre;LSL-KRAS*^{G12D}*;Ink4a/Arf*$^{lox/lox}$ mice [60], 165 proteins were identified that were dramatically more abundant in the plasma of tumor-bearing compared to control mice. From these, a panel of five proteins was measured in healthy humans and was found to predict the development of pancreatic cancer up to a year prior to clinical diagnosis [82]. These important findings suggest that endogenous murine models of pancreatic cancer have the potential to identify plasma biomarkers of early pancreatic cancer that can be extrapolated to humans. The difficulty in detecting early human pancreatic neoplasia, and therefore in obtaining plasma from such individuals, makes these type of approaches particularly exciting.

Mouse PDA models should also help to identify potential therapeutic targets, for example using exciting new technologies such as transposon-mediated forward genetics. Transposons are sequences of DNA capable of mobilizing to different positions within the genome of a single cell after excision by transposase. The *Sleeping Beauty* transposon contains splice acceptors in both orientations flanked by polyadenylation signals such that it can cause loss of function mutations in tumor suppressor genes. The incorporation of sequences from the murine stem cell virus promoter/enhancer regions also allows it to promote over-expression of proto-oncogenes [83]. Introducing this system into existing murine models of pancreatic cancer could identify genes that co-operate with *KRAS*^{G12D} as well as potentially identifying new drug targets.

Finally, murine cancer models provide an accessible platform for the evaluation of therapeutic agents. In addition to the genetic abnormalities described above, a multitude of molecular pathways are altered in human PDA and several of these have also been found to be activated in pancreatic pre-neoplasms in the murine models described here. Examples include cyclo-oxygenase 2 (COX2), matrix metalloproteinase 9, and the Notch and Hedgehog developmental signaling pathways [59]. Drugs capable of inhibiting each of these pathways exist at various stages of development. The ready availability of murine cancer models should enable the evaluation of these and other novel agents with the ultimate aim of facilitating translation of the most promising agents to the clinic, such that patient benefit is maximized.

Key Research Points

- Pancreatic adenocarcinoma is characterized by a well-defined series of genetic events
- *KRAS* mutations are found in 95% of PDA and are the earliest change noted in PanINs
- Pre-invasive neoplasms include PanIN, MCN and IPMN
- Co-operating mutations in addition to mutant *KRAS* are required for malignant progression
- Additional mutations determine malignant histology
- Endogenous murine models of PDA utilize:
  - pancreas-specific promoters
  - site-specific recombinase enzymes such as *Cre*

Future Scientific Directions + Clinical Implications

- **Improving animal models:**
  - Combining site-specific recombinases
  - Using drug-inducible systems
  - Incorporating forward genetic approaches, eg., transposases
- **Exploiting existing models:**
  - Investigating cancer stem cells
  - Discovering novel biomarkers
  - Testing new and existing therapies

References

1. CancerStats: Pancreatic cancer-UK. Cancer Research UK. 2006. *http://intranet.cancerresearchuk.org/multimedia/pdfs/pc_pancreas_pdf_march_2006.*
2. Mueller MM, Fusenig NE: Friends or foes - bipolar effects of the tumour stroma in cancer. Nature Rev 2004;4:839–849.
3. Frese KK, Tuveson DA: Maximizing mouse cancer models. Nat Rev 2007;7:645–658.
4. Caldas C, Kern SE: K-ras mutation and pancreatic adenocarcinoma. Int J Pancreatol 1995;18:1–6.
5. Almoguera C, Shibata D, Forrester K, Martin J, Arnheim N, Perucho M: Most human carcinomas of the exocrine pancreas contain mutant c-K-ras genes. Cell 1988;53:549–554.
6. Hilgers W, Kern SE: Molecular genetic basis of pancreatic adenocarcinoma. Genes Chromosomes Cancer 1999;26:1–12.
7. Maitra A, Hruban RH: Pancreatic cancer. Annual Rev Pathol 2008;3:157–188.
8. Schutte M, Hruban RH, Geradts J, Maynard R, Hilgers W, Rabindran SK, Moskaluk CA, Hahn SA, Schwarte-Waldhoff I, Schmiegel W, et al.: Abrogation of the Rb/p16 tumor-suppressive pathway in virtually all pancreatic carcinomas. Cancer Res 1997;57:3126–3130.
9. Redston MS, Caldas C, Seymour AB, Hruban RH, da Costa L, Yeo CJ, Kern SE: p53 mutations in pancreatic carcinoma and evidence of common involvement of homocopolymer tracts in DNA microdeletions. Cancer Res 1994;54:3025–3033.
10. Rozenblum E, Schutte M, Goggins M, Hahn SA, Panzer S, Zahurak M, Goodman SN, Sohn TA, Hruban RH, Yeo CJ, Kern SE: Tumor-suppressive pathways in pancreatic carcinoma. Cancer Res 1997;57:1731–1734.
11. Maitra A, Adsay NV, Argani P, Iacobuzio-Donahue C, De Marzo A, Cameron JL, Yeo CJ, Hruban RH: Multicomponent analysis of the pancreatic adenocarcinoma progression model using a pancreatic intraepithelial neoplasia tissue microarray. Mod Pathol 2003;16:902–912.
12. Yokoyama M, Yamanaka Y, Friess H, Buchler M, Korc M: p53 expression in human pancreatic cancer correlates with enhanced biological aggressiveness. Anticancer Res 1994;14:2477–2483.
13. Hahn SA, Schutte M, Hoque AT, Moskaluk CA, da Costa LT, Rozenblum E, Weinstein CL, Fischer A, Yeo CJ, Hruban RH, Kern SE: DPC4, a candidate tumor suppressor gene at human chromosome 18q21.1. Science 1996;271:350–353.
14. Jones S, Zhang X, Parsons DW, Lin JC, Leary RJ, Angenendt P, Mankoo P, Carter H, Kamiyama H, Jimeno A, et al.: Core signaling pathways in human pancreatic cancers revealed by global genomic analyses. Science 2008;321:1801–1806.
15. Maitra A, Fukushima N, Takaori K, Hruban RH: Precursors to invasive pancreatic cancer. Adv Anat Pathol 2005;12:81–91.
16. Pour P, Kruger FW, Althoff J, Cardesa A, Mohr U: Effect of beta-oxidized nitrosamines on syrian hamsters. III. 2,2′-Dihydroxydi-n-propylnitrosamine. J Natl Cancer Inst 1975b;54:141–146.
17. Pour P, Althoff J, Kruger F, Schmahl D, Mohr U: Induction of pancreatic neoplasms by 2,2′-dioxopropyl-N-propylnitrosamine. Cancer Lett 1975a;1:3–6.
18. Levitt M, Harris C, Squire R, Wenk M, Mollelo C, Springer S: Experimental pancreatic carcinogenesis. II. Lifetime carcinogenesis studies in the outbred Syrian golden hamster with N-nitroso-bis(2-hydroxypropyl)amine. J Natl Cancer Inst 1978;60:701–705.
19. Pour P, Althoff J, Gingell R, Kupper R, Kruger F, Mohr U: N-nitroso-bis(2-acetoxypropyl)amine as a further pancreatic carcinogen in Syrian golden hamsters. Cancer Res 1976;36:2877–2884.
20. Pour P, Althoff J, Kruger FW, Mohr U: A potent pancreatic carcinogen in Syrian hamsters:

N-nitrosobis(2-oxopropyl)amine. J Natl Cancer Inst 1977;58:1449–1453.

21. Dissin J, Mills LR, Mains DL, Black O, Jr., Webster PD, 3rd: Experimental induction of pancreatic adenocarcinoma in rats. J Natl Cancer Inst 1975;55:857–864.

22. Longnecker DS, Curphey TJ: Adenocarcinoma of the pancreas in azaserine-treated rats. Cancer Res 1975;35:2249–2258.

23. Osvaldt AB, Wendt LR, Bersch VP, Backes AN, de Cassia ASR, Edelweiss MI, Rohde L: Pancreatic intraepithelial neoplasia and ductal adenocarcinoma induced by DMBA in mice. Surgery 2006;140: 803–809.

24. Levitt MH, Harris CC, Squire R, Springer S, Wenk M, Mollelo C, Thomas D, Kingsbury E, Newkirk C: Experimental pancreatic carcinogenesis. I. Morphogenesis of pancreatic adenocarcinoma in the Syrian golden hamster induced by N-nitroso-bis(2-hydroxypropyl)amine. Am J Pathol 1977;88:5–28.

25. Pour P, Althoff J: The effect of N-nitrosobis(2-oxopropyl)amine after oral administration to hamsters. Cancer Lett 1977;2:323–326.

26. Pour PM: Experimental pancreatic cancer. Am J Surg Pathol 1989;13:Suppl 1, 96–103.

27. Chang KW, Laconi S, Mangold KA, Hubchak S, Scarpelli DG: Multiple genetic alterations in hamster pancreatic ductal adenocarcinomas. Cancer Res 1995;55:2560–2568.

28. Hotz HG, Hines OJ, Foitzik T, Reber HA: Animal models of exocrine pancreatic cancer. Int J Colorectal Dis 2000;15:136–143.

29. Rao MS: Animal models of exocrine pancreatic carcinogenesis. Cancer Metastasis Rev 1987;6:665–676.

30. Pour P, Salmasi S, Runge R, Gingell R, Wallcave L, Nagel D, Stepan K: Carcinogenicity of N-nitrosobis(2-hydroxypropyl)amine and N-nitrosobis(2-oxopropyl)amine in MRC rats. J Natl Cancer Inst 1979;63:181–190.

31. Bockman DE, Black O, Jr., Mills LR, Mainz DL, Webster PD, 3rd: Fine structure of pancreatic adenocarcinoma induced in rats by 7,12-dimethylbenz(a)anthracene. J Natl Cancer Inst 1976;57:931–936.

32. Longnecker DS, Roebuck BD, Yager JD, Jr., Lilja HS, Siegmund B: Pancreatic carcinoma in azaserine-treated rats: induction, classification and dietary modulation of incidence. Cancer 1981;47: 1562–1572.

33. Schaeffer BK, Zurlo J, Longnecker DS: Activation of c-Ki-ras not detectable in adenomas or adenocarcinomas arising in rat pancreas. Mol Carcinog 1990;3:165–170.

34. Wendt LR, Osvaldt AB, Bersch VP, Schumacher Rde C, Edelweiss MI, Rohde L: Pancreatic intraepithelial neoplasia and ductal adenocarcinoma induced by DMBA in mice: effects of alcohol and caffeine.

Acta cirurgica brasileira/Sociedade Brasileira para Desenvolvimento Pesquisa em Cirurgia 2007;22: 202–209.

35. Bersch VP, Osvaldt AB, Edelweiss MI, Schumacher RD, Wendt LR, Abreu LP, Blom CB, Abreu GP, Costa L, Piccinini P, Rohde L: Effect of Nicotine and Cigarette Smoke on an Experimental Model of Intraepithelial Lesions and Pancreatic Adenocarcinoma Induced by 7,12-Dimethylbenzanthracene in Mice. Pancreas.2008;38(1):65–70.

36. Erill N, Cuatrecasas M, Sancho FJ, Farre A, Pour PM, Lluis F, Capella G: K-ras and p53 mutations in hamster pancreatic ductal adenocarcinomas and cell lines. Am J Pathol 1996;149:1333–1339.

37. Egami H, Tomioka T, Tempero M, Kay D, Pour PM: Development of intrapancreatic transplantable model of pancreatic duct adenocarcinoma in Syrian golden hamsters. Am J Pathol 1991;138:557–561.

38. Hotz HG, Reber HA, Hotz B, Foitzik T, Buhr HJ, Cortina G, Hines OJ: An improved clinical model of orthotopic pancreatic cancer in immunocompetent Lewis rats. Pancreas 2001;22:113–121.

39. Tan MH, Chu TM: Characterization of the tumorigenic and metastatic properties of a human pancreatic tumor cell line (AsPC-1) implanted orthotopically into nude mice. Tumour Biol 1985;6:89–98.

40. Mohammad RM, Al-Katib A, Pettit GR, Vaitkevicius VK, Joshi U, Adsay V, Majumdar AP, Sarkar FH: An orthotopic model of human pancreatic cancer in severe combined immunodeficient mice: potential application for preclinical studies. Clin Cancer Res 1998;4:887–894.

41. Marincola FM, Drucker BJ, Siao DY, Hough KL, Holder WD, Jr.: The nude mouse as a model for the study of human pancreatic cancer. J Surg Res 1989;47:520–529.

42. Fu X, Guadagni F, Hoffman RM: A metastatic nude-mouse model of human pancreatic cancer constructed orthotopically with histologically intact patient specimens. Proc Natl Acad Sci USA 1992;89:5645–5649.

43. Swift GH, Hammer RE, MacDonald RJ, Brinster RL: Tissue-specific expression of the rat pancreatic elastase I gene in transgenic mice. Cell 1984;38:639–646.

44. Ornitz DM, Palmiter RD, Hammer RE, Brinster RL, Swift GH, MacDonald RJ: Specific expression of an elastase-human growth hormone fusion gene in pancreatic acinar cells of transgenic mice. Nature 1985;313:600–602.

45. Ornitz DM, Hammer RE, Messing A, Palmiter RD, Brinster RL: Pancreatic neoplasia induced by SV40 T-antigen expression in acinar cells of transgenic mice. Science 1987;238:188–193.

46. Quaife CJ, Pinkert CA, Ornitz DM, Palmiter RD, Brinster RL: Pancreatic neoplasia induced by ras

expression in acinar cells of transgenic mice. Cell 1987;48:1023–1034.

47. Sandgren EP, Quaife CJ, Paulovich AG, Palmiter RD, Brinster RL: Pancreatic tumor pathogenesis reflects the causative genetic lesion. Proc Natl Acad Sci USA 1991;88:93–97.

48. Sandgren EP, Luetteke NC, Palmiter RD, Brinster RL, Lee DC: Overexpression of TGF alpha in transgenic mice: induction of epithelial hyperplasia, pancreatic metaplasia, and carcinoma of the breast. Cell 1990;61:1121–1135.

49. Schmid RM, Kloppel G, Adler G, Wagner M: Acinar-ductal-carcinoma sequence in transforming growth factor-alpha transgenic mice. Ann NY Acad Sci 1999;880:219–230.

50. Grippo PJ, Nowlin PS, Demeure MJ, Longnecker DS, Sandgren EP: Preinvasive pancreatic neoplasia of ductal phenotype induced by acinar cell targeting of mutant Kras in transgenic mice. Cancer Res 2003;63:2016–2019.

51. Brembeck FH, Schreiber FS, Deramaudt TB, Craig L, Rhoades B, Swain G, Grippo P, Stoffers DA, Silberg DG, Rustgi AK: The mutant K-ras oncogene causes pancreatic periductal lymphocytic infiltration and gastric mucous neck cell hyperplasia in transgenic mice. Cancer Res 2003;63:2005–2009.

52. Kim SK, MacDonald RJ: Signaling and transcriptional control of pancreatic organogenesis. Curr Opin Genet Dev 2002;12:540–547.

53. Ahlgren U, Jonsson J, Edlund H: The morphogenesis of the pancreatic mesenchyme is uncoupled from that of the pancreatic epithelium in IPF1/PDX1-deficient mice. Development 1996;122:1409–1416.

54. Kawaguchi Y, Cooper B, Gannon M, Ray M, MacDonald RJ, Wright CV: The role of the transcriptional regulator Ptf1a in converting intestinal to pancreatic progenitors. Nat Genet 2002;32:128–134.

55. Offield MF, Jetton TL, Labosky PA, Ray M, Stein RW, Magnuson MA, Hogan BL, Wright CV: PDX-1 is required for pancreatic outgrowth and differentiation of the rostral duodenum. Development 1996;122:983–995.

56. Krapp A, Knofler M, Ledermann B, Burki K, Berney C, Zoerkler N, Hagenbuchle O, Wellauer PK: The bHLH protein PTF1-p48 is essential for the formation of the exocrine and the correct spatial organization of the endocrine pancreas. Genes Dev 1998;12:3752–3763.

57. Lakso M, Sauer B, Mosinger B, Jr., Lee EJ, Manning RW, Yu SH, Mulder KL, Westphal H: Targeted oncogene activation by site-specific recombination in transgenic mice. Proc Natl Acad Sci USA 1992;89:6232–6236.

58. Jackson EL, Willis N, Mercer K, Bronson RT, Crowley D, Montoya R, Jacks T, Tuveson DA: Analysis of lung tumor initiation and progression using conditional expression of oncogenic K-ras. Genes Dev 2001;15:3243–3248.

59. Hingorani SR, Petricoin EF, Maitra A, Rajapakse V, King C, Jacobetz MA, Ross S, Conrads TP, Veenstra TD, Hitt BA, et al.: Preinvasive and invasive ductal pancreatic cancer and its early detection in the mouse. Cancer Cell 2003;4:437–450.

60. Aguirre AJ, Bardeesy N, Sinha M, Lopez L, Tuveson DA, Horner J, Redston MS, DePinho RA: Activated Kras and Ink4a/Arf deficiency cooperate to produce metastatic pancreatic ductal adenocarcinoma. Genes Dev 2003;17:3112–3126.

61. Hustinx SR, Leoni LM, Yeo CJ, Brown PN, Goggins M, Kern SE, Hruban RH, Maitra A: Concordant loss of MTAP and p16/CDKN2A expression in pancreatic intraepithelial neoplasia: evidence of homozygous deletion in a noninvasive precursor lesion. Mod Pathol 2005;18:959–963.

62. Bardeesy N, Aguirre AJ, Chu GC, Cheng KH, Lopez LV, Hezel AF, Feng B, Brennan C, Weissleder R, Mahmood U, et al.: Both p16(Ink4a) and the p19 (Arf)-p53 pathway constrain progression of pancreatic adenocarcinoma in the mouse. Proc Natl Acad Sci USA 2006a 103:5947–5952.

63. Olivier M, Eeles R, Hollstein M, Khan MA, Harris CC, Hainaut P: The IARC TP53 database: new online mutation analysis and recommendations to users. Hum Mutat 2002;19:607–614.

64. Hingorani SR, Wang L, Multani AS, Combs C, Deramaudt TB, Hruban RH, Rustgi AK, Chang S, Tuveson DA: Trp53R172H and KrasG12D cooperate to promote chromosomal instability and widely metastatic pancreatic ductal adenocarcinoma in mice. Cancer Cell 2005;7:469–483.

65. Guerra C, Schuhmacher AJ, Canamero M, Grippo PJ, Verdaguer L, Perez-Gallego L, Dubus P, Sandgren EP, Barbacid M: Chronic pancreatitis is essential for induction of pancreatic ductal adenocarcinoma by K-Ras oncogenes in adult mice. Cancer Cell 2007;11:291–302.

66. Malka D, Hammel P, Maire F, Rufat P, Madeira I, Pessione F, Levy P, Ruszniewski P: Risk of pancreatic adenocarcinoma in chronic pancreatitis. Gut 2002;51:849–852.

67. Hansel DE, Kern SE, Hruban RH: Molecular pathogenesis of pancreatic cancer. Annu Rev Genomics Hum Genet 2003;4:237–256.

68. Howe JR, Roth S, Ringold JC, Summers RW, Jarvinen HJ, Sistonen P, Tomlinson IP, Houlston RS, Bevan S, Mitros FA, et al.: Mutations in the SMAD4/DPC4 gene in juvenile polyposis. Science (New York, NY 1998;280:1086–1088.

69. Bierie B, Moses HL: Tumour microenvironment: TGFbeta: The molecular Jekyll and Hyde of cancer. Nat Rev 2006;6:506–520.

70. Takaku K, Miyoshi H, Matsunaga A, Oshima M, Sasaki N, Taketo MM: Gastric and duodenal polyps in Smad4 (Dpc4) knockout mice. Cancer Res 1999;59:6113–6117.

71. Bardeesy N, Cheng KH, Berger JH, Chu GC, Pahler J, Olson P, Hezel AF, Horner J, Lauwers GY, Hanahan D, DePinho RA: Smad4 is dispensable for normal pancreas development yet critical in progression and tumor biology of pancreas cancer. Genes Dev 2006b;20:3130–3146.

72. Iacobuzio-Donahue CA, Klimstra DS, Adsay NV, Wilentz RE, Argani P, Sohn TA, Yeo CJ, Cameron JL, Kern SE, Hruban RH: Dpc-4 protein is expressed in virtually all human intraductal papillary mucinous neoplasms of the pancreas: comparison with conventional ductal adenocarcinomas. Am J Pathol 2000;157:755–761.

73. Izeradjene K, Combs C, Best M, Gopinathan A, Wagner A, Grady WM, Deng CX, Hruban RH, Adsay NV, Tuveson DA, Hingorani SR: Kras (G12D) and Smad4/Dpc4 haploinsufficiency cooperate to induce mucinous cystic neoplasms and invasive adenocarcinoma of the pancreas. Cancer Cell 2007;11:229–243.

74. Zhang Z, Wang Y, Vikis HG, Johnson L, Liu G, Li J, Anderson MW, Sills RC, Hong HL, Devereux TR, et al.: Wildtype Kras2 can inhibit lung carcinogenesis in mice. Nat Genet 2001;29:25–33.

75. van Heek NT, Meeker AK, Kern SE, Yeo CJ, Lillemoe KD, Cameron JL, Offerhaus GJ, Hicks JL, Wilentz RE, Goggins MG, et al.: Telomere shortening is nearly universal in pancreatic intraepithelial neoplasia. Am J Pathol 2002;161:1541–1547.

76. Leach SD: Epithelial differentiation in pancreatic development and neoplasia: new niches for nestin and Notch. J Clin Gastroenterol 2005;39:S78–S82.

77. Li C, Heidt DG, Dalerba P, Burant CF, Zhang L, Adsay V, Wicha M, Clarke MF, Simeone DM: Identification of pancreatic cancer stem cells. Cancer Res 2007;67:1030–1037.

78. O'Brien CA, Pollett A, Gallinger S, Dick JE: A human colon cancer cell capable of initiating tumour growth in immunodeficient mice. Nature 2007;445:106–110.

79. Ricci-Vitiani L, Lombardi DG, Pilozzi E, Biffoni M, Todaro M, Peschle C, De Maria R: Identification and expansion of human colon-cancer-initiating cells. Nature 2007;445:111–115.

80. Hermann PC, Huber SL, Herrler T, Aicher A, Ellwart JW, Guba M, Bruns CJ, Heeschen C: Distinct populations of cancer stem cells determine tumor growth and metastatic activity in human pancreatic cancer. Cell Stem Cell 2007;1:313–323.

81. Hess V, Glimelius B, Grawe P, Dietrich D, Bodoky G, Ruhstaller T, Bajetta E, Saletti P, Figer A, Scheithauer W, Herrmann R: CA 19–9 tumour-marker response to chemotherapy in patients with advanced pancreatic cancer enrolled in a randomised controlled trial. lancet Oncol 2008;9:132–138.

82. Faca VM, Song KS, Wang H, Zhang Q, Krasnoselsky AL, Newcomb LF, Plentz RR, Gurumurthy S, Redston MS, Pitteri SJ, et al.: A mouse to human search for plasma proteome changes associated with pancreatic tumor development. PLoS Med 2008;5:e123.

83. Collier LS, Carlson CM, Ravimohan S, Dupuy AJ, Largaespada DA: Cancer gene discovery in solid tumours using transposon-based somatic mutagenesis in the mouse. Nature 2005;436:272–276.

21 Principles and Applications of Microarray Gene Expression in Pancreatic Cancer

Malte Buchholz · Thomas M. Gress

1	Introduction to DNA Array Technology	498
2	DNA Arrays in Pancreatic Oncology	500
2.1	Candidate Gene Selection	500
2.2	Class Prediction and Class Discovery	503
3	Future Perspectives	505

J. P. Neoptolemos, R. Urrutia, J. L. Abbruzzese, M. W. Büchler (eds.), *Pancreatic Cancer*,
DOI 10.1007/978-0-387-77498-5_21, © Springer Science+Business Media, LLC 2010

Abstract: Like most other malignancies, pancreatic cancer is a polygenic disease arising from the accumulation of multiple genetic and epigenetic defects in the affected cells. DNA arrays offer the possibility to monitor the expression levels of thousands of mRNA transcripts simultaneously in a single assay, making them ideal tools to study the complex network of transcriptional changes that are associated with the malignant transformation of normal cells. Expression profiling analyses are rapidly expanding our knowledge of pancreatic cancer biology, laying the basis for the development of more sophisticated diagnostic procedures and more effective treatment modalities. Moreover, microarrays can directly be employed as highly sophisticated diagnostic tools in the clinic, enabling the extraction of much more detailed and differentiated diagnostic information from biopsy samples than single molecular markers or conventional diagnostic procedures can provide.

1   Introduction to DNA Array Technology

Microarrays have rapidly become the leading technology in high throughput molecular research. Although applications and protocols vary widely, the basic principle is the same for all microarray formats. Capture molecules which are specific for individual target molecules are immobilized on solid support matrices in miniaturized and highly ordered arrays. For analysis of complex biological samples, the samples are globally tagged with traceable labels (see below) and dispensed onto the microarrays. Under appropriate incubation conditions, individual labeled target molecules will be bound by their specific capture molecules, generating a traceable signal at the corresponding spot on the microarray, the intensity of which is proportional to the amount of labeled target molecule present in the biological sample.

This basic principle, implemented in a myriad of different technological approaches, is today being used for the high-throughput application of very different types of analyses. Microarrays of genomic DNA sequences are used in comparative genomic analyses aimed at the genome-wide identification of chromosomal imbalances (commonly referred to as Matrix- or Array-CGH). Recently, so-called tiling arrays have become available, which cover the entire human genome in overlapping short oligonucleotide sequences, providing an extremely high-resolution tool for the detection of disease-associated mutations or single nucleotide polymorphisms (SNPs). The development of peptide- and antibody arrays has reached a stage where these tools are now ready for routine application in high-throughput proteome research. A very recently developed application is the high-content evaluation of chromatin immunoprecipitation (ChIP) experiments using genomic DNA arrays (so-called ChIP-on-chip), which provides a comprehensive view of promoter sequences bound by a specific transcription factor at a given time point. The "classic" application of microarray technology, however, is gene expression profiling for the simultaneous assessment of transcript levels of up to several tens of thousands of genes in a single experiment. Since this is the most advanced and most widely used application of microarray technology to date, this chapter will mainly focus on principles and applications of different implementations of DNA array technology in pancreatic cancer research and patient management.

As mentioned above, the production of any type of microarray consists of immobilization of specific capture molecules in a highly ordered array on solid support media. In the case of DNA microarrays, these capture molecules are representative segments of all genes which are intended to be analyzed in the microarray experiments. The gene segments are usually prepared in the form of denatured cDNA fragments or long oligonucleotides (50–80mers), stored in microtiter plates and transferred to glass slides, nylon membranes or (less commonly) plastic supports using robotic devices (❯ *Fig. 21-1*). Alternatively, short oligonucleotides can be synthesized in situ on the array surface. In this case, each gene is represented by several different sequences to compensate for the short length of the individual oligonucleotides. The term "DNA Chips" was originally coined to describe a type of in situ oligonucleotide arrays that is manufactured by Affymetrix Inc. using photolithographic techniques developed for the computer chip industry.

For expression profiling analyses, the complete mRNA pool of a tissue or cell type is prepared and labeled using either radioactive isotopes (nylon membrane arrays), fluorescent dyes (glass arrays) or biotynilated nucleotides (Affymetrix GeneChips). During the subseqent hybridization step, the labeled transcripts pair with their immobilized counterparts on the array and can be detected using phosphorimager (radioactive labeling) or laser scanning (fluorescent labeling) technologies. Biotynilated probes hybridized to Affymetrix GeneChip arrays are detected indirectly using Streptavidine-coupled enzymes and corresponding chemiluminescence substrates. The resulting signals on the array are quantified and serve as a measure for the relative abundance of the corresponding genes in the analyzed sample.

⬛ Fig. 21-1

Production of "spotted" arrays. Nucleic acids, antibodies or polypeptides are stored in microtiter plates and transferred to support media (e.g., glass slides or nylon membranes) by robotic devices using high precision "pin tools". The resulting arrays are probed with labeled mRNA or protein preparations to measure the abundance of the corresponding transcripts or proteins in the tissue or cell type of interest.

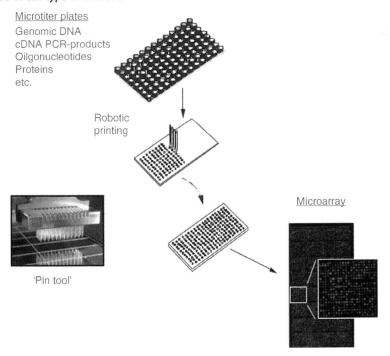

2   DNA Arrays in Pancreatic Oncology

Like most other malignancies, pancreatic cancer is a complex disease arising from the accumulation of a multitude of genetic and epigenetic defects in the affected cells. Among well-established hallmark features of PDAC are mutations in the K-ras and HER2/neu oncogenes as well as the p53, p16INK4a, and SMAD4/DPC4 tumor suppressor genes (for an overview, see [1, 2]). In addition to mutations, malignant transformation of normal pancreatic cells is associated with sometimes dramatic changes in expression levels of a vast number of genes. DNA arrays with their potential to assess the mRNA levels of thousands of genes simultaneously are ideal tools to study these profound transcriptional changes in a highly efficient manner.

Within the framework of translational research in oncology, the use of DNA arrays can broadly be divided into three general categories: Candidate gene selection, class prediction and class discovery. While the first aims at identifying individual genes which may serve as new diagnostic or therapeutic targets, the latter two applications comprise the analysis of complex gene expression patterns to assign clinical samples to known disease entities or to define new disease subtypes which were previously not recognizable using classical diagnostic procedures (◉ *Fig. 21-2*).

2.1   Candidate Gene Selection

From a data analysis point of view, this category is the most straightforward application of microarray technology. Expression profiles of cancerous tissues are compared with profiles of non-cancerous tissues from the same organ using statistical tests to identify genes which are predominantly or exclusively expressed in the malignant state. However, caution has to be exercised when interpreting the results of comparative microarray studies, since the greatest strength of microarrays, i.e., the ability to measure thousands of genes simultaneously, also poses some systematic problems. Since genome-wide microarray studies are usually very costly, relatively few samples are usually analyzed, leading to a situation where many thousand genes are queried in few representative samples. For statistical reasons, such experiments will tend to produce many false positive calls if the results are not carefully controlled for the effects of the "multiple testing" character of the analysis, e.g., by computing false discovery rates and adjusting the results accordingly. In addition, further exploitation of the results is complicated by the fact that several hundreds or thousands of genes may effectively change their expression levels upon malignant transformation of a normal cell. In the case of pancreatic cancer, more than 2,000 genes have to date been reported to be differentially expressed in cancer compared to normal or inflammatory tissues (a comprehensive view of gene expression profiles in pancreatic tissues is offered by the Pancreatic Expression Database, hosted at http://www.pancreasexpression.org/). Thus, additional strategies have to be applied to select the most promising candidates for further in-depth characterization. While well-annotated genes can be screened for known characteristics enabling the development of new diagnostic tests or new treatment modalities, unknown genes or EST's have to be characterized in additional series of in vitro and/or in vivo experiments to select the most suitable target genes. To this end, the genes can for example be assembled on specialized candidate gene arrays, which due to the limited number of genes are both more affordable and easier to analyze than comprehensive "whole genome" arrays.

☐ Fig. 21-2

DNA arrays in pancreatic oncology. Global gene expression profiling of tumor tissue and non-malignant tissue samples from the same site form the basis for the discovery of potential new diagnostic and therapeutic targets (candidate gene selection), the definition of previously unrecognized, clinically distinct disease subtypes (class discovery) and the development of specialized arrays for sophisticated cancer diagnostics (class prediction).

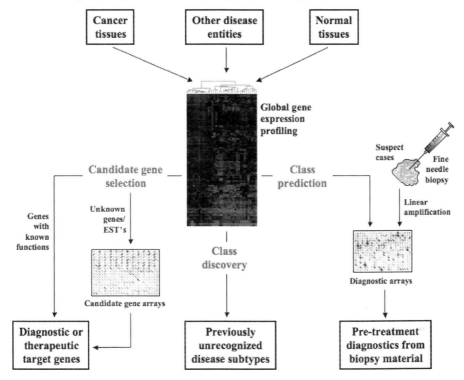

The candidate gene arrays can then be used in larger series of experiments using model systems modulating important characteristics of tumor cells (invasive and metastatic potential, escape from growth control, resistance to chemotherapeutic agents, escape from programmed cell death etc.) to provide a better basis for the selection of genes with central roles in tumorigenesis (◉ *Fig. 21-2*).

Using a variety of different selection strategies, different groups have already identified a number of promising new candidate genes which may potentially serve as novel molecular diagnostic markers of pancreatic cancer. One of these is the *KH homology domain containing protein overexpressed in cancer* (KOC), also known as *insulin-like growth factor 2 mRNA binding protein 3* (IGF2BP3). KOC is an oncofetal RNA-binding protein that is thought to be involved in the posttranscriptional regulation of cell proliferation during embryogenesis. It is strongly overexpressed in pancreatic cancer, while its expression in normal adult tissues appears to be limited to the placenta [3]. In a study by Mueller et al., detection of KOC mRNA by RT-PCR in a series of 41 fine needle aspiration biopsy (FNAB) samples from different abdominal lesions resulted in a sensitivity and specificity for the detection of malignancy of 93% and 83%, respectively [4]. In a subsequent study examining immunohistochemical KOC staining patterns in surgically resected pancreatic tissues, strong staining was observed in 97% of invasive carcinomas (PDAC, papillary-mucinous carcinomas and mucinous cystadenocarcinomas) as well as the majority of advanced PanIN lesions, while staining was weak or absent in all benign cells and tissues [5]. Finally, a recent study by Zhao et al. on immunohistochemical detection of KOC expression on FNAB samples demonstrated a sensitivity and specificity of 88% and 100%, respectively, for the KOC immune staining alone, and 95% and 100% for the combination of cytology and KOC staining [6].

Another candidate with high diagnostic potential is S100P, a member of the S100 family of calcium-binding proteins. S100P has been reported to be overexpressed in pancreatic cancer as compared to chronic pancreatitis and normal pancreas in several independent microarray studies, and importantly was also found to be overexpressed in precursor lesions of pancreatic cancer, so-called pancreatic intraepithelial neoplasias (PanINs) [7]. Immunohistochemical analysis of a series of pancreatic cancer and PanIN tissues demonstrated S100P to be expressed in 31% of PanIN-2 lesions, 41% of PanIN-3 lesions, and 92% of invasive PDAC specimens [8]. Together, these results suggest that S100P may be suitable to serve as an early marker of malignancy. A recent study on the immunohistochemical detection of S100P in FNAB samples [9] as well as one study on the detection of S100P mRNA in pancreatic juice [10] support the notion that this gene may emerge as a sensitive, specific, and early marker for pancreatic cancer in biopsy material.

An example for a novel potential therapeutic target for pancreatic cancer treatment selected on the basis of functional annotation of microarray results is the tight junction protein Claudin-4, which was found to be ectopically expressed by pancreatic cancer cells in many patient samples. This protein is normally located on the surface of intestinal epithelial cells and has previously been demonstrated to serve as the receptor of the *Clostridium perfringens* enterotoxin (CPE), the causative agent of many food poisonings. CPE exerts an acute cytotoxic effect on Claudin-4 expressing cells by disrupting the cell membrane and destroying ion gradients, while cells not expressing Claudin-4 remain completely unaffected. Since the protein is absent from healthy pancreatic cells, CPE can be locally administered to selectively kill Claudin-4 expressing cancer cells, as has successfully been demonstrated in animal experiments using subcutaneously implanted pancreatic tumors in immunodeficient nude mice [11].

In addition to these examples, which are already relatively close to clinical applications, microarray experiments have been the starting point of countless studies in recent years where differentially expressed genes have been scrutinized in detail for their functional roles in pancreatic cancer. The results of these studies have already provided, and continue to provide, significant improvements to our understanding of very basic aspects of pancreatic cancer biology, from organization and cross-talk of oncogenic signaling cascades to molecular determinants of drug resistance, and from mediators of invasion and metastasis to mechanisms of tumor-host-interactions. An exciting new development in the field of array technologies which has the potential to significantly speed up the process of functionally characterizing candidate genes is the invention of so-called transfected cell microarrays, also known as reverse transfection microarrays [12]. The principle of this technique is to array fluorescence-tagged cDNA expression constructs of the genes of interest, together with transfection reagents, onto microscope slides. Cultured cells seeded onto the slides take up the expression constructs, resulting in overexpression of the corresponding gene in the cells. The reverse effect, i.e., knock-down of the genes of interest, can be achieved by arraying

■ Fig. 21-3

Principle of "reverse transfection array" technology. Expression constructs or siRNAs together with transfection reagents are arrayed onto microscope slides and cells are seeded onto the arrays. Cells take up the DNA, resulting in overexpression or knock-down of the genes of interest. The right side of the figure shows 20 spots of HEK293 cells transfected with EGFP expression constructs (*upper panel*) and details of subcellular localization of different candidate genes transfected as EYFP fusion constructs (*lower panel*).

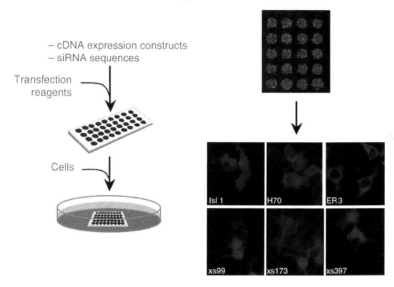

siRNAs directed against the genes onto the slides (◑ *Fig. 21-3*). A large number of different functional assays can be performed in this format, including assays for subcellular localization, morphological changes, proliferation-, migration-, apoptosis- and differentiation assays, thus generating data for many candidate genes in parallel. Automated microscope systems and image analysis algorithms assist in further increasing the throughput in these high-content functional screens.

2.2 Class Prediction and Class Discovery

A principally different approach to using expression profiling for diagnostic purposes, in contrast to using comparative studies to identify individual diagnostic markers, is to try to identify complex patterns within gene expression profiles that are associated with the presence or absence of known diseases or disease subtypes (class prediction) or that will even allow to define previously unrecognized disease subtypes associated with a characteristic prognosis, response to therapy, risk of relapse etc (class discovery). It is readily conceivable that the simultaneous analysis of many genes in parallel can potentially deliver much more comprehensive and detailed information than the analysis of individual markers. Indeed, a number of studies with different types of tumors have early on demonstrated the power of DNA array analyses in differentiating between tumor types and subtypes. Correct assignment of tumor samples to well-defined disease entities according to typical expression profiles (class prediction) had first been demonstrated for the differentiation between acute myeloid leukemia (AML) and acute lymphoblastic leukemia (ALL) [13] as well as the different types of small round blue-cell tumors of childhood [14]. The definition of new distinct tumor subtypes that are indistinguishable by conventional diagnostic methods through microarray analyses (class discovery) was first described for breast cancer and diffuse large B-cell lymphomas, where molecular tumor subtypes with markedly differing prognoses were identified, respectively [15,16]. As mentioned above, a multitude of high-content screening analyses have also been conducted on pancreatic tissues, both on the genome [17–20] as well as the transcriptome level [7,21–33]. These studies have identified a multitude of differences between malignant and benign processes in the pancreas and, moreover, have demonstrated that different entities of malignant tumors of the pancreas are associated with distinct expression profiles. However, as already noted for comparative gene expression analyses, interpretation of microarray results is not trivial, and classification of clinical or biological samples based on complex gene expression profiles presents a number of potential pitfalls. Since the number of genes analyzed in a microarray study usually far exceeds the number of samples available for analysis, great care must be taken to prevent "overfitting" of classifying algorithms to individual datasets (i.e., basing the classification of samples on random features of the specific samples in the analysis, instead of features which are truly characteristic of the class or entity the sample belongs to). The higher the number of genes and the lower the number of samples in the analysis, the greater the danger that a given set of samples (which are used as representatives of a diagnostic class) will by chance share a set of gene expression features which may distinguish them from the other samples in this particular analysis, but which are not representative of the diagnostic class in general [34]. When using large scale microarrays for classification, it is therefore imperative to employ mathematical methods such as principal component analysis (PCA) to reduce the dimensionality of the datasets, and to carefully control for overfitting artifacts e.g., by performing cross-validation experiments or by testing the newly defined algorithms on independent test datasets.

Another way to reduce the complexity (and at the same time the costs) of microarray analyses in diagnostics is to develop specialized, small-scale arrays with limited numbers of selected genes which have a high probability of yielding useful information. Van de Vijver et al. have used the results of their breast cancer expression profiling experiments to develop a microarray containing 70 selected genes which they now use in the routine stratification of patients for adjuvant therapy after surgery [35]. In the context of pancreatic cancer diagnostics, our own group has previously designed a specialized 588 feature cDNA array for differential diagnosis of pancreatic tumors. In a proof-of-principle study with 62 pancreatic tissue samples, including 16 fine needle aspiration biopsy (FNAB) samples, it was demonstrated that a 169 gene expression signature obtained with this array in conjunction with a specifically developed classification algorithm is suitable to distinguish between PDAC and non-malignant processes with > 95% diagnostic accuracy [36]. Currently, these studies are being extended to the analysis of additional tumor types in order to develop a multiclass classification system for the comprehensive diagnosis of different malignancies in the pancreas. Preliminary results show that ampullary cancers as well as distant bile duct tumors, which can be very difficult to differentiate from PDAC with conventional diagnostic procedures, have very distinct diagnostic array expression signatures and can readily be distinguished from both PDAC and benign pancreas samples.

3   Future Perspectives

The vast majority of DNA array studies in oncology, including pancreatic cancer research, have so far been conducted in basic research settings or in the form of retrospective studies using archived tissue specimens. A number of challenges have to be met before the promising results of these studies can be transferred to clinical practice. Standardization of results across different technological platforms is an important and largely unsolved issue. Also, due to the enormous technical and financial expense of large scale DNA array experiments, most studies have been limited to rather small sample sizes, requiring validation of the results in larger sample sets. However, DNA array technology undoubtedly has the potential to greatly impact cancer patient management in the future, both directly through clinical application of microarray technology as well as indirectly by significantly accelerating basic and applied pancreatic cancer research. Expression profiling analyses of cancer tissues and tumor model systems are rapidly expanding our knowledge of cancer cell biology, providing valuable clues for the development for new diagnostic and therapeutic principles. Analyses of precursor lesions help to elucidate the chain of molecular events that lead to the formation and progression of tumors and will likely improve our means of screening for developing tumors. Moreover, DNA microarrays have the potential to directly serve as a highly sophisticated diagnostic tools in the clinic, not only providing information on the tumor type, but also the predicted metastatic potential, response to therapy, risk of relapse etc., thus setting the stage for therapeutic regimens custom tailored to the individual tumor patient.

Key Research Points

- DNA microarrays are mainly used in three types of analysis:
- *Candidate gene selection:* Identification of genes with significantly different expression levels in cancer versus control tissues. Selection of individual genes for subsequent detailed characterization.
- *Class prediction:* Identification of complex gene expression patterns which distinguish known disease entities and which can be used for molecular diagnostic approaches.
- *Class discovery:* Identification and definition of new disease subtypes which are not recognizable using conventional diagnostic procedures based on the analysis of gene expression patterns.

Future Scientific Directions

- Results from experimental, retrospective studies with limited numbers of samples will have to be validated in large, controlled prospective studies.
- In addition to comprehensive, multiclass differential diagnosis of different entities of pancreatic tumors, further development of specialized diagnostic arrays and algorithms is aimed at providing detailed prognostic information for the individual patient.

References

1. Ghaneh P, Costello E, Neoptolemos JP: Biology and management of pancreatic cancer. Gut 2007; 56:1134–1152.

2. Li D, Xie K, Wolff R, Abbruzzese JL: Pancreatic cancer. Lancet 2004;363:1049–1057.

3. Mueller-Pillasch F, Pohl B, Wilda M, Lacher U, Beil M, Wallrapp C, Hameister H, Knochel W, Adler G, Gress TM: Expression of the highly conserved RNA binding protein KOC in embryogenesis. Mech Dev 1999;88:95–99.

4. Mueller F, Bommer M, Lacher U, Ruhland C, Stagge V, Adler G, Gress TM, Seufferlein T: KOC is a novel molecular indicator of malignancy. Br J Cancer 2003;88:699–701.

5. Yantiss RK, Woda BA, Fanger GR, Kalos M, Whalen GF, Tada H, Andersen DK, Rock KL, Dresser K: KOC (K homology domain containing protein overexpressed in cancer): a novel molecular marker that distinguishes between benign and malignant lesions of the pancreas. Am J Surg Pathol 2005;29:188–195.

6. Zhao H, Mandich D, Cartun RW, Ligato S: Expression of K homology domain containing protein overexpressed in cancer in pancreatic FNA for diagnosing adenocarcinoma of pancreas. Diagn Cytopathol 2007;35:700–704.

7. Buchholz M, Braun M, Heidenblut A, Kestler HA, Kloppel G, Schmiegel W, Hahn SA, Luttges J, Gress TM: Transcriptome analysis of microdissected pancreatic intraepithelial neoplastic lesions. Oncogene 2005;24:6626–6636.

8. Dowen SE, Crnogorac-Jurcevic T, Gangeswaran R, Hansen M, Eloranta JJ, Bhakta V, Brentnall TA, Luttges J, Kloppel G, Lemoine NR: Expression of S100P and its novel binding partner S100PBPR in early pancreatic cancer. Am J Pathol 2005;166:81–92.

9. Deng H, Shi J, Wilkerson M, Meschter S, Dupree W, Lin F: Usefulness of S100P in diagnosis of adenocarcinoma of pancreas on fine-needle aspiration biopsy specimens. Am J Clin Pathol 2008;129:81–88.

10. Ohuchida K, Mizumoto K, Egami T, Yamaguchi H, Fujii K, Konomi H, Nagai E, Yamaguchi K, Tsuneyoshi M, Tanaka M: S100P is an early developmental marker of pancreatic carcinogenesis. Clin Cancer Res 2006;12:5411–5416.

11. Michl P, Buchholz M, Rolke M, Kunsch S, Lohr M, McClane B, Tsukita S, Leder G, Adler G, Gress TM: Claudin-4: a new target for pancreatic cancer treatment using *Clostridium perfringens* enterotoxin. Gastroenterology 2001;121:678–684.

12. Ziauddin J, Sabatini DM: Microarrays of cells expressing defined cDNAs. Nature 2001;411:107–110.

13. Golub TR, Slonim DK, Tamayo P, Huard C, Gaasenbeek M, Mesirov JP, Coller H, Loh ML, Downing JR, Caligiuri MA, Bloomfield CD, Lander ES: Molecular classification of cancer: class discovery and class prediction by gene expression monitoring. Science 1999;286:531–537.

14. Khan J, Wei JS, Ringner M, Saal LH, Ladanyi M, Westermann F, Berthold F, Schwab M, Antonescu CR, Peterson C, Meltzer PS: Classification and diagnostic prediction of cancers using gene expression profiling and artificial neural networks. Nat Med 2001;7:673–679.

15. Van't Veer LJ, Dai H, van de Vijver MJ, He YD, Hart AA, Mao M, Peterse HL, van der KK, Marton MJ, Witteveen AT, Schreiber GJ, Kerkhoven RM, Roberts C, Linsley PS, Bernards R, Friend SH: Gene expression profiling predicts clinical outcome of breast cancer. Nature 2002;415:530–536.

16. Alizadeh AA, Eisen MB, Davis RE, Ma C, Lossos IS, Rosenwald A, Boldrick JC, Sabet H, Tran T, Yu X, Powell JI, Yang L, Marti GE, Moore T, Hudson J, Jr., Lu L, Lewis DB, Tibshirani R, Sherlock G, Chan WC, Greiner TC, Weisenburger DD, Armitage JO, Warnke R, Staudt LM: Distinct types of diffuse large B-cell lymphoma identified by gene expression profiling [see comments]. Nature 2000;403:503–511.

17. Harada T, Chelala C, Bhakta V, Chaplin T, Caulee K, Baril P, Young BD, Lemoine NR: Genome-wide DNA copy number analysis in pancreatic cancer using high-density single nucleotide polymorphism arrays. Oncogene 2008;27:1951–1960.

18. Harada T, Baril P, Gangeswaran R, Kelly G, Chelala C, Bhakta V, Caulee K, Mahon PC, Lemoine NR: Identification of genetic alterations in pancreatic cancer by the combined use of tissue microdissection and array-based comparative genomic hybridisation. Br J Cancer 2007;96:373–382.

19. Nowak NJ, Gaile D, Conroy JM, McQuaid D, Cowell J, Carter R, Goggins MG, Hruban RH, Maitra A: Genome-wide aberrations in pancreatic

adenocarcinoma. Cancer Genet Cytogenet 2005;161: 36–50.

20. Holzmann K, Kohlhammer H, Schwaenen C, Wessendorf S, Kestler HA, Schwoerer A, Rau B, Radlwimmer B, Dohner H, Lichter P, Gress T, Bentz M: Genomic DNA-chip hybridization reveals a higher incidence of genomic amplifications in pancreatic cancer than conventional comparative genomic hybridization and leads to the identification of novel candidate genes. Cancer Res 2004;64: 4428–4433.

21. Gress TM, Muller-Pillasch F, Geng M, Zimmerhackl F, Zehetner G, Friess H, Buchler M, Adler G, Lehrach H: A pancreatic cancer-specific expression profile. Oncogene 1996;13:1819–1830.

22. Han H, Bearss DJ, Browne LW, Calaluce R, Nagle RB, Von Hoff DD: Identification of differentially expressed genes in pancreatic cancer cells using cDNA microarray. Cancer Res 2002;62:2890–2896.

23. Crnogorac-Jurcevic T, Efthimiou E, Capelli P, Blaveri E, Baron A, Terris B, Jones M, Tyson K, Bassi C, Scarpa A, Lemoine NR: Gene expression profiles of pancreatic cancer and stromal desmoplasia. Oncogene 2001;20:7437–7446.

24. Crnogorac-Jurcevic T, Efthimiou E, Nielsen T, Loader J, Terris B, Stamp G, Baron A, Scarpa A, Lemoine NR: Expression profiling of microdissected pancreatic adenocarcinomas. Oncogene 2002;21: 4587–4594.

25. Iacobuzio-Donahue CA, Maitra A, Olsen M, Lowe AW, Van Heek NT, Rosty C, Walter K, Sato N, Parker A, Ashfaq R, Jaffee E, Ryu B, Jones J, Eshleman JR, Yeo CJ, Cameron JL, Kern SE, Hruban RH, Brown PO, Goggins M: Exploration of global gene expression patterns in pancreatic adenocarcinoma using cDNA microarrays. Am J Pathol 2003;162: 1151–1162.

26. Iacobuzio-Donahue CA, Maitra A, Shen-Ong GL, van HT, Ashfaq R, Meyer R, Walter K, Berg K, Hollingsworth MA, Cameron JL, Yeo CJ, Kern SE, Goggins M, Hruban RH: Discovery of novel tumor markers of pancreatic cancer using global gene expression technology. Am J Pathol 2002;160: 1239–1249.

27. Grutzmann R, Foerder M, Alldinger I, Staub E, Brummendorf T, Ropcke S, Li X, Kristiansen G, Jesnowski R, Sipos B, Lohr M, Luttges J, Ockert D, Kloppel G, Saeger HD, Pilarsky C: Gene expression profiles of microdissected pancreatic ductal adenocarcinoma. Virchows Arch 2003;443:508–517.

28. Grutzmann R, Pilarsky C, Ammerpohl O, Luttges J, Bohme A, Sipos B, Foerder M, Alldinger I, Jahnke B,

Schackert HK, Kalthoff H, Kremer B, Kloppel G, Saeger HD: Gene expression profiling of microdissected pancreatic ductal carcinomas using high-density DNA microarrays. Neoplasia 2004;6: 611–622.

29. Jin G, Hu XG, Ying K, Tang Y, Liu R, Zhang YJ, Jing ZP, Xie Y, Mao YM: Discovery and analysis of pancreatic adenocarcinoma genes using cDNA microarrays. World J Gastroenterol 2005;11:6543–6548.

30. Logsdon CD, Simeone DM, Binkley C, Arumugam T, Greenson JK, Giordano TJ, Misek DE, Kuick R, Hanash S: Molecular profiling of pancreatic adenocarcinoma and chronic pancreatitis identifies multiple genes differentially regulated in pancreatic cancer. Cancer Res 15-5-2003;63:2649–2657.

31. Nakamura T, Furukawa Y, Nakagawa H, Tsunoda T, Ohigashi H, Murata K, Ishikawa O, Ohgaki K, Kashimura N, Miyamoto M, Hirano S, Kondo S, Katoh H, Nakamura Y, Katagiri T: Genome-wide cDNA microarray analysis of gene expression profiles in pancreatic cancers using populations of tumor cells and normal ductal epithelial cells selected for purity by laser microdissection. Oncogene 2004;23:2385–2400.

32. Prasad NB, Biankin AV, Fukushima N, Maitra A, Dhara S, Elkahloun AG, Hruban RH, Goggins M, Leach SD: Gene expression profiles in pancreatic intraepithelial neoplasia reflect the effects of Hedgehog signaling on pancreatic ductal epithelial cells. Cancer Res 2005;65:1619–1626.

33. Friess H, Ding J, Kleeff J, Fenkell L, Rosinski JA, Guweidhi A, Reidhaar-Olson JF, Korc M, Hammer J, Buchler MW: Microarray-based identification of differentially expressed growth- and metastasis-associated genes in pancreatic cancer. Cell Mol Life Sci 2003;60:1180–1199.

34. Cover TM: Geometrical and statistical properties of systems of linear inequalities with applications in pattern recognition. IEEE Trans Electronic Computer 1965;14:326–334.

35. Van de Vijver MJ, He YD, Van't Veer LJ, Dai H, Hart AA, Voskuil DW, Schreiber GJ, Peterse JL, Roberts C, Marton MJ, Parrish M, Atsma D, Witteveen A, Glas A, Delahaye L, Van der Velde T, Bartelink H, Rodenhuis S, Rutgers ET, Friend SH, Bernards R: A gene-expression signature as a predictor of survival in breast cancer. N Engl J Med 2002;347: 1999–2009.

36. Buchholz M, Kestler HA, Bauer A, Bock W, Rau B, Leder G, Kratzer W, Bommer M, Scarpa A, Schilling MK, Adler G, Hoheisel JD, Gress TM: Specialized DNA arrays for the differentiation of pancreatic tumors. Clin Cancer Res 2005;11:8048–8054.

22 Principles and Applications of Proteomics in Pancreatic Cancer

Sarah Tonack · John Neoptolemos · Eithne Costello

1	*Introduction*	*510*
2	*Considerations Regarding Samples*	*510*
2.1	Choice of Sample	510
2.2	What Control Samples Should Be Considered?	512
3	*Simplification of Samples Prior to Analysis: Prefractionation Techniques*	*516*
3.1	Serum and Plasma Fractionation Techniques	516
3.1.1	Albumin and Immunoglobulin Removal	516
3.1.2	High Abundance Protein Depletion	518
3.1.3	Protein Normalization	518
4	*Proteomic Techniques*	*518*
4.1	Gel Based Approaches	518
4.1.1	Two Dimensional Gel Electrophoresis	518
4.1.2	Differential In-Gel Electrophoresis (DIGE)	520
5	*Quantitative LC-MS/MS Approaches*	*521*
5.1	Isotope-Coded Affinity Tags (ICAT)	521
5.2	Isobaric Tags for Relative and Absolute Quantification (iTRAQ)	523
5.3	Stable Isotope Labeling with Amino Acids in Cell Culture (SILAC)	524
5.4	Isotopic Labeling of Cysteine Residues with Acrylamide	525
6	*Surface Enhanced Laser Desorption Ionization (SELDI)*	*525*
7	*Autoimmunoantibody Approaches*	*527*
8	*Microarray Analysis*	*528*
9	*Limitations and Cautionary Notes*	*528*
10	*Conclusion*	*529*

J. P. Neoptolemos, R. Urrutia, J. L. Abbruzzese, M. W. Büchler (eds.), *Pancreatic Cancer*,
DOI 10.1007/978-0-387-77498-5_22, © Springer Science+Business Media, LLC 2010

Abstract: The proteome is the complete set of proteins expressed in a subcellular or cellular compartment, tissue, biological fluid, or organism. It is estimated that there are some 250,000–300,000 human proteins, encoded from 20,000 to 25,000 genes. The discrepancy between the number of genes and the number of proteins is due in part to alternative gene splicing and post-translational modification of proteins.

The proteome is dynamic and changes in response to both intracellular and extracellular signaling. Therefore, comparisons of protein profiles from normal and malignant pancreatic cells, or cells from distinct histological stages that occur during the development of pancreatic cancer provide opportunities for further understanding the pathogenesis of this tumor type. Moreover, such analyses as well as detailed proteomic studies of body fluids, such as pancreatic juice, serum, plasma or urine will likely facilitate the elucidation of new biomarkers for the diagnosis, or management of this disease.

Although proteomic technologies have been rapidly advancing for a number of years, the last decade in particular has seen developments that enable the simultaneous study of large numbers of proteins in a single experiment or set of experiments. In this chapter, the proteomic-based approaches that are most commonly used to analyze pancreatic cancer specimens are reviewed. The range of sample types that have been subjected to analysis, including samples from animal models of pancreatic cancer are discussed, along with examples of proteins that have been identified in these studies.

1   Introduction

Proteomic analysis may be undertaken to catalog the proteins expressed in a given tissue or body fluid. Alternatively, comparative analysis of more than one sample type may be performed, e.g., pancreatic cancer versus disease control samples for the discovery of differences that provide insight into the disease or ultimately lead to biomarkers for that disease. Biomarkers are biological characteristics of a disease that can inform the diagnosis, prognosis or therapy. For biomarkers to be useful clinically, they should be sensitive and specific. However, they also need to be straightforward and inexpensive to measure.

A typical proteomic workflow is presented in ❯ *Fig. 22-1*. Samples from a variety of sources are suitable and may be pre-fractionated to less complex fractions prior to analysis. The proteins or peptides within each fraction may then be examined by a number of techniques, any one of which provides data on only a small portion of the proteome. Differentially expressed proteins or candidate biomarkers are identified, and results validated, usually by immunohistochemical techniques. For biomarker development, a large scale trial is ultimately essential to test the validity of the biomarker.

2   Considerations Regarding Samples

2.1   Choice of Sample

Global proteomic profiling has been performed on normal and malignant pancreatic tissue, as well as pancreatic juice, blood and urine from patients with pancreatic cancer (reviewed in [1–3]). Examples of proteins that have been detected using a variety of proteomic approaches

⬛ Fig. 22-1

Typical proteomic workflow. Samples from a variety of different sample types are suitable for analysis. They may be subjected to pre-fractionation, following which, proteins or peptides within each fraction may then be examined by a number of techniques. Any one of these techniques provides data on only a small portion of the proteome. Differentially expressed proteins or candidate biomarkers are identified, and results validated, usually by techniques, such as ELISA or immunohistochemistry. For biomarker development, a large scale trial is ultimately essential to test the validity of the biomarker.

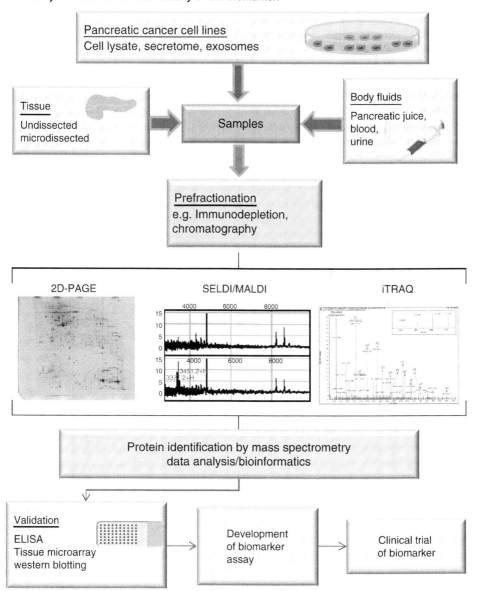

are presented in ❯ *Table 22-1*. While specific experiments and their outcomes are discussed in greater detail below, it is worth considering here some important factors governing the choice of sample for proteomic analysis. Blood represents an excellent potential source of biomarkers [4] as it is minimally invasive to obtain and clinical laboratories have experience of performing blood tests for specified proteins. Moreover, such tests are not necessarily prohibitively expensive. However, blood contains a relatively small number of highly abundant proteins, the presence of which can make it difficult to detect and quantify less abundant proteins. The proportion of blood taken up by high abundance proteins such as albumin and immunoglobulins is illustrated in ❯ *Fig. 22-2*. For optimal protein detection in blood, certain proteomic protocols benefit from prior fractionation and processing of blood. Some of the fractionation procedures applied to blood are described in detail later.

Pancreatic juice may be a richer source of pancreatic-specific biomarkers than blood, since juice is in direct contact with the pancreas. However, obtaining pancreatic juice is more complex than obtaining blood, and can cause unwanted side-effects. Juice sampling by endoscopic retrograde cholangiopancreatography (ERCP) carries the risk of pancreatitis in an estimated 4–7% of cases [5–7]. Analysis of pancreatic juice is therefore most likely to be restricted to screening of individuals at high risk of developing pancreatic cancer. With improved detection techniques analysis of pancreatic juice from the duodenum following pancreas stimulation with i.v. secretin may offer better prospects for screening.

Proteomic studies of whole pancreatic tissue [8–12] as well as microdissected compartments [13,14] have been undertaken. While laser capture microdissection techniques allow one to overcome issues of tissue heterogeneity, they can be labor intensive and time consuming. The nature of proteins found to be differentially expressed largely determines whether those proteins are likely to become valuable biomarkers. For example, proteins whose tissue levels can inform a patient's likelihood to respond to particular treatments are very sought after. Moreover tissue proteins that are secreted and therefore likely to be found in blood or juice are also desirable. Projects specifically studying proteins secreted from pancreatic cancer cell lines [15,16] or exosomes [17] have been undertaken. Analysis of urine has also been explored as a potential source of biomarkers [18]. Finally, genetically engineered mouse models of pancreatic cancer have been the subject of proteomic analysis for the detection of candidate markers relevant to human cancer [19,20].

In summary, the suitability of many sample types for proteomic analysis has been demonstrated and the choice of sample type will depend ultimately on the goals of individual experiments. However, practical reasons will also dictate the types of experiments that are undertaken. Pancreatic cancer tissue, whilst hugely valuable, can be a very scarce resource which is not available at all institutes. Similarly, good collections of plasma/serum or pancreatic juice are not widely available.

2.2   What Control Samples Should Be Considered?

Proteomic analyses that are aimed at identifying biomarkers that facilitate diagnosis need to carefully consider the control sample sets included in the early stages of the experiments and at the later validation stages. Currently, Carbonic Anhydrase 19–9 (CA19–9, sialylated Lewis antigen) [21,22] is the only biomarker commonly used in the clinical setting as a diagnostic tool for the preliminary evaluation of patients with suspected pancreatic cancer [23]. This marker is also valuable in predicting clinical course in both resected and advanced cases,

Table 22-1

Some notable examples of proteins emerging from proteomic-based research. Please note, this list is not exhaustive

Protein Name	Detected in	Function	Method used	Citation
Annexin A2	Tissue	Annexins are cellular proteins that bind the phospholipid membrane in a calcium dependent manner	ICAT	[45]
	Tissue		2-DE	[12]
Annexin A4	Tissue		LC-MS/MS	[73]
Annexin A5	Pancreatic Juice			
CEACAM-1	Serum		cDNA Microarray	[74]
CEACAM-5	Pancreatic Juice		LC-MS/MS	[73]
CEACAM-6	Tissue		Gene silencing	[75]
Cathepsin D	Tissue	Belongs to the aspartyl proteases	2-DE	[12]
CapG	Tissue	Actin capping proteins	2-DE of LCM- procured protein	[76]
Gelsolin	Tissue			
ITIH1	Serum	Inter-alpha inhibitor proteins are trypsin inhibitor proteins involved in hyaluronan metabolism	SELDI	[54]
ITIH2	Serum			
ITIH4	Serum			
MnSOD	Tissue	Manganese superoxide dismutase is a mitochondrial matrix protein	2-DE	[12]
MIC-1	Serum	Macrophage inhibitory cytokine 1	2-DE and SELDI	[77]
MUC1	Pancreatic Juice	Mucin-1 is also known as the tumor associated mucin, whereas Mucin-4 as the pancreatic adenocarcinoma mucin	LC-MS/MS	[73]
	Tissue (immunostaining)		IHC	[78]
MUC4	Tissue		IHC	[79,80]
Osteopontin	Serum	Osteopontin is a glycoprotein, also known as secreted phosphoprotein 1	2-DE and SELDI	[81]

■ Table 22-1 (**continued**)

Protein Name	Detected in	Function	Method used	Citation
Regenerating islet-derived 3 alpha (HIP/PAP; REG3)	Pancreatic juice	Pancreatic islet secretory proteins	2-DE and SELDI	[51]
			Differential isotope labeling	[19]
				[82]
				[45]
				[45]
	Serum		ELISA	[73]
			ICAT	
			ICAT	
	Serum		LC-MS/MS	
	Tissue			
	Pancreatic Juice			
REG1	Pancreatic Juice			
REG4				
S100A6	Laser dissected tissue	S100 proteins belong to a multigen family of calcium binding proteins	2-DE	[14]
			2-DE	[12]
			cDNA Microarray	[83]
S100A8	Tissue			
	Pancreatic Juice			
S100P	Tissue			
Galectin-3	Pancreatic Juice	Beta-galactoside binding proteins	LC-MS/MS	[73]

■ Fig. 22-2

The protein composition of blood is presented. The proportion of blood taken up by highly abundant proteins is illustrated, as is the fraction remaining after depletion of abundant proteins has been undertaken.

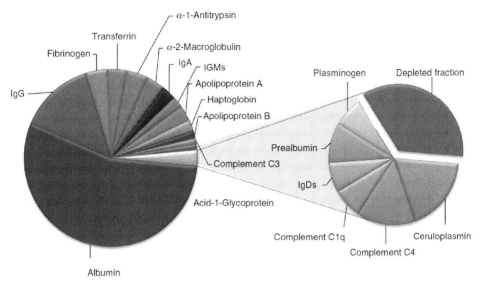

however, it is neither sufficiently sensitive nor specific for sole use as a screening tool for early detection of pancreatic cancer [24]. For clinicians, a biomarker or group of biomarkers that could aid in the distinction between patients with pancreatic cancer and those with benign diseases of the pancreas would be a remarkable advance. Diseases such as chronic pancreatitis or biliary tract stones can cause similar symptoms to those of pancreatic cancer. Moreover, high-resolution computed tomography (CT) imaging cannot always distinguish chronic pancreatitis from pancreatic cancer. An estimated 10% of patients operated for suspected pancreatic malignancy are found to have benign disease following histopathological assessment [25]. Thus experiments undertaken for the analysis of samples such as plasma/serum or juice for biomarkers of pancreatic cancer will benefit from inclusion of patients with chronic pancreatitis, so as to maximize the possibility of finding markers that are cancer-specific, and not present due to pancreatitis. Similarly, when analyzing plasma or serum from patients with pancreatic cancer, it is worth taking into consideration that some of these patients may have obstruction of the distal common bile duct that can result in jaundice. The effect is significant derangement of liver function which may also be associated with secondary biliary bacterial sepsis [acute cholangitis]. Thus, altered levels of some proteins may reflect the presence of jaundice rather than that of cancer [26], and this may need to be carefully accounted for either by analyzing patients with and without jaundice or by considering the potential confounding effects of jaundice during validation steps. Of note, elevated CA19–9 levels are also seen in some patients with pancreatitis or in patients with biliary duct obstruction. When comparing protein profiles of pancreatic bulk undissected cancer tissue, some groups have used bulk undissected normal tissue as a control [11,27], whist other groups have included tissue affected by chronic pancreatitis [9,12]. In other cases, laser capture microdissection (LCM) has been undertaken to enrich for tumor cells, benign ductal epithelial or stromal components [13,14].

3   Simplification of Samples Prior to Analysis: Prefractionation Techniques

Depending on the sample type, different methods to simply the proteome or purify specific cell types can be applied. Cell and tissue samples can be fractionated into subproteomes e.g., nuclear, cytoplasmic, or membrane fractions. As mentioned above, tissue material can be successfully dissected [13,14] such that tumor cells, benign ductal cells or stromal elements may be analyzed separately.

3.1   Serum and Plasma Fractionation Techniques

Blood, in the form of serum or plasma, is one of the most difficult samples to investigate using proteomic approaches. This is in part due to the fact that the proteome of blood contains an enormous concentration range, consisting of a limited number of highly abundant proteins which can mask the detection of the lower abundance proteins (❯ *Fig. 22-2*). The low abundance proteins are however, of special interest as they are likely to include potential biomarkers, which will in some cases be tissue-specific leakage factors. To overcome the complexity of this proteome, fractionation steps prior to analysis are required. During recent years a number of different approaches have been applied to normalize or deplete the high abundance proteins, enabling in-depth analysis of proteins present at lower levels. Some of the approaches taken to simply plasma/blood prior to proteomic analysis are presented schematically in ❯ *Fig. 22-3* and are reviewed below.

3.1.1   Albumin and Immunoglobulin Removal

The original procedures for the simplification of blood were focused on the removal of the most abundant serum protein, albumin. In the 1970s, early approaches were based on dye-ligand affinity chromatography. Cibacron Blue 3GA, a triazine dye, also known as blue dextran was used for identifying proteins which possess a dinucleotide fold, a structure which forms the binding sides for substrates and effectors in a wide range of proteins [28]. It was found that Cibacron Blue bound efficiently to albumin and could be used for the selective removal of albumin [29]. Further studies revealed that Cibacron Blue has highest affinity for human albumin, binding only inefficiently to albumin from other mammalian species. The dye interacts strongly with the bilirubin binding sites of human albumin, probably simulating a bilirubin like structure. Further fatty acids also bind to Cibacron Blue lowering the amount of free interaction sites with albumin [30]. These data suggest that the dye should be used carefully, where no implications from high bilirubin levels as well as fatty acids are a cause for concern. Nowadays Cibacron Blue is still in use for albumin depletion and is available in different formats, depending on the application.

■ Fig. 22-3

Approaches for the simplification of plasma/blood prior to proteomic analysis.

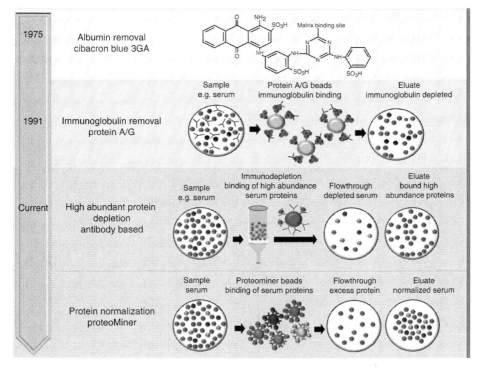

Further improvements were observed in 1991 by combining the use of Cibacron Blue with Protein A and Protein G binding columns (❯ *Fig. 22-3*). Protein A is a bacterial surface protein originally found on *Staphylococcus aureus*. It possesses the ability to bind immunoglobulins (IgG's). Similarly Protein G is an immunoglobulin binding protein from *Streptococcus*, although it has different binding specificities compared to protein A [31]. Nowadays Proteins A and G as well as L are available in different formats ranging from simple centrifugal spin filters for immunoglobulin removal to more sophisticated HPLC columns [32]. Moreover, recombinant forms of Protein A/G and A/G/L are available as well as mixtures of Protein A with Cibacron Blue for simultaneous albumin and immunoglobulin depletion. As proteomic approaches advanced, additional high abundance protein depletion methods were introduced based on antibodies against specific proteins. Firstly, anti-human serum albumin (HSA) antibody based approaches were introduced. A comparison of Cibacron Blue with anti-HSA columns and Protein G immunoglobulin depletion has shown that each approach works well. However, the combination of albumin and immunoglobulin removal was particularly useful in allowing the detection of lower abundance proteins [33]. As a result the range of high abundance proteins that could be removed using antibody-based depletion columns was increased.

3.1.2 High Abundance Protein Depletion

There are a number of different antibody-based high abundant depletion columns on the market. Most are produced in practical small-scale centrifuge spin filter format as well as in liquid chromatography (LC)-formats. Examples of columns in common use currently include "Multiple Affinity Removal System" (MARS) by Agilent, the "Proteomelab IgY" by Beckman-Coulter, several IgY columns by Genway Biotech and the "ProteoPrep 20 Immunodepletion kit" by Sigma Aldrich. The MARS system was first introduced in 2005 for the depletion of six high abundance proteins, and since 2007 is available for the depletion of fourteen high abundance proteins. The technology of all of these different high abundance protein depletion columns is based on specific antibodies bound to resin or agarose beads which bind the high abundance proteins in serum/plasma samples. Immunodepletion approaches are a major advance in the improvement of low abundance protein detection (◉ *Fig. 22-3*). A further approach, recently introduced is the Supermix System by Genway Biotech, which allows a further immunodepletion step of medium abundance proteins.

3.1.3 Protein Normalization

As the immunodepletion methods are specifically removing high or medium abundance proteins, an alternative approach relies on protein normalization. Protein normalization, introduced by BioRad as "ProteoMiner Protein Enrichment" is based on a large, highly diverse library of hexapeptides, which are bound to chromatography beads. Theoretically, highly abundant proteins saturate their hexapeptide binding partners, whereas proteins of lower abundance will not. The flowthrough from this column represents the non bound highly abundant proteins, while the eluted fraction represents serum/plasma where the concentration of proteins has been normalized (◉ *Fig. 22-3*). In that normalized serum, the huge dynamic range of the different proteins is normalized. It was shown that the normalization of serum proteins reveals new low abundance proteins [34].

4 Proteomic Techniques

Proteomic approaches for analyzing different whole or prefractionated sample types, range from the two dimensional gel electrophoresis, developed in the 1970s to the recently introduced liquid chromatography based isobaric tags for relative and absolute quantification (iTRAQ). An overview of the different methods used in pancreatic cancer proteomics is given below.

4.1 Gel Based Approaches

4.1.1 Two Dimensional Gel Electrophoresis

The best known and most widely applied proteomic technique for investigating differences between samples is two-dimensional gel electrophoresis (2-DE; ◉ *Fig. 22-4*). First described by P.H. O'Farrell and J. Klose in 1975 and further improved by Görg and co-workers, it still

Fig. 22-4

Two dimensional gel electrophoresis and its application within proteomic protocols.

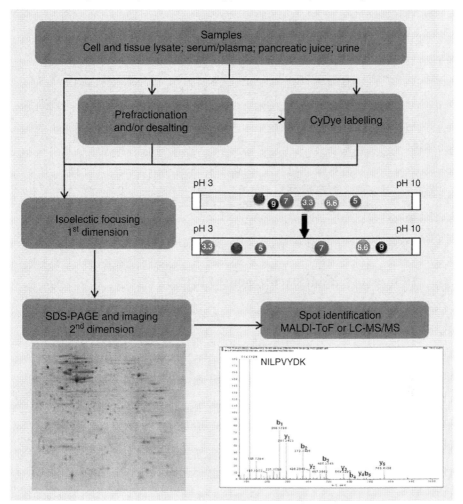

provides a powerful method today [35,36]. In recent years it has proven valuable in the detection of posttranslational modifications of proteins. Limitations in sample preparation include the relatively high quantity of protein that is needed. This is especially challenging when sample quantities are restricted or samples have been fractionated into sub-proteomes. The analysis, by 2-DE, of complex samples such as plasma/serum benefit from fractionation, as a much higher resolution of lower abundance proteins is achieved. Samples such as urine, which are defined by high salt concentrations or low protein levels, require buffer exchange and/or concentration. Several methods for these steps are available including precipitation or ultrafiltration.

The first phase of the 2D approach consists of isoelectric focusing (IEF), separating the proteins according to their charge (● Fig. 22-4). Proteins are then separated in the second dimension according to their molecular weight (❯ *Fig. 22-4*) using SDS-polyacrylamide gel electrophoresis (SDS-PAGE). Nowadays IEF is achieved using manufactured immobilized pH gradient (IPG) gel strips, which are available in several pH ranges. Samples are usually applied whilst the strips are rehydrated. The second dimension, SDS-PAGE, can vary from single percentage gels to gradient gels which zoom into the molecular weight regions displaying proteins of greatest interest. Standard staining procedures include silver staining and colloidal Coomassie Blue. Silver staining is quite sensitive, detecting typically 2–4 ng protein. If identification of proteins is desired, then a mass spectrometry (MS)-compatible silver stain needs to be used. Colloidal Coomassie Blue can detect proteins in the range of 8–50 ng, and the stain is MS-compatible. Fluorescent staining dyes are also available. A recent study compared fluorescent stains including Sypro Ruby, Deep Purple and alternatives such as Rubeo and Flamingo [37]. SYPRO Ruby is as sensitive as silver stain and has the advantage of being linear over a wide concentration range, which silver stain lacks.

Spots of interest on gels can be dissected out, digested into peptides and analyzed using MS. As the databases on protein and peptide information increased greatly in recent years, good coverage of the proteome is available, which allows efficient identification of the gel spots.

4.1.2 Differential In-Gel Electrophoresis (DIGE)

The introduction of fluorescent stains (❯ *Fig. 22-4*) into proteomic analyses has improved 2-DE in sensitivity, reproducibility and quantification [38]. Furthermore it allows easier access to methods like differential in-gel electrophoresis (DIGE), which was developed by Ünlü et al. in 1997 [39]. This multiplex approach allows the loading of two protein mixtures from different samples, labeled with different fluorescent dyes onto one gel. The fluorophores which can be used for the labeling are cyanine dyes, Alexa fluor dyes, infrared dyes and DyLights. The most commonly used dyes are the cyanine dyes Cy2, Cy3 and Cy5 which can be differentiated by their different absorbance and emission spectra. Two different DIGE approaches have been described. They use minimal or saturation Cy dyes respectively. In the case of minimal labeling, the ratio of dye to protein is kept very low. This is achieved by labeling only lysine residues of proteins. Minimal dyes are conjugated with a N-hydroxysuccinimidyl (NHS)-ester, which covalently binds to the ε–amines of lysine residues by building an amide bond. Using saturation labeling, dyes bind all available cysteine groups, obtaining a high ratio of dye to protein. These dyes are conjugated with a maleimide reactive group, which covalently binds to the thiol group of cysteines, forming a thioether linkage. Succinimidyl esters are commonly used as linkers between cyanine dyes and proteins. The samples are combined after labeling and then applied to a 2D-gel. After 2D-PAGE the gels are scanned using fluorescent imagers capable of scanning through a wide range of the spectra. The scanned gels for each dye are overlaid and differences in fluorescence intensities quantified.

Proteomic profiling of pancreatic cancer tissue, serum, pancreatic juice and urine samples have all been undertaken using 2D-PAGE. Notable examples of these studies are reviewed below. Tian et al. investigated pancreatic juice samples using 2D and DIGE analysis. Their study identified 14 differentially regulated proteins, the most promising of which was matrix metalloprotease 9, which was up regulated in pancreatic cancer samples [40]. Serum/plasma has been investigated by a number of groups. Bloomston et al. used high-resolution two-dimensional gel electrophoresis to compare serum from 32 normal and 30 pancreatic cancer patients, resolving around 1750 proteins spots per sample [41]. The study found nine protein spots that could effectively separate cancer from normal controls, one of which was identified as fibrinogen gamma and further validated. Deng et al. included patients with chronic pancreatitis as well as healthy controls and pancreatic cancer patients in their 2D analysis of plasma [43]. They reported finding mostly highly abundant proteins and observed that haptoglobin (Hp) beta chain and leucine-rich alpha2 glycoprotein were up-regulated slightly in plasma from pancreatic cancer. DIGE has been applied to plasma analysis of pancreatic cancer patients before and after surgery for the removal of the tumor [42, 43]. A group of proteins which changed consistently in plasma following complete resection of pancreas tumor was identified, including Complement component 3, vitamin D binding protein, apolipoprotein A IV.

5   Quantitative LC-MS/MS Approaches

In recent years new multidimensional protein identification and quantification technologies have been established. In the case of protein or peptide fractionation by two-dimensional liquid chromatography, as the name suggests, a combination of two different affinity columns is used. The first dimension can, for example, consist of a cation or anion exchange chromatography column, fractionating the complex sample on the basis of protein or peptide charge. Usually, the second phase comprises on-line reverse-phase high-performance liquid chromatography (RP-HPLC), where the protein or peptide fractions from the first dimension are further sub-divided by their molecular weight. Generally, in the case of peptides, the second phase uses a nano-LC column which is coupled online to a tandem mass spectrometer (MS/MS). This configuration is very powerful as it allows identification of a cellular proteome without using a gel based approach. Moreover, it can be setup such that it runs in a fully automated manner. Comparison of different protein quantities in different biological samples can be achieved using methods such as ICAT, iTRAQ or SILAC. The principles behind these techniques are described in detail below, and displayed schematically in ⊙ *Fig. 22-5*.

5.1   Isotope-Coded Affinity Tags (ICAT)

In 1999 a gel-free protein quantification method using stable isotopes was introduced (reviewed in [44]). Isotope-coded affinity tag (ICAT) labels exist in two forms (⊙ *Fig. 22-5*), heavy or light. Each tag consists of three different groups, a thiol-specific reactive group, which targets the thiol groups of cysteines, a biotin group, which can be used for purification purposes, and a linker placed between the thiol reactive and biotin group. This linker is an important part of the tag, discriminating between the heavy and light forms of the label. The light form has hydrogen atoms (instead of deuterium) incorporated into the linker (d0), while the heavy form contains deuterium atoms (d8). A new cleavable version of the ICAT label is available, which uses carbon-13 atoms instead of deuterium atoms. The mass difference between the original light and heavy form is 8 daltons (Da), while the mass difference of the new form is 9 Da. ICAT labeling can be used with a variety of different sample types. For pancreatic cancer biomarker discovery, tissue as well as pancreatic juice has been investigated. Chen et al. used ICAT to compare the protein profile from pancreatic cancer tissue with that of normal pancreatic tissue [45]. They also compared protein profiles of pooled pancreatic juice (from ten benign disease control patients) with juice from a pancreatic cancer patient and a

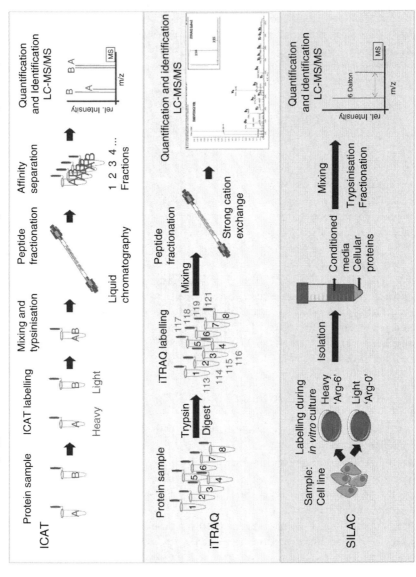

☐ Fig. 22-5

Schematic representation of three widely applied methods for the relative and absolute quantification of biological samples.

patient with chronic pancreatitis [46,47]. In all three publications the cleavable ICAT reagent was used. The principles behind the experimental protocol are as follows: Firstly, the two protein mixtures (e.g., proteins from cancer and normal tissue) are labeled separately, one with the heavy label, the other with the light label. Ideally the label is covalently bound to every cysteine of the proteins in the mixture. In the next step the two protein mixtures are combined, trypsin digested into peptides and fractionated by cation exchange chromatography. This step allows a simplification of the complex sample as well as removal of the reagents used during labeling, such as sodium dodecyl sulphate (SDS), excess ICAT label and trypsin. The ICAT labeled peptides from these fractions are purified by their biotin tag using an avidin affinity chromatography. This step allows a major simplification of mixture as only 26.6% of trypsin digested peptides contain cysteines, and only these peptides will be selected at this point. These peptides nonetheless represent 96.1% of human proteins. Finally the purified ICAT-labeled peptide fractions are applied to a microcapillary HPLC coupled online to MS/MS. The paired light and heavy labeled peptides elute from the HPLC at the same time, but the mass difference of 9 DA is detected as two signals in the scanning MS. If a peptide is detected in the first MS it will be fragmented in the second MS into its ion spectrum. This supplies information about the peptide's amino acid sequence, which can then be searched against a protein database, and the protein to which this peptide belongs, identified. In this manner ICAT allows the quantification of the relative abundance of proteins from two different sample mixtures.

ICAT studies have demonstrated the detection of approximately 1,000–2,000 proteins. Considering that a mammalian cell has an average of 10,000 different proteins, only 10–20% of this proteome is analyzed by ICAT. Chen et al. identified 656 proteins in pancreatic tissue, covering approximately 6.5% of the investigated proteome. It is most likely, that potential pancreatic cancer biomarkers have been missed, due to these limitations. From these 656 proteins, 151 were altered in abundance between cancer and control. The group further validated the potential markers annexin A2, cathepsin D and integrin β1. From pancreatic juice Chen et al. identified a total of 105 proteins including insulin-like growth factor binding protein-2 which was found to be upregulated in cancer and validated by Western blotting. These researchers additionally identified differential levels of plasminogen, neural cell adhesion molecule L1 and caldecrin, although these were not further validated.

5.2   Isobaric Tags for Relative and Absolute Quantification (iTRAQ)

A major limitation of ICAT is that only two samples can be compared to each other at a time. This constraint was overcome with the introduction of a new technology, namely isobaric tag for relative and absolute quantitation (iTRAQ). iTRAQ was a major breakthrough in quantitative proteomics, as it allows a simultaneous relative quantification of up to four (4-PLEX) and more recently eight (8-PLEX) different samples (⊙ Fig. 22-5). It gives the investigator the possibility to include additional appropriate controls, or internal duplicates of one sample. iTRAQ can be used with a variety of different samples. Different kits are available for investigating tissue or serum/plasma samples. To use iTRAQ with serum or plasma a fractionation step, such as high abundance protein depletion, is recommended. The iTRAQ label itself consists of three elements, a reporter group, a balance group and a peptide reactive group. The reporter group is important as this group has different masses (for the 4-PLEX 114.1, 115.1, 116.1 and 117.1 and for the 8-PLEX an additional 113.1, 118.1, 119.1 and 121.1). In the second part of the tandem MS/MS procedure during the peptide sequencing, these reporter groups are ionized and their relative quantities measured by their intensities. The balance group has a neutral mass loss ranging from 31 to 28 Da for the 4-PLEX. This means that the 114 label contains the 31 mass balance group, whereas the 116 label contains the 29 mass balance group, ensuring that every label maintains a total mass of 145 Da. Thus, the labels are indistinguishable by mass and can only be differentiated by collision-induced dissociation through the release of their reporter ion group.

The peptide reactive group of the label is used to react with the N-terminal groups of peptides. Using iTRAQ, the first important point is that samples must be free of primary amines and buffered in an iTRAQ-compatible buffer, such as 0.5 M triethylammoniumbicarbonate at pH 8.5. Ideally, samples containing 100 μg protein, are each denatured, reduced and alkylated, then trypsin digested and labeled with individual iTRAQ labels. After the labeling reaction, samples with different labels are combined and fractionated using strong cation exchange chromatography. The resulting fractions are then analyzed using nano reverse phase chromatography coupled with MS/MS. Although peptides from different samples are labeled with different iTRAQ labels, they elute together as the mass of the iTRAQ label is always the same. As stated above, it is only in the second phase of MS/MS that collision-induced dissociation allows the labels to be distinguished and quantified. Thus at this stage, a given peptide from a cancer and a healthy control sample respectively can be distinguished and the relative quantities of each determined. To date, no studies on pancreatic cancer using iTRAQ have been reported. However, this is a relatively new technology and a number of studies using this approach are anticipated.

5.3   Stable Isotope Labeling with Amino Acids in Cell Culture (SILAC)

The quantitative approaches already described, i.e., 2D-PAGE-based, ICAT and iTRAQ all share a common feature. The labeling of proteins/peptides occurs after proteins have been harvested or extracted. By contrast, the SILAC approach (Fig. 22-5) is different, because proteins are labeled in vivo. Therefore, the focus of SILAC experiments is cell culture-based. Like ICAT, the SILAC technique uses a heavy and light label [48]. Mammalian cell cultures, as well as bacterial and yeast cultures are all suitable starting points for SILAC experiments. As there are many different pancreatic cell lines available, this technique should be considered. Gronborg et al. studied the Panc-1 cell line derived from a human pancreatic ductal adenocarcinoma and immortalized human pancreatic ductal epithelial cells, HPDE representing an in vitro surrogate for human ductal epithelium [15]. The aim of this study was to investigate and quantify the difference in the secretome of both pancreas derived cell lines. For qualitative analysis, normal LC-MS/MS or SELDI approaches are appropriate, however SILAC offers the possibility of including a quantitative measurement. Using SILAC, two groups of cells are cultured separately in similar culture media. The culture media for one group, however contains unmodified or "light," L-leucine, while the second group are exposed to "heavy" deuterated L-leucine in their medium. Other essential amino acids may be used in SILAC experiments. Gronborg et al. [15] used a mix of heavy $[^{13}C_6]$Arginine and $[^{13}C_6]$Lysine, to maximize the incorporation into protein of the heavy amino acids. After culturing the cells in light and heavy media, the cells were harvested and protein extracted and/or fractionated. This can be done for both groups alone or combined. In the study by Gronborg et al. the researchers were interested in secretome changes [15]. Therefore they harvested conditioned media, concentrated it, evaluated the quantities of heavy and light protein and then combined matched protein quantities. For fractionation and quantification LC-MS/MS analysis is generally used. Gronborg et al. took a slightly different approach, separating the secreted proteins by 1D-PAGE and sectioned the resulting gel into 25 bands, which were subsequently in-gel digested and analyzed by automated nanoflow LC-MS/MS. From 195 proteins identified, they further validated, by Western blotting, proteins that were upregulated in the Panc-1 secretome compared to the HPDE secretome. These included monocyte chemotactic protein 1, cathepsin B, cathepsin D, apolipoprotein E, L1 cell adhesion molecule isoform 1, and Mac-2-binding protein. They also identified a number of proteins that were less abundant in the Panc-1 secretome compared to the HPDE secretome, including secretory leukocyte protease inhibitor and insulin-like growth factor binding protein-7. In addition, the tissue levels of a number of proteins, found by SILAC to be differentially present in the secretomes under consideration, were examined using pancreatic cancer tissue microarrays. These included, CD9, perlecan, stromal cell derived factor 4 and apolipoprotein E.

5.4 Isotopic Labeling of Cysteine Residues with Acrylamide

The group of Hanash et al. recently compared the plasma profiles of a genetically engineered mouse model of pancreatic cancer at different stages in the development of pancreatic cancer [19]. Plasma from control animals was compared with plasma from animals with early lesions (PanIN) or advanced cancer. Samples were depleted of three highly abundant proteins (albumin, IgG, and transferrin) and whole proteins then differentially labeled with heavy or light deuterated isotopes of acrylamide. The heavy and light labeled samples were then mixed and subjected to anion-exchange chromatography. Fractions collected from this first dimension were then subjected to reversed-phase chromatography, the second dimension, and aliquots of the collected fractions were either separated for mass-spectrometry shotgun analysis or alternatively, digested with trypsin and analyzed by mass spectrometry. This analysis led to the identification of 1,442 plasma proteins, with quantification data on 621 proteins. Of these, 165 proteins were found to be up-regulated in cancer samples or PanIN or both compared to controls. Strict criteria were applied for the selection of candidates for follow-up by immmunohistochemistry (IHC) or ELISA on mouse plasma samples. Examples include CD166 antigen precursor (ALCAM), receptor-type tyrosine-protein PTPRG, and TIMP1, and tenascin C (TNC) which were validated by IHC. Elevated circulating levels of ICAM1, and TIMP1 were found in mice with pancreatic cancer. Notably, TIMP1 was also elvevated in PanIN plasma samples. A very important element of this study was the evaluation of a panel of markers, including LCN2, REG1A, REG3, TIMP1, and IGFBP4, in patients with very early cancers. This panel performed slightly better in comparison to CA19–9. However, when the panel was combined with CA19–9 significantly improved discrimination between early stage (pre-diagnostic) sera and matched controls was achieved.

6 Surface Enhanced Laser Desorption Ionization (SELDI)

SELDI, a chip based sample fractionation technique coupled with MALDI-TOF analysis, has had a considerable impact on pancreatic cancer shotgun proteomics. SELDI (◉ *Fig. 22-6*) can be used with any sample type, including cells, serum, plasma and pancreatic juice. In contrast to other approaches SELDI requires relatively little protein. For example protein from around

☐ Fig. 22-6

Schematic representation of Surface Enhanced Laser Desorption Ionization (SELDI).

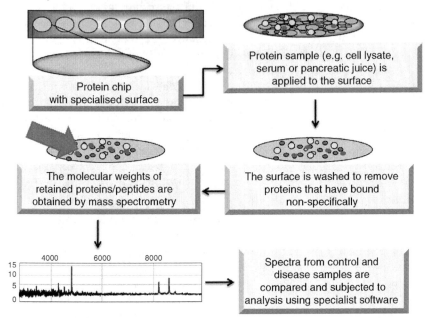

25 to 100 cells is sufficient for SELDI, whereas other methods require higher quantity (~50,000 cells are needed for a 2D-PAGE) [49]. The individual chips used as part of the SELDI process have different surfaces, which play an important role during processing of the samples. The surface structure determines different aspects such as fractionation, amplification and extraction. Commonly used chips include normal phase silica (NP) chips which capture generic proteins, weak or strong anion or cation exchange, hydrophobic surfaces, immobilized metal affinity-capture, preactivated surfaces with reactive carbonyl diimidazole moieties or epoxy groups [50]. Depending on the chip used, complex proteomic samples, such as whole cell or tissue protein lysate, as well as serum or plasma is fractionated so that only proteins that efficiently bind to the chip surface will be detected subsequently during MALDI analysis. After the binding/ fractionation step a thorough washing step is required in order to reduce non-specific protein binding to the chip surface. Proteins are then mixed with the MALDI matrices and their masses are determined using a linear Time Of Flight MS or MS/MS. Depending on the sample origin, for example cancer or normal, a different protein profile is obtained. The bottleneck of this approach is that whilst good differentiation between different samples is achieved, the identity of individual proteins/biomarkers is not learned as part of the SELDI process.

One of the first SELDI studies aimed at the detection of pancreatic cancer specific biomarkers led to identification in pancreatic juice of the protein, regenerative islet derived 3 alpha (REG3A, also known as hepatocarcinoma-intestine-pancreas/pancreatitis-associated protein 1) [51]. REG3A is a pancreatic secretory protein, with possible roles in cell proliferation and or differentiation. It is differentially regulated during pancreatic inflammation, cancer and also liver carcinogenesis and was identified in juice samples using an immobilized metal affinity capture (IMAC3) chip. An immunoassay chip conjugated with REG3A was employed for further evaluation [51]. Of note, this protein was one of the proteins detected in the plasma of mice with pancreatic cancer, described above. Other chip types have also been used in association with pancreatic cancer specimens. Sasaki et al. identified the C-terminal peptide of the putative tumor suppressor protein DMBT1 in the secretomes of pancreatic cancer cell lines using a C16 hydrophobic interaction chip [52]. As the serum proteome is difficult to analyze, even the SELDI approach benefits from prior sample fractionation. Koopman et al. divided the proteome into six fractions by anion exchange chromatography. Fractions were then immobilized on metal affinity capture-coupled with copper chips (IMAC-Cu$^+$) or weak cation exchange chips. The outcome of the study was a minimum set of protein peaks with the ability to discriminate between pancreatic cancer patients, nonmalignant pancreatic disease patients and healthy controls [53]. In another serum study, SELDI was used to investigate the fragmentation of the serum protein inter-α-trypsin inhibitor heavy chain 4 (ITIH4) [54]. Ehmann et al. analyzed serum samples using similar chips to those used by Koopman et al. and found that the levels of apolipoprotein AI and AII as well as transthyretin are decreased in pancreatic cancer [55]. Beside serum and pancreatic juice, pancreatic cyst fluid was also investigated from patients with pancreatic ductal adenocarcinoma, non-carcinoma, intraductal papillary mucinous neoplasm, pseudocysts and patients with no evidence of malignancy. For analysis a hydrophobic (H50) protein chip was used [56]. A differentiation between cancer and non-malignant controls was achieved by using a profile of 12 protein peaks for discrimination.

7 Autoimmunoantibody Approaches

Tumor specific antibodies for several cancers have been documented [57,58]. Detecting tumor proteins that have provoked an immune response (tumor antigens) or the antibodies that have been raised against them (autoantibodies) may provide a method for sensitive and specific diagnosis and potential targets for immunotherapy. The first "shotgun" proteomic method applied for the systematic identification of tumor antigens was named serological analysis of recombinant cDNA expression libraries (SEREX) [57]. Using the SEREX approach, a cDNA expression library from tumor cell lines or tissue is screened using patient sera for the detection of antibody reactivity against tumor proteins in that sera. The SEREX method has been applied for the detection of antibody-based reactivity to expressed cDNAs from a pancreatic cancer cell line, and has led to the identification of 18 potential antigens [59].

In recent years the SEREX approach has been combined with 2D-PAGE technology. This method is referred to as serological proteome analysis (SERPA) [60] or combination of proteome analysis and SEREX (PROTEOMEX) [61]. SERPA involves resolving proteins by 2D-PAGE, transferring them onto a nitrocellulose membrane and probing the membrane with patient sera (normal or cancer). Proteins bound to primary human antibodies (autoantibodies) are revealed using a conjugated secondary anti human IgM or IgG antibody. The corresponding protein spots are visualized by autoradiography, the spots localized, and picked from a second, matching 2D-PAGE and analyzed by mass spectrometry. Hong et al. applied this protocol using total protein from Panc-1 cells and sera from patients with pancreatic cancer, chronic pancreatitis or healthy individuals. This led to the identification of calreticulin isoforms 1 and 2 [62]. Tomaino et al. performed similar experiments using three pancreatic cancer cell lines: CFPAC-1 (metastatic), MiaPaca-2 (undifferentiated) and BxPC-3 (poorly differentiated). The sera were from patients with pancreatic cancer and, as controls, patients with chronic pancreatitis and other malignant diseases. The most promising results included an autoimmunresponse to keratin type 1 cytoskeletal 10 and cofilin-1 [63].

8   Microarray Analysis

Protein microarrays have been introduced and are becoming a compelling alternative platform for proteomic analysis. Improvements in sensitivity have been reported along with expansion of the number of antibodies spotted on arrays which raises the number of quantifiable proteins in a sample. Both complex protein mixtures and prefractionated protein mixtures from cells, serum/plasma can be used. Currently a range of protein microarrays are in use. There are four basic types including (1) interaction partner identification, (2) a fixed-analyte free-detector combination, (3) a fixed-detector free analyte combination and (4) a combination of (2) and (3) (for a detailed review see [64]). Antibody microarrays can be used in a forward phase approach, where different antibody "detectors" are spotted onto the array and probed with proteins (type c) or reverse phase, where the cell lysates or serum "analyte" are spotted onto the array (type b). Orchekowski et al. used a forward phase approach for identifying differentially expressed PDAC proteins, using 90 different spotted antibodies [65]. The antibodies were spotted on the array, whereas the serum samples were labeled with a fluorescent dye. Serum samples from patients with pancreatic cancer, benign pancreatic disease and healthy control subjects were used as probes. Samples were labeled with either N-hydroxysuccinimide-biotin or N-hydroxysuccinimide-digoxigenin. All samples labeled with the digoxigenin were combined and used as a standard on each array. Using this approach, the researchers were able to identify differentially expressed proteins, which were already described as being regulated (e.g., C-reactive protein, α-1-antitrypsin, cathepsin D). This study demonstrated that it is possible to distinguish cancer samples from healthy controls or benign disease using antibody microarrays [65]. A different labeling approach was used by Hamelinck et al. [66] who also investigated pancreatic cancer serum samples against controls. Samples were labeled with the fluorescent dyes Cy3 and Cy5 coupled with N-hydroxysuccinimide for protein binding. Cy5 labeled samples were pooled and served as a standard. An upregulation of C-reactive protein, a1-antichymotrypsin and α1-antitrypsin and decreased amounts of complement C4 and C3, transferrin and cathepsin D were observed. In a recent study by Ingvarrson et al. 129 human recombinant scFc antibodies against sixty different proteins were obtained and spotted onto microarrays [67]. The group used this platform to analyze nonfractionated, directly labeled, whole human serum proteomes, resulting in a protein signature based on 19 nonredundant analytes, that discriminated between pancreatic cancer patients and healthy subjects. Using an alternative approach, lysates from pancreatic cancer cell lines with either mutated p53 (Capan 1, CF, E6E7, PANC-1, Miapaca2) or p53 null (ASPC-1) were spotted onto array slides and probed with antibodies specific for 52 different signaling proteins [68]. The study in question was part of a larger study examining transduction signaling in cancer. A number of signaling pathways unique to different cancers were observed. Pancreatic cancer was the only type of cancer where the epidermal growth factor receptor (EGFR) signaling pathway was significantly differentially expressed.

9   Limitations and Cautionary Notes

It is worth remembering that no single proteomic approach or platform will allow complete proteome coverage and if extensive coverage is desired, then the use of a variety of complementary approaches may be necessary. Moreover, as is true for many other types of analyses, the quality of the data obtained will depend on the nature of the samples studied. Where possible, standard operating procedures for the collection, storage, processing and analysis of samples should be developed and adhered to, and samples in all study groups should be treated in a uniform way, so as to minimize the effects of external influences on protein profiles [69]. The importance of including appropriate disease control patients in experiments has been mentioned earlier in this chapter, as have limitations associated with the various techniques that have been described. Finally, the reader is referred an excellent review on the threats (including bias) to the validity of data in clinical biomarker research [70], and proposals for improving the reliability with which good biomarkers are discovered, validated and further developed [71,72].

10   Conclusion

Whist much progress has been made in applying a range of techniques to pancreatic cancer samples, the challenge now is to follow-up on these initial findings. Interrogating the less readily accessible, lower abundance proteome is particularly important. Moreover, implementing large-scale validation studies to develop potential markers, antigens and targets that come out of such research will be vital if they are to be successfully translated into the clinic.

Key Research Points

- The proteome is the complete set of proteins expressed in a subcellular or cellular compartment, tissue, biological fluid, or organism. Proteomics, the study of the proteome, complements genomic studies. It enables the examination of proteins both quantitatively and qualitatively, including post-translational modifications.
- Major advances in technology, including the reproducibility of two dimensional gel electrophoresis, and developments in mass spectrometry as well as bioinformatics have greatly enhanced proteomic studies. Innovations, such as isotope-coded affinity tags (ICAT), isobaric tags for relative and absolute quantification (iTRAQ), and stable isotope labeling with amino acids in cell culture (SILAC) facilitate quantitative measurements of protein levels and have marked real progress.
- Much knowledge has been gained also on how to simplify samples prior to analysis, such that in-depth proteomic analysis is possible. All of these advances have resulted in an increased understanding of the pathogenesis of many diseases and opportunities for biomarker discovery.
- With respect to pancreatic cancer, proteomic analysis, using a variety of techniques, has been applied to human tissue, plasma/serum, pancreatic juice and urine. Moreover the application of animal models of pancreatic cancer for the detection of biomarkers relevant to human cancer has also been undertaken. Differentially expressed proteins in all of the above sample types have been reported, and arising from these analyses, a number of potential biomarkers have been suggested.

Future Scientific Directions

- Proteomic analysis already undertaken on pancreatic cancer samples has helped elaborate the biology of this disease. Moreover, it has also provided insight into potential biomarker panels for earlier diagnosis.
- The challenge ahead is to build on this initial work. Mining deeper into the proteome, accessing the lower abundance proteome will likely provide the best opportunities for cancer-specific markers. Where they are lacking, high throughput assays need to be developed for candidate biomarkers that are identified. Large-scale validation studies to develop potential markers, antigens and targets need to be undertaken to translate the outcomes of proteomic studies into the clinic.
- Whist the focus of attention currently is on biomarker discovery, future research can look towards further unraveling of the biology of pancreatic cancer through, for example, examining specific subproteomes, such as the phosphoproteome.

Clinical Implications

- Currently, there is only one blood-borne biomarker in routine clinical practice that is used in association with pancreatic cancer. This is the Carbonic Anhydrase 19–9 (CA19–9, sialylated Lewis antigen). Although this marker is helpful in predicting clinical course, it lacks adequate sensitivity and specificity for sole use in diagnosis and it provides unreliable information on the likelihood of treatment response.
- For pancreatic cancer, a major obstacle to better treatment and improved outcome is the difficulty in diagnosing the disease early. Accurate biomarkers are crucial for facilitating earlier diagnosis. They are also essential for enhancing the effectiveness of current therapeutic options as well as the evaluation of tumor responsiveness in emerging early drug trial designs.
- Proteomic analysis has the power to detect such markers. Indeed, we are already seeing the identification of potential markers that will facilitate earlier diagnosis. However much commitment of effort will be needed to validate and develop markers that emerge from proteomic studied such that they are translated into clinical practice.

References

1. Aspinall-O'Dea M, Costello E: The pancreatic cancer proteome – recent advances and future promise. Proteomics Clin Appl 2007;1(9):1066–1079.
2. Chen R, Pan S, Aebersold R, Brentnall T: Proteomics studies of pancreatic cancer. Proteomics Clin Appl 2007;1(12):1582–1591.
3. Grantzdorffer I, Carl-McGrath S, Ebert MP, Rocken C: Proteomics of pancreatic cancer. Pancreas 2008;36(4):329–336.
4. Hanash SM, Pitteri SJ, Faca VM: Mining the plasma proteome for cancer biomarkers. Nature 2008; 452(7187):571–579.
5. Loperfido S, Angelini G, Benedetti G, et al.: Major early complications from diagnostic and therapeutic ERCP: a prospective multicenter study. Gastrointest Endosc 1998;48(1):1–10.
6. Suissa A, Yassin K, Lavy A, et al.: Outcome and early complications of ERCP: a prospective single center study. Hepatogastroenterology 2005;52(62):352–355.
7. Vandervoort J, Soetikno RM, Tham TC, et al.: Risk factors for complications after performance of ERCP. Gastrointest Endosc 2002;56(5):652–656.
8. Chen YI, Donohoe S, et al.: Pancreatic cancer proteome: the proteins that underlie invasion, metastasis,

and immunologic escape. Gastroenterology 2005; 129(4):1187–1197.

9. Crnogorac-Jurcevic T, Gangeswaran R, Bhakta V, et al.: Proteomic analysis of chronic pancreatitis and pancreatic adenocarcinoma. Gastroenterology 2005;129(5):1454–1463.

10. Hu L, Evers S, Lu ZH, Shen Y, Chen J: Two-dimensional protein database of human pancreas. Electrophoresis 2004;25(3):512–518.

11. Lu Z, Hu L, Evers S, Chen J, Shen Y: Differential expression profiling of human pancreatic adenocarcinoma and healthy pancreatic tissue. Proteomics 2004;4(12):3975–3988.

12. Shen J, Person MD, Zhu J, Abbruzzese JL, Li D: Protein expression profiles in pancreatic adenocarcinoma compared with normal pancreatic tissue and tissue affected by pancreatitis as detected by two-dimensional gel electrophoresis and mass spectrometry. Cancer Res 2004;64(24):9018–9026.

13. Sheikh AA, Vimalachandran D, Thompson CC, et al.: The expression of S100A8 in pancreatic cancer-associated monocytes is associated with the Smad4 status of pancreatic cancer cells. Proteomics 2007;7(11):1929–1940.

14. Shekouh A, Thompson C, Prime W: et al.: Application of laser capture microdissection combined with two-dimensional electrophoresis for the discovery of differentially regulated proteins in pancreatic ductal adenocarcinoma. Proteomics 2003; 3(10):1988–2001.

15. Gronborg M, Kristiansen TZ, Iwahori A, et al.: Biomarker discovery from pancreatic cancer secretome using a differential proteomic approach. Mol Cell Proteomics 2006;5(1):157–171.

16. Mauri P, Scarpa A, Nascimbeni AC, et al.: Identification of proteins released by pancreatic cancer cells by multidimensional protein identification technology: a strategy for identification of novel cancer markers. FASEB J 2005;19(9):1125–1127. doi:10.1096/fj.04–3000fje.

17. Ristorcelli E, Beraud E, Verrando P, et al.: Human tumor nanoparticles induce apoptosis of pancreatic cancer cells. FASEB J 2008;22(9):3358–3369.

18. Kojima K, Asmellash S, Klug CA, Grizzle WE, Mobley JA, Christein JD: Applying proteomic-based biomarker tools for the accurate diagnosis of pancreatic cancer. J Gastrointest Surg 2008;12(10):1683–1690.

19. Faca VM, Song KS, Wang H, et al.: A mouse to human search for plasma proteome changes associated with pancreatic tumor development. PLoS Med 2008;5(6):e123.

20. Hingorani SR, Petricoin EF, Maitra A: et al.: Preinvasive and invasive ductal pancreatic cancer and its early detection in the mouse. Cancer Cell 2003;4(6):437–450.

21. Koprowski H, Steplewski Z, Mitchell K, Herlyn M, Herlyn D, Fuhrer P: Colorectal carcinoma antigens detected by hybridoma antibodies. Somatic Cell Genet 1979;5(6):957–971.

22. Koprowski H, Herlyn M, Steplewski Z, Sears HF: Specific antigen in serum of patients with colon carcinoma. Science (New York, NY) 1981;212 (4490):53–55.

23. Locker GY, Hamilton S, Harris J, et al.: ASCO 2006 update of recommendations for the use of tumor markers in gastrointestinal cancer. J Clin Oncol 2006;24(33):5313–5327.

24. Goonetilleke KS, Siriwardena AK: Systematic review of carbohydrate antigen (CA 19–9) as a biochemical marker in the diagnosis of pancreatic cancer. Eur J Surg Oncol 2007;33(3):266–270.

25. Alexakis N, Halloran C, Raraty M, Ghaneh P, Sutton R, Neoptolemos JP: Current standards of surgery for pancreatic cancer. Br J Surg 2004;91(11):1410–1427.

26. Yan L, Tonack S, Smith R, et al.: Confounding effect of obstructive jaundice in the interpretation of proteomic plasma profiling data for pancreatic cancer. J Proteome Res 2009;8(1):142–148.

27. Chen R, Brentnall TA, Pan S, et al.: Quantitative proteomics analysis reveals that proteins differentially expressed in chronic pancreatitis are also frequently involved in pancreatic cancer. Mol Cell Proteomics 2007;6(8):1331–1342.

28. Thompson ST, Cass KH, Stellwagen E: Blue dextran-sepharose: an affinity column for the dinucleotide fold in proteins. Proc Natl Acad Sci USA 1975; 72(2):669–672.

29. Miribel L, Gianazza E, Arnaud P: The use of dye-ligand affinity chromatography for the purification of non-enzymatic human plasma proteins. J Biochem Biophys Methods 1988;16(1):1–15.

30. Leatherbarrow RJ, Dean PD: Studies on the mechanism of binding of serum albumins to immobilized cibacron blue F3G A. Biochem J 1980;189(1):27–34.

31. Sjobring U, Bjorck L, Kastern W: Streptococcal protein G. Gene structure and protein binding properties. J Biol Chem 1991;266(1):399–405.

32. Wang YY, Cheng P, Chan DW: A simple affinity spin tube filter method for removing high-abundant common proteins or enriching low-abundant biomarkers for serum proteomic analysis. Proteomics 2003;3(3):243–248.

33. Govorukhina NI, Keizer-Gunnink A, van der Zee AGJ, de Jong S, de Bruijn HWA, Bischoff R: Sample preparation of human serum for the analysis of tumor markers: Comparison of different approaches for albumin and [gamma]-globulin depletion. J Chromatogr A 2003;1009(1–2):171–178.

34. Sennels L, Salek M, Lomas L, Boschetti E, Righetti PG, Rappsilber J: Proteomic analysis of human

blood serum using peptide library beads. J Proteome Res 2007;6(10):4055–4062.

35. O'Farrell PH: High resolution two-dimensional electrophoresis of proteins. J Biol Chem 1975;250 (10):4007–4021.

36. Gorg A, Obermaier C, Boguth G, et al.: The current state of two-dimensional electrophoresis with immobilized pH gradients. Electrophoresis 2000; 21(6):1037–1053.

37. Harris LR, Churchward MA, Butt RH, Coorssen JR: Assessing detection methods for gel-based proteomic analyses. J Proteome Res 2007;6(4):1418–1425.

38. Riederer BM: Non-covalent and covalent protein labeling in two-dimensional gel electrophoresis. J Proteomics 2008;71(2):231–244.

39. Unlu M, Morgan ME, Minden JS: Difference gel electrophoresis: a single gel method for detecting changes in protein extracts. Electrophoresis 1997; 18(11):2071–2077.

40. Tian M, Cui YZ, Song GH, et al.: Proteomic analysis identifies MMP-9, DJ-1 and A1BG as overexpressed proteins in pancreatic juice from pancreatic ductal adenocarcinoma patients. BMC Cancer 2008;8:241.

41. Bloomston M, Zhou JX, Rosemurgy AS, Frankel W, Muro-Cacho CA, Yeatman TJ: Fibrinogen {gamma} Overexpression in pancreatic cancer identified by large-scale proteomic analysis of serum samples. Cancer Res 2006;66(5):2592–2599.

42. Lin Y, Goedegebuure PS, Tan MCB, et al.: Proteins associated with disease and clinical course in pancreas cancer: a proteomic analysis of plasma in surgical patients. J Proteome Res 2006;5(9):2169–2176.

43. Deng R, Lu Z, Chen Y, Zhou L, Lu X: Plasma proteomic analysis of pancreatic cancer by 2-dimensional gel electrophoresis. Pancreas 2007;34(3):310–317.

44. Shiio Y, Aebersold R: Quantitative proteome analysis using isotope-coded affinity tags and mass spectrometry. Nat Protoc 2006;1(1):139–145.

45. Chen R, Yi EC, Donohoe S, et al.: Pancreatic cancer proteome: the proteins that underlie invasion, metastasis, and immunologic escape. Gastroenterology 2005;129(4):1187–1197.

46. Chen R, Pan S, Cooke K, et al.: Comparison of pancreas juice proteins from cancer versus pancreatitis using quantitative proteomic analysis. Pancreas 2007;34(1):70–79.

47. Chen R, Pan S, Yi EC, et al.: Quantitative proteomic profiling of pancreatic cancer juice. Proteomics 2006;6(13):3871–3879.

48. Ong SE, Foster LJ, Mann M: Mass spectrometric-based approaches in quantitative proteomics. Methods (San Diego, Calif) 2003;29(2):124–130.

49. Roboz J: Mass spectrometry in diagnostic oncoproteomics. Cancer Invest 2005;23(5):465–478.

50. Merchant M, Weinberger SR: Recent advancements in surface-enhanced laser desorption/ionization-time of flight-mass spectrometry. Electrophoresis 2000;21(6):1164–1177.

51. Rosty C, Christa L, Kuzdzal S, et al.: Identification of hepatocarcinoma-intestine-pancreas/pancreatitis-associated protein I as a biomarker for pancreatic ductal adenocarcinoma by protein biochip technology. Cancer Res 2002;62(6):1868–1875.

52. Sasaki K, Sato K, Akiyama Y, Yanagihara K, Oka M, Yamaguchi K: Peptidomics-based approach reveals the secretion of the 29-residue COOH-terminal fragment of the putative tumor suppressor protein DMBT1 from pancreatic adenocarcinoma cell lines. Cancer Res 2002;62(17):4894–4898.

53. Koopmann J, Zhang Z, White N, et al.: Serum diagnosis of pancreatic adenocarcinoma using surface-enhanced laser desorption and ionization mass spectrometry 10.1158/1078-0432.CCR-1167-3. Clin Cancer Res 2004;10(3):860–868.

54. Song J, Patel M, Rosenzweig CN, et al.: Quantification of fragments of human serum inter-alpha-trypsin inhibitor heavy chain 4 by a surface-enhanced laser desorption/ionization-based immunoassay. Clin Chem 2006;52(6):1045–1053.

55. Ehmann M, Felix K, Hartmann D, et al.: Identification of potential markers for the detection of pancreatic cancer through comparative serum protein expression profiling. Pancreas 2007;34(2):205–214.

56. Scarlett CJ, Samra JS, Xue A, Baxter RC, Smith RC: Classification of pancreatic cystic lesions using SELDI-TOF mass spectrometry. ANZ J Surg 2007;77(8):648–653.

57. Sahin U, Tureci O, Schmitt H, et al.: Human neoplasms elicit multiple specific immune responses in the autologous host. Proc Natl Acad Sci USA 1995;92(25):11810–11813.

58. Scanlan MJ, Chen YT, Williamson B, et al.: Characterization of human colon cancer antigens recognized by autologous antibodies. Int J Cancer 1998;76(5):652–658.

59. Nakatsura T, Senju S, Yamada K, Jotsuka T, Ogawa M, Nishimura Y: Gene cloning of immunogenic antigens overexpressed in pancreatic cancer. Biochem Biophys Res Commun 2001;281(4):936–944.

60. Klade CS, Voss T, Krystek E, et al.: Identification of tumor antigens in renal cell carcinoma by serological proteome analysis. Proteomics 2001; 1(7):890–898.

61. Seliger B, Kellner R: Design of proteome-based studies in combination with serology for the identification of biomarkers and novel targets. Proteomics 2002;2(12):1641–1651.

62. Hong SH, Misek DE, Wang H, et al.: An autoantibody-mediated immune response to

calreticulin isoforms in pancreatic cancer. Cancer Res 2004;64(15):5504–5510.

63. Tomaino B, Cappello P, Capello M, et al.: Autoantibody signature in human ductal pancreatic adenocarcinoma. J Proteome Res 2007;6(10):4025–4031.

64. Spurrier B, Honkanen P, Holway A, et al.: Protein and lysate array technologies in cancer research. Biotechnol Adv 2008;26(4):361–369.

65. Orchekowski R, Hamelinck D, Li L, et al.: Antibody microarray profiling reveals individual and combined serum proteins associated with pancreatic cancer. Cancer Res 2005;65(23):11193–11202.

66. Hamelinck D, Zhou H, Li L, et al.: Optimized normalization for antibody microarrays and application to serum-protein profiling. Mol Cell Proteomics 2005;4(6):773–784.

67. Ingvarsson J, Wingren C, Carlsson A, et al.: Detection of pancreatic cancer using antibody microarray-based serum protein profiling. Proteomics 2008;8(11):2211–2219.

68. Mendes KN, Nicorici D, Cogdell D, et al.: Analysis of signaling pathways in 90 cancer cell lines by protein lysate array. J Proteome Res 2007;6(7):2753–2767.

69. Rai AJ, Vitzthum F: Effects of preanalytical variables on peptide and protein measurements in human serum and plasma: implications for clinical proteomics. Expert Rev Proteomics 2006; 3(4):409–426.

70. Ransohoff DF: Bias as a threat to the validity of cancer molecular-marker research. Nat Rev Cancer 2005;5(2):142–149.

71. Ransohoff DF: How to improve reliability and efficiency of research about molecular markers: roles of phases, guidelines, and study design. J Clin Epidemiol 2007;60(12):1205–1219.

72. Ransohoff DF: The process to discover and develop biomarkers for cancer: a work in progress. J Natl Cancer Inst 2008;100(20):1419–1420.

73. Gronborg M, Bunkenborg J, Kristiansen TZ, et al.: Comprehensive proteomic analysis of human pancreatic juice. J Proteome Res 2004;3(5):1042–1055.

74. Simeone DM, Ji B, Banerjee M, et al.: CEACAM1, a novel serum biomarker for pancreatic cancer. Pancreas 2007;34(4):436–443.

75. Duxbury MS, Matros E, Clancy T, et al.: CEACAM6 is a novel biomarker in pancreatic adenocarcinoma and PanIN lesions. Ann Surg 2005;241(3):491–496.

76. Thompson CC, Ashcroft FJ, Patel S, et al.: Pancreatic cancer cells overexpress gelsolin family-capping proteins, which contribute to their cell motility. Gut 2007;56(1):95–106.

77. Koopmann J, Buckhaults P, Brown DA, et al.: Serum macrophage inhibitory cytokine 1 as a marker of pancreatic and other periampullary cancers. Clin Cancer Res 2004;10(7):2386–2392.

78. Roberts PF, Burns J: A histochemical study of mucins in normal and neoplastic human pancreatic tissue. J Pathol 1972;107(2):87–94.

79. Balague C, Gambus G, Carrato C, et al.: Altered expression of MUC2, MUC4, and MUC5 mucin genes in pancreas tissues and cancer cell lines. Gastroenterology 1994;106(4):1054–1061.

80. Jhala N, Jhala D, Vickers SM, et al.: Biomarkers in diagnosis of pancreatic carcinoma in fine-needle aspirates. Am J Clin Pathol 2006;126(4):572–579.

81. Koopmann J, Fedarko NS, Jain A, et al.: Evaluation of osteopontin as biomarker for pancreatic adenocarcinoma. Cancer Epidemiol Biomarkers Prev 2004;13(3):487–491.

82. Satomura Y, Sawabu N, Mouri I, et al.: Measurement of serum PSP/reg-protein concentration in various diseases with a newly developed enzyme-linked immunosorbent assay. J Gastroenterol 1995;30 (5):643–650.

83. Ohuchida K, Mizumoto K, Egami T, et al.: S100P is an early developmental marker of pancreatic carcinogenesis. Clin Cancer Res 2006;12(18): 5411–5416.

23 Tumor-Stromal Interactions in Invasion and Metastases

Mert Erkan · Irene Esposito · Helmut Friess · Jörg Kleeff

1   The Microenvironment of Pancreatic Ductal Adenocarcinoma 536

2   Inflammation and Cancer 538

3   Inflammation and Pancreatic Cancer 539

4   Pancreatic Stellate Cells: Producers of Desmoplasia in Pancreatic Cancer 540

5   Mutual Interactions of Pancreatic Cancer and Stellate Cells 544

6   Neoangiogenesis in Pancreatic Cancer 545

7   The Impact of the Tumor Microenvironment on Initiating Pancreatic Cancer
    Invasion and Metastasis 547

8   Perineural Invasion in Pancreatic Ductal Adenocaricnoma 552

9   Assessment of the Stromal Contribution to Pancreatic Cancer Behavior:
    The Activated Stroma Index 555

10 Targetting Pancreatic Cancer – Stroma Interactions as a Therapy Option 556

J. P. Neoptolemos, R. Urrutia, J. L. Abbruzzese, M. W. Büchler (eds.), *Pancreatic Cancer*,
DOI 10.1007/978-0-387-77498-5_23, © Springer Science+Business Media, LLC 2010

Abstract: Pancreatic ductal adenocarcinoma is characterized by "tumor desmoplasia," a remarkable increase in connective tissue that penetrates and envelopes the neoplasm. Although excessive desmoplasia also occurs in breast and prostate cancers, it is rarely observed in other tumors of the pancreas. Desmoplastic reaction consists of abundant fibrous tissue composed of extracellular matrix proteins, new blood vessels, inflammatory and stellate cells. After their isolation a decade ago, it is now clear that pancreatic stellate cells produce this highly fibrotic microenvironment of pancreatic cancer. Through secretion of growth factors and cytokines, cancer cells can activate the stellate cells within their immediate vicinity. Moreover, the interactions between the inflammatory cells, stellate cells and cancer cells sustain the activity of the stromal reaction. Once activated, pancreatic stellate cells can also perpetuate their own activity by forming autonomous feedback loops. Experimental data is emerging that there is a symbiotic relationship between pancreatic adenocarcinoma cells and pancreatic stellate cells that results in an overall increase in the growth rate of the tumor. Similarly, recent evidence supports an active protumorigenic role of inflammatory cells in the development and progression of pancreatic cancer. Nevertheless, despite abundant experimental evidence, the exact role of the stromal component of the tumor mass in human cancer progression in vivo is not yet fully clarified. Recently however, the ratio of the tumor desmoplasia to the amount of activated stellate cells was identified as an independent prognostic marker with an impact on patient survival equivalent to that of the lymph node status of the pancreatic cancer. Likewise, the number of tumor infiltrating macrophages and mast cells correlate with the microvessel density and aggressiveness of the pancreatic ductal adenocarcinoma. Although the mechanisms behind these important observations have to be elucidated individually, one possible fundamental biologic explanation could be made through a selection process leading to the evolution of cancer cells. Carcinogenesis requires tumor populations to surmount distinct microenvironmental proliferation barriers that arise in the adaptive landscapes of normal and premalignant populations growing from epithelial surfaces. Therefore, somatic evolution of invasive cancer could be viewed as a sequence of phenotypical adaptations to these barriers, highlighting the importance of tumor microenvironment on cancer behavior.

For the clarity of understanding, while analyzing the tumor-stromal interaction and its impact on invasion and metastases, the authors will focus only on pancreatic ductal adenocarcinoma (PDAC) and not on other neoplasms of the pancreas.

1   The Microenvironment of Pancreatic Ductal Adenocarcinoma

The densely fibrotic stroma of pancreatic ductal adenocarcinoma is characterized by a complex interaction between normal exocrine and endocrine cells of the pancreas, invading tumor cells, and an activated stroma composed of stellate cells, inflammatory cells, proliferating endothelial cells, with an altered extracellular matrix that distorts the normal architecture of the gland. Damaged/stressed cellular populations within the pancreas, as well as cytokines and growth factors released by inflammatory cells, platelets and neoplastic cells, can activate pancreatic stellate cells through various mechanisms. Compared to the normal parts of the parenchyma, the fibrotic parts of the stroma are also hypoxic [1,2]. Recently Masamune et al. (2008) have shown that hypoxia activates stellate cells [3]. Therefore, activation of PSC at the invasive front of the reactive stroma possibly creates a vicious cycle where abundance of cytokines and fibrosis around the capillaries in the periacinar spaces interfere with tissue oxygenation and the consequent hypoxia further activates PSC, thereby propagating the chronic pancreatitis like changes beyond the actual tumor [3,4]. It is likely that the activated stroma forming the tumor microenvironment in pancreatic ductal adenocarcinoma on one side supports the tumor growth through production of several growth factors and cytokines while on the other side applies a selection pressure on cancer cells leading to the evolution of aggressive clones. This selection process eventually promotes cancer growth and invasion through mechanisms likely to include apoptosis resistance and genomic instability.

At the molecular level, stroma production is facilitated by the abundance of growth factors including fibroblast growth factors, epidermal growth factors, transforming growth factor–ß (TGF-ß), platelet derived growth factors, connective tissue growth factor, nerve growth factors and proangiogenic factors like vascular endothelial growth factor (VEGF). These factors are secreted not only by cancer cells but also by inflammatory cells and stellate cells that influence the composition of the stroma by modulating its production and turnover. Proliferating fibroblasts and pancreatic stellate cells produce and deposit collagens and fibronectin, which are shown to support tumor growth and increase chemoresistance in vitro [3–5]. As shown to occur in other epithelial cancers, inflammatory cells and macrophages produce chemokines and cytokines that have not only protumorigenic attributes but also activate pancreatic stellate cells and contribute to the tumor supportive milieu of PDAC by indirect mechanisms [6–8]. For example, although tumor cells can secrete VEGF themselves, stromal and inflammatory cells are the principal sources of host-derived VEGF [9,10].

According to standard reasoning, primary epithelial tumors that are initially separated from underlying vessels by the basement membrane eventually become hypoxic as they outgrow the ambient vascular supply [11,12]. Without accompanying neoangiogenesis, tumors cannot exceed 1–2 mm in diameter [13,14]. Studies on wound healing and tissue regeneration have shown that angiogenesis and extracellular matrix production are inter-related physiologic responses where several molecules have bimodal functions. Therefore the early tumor microenvironment is associated with an increased number of stromal cells, enhanced capillary density, and type-I-collagen and fibrin deposition [4,15–17]. On the other hand, several artificial models in which tumor cells are seeded into initially avascular spaces (i.e., subcutaneous, cornea pocket, vitreous) prove that hypoxic tumor cells induce angiogenic in-growth by secretion of neoangiogenic substances such as vascular endothelial growth factor VEGF and angiopoietin-2 [12,18]. Such manipulation of the microenvironment allows further growth of the initial tumor [12,15]. Interestingly, although both pancreatic cancer and stellate cells secrete proangiogenic factors, pancreatic ductal adenocarcinoma is a scirrhous and hypoxic tumor. This hypoxic microenvironment possibly contributes to the aggressive nature of the disease by creating genetic instability, selecting more aggressive tumor phenotypes and increasing chemo-radioresistance [4,11,19,20].

Another unique property of PDAC microenvironment is the commonly encountered nerve alterations. Schwann cells around the damaged nerve fibres, pancreatic cancer cells and inflammatory cells all produce nerve growth factors which not only enlarge the calibre of the nerve fibres but also act as chemoattractants for the cancer cells. Therefore these intra-pancreatic neuro-cancer interactions may theoretically pave the way for extrapancreatic perineural invasion along the major abdominal vessels which eventually preclude curative resections [21,22].

2   Inflammation and Cancer

A relationship between inflammation and cancer was hypothesized by Rudolph Virchow back in the 1850s [23]. Epidemiological, clinical and experimental evidence has then contributed to support and further elucidate the functional role of inflammatory cells in tumor progression [6]. Accordingly, malignant tumors are nowadays considered as "wounds that do not heal" [24], where microenvironment-derived growth promoting factors sustain the survival and proliferation of initiated cells.

Infection-driven persistent inflammation is involved in the pathogenesis of about 15% of tumors worldwide, as in the case of *Helicobacter pylori*-induced gastritis and stomach cancer or of viral chronic hepatitis and hepatocellular carcinoma. Moreover, a clear relationship between a chronic persistent inflammatory condition and cancer has been established for other human tumors, such as ulcerative colitis and colon carcinoma or chronic pancreatitis and pancreatic cancer [25]. Important evidence that connects inflammation and cancer comes from epidemiological studies showing how long-term usage of anti-inflammatory drugs significantly reduces cancer risk, at least in some tumor types [26]. Morphological observations and expression analyzes in human cancer tissues, as well as studies on oncogene-driven tumors in transgenic mice over the last decades have contributed to identify the non malignant cell types that act as major players in modifying the tumor microenvironment. Moreover, the molecular pathways that connect inflammation and cancer are currently being elucidated.

All components of the innate (e.g., macrophages, dendritic cells, mast cells, granulocytes) and adaptive immunity (B- and T-lymphocytes) are present in the tumor microenvironment, although in different proportions and with different – and sometimes probably opposite functions [27]. Cells of the innate immunity are recruited to tumor sites by growth factors and chemokines that are often produced by the cancer cell themselves, including colony-stimulating factor-1 (CSF-1), CC chemokines (CCL2, CCL3, CCL4, CCL5, CCL8), transforming growth factor β-1, vascular endothelial growth factor In return, inflammatory cells produce mediators that contribute to cancer growth, invasion and metastasis [8]. Tumor-associated macrophages (TAM) exhibit a distinct phenotype that share many characteristics with M2-polarized macrophages and influence every step of tumor progression [28]. An accumulation of macrophages has been described in the basal membrane region of preinvasive epithelial lesions of the breast, where they express proteolytic enzymes like cathepsin B or urokinase plasminogen activator (uPA) and its receptor (uPAR) and facilitate stroma invasion [29]. Growth of invasive tumors can be further stimulated by a number of growth and survival factors (EGF, TGFβ-1, bFGF, HGF, VEGF, IL-8, TNF-α) that directly affect cancer cells or promote angiogenesis. In addition, TAM seem to be particularly relevant for the establishment of distant metastases, since absence of CSF-1 in transgenic mice susceptible to the development of mammary cancer (PyMT mice) significantly reduces the frequency of lung metastases, whereas the metastatic potential is restored by restoration of CSF-1 expression and macrophage recruitment [30]. Experimental evidence further exists that macrophages can contribute both to the release of cancer cells from primary tumor sites and to the growth of metastases at secondary sites [31]. Moreover, monocyte-derived osteoclasts at the tumor-bone interface play an important role in breast cancer metastasis-induced osteolysis through the production of cathepsin G [32]. The protumorigenic activity of TAM and other immune cells in human neoplasms is further supported by clinical studies reporting a correlation between inflammatory cell infiltration and unfavorable prognosis, which has been shown for instance in breast, prostate, endometrial and bladder cancer [33]. However, the tumor type and the type and location of infiltrating cells seems to be critical in this respect, since the accumulation of different subtypes of T-lymphocytes positively influences the prognosis of patients affected by colorectal cancer [34].

In this respect, another important aspect of the interactions between cancer cells and inflammatory cells in tumor development and progression is the immunomodulatory function exerted by tumor cells on immune cells. Cancer cells produce soluble factors (e.g., IL-10) that induce the M2 phenotype of infiltrating macrophages, thus impairing their cytotoxic and antigen- presenting phenotype in favor of a profibrotic and proangiogenetic one [28,35]. On the other hand, TAM produce chemokines like CCL22 that attract $CD4^+CD25^+FOXP3^+$ regulatory T-cells into tumors, where they further suppress tumor-specific T-cell responses, as it has been shown for ovarian cancer [36]. Myeloid- derived suppressor cells $(CD11b^+Gr-1^+)$ are additional cells of the innate immunity that accumulate in tumors and induce lymphocyte dysfunctions [37].

3   Inflammation and Pancreatic Cancer

Inflammatory cells are part of the stromal reaction that characterizes pancreatic cancer, a fact that highlights the close relation between a chronic inflammatory condition and this tumor. Indeed, similarities between the stroma composition in chronic pancreatitis and pancreatic cancer further emphasize the pathogenetic link between them [38]. Macrophages, mast cells, neutrophils, dendritic cells, B- and T-lymphocytes have all been described in the stroma of pancreatic cancer [9,39]. However, only a few experimental studies exploited the functional role of immune cells in the biology of pancreatic ductal adenocarcinoma. Mast cells have been shown to accumulate in the pancreas of patients affected by chronic pancreatitis of different etiologies, where they might undergo an IgE-mediated activation [40]. Moreover, mast cells and macrophages infiltrate the stroma of pancreatic cancer and, together with the cancer cells, they express pro-angiogenic and pro-lymphangiogenic factors, namely VEGF-A, bFGF and VEGF-C, which potentially influence the invading and metastatic ability of pancreatic cancer [9,39]. Interestingly, the number of mast cells and macrophages showed a positive correlation with the microvessel count and mast cell/macrophage-rich tumors with high microvessel density displayed a tendency for a worse prognosis[9]. Intrapancreatic mast cells express stem cell factor (SCF), which is the main mast cell maturation, differentiation and growth factor. SCF binds the tyrosine-kinase receptor KIT (CD117) and a SCF-KIT dependent growth/migration promoting autocrine loop has been demonstrated in colon, stomach and lung cancer cell lines [41]. Although pancreatic cancer cells express KIT, no growth promoting effect of SCF on pancreatic cancer cell lines could be demonstrated in vitro [39]. Intrapancreatic mast cells express the neutral proteases tryptase and chymase and belong therefore to the so-called MC_{TC} or connective tissue-type mast cells, which are otherwise mainly found in the skin and the intestinal submucosa [39]. Interestingly, an increased number of MC_{TC} has been described in livers with metastases from gastrointestinal cancers, including pancreatic cancer [42]. In addition to their role in promoting an angiogenic phenotype, mast cells are also probably involved in the establishment of the stromal reaction in primary and metastatic pancreatic cancer. Mast cell-derived tryptase, TGFβ-1 and TNF-α have been shown to activate fibroblasts and promote collagen synthesis [43,44]; moreover a functional interaction between mast cells and stellate cells has been described in the pathogenesis of liver fibrosis [45] and the accumulation of activated stellate cells is accompanied by an increased mast cell degranulation in chronic pancreatitis [46]. Macrophages are likely to be attracted into pancreatic cancer tissues by cancer cells and stellate cells, for instance through the production of monocyte chemotactic protein (MCP)-1/CCL2 [47]. Tissue macrophages are then involved in tumor angiogenesis and invasion [9]. Chemokines like macrophage inflammatory protein (MIP)-3α and proteolytic enzymes like matrix metalloproteinases (MMPs) are likely to be involved in the process of invasion and metastases [8,48]. Human macrophage metalloelastase (HME, also named MMP-12) accumulation in pancreatic cancer tissue has further been shown to bear a prognostic significance in patients affected by pancreatic cancer [49]. An invasive front of neutrophil granulocytes has been reported at the invasive edge of pancreatic ductal adenocarcinoma, where they produce TGFβ-1, which further affects the stromal reaction that accompanies pancreatic cancer [50]. On the other hand, ductal adenocarcinomas with a high number of CD4/CD8-positive tumor-infiltrating lymphocytes (TIL) had a significantly better prognosis than cases with only CD4-positive or only CD8-positive lymphocyte infiltration and the CD4/CD8 +/+ status was negatively correlated with TNM stage [51]. However, a progressive decrease in the number of infiltrating cytotoxic T-cells has been reported during the progression of preinvasive lesions, such as pancreatic intraepithelial neoplasia (PanIN) and intraductal papillary-mucinous neoplasms (IPMN) [52]. Conversely, a progressive increase in the number of $FOXP3^+CD4^+CD25^*$ regulatory T cells (T_{REG}) in pancreatic cancer progression, as well as a significantly higher prevalence of T_{REG} in cancer tissues compared with the nonneoplastic stroma has been observed [52]. Tumor-derived endothelial cells seem to be involved in the selective transmigration of T_{REG} into pancreatic cancer tissues through a high expression of addressins, such as mucosal addressin cell adhesion molecule-1 (MAdCAM-1), vascular cell adhesion molecule-1 (VCAM-1), CD62-E and CD166 [53].

Taken together, recent evidence supports an active protumorigenic role of inflammatory cells in the development and progression of human neoplasms [6]. Due to its extensive desmoplastic stromal reaction and its causal relationship with a chronic inflammatory condition, pancreatic cancer is an ideal candidate for the investigation of the interactions between inflammatory cells, stromal cells and tumor cells in the process of neoplastic progression, invasion and metastasis. Morphological and clinical data and the characterization of the dynamic of the immune reaction in a genetically defined mouse model of pancreatic ductal adenocarcinoma support the involvement of the innate and adaptive immunity in all phases of pancreatic cancer progression [54]. Functional studies aiming at clarifying the molecular mechanisms of the recruitment of the immune cells into the tumor tissue and of their interactions with other stromal cells and the cancer cells are needed in order to define potential future therapeutic targets.

4 Pancreatic Stellate Cells: Producers of Desmoplasia in Pancreatic Cancer

In recent years, researchers studying the pathogenesis of PDAC have turned their attention to the desmoplastic reaction found in the majority of pancreatic cancers [55]. As previously shown in breast and prostate cancers, it is possible that interactions between stromal cells and tumor cells influence both the progression of the cancer and influence tumor responses to conventional therapies.

Mollenhauer et al. (1987) were among the first to report that there was a remarkable increase in interstitial fibrotic component in PDAC [56]. This observation predates the identification of the pancreatic stellate cells with almost two decades. Although hepatic stellate cells were first described by Karl von Kupffer in 1876 as Sternzellen (stellate cells), similar fat-storing cells in the pancreas were first observed with the use of autofluorescence and electron microscopy in 1982 [57,58]. These cells were identified when rats were given vitamin A, because cells with cytoplasmic fat droplets, such as HSCs, become autofluorescent when vitamin A accumulates in these droplets [58].

Although pancreatic cancer cells can produce several components of the extracellular matrix (ECM) including collagen types I, III, and IV, fibronectin, laminin, and vitronectin in vitro and in vivo, they predominantly stimulate pancreatic stellate cells to synthesize the excessive fibrotic tissue composed mostly of collagen type I, III and fibronectin [4,55,59]. Using in situ hybridization Gress et al. (1998) have demonstrated that transcripts coding for collagens were associated with spindle-shaped cells in pancreatic cancer tissue [60]. These early observations have been substantiated when in 1998 two independent research groups separately identified and cultivated pancreatic stellate cells from human and rat pancreatic tissues and validated their fibrogenic properties in vitro [61,62]. Stellate cells derive their name from their shape (stella in Latin means "a star") and are also present in several other organs, including the kidney, lung and liver [57]. Pancreatic stellate cells (PSC) are myofibroblast-like cells found in the periacinar spaces in the normal pancreas and have long cytoplasmic processes that encircle the base of the acinus like the pericytes around the breast acini. In their quiescent state, pancreatic stellate cells comprise approximately 4% of the pancreatic cell population. They can also be found in perivascular and periductal regions of the pancreas and serve as key participants in the pathobiology of the major disorders of the exocrine pancreas, i.e., chronic pancreatitis and pancreatic cancer [58,61,62]. In these disorders, PSC participate in disease pathogenesis after transforming from a quiescent state into an "activated" state (also known as a "myofibroblastic" state). This activation process is accompanied by a loss of the characteristic retinoid-containing fat droplets in their cytoplasm. The antifibrogenic effects of vitamin A suggest that retinoids are not mere markers of the quiescent state of pancreatic stellate cells, but may act as a switch between the activated and quiescent state through their nuclear receptors. Most investigators agree that stellate cells are similar to myofibroblasts found in other tumor stroma including breast and prostate cancer. Both stellate cells and myofibroblasts stain positive for alpha smooth muscle actin when activated; however, stellate cells express glial fibrillary acidic protein or desmin, which distinguishes them from other myofibroblasts [63]. On the other hand, PSC are regulated by autocrine and paracrine stimuli and share many features with their hepatic counterparts, studies of which have helped further our understanding of PSC biology [57].

By morphologic and functional studies as well as their transcriptome analysis, these cells are found to be almost identical to hepatic stellate cells and possibly share a common origin [64]. Their similarities also extend to pathways of fibrogenesis, including similar roles of cytokines, growth factors and alcohol metabolites [57,64]. Nevertheless the fundamental differences in their microenvironments could condition these cells to respond differently to injury and cancer [64]. For example, in contrast to hepatocellular carcinoma, desmoplasia is a typical feature of pancreatic ductal adenocarcinoma. This difference is speculated to be due to the release potent fibrogenic mediators by pancreatic cancer cells rather then the differences of hepatic and pancreatic stellate cells [4,55,64]. This argument is further corroborated by the observation that excessive desmoplasia is rarely seen in other tumors of the pancreas.

As of today there is no clear consensus on the origin of PSC, since activated PSC express not only markers of mesenchymal cells but also of muscle cells and neural cells. Judging by these markers, it is likely that upon activation they are transformed from their quiescent precursors, or recruited from local fibroblasts, bone marrow derived cells as well as from epithelial cells through epithelial-mesenchymal transformation [15,17,57,64,65] ◉ Table 23-1, ◉ Fig. 23-1.

■ Table 23-1

Typical features of quiescent and activated pancreatic stellate Cells

Typical feature	Quiescent PSC	Activated PSC
Periacinar localization	+	++
Presence in fibrotic areas	–	++
Retinoid containing fat droplets	++	–
Mitotic index	–/+	++
α-SMA expression	–/+	++
Vimentin expression	++	++
Desmin expression	+	+
GFAP expression	+	+
Nestin expression	+	++
Periostin expression	–/+	++
PDGF-R expression	–/+	++
TGFß-R expression	–/+	++
ICAM-1 and VCAM-1 expression	–/+	++
MMP/TIMP/EMMPRIN production	–/+	++
ECM synthesis: (Collagens, Fibronectin, Periostin, Decorin)	–/+	++
Phagocytosis	unknown	+
Angiogenic activity: VEGF, angiopoietin-II, production	unknown	+
Growth factor/cytokine production: (FGFs, PDGFs, TGFß1, CTGF, HGF, IL1ß, IL-6, IL-8, RANTES, TNFα, MCP-1)	–/+	++

Although in acute pancreatitis PSC activity is transient, their persistent activity in chronic inflammation and PDAC can impair organ function due to their excessive contraction and abundant extracellular matrix protein deposition. It is also becoming clearer that myofibroblast like cells found in the activated stroma of epithelial tumors significantly impact tumor behavior [65]. As of today the most extensively studied attribute of PSC is the production of the abundant ECM in the diseased pancreas.

Although a fibrotic matrix was initially regarded as a host barrier against tumor invasion, it has become evident that it can modulate and even initiate tumorigenesis [66,67]. In fact, the ECM influences growth, differentiation, survival and motility of cells both by providing a physical scaffold and by acting as a reservoir for soluble mitogens, and cancer cells are believed to exploit this tumor-supportive microenvironment[15]. The replacement of the normal parenchyma by excessive desmoplastic tissue rich in collagen and fibronectin ostensibly plays a role in the aggressive behavior of PDAC. Normally, the collagen type IV-rich basement membrane, which separates epithelial cells from the interstitial matrix, exerts inhibitory effects on both cancer cells and stellate cells [68,69]. In various tumors, including PDAC, breaching of the basement membrane is a critical step in tumor progression. This step brings malignant cells into direct contact with ECM proteins such as fibrillary collagens, supporting their growth and contributing to their chemo-resistance [4,5,68]. One role of the desmoplasia is to promote survival and prevent apoptosis of the tumor cells through a direct action of ECM proteins on the tumor cells [4,55,57]. The prosurvival effects of the ECM proteins laminin and

■ Fig. 23-1

Immunofluorescence analysis of pancreatic stellate cells for specific activation markers and extracellular proteins: (a) The typical activation marker for PSC; intracytoplasmic alpha-smooth muscle actin filaments appear red while the DAPI stained nucleus appears blue, 400x magnification. (b) The actin cytoskeleton of the PSC appears green while the perinuclear vimentin filaments appear red, and the DAPI stained nucleus appears blue, 400x magnification. (c) Activated PSC express high levels of PDGF-2 receptor (green), 200x magnification. When the PSC are activated they produce significant amounts of (d) collagen type-I (green), 200x magnification, (e) fibronectin (green), 100x magnification, and (f) periostin (green), 200x magnification.

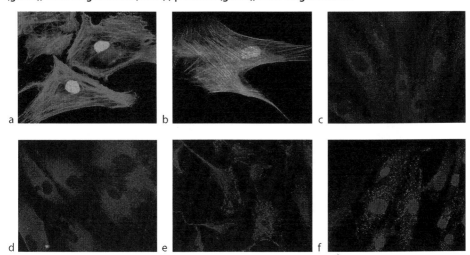

fibronectin are mediated through their integrin receptors, which are expressed by the tumor cells. In addition, the effects of fibronectin seem to be mediated through transactivation of IGF-1. Overall, these interactions lead to the activation of prosurvival and progrowth signaling pathways in pancreatic tumor cells [55,70].

Moreover, when in direct contact with stromal cells, cancer cells stimulate the production of several proteins from the PSC which amplify the aggressive behavior of the cancer cells. For example, periostin is a proangiogenic and profibrogenic ECM protein secreted exclusively by PSC in the pancreas [4]. Periostin does not only increase tumor growth and therapy resistance, but it also perpetuates the PSC activity thereby sustaining the activity of stromal component of the tumor mass [4].

Another example is the extracellular matrix metalloproteinase inducer (EMMPRIN) [10,71]. Due to its ability to stimulate the synthesis of collagenase–1 (MMP1) in fibroblasts, EMMPRIN was designated as tumor collagenase stimulating factor[65]. EMMPRIN expression is increased in tumors such as bladder carcinoma, lung carcinoma, glioma, melanoma, lymphoma and pancreatic cancer and correlates with tumor size, stage, and prognosis in primary breast and ovarian cancer [65]. In addition, EMMPRIN also plays a role in tumor invasion, angiogenesis, apoptosis and chemoresistance [10,65,71]. Schneiderhan et al. (2007) have shown that the pancreas carcinoma cell lines MiaPaCa2, Panc1, and SW850 express EMMPRIN on their cell surface [71]. Co-culture of these pancreatic cancer cell lines with human PSC indicates a strong expression of EMMPRIN on the surface of carcinoma cells, whereas PSC are almost negative for EMMPRIN. In addition, zymography and Immunoblot analyzes have shown that tumor cell supernatant of these pancreas carcinoma cell lines induce MMP-2 synthesis of cultured PSC. Furthermore, immunodepletion of EMMPRIN in carcinoma cell supernatants significantly reduced MMP-1 and MMP-2 synthesis in cultured PSC, demonstrating that the pancreas carcinoma cell lines induce MMP synthesis in stellate cells via soluble EMMPRIN [71]. Taken together, these data show that PSC not only produce and deposit the ECM in pancreatic cancer but are also actively regulating its turnover.

Unfortunately, as it will be discussed later in detail, in vitro experimental setups which analyze the effect of one particular component of the ECM on cultured cancer cells are inadequate to recapitulate the combined effect of the tumor microenvironment in vivo. Nevertheless, uncoupling pancreatic stellate-cancer cell interactions could be an option to mitigate the tumor supportive microenvironment in pancreatic ductal adenocarcinoma, which ostensibly contributes to the aggressive behavior of this malignancy.

5   Mutual Interactions of Pancreatic Cancer and Stellate Cells

Evidence is emerging that there is a symbiotic relationship between pancreatic adenocarcinoma cells and PSC that results in an overall increase in the rate of tumor growth as well as its metastatic spread [4,55,70]. Based on the intimate association between PSC and cancer cells in tissues, several in vitro and animal experiments were conducted to elucidate their interactions [4,55,57,70]. Taken together, these studies indicate that a tumor-supportive microenvironment is created as pancreatic cancer cells (PCC) activate PSC. For example, culture supernatants from human pancreatic tumor cell lines stimulate PSC proliferation, motility and production of ECM proteins as well as MMPs and TIMPs that regulate the ECM turnover which is instrumental for tumor angiogenesis and metastasis [4,15,55,57,70].The most potent mitogenic and fibrogenic stimulants for PSC identified are platelet derived growth factor (PDGF)s, FGF-2 and TGF-ß1 [57,65,72]. Bachem et al. (2005) have reported that the inductive effect of pancreatic cancer cells on ECM protein synthesis by PSC may be mediated by TGF-ß1 and FGF-2 [55] while cancer cells increase the motility of the PSC via PDGF secretion [70,71]. In return, collagen type-I, -III, -IV, fibronectin, laminin and periostin produced by PSC increase pancreatic cancer cell growth and promote resistance to hypoxia, as well as to chemotherapeutics like 5FU, gemcitabine, cisplatin and doxorubicin [4,5].

Interestingly, the effects of growth factors secreted by cancer and inflammatory cells on production of extracellular matrix proteins by stellate cells can not be simplified as positive or negative. In order to compare the effects of known growth factors on stellate cells' synthetic and secretory capacity for various extracellular matrix proteins, Erkan et al. (2007) have analyzed PSC cell lysates and supernatants by Immunoblot analysis [4] and showed that the same growth factors may have opposite effect on the production of different ECM proteins. For example as reported for various other myofibroblastic cells, TGF-ß1 and BMP-2 were the strongest stimulants of α-SMA expression. Surprisingly however, although PDGF-bb and FGF-2 almost eliminated collagen type-I and α-SMA expression in pancreatic stellate cells, they were the most potent secretagogues for periostin and fibronectin, respectively [4]. These results highlight that the complex milieu of the pancreatic cancer microenvironment is difficult to recapitulate in simple in vitro settings and that the interaction between the cancer cells, stromal cells and inflammatory cells is very dynamic.

To determine whether the observed in vitro interactions between tumor cells and PSC are relevant to the in vivo situation, researchers have turned to animal models of pancreatic cancer. Using subcutaneous xenografts of a human pancreatic cancer cell line in nude mice, Bachem et al. (2005) were the first to show that the rate of tumor growth in mice injected with a mixture of cancer cells and PSC was significantly greater than that in mice injected with cancer cells alone [55]. Although this study provides important information, the relatively early time points taken to analyze the results makes the conclusions suboptimal for interpretation. Moreover as Vonlaufen et al. (2008) recently argued, subcutaneous tumor models provide useful data but are somewhat limited because they do not allow an assessment of tumor behavior within the organ of interest and cannot be used to assess processes such as distant metastasis of the cancers under study [70]. Therefore in a recent study, by using an orthotopic model of pancreatic cancer produced by injection of a suspension of pancreatic cancer cells with and without PSC into the tail of the pancreas of nude mice the authors tried to overcome the limitations of subcutaneous models and aim to examine tumor growth, local invasion, and distant metastasis [70]. This study took a more physiologic approach because so far most of the orthotopic models of pancreatic cancer described in the literature have only assessed tumors produced after injection of pancreatic cancer cells alone [73,74]. Even where pancreatic tumors were produced in nude mouse pancreas by implantation of small pieces of human pancreatic cancer tissue, the stromal component of pancreatic cancers has largely been ignored. Although using human cancer and human stellate cells in nude mice may still bring some bias due to species specific differences, the results of Vonlaufen et al. (2008) are the first to assess the interactions between tumor cells and the stromal component of pancreatic cancer in a relatively physiologically representative in vivo situation. Vonlaufen et al. (2008) showed that, compared with mice receiving MiaPaCa-2 human pancreatic cancer cells alone, mice injected with human PSC and MiaPaCa-2 cells exhibited (a) increased tumor size and regional and distant metastasis (50% more), (b) significantly more fibrotic bands (desmoplasia) containing activated PSC within tumors, and (c) increased cancer cell numbers [70]. Their in vitro studies confirmed that, in the presence of pancreatic cancer cells, PSC migration was significantly increased. Furthermore, human PSC secretions induced the proliferation and migration, but inhibited the apoptosis, of MiaPaCa-2and Panc-1 cells. The proliferative effect of human PSC secretions on pancreatic cancer cells was inhibited in the presence of neutralizing antibody to platelet-derived growth factor [70].

In line with our unpublished observations, perhaps the most interesting finding in this study is that pancreatic cancer cells not only activate and recruit local (mouse) PSC but also liver metastasis of PDAC showed the presence of α-SMA-positive cells that were positive for human nuclear antigen, suggesting that spread of pancreatic cancer to distant sites may involve not only cancer cells but also stromal cells [70]. These findings may bring a new dimension in the discussion that has been ongoing and challenging ever since Paget (1889) first introduced the "seed and soil hypothesis" over a century ago [75].

6   Neoangiogenesis in Pancreatic Cancer

Many of the signals driving the proliferation and invasion of carcinoma cells originate from the stromal cell component of the tumor mass [15,76]. For example, tumor angiogenesis begins by mutual stimulation between tumor cells and endothelial cells by paracrine mechanisms. It is a known phenomenon that cancer clones that acquire the ability to co-opt their normal neighbors to provide support at earlier stages of their malignant transformation have a survival advantage [4,15,57]. Accordingly, stromal cells may depart from normalcy, co-evolving with their malignant neighbors in order to sustain the growth of the latter [4,15,77]. As tumors grow, further angiogenesis requires tumor cells or stromal cells to release stimulatory factors and endothelial cells to respond to them such that endothelial and stromal cells can release proteolytic enzymes to degrade the extracellular matrix for migration and proliferation [57,63,72]. In clinical studies of pancreatic cancer, angiogenesis is closely correlated with rapid tumor growth and a poorer prognosis [63].

As also shown in other tumors, inflammatory and stellate cells within the pancreatic cancer stroma are important mediators of angiogenesis by release of vascular endothelial growth factor [10,63,64,72] making them important players in tumor angiogenesis. As proven by the needle measurement of tissue oxygen pressure, the fibrotic stroma of the pancreatic ductal adenocarcinoma is hypoxic compared to the normal parenchyma around it [1]. The cellular response to hypoxia is largely mediated by the transcription factor, hypoxia-inducible factor (HIF)-1, which is a heterodimer protein composed of α and β subunits. While HIF-1β protein is constitutively expressed under normoxia, HIF-1α is unstable under normoxia due to an oxygen-dependent degradation involving an ubiqutin-proteasomal pathway [78]. HIF-1α is an oxygen-sensitive partner, as it is accumulated under hypoxia, translocates to the nucleus, and transactivates a variety of genes including VEGF [78]. Reiser-Erkan et al. (2008) have shown that there is a significant accumulation of HIF-1α both in the pancreatic cancer and stellate cells [2]. ⊙ *Fig. 23-2*. In solid tumors including cervix and pancreatic cancers, hypoxia is associated with poor prognosis, resistance to chemotherapy and radiation therapy, and increased metastatic potential. These effects are attributable in part to the hypoxia-induced

◘ Fig. 23-2

Expression of Hypoxia-inducible factor-1 as a marker tissue hypoxia in pancreatic cancer:
Hypoxia-inducible factor-1 is a transcription factor that responds to changes in available oxygen
in the cellular environment. It is the master regulator of hypoxic responses. The alpha subunit of
HIF-1 undergoes a rapid degradation by the proteasome under normoxic conditions. In hypoxic
conditions however, HIF-1 degradation is inhibited, resulting in the accumulation of the
transcription factor (brown staining). In pancreatic cancer, HIF-1 expression assessed by
immunohistochemistry, not only increases in the cancer cells (a, arrows, 200x magnification), but
also in the stellate cells found in the immediate vicinity of them cells as well as in the areas of
peritumoral chronic pancreatitis like changes (b, 200x magnification) clearly demonstrating the
reduction of tissue oxygenation.

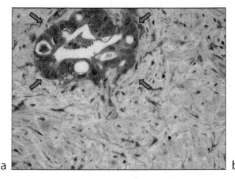
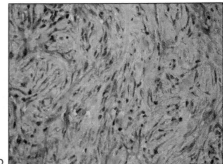

a   b

expression of proangiogenic factors such as VEGF in pancreatic cancer cells. Recently, pancreatic stellate cells have been shown to participate in neoangiogenesis by robust production of strong proangiogenic factors like VEGF, FGF, PDGF and periostin[3,4,10]. On the other hand VEGF, FGF, PDGF and periostin are also known to activate stellate cells, increase their proliferation, motility and synthetic capacity [3,4,55,63,64,79]. Therefore, these factors might operate as hypoxia-dependent, autocrine and paracrine factors which are able to stimulate migration and recruit profibrogenic PSC into the areas of cancer and inflammation. Given that cancer cells, stellate and inflammatory cells are all known to secrete proangiogenic factors, it is difficult to explain why pancreatic ductal adenocarcinoma is still a hypoxic tumor. Generally it is an oversimplification to translate in vitro data where single factors are analyzed artificially into in vivo setting where multiple factors interact. Nonetheless, one possible explanation could be that angiogenesis and fibrogenesis are interrelated phenomena, where stimulants like cancer cells and hypoxia activate PSC whose dominant response is more fibrogenic than angiogenic. Moreover, Jain et al. (1987) have shown that, as the number of tumor cells within a fibrotic stroma increase, capillary perfusion decreases reciprocally due to increasing tissue pressure [80]. Similarly, secondary to excessive PSC growth and ECM deposition, the capillaries are probably compressed, hindering blood perfusion of the normal pancreas. Therefore, on the invasive front of the activated stroma, continuous activation of PSC in the periacinar spaces and the subsequent deposition of ECM proteins around a fine capillary network may physically cause tissue hypoxia by hindering the blood circulation and oxygen diffusion.

Another possible explanation could be that pancreatic cancer cells do not only secrete proangiogenic factors, but also antiangiogenic factors like angiostatin and endostatin [81]. According to Folkman (2006), primary tumors secrete these antiangiogenic factors in order to suppress the growth of metastatic clones to prevent rivalry in host derived resources [81].

Independent of the exact reasons, it is plausible that this already hypovascular microenvironment may be a reason that antiangiogenic therapies generally fail in pancreatic ductal adenocarcinoma [82].

7   The Impact of the Tumor Microenvironment on Initiating Pancreatic Cancer Invasion and Metastasis

Over the past decade, seminal papers by Fearon, Vogelstein, Hanahan and Weinberg [11,20,83] have resulted in a powerful iconography to describe the molecular etiopathology and essential characteristics of cancer. This process of accumulating genetic and epigenetic changes during carcinogenesis is often described as "somatic evolution" because it is generally a prolonged, multistep process in which genotypes and phenotypes are sequentially generated and selected, ultimately leading to emergence of a malignant population.

Among these advantageous phenotypes are the acquisition of the constituive mitogenic signals, apoptosis resistance and ability to induce neoangiogenesis [11]. Subsequently, individual cells in these large cell populations acquire yet more mutant allelles that enable them to metastasize to seed new colonies at distant sites. Therefore according to the prevailing hypothesis metastasis is the end stage of a progressive disease that happens with a long latency [11].

There is a tremendous body of literature that supports the hypothesis that cancer results from the slow accumulation of mutations that eventually give rise to rare variant cells with invasive and metastatic potential. Accordingly, several progression models for various cancers have been proposed. In breast cancer this progression consists of atypical ductal hyperplasia, preinvasive ductal carcinoma in situ, and invasive ductal carcinoma [67]. For familial colorectal cancer the histopathologic progression, as well as the progression of genetic alterations, has been defined in the classical adenoma-carcinoma sequence of Fearon and Vogelstein (1990) [83]. More recently, the histopathologic progression with corresponding genetic mutation profiles have been described for Barrett's esophageal cancer and from PanIN leasions to invasive pancreatic ductal adenocarcinoma [67,84]. According to these models, cancer progression from premalignancy to malignancy is slow, which is consistent with a natural selection model in which multiple mutations are required in order to reach full metastatic potential. Nevertheless, even when the cells reach this metastatic potential, "successful metastasis" is a relatively rare event.

Tarin et al. (1984) have analyzed patients who had metastatic spread of a variety of primary cancers to the peritoneal cavity that were fitted with peritoneovenous shunts [85]. By this palliative operation, as the symptoms of increased abdominal pressure were alleviated by draining ascites fluid directly into the central venous system, viable metastatic cells were also inevitably drained into the blood stream. In this abnormal setting, several initial obstacles of metastasis that the primary cells have to overcome are circumvented. For example metastatic cells floating in the ascites fluid do not need to detach, invade and gain access to the local vessels or lymphatics [67]. Therefore, theoretically the frequency of metastatic spread should increase dramatically. Accordingly, based on blood samples taken from 16 peritoneovenous shunt bearing patients, it was estimated that on average 2×10^7 viable cells were present per 20 ml blood, of which approximately 1 in 10^4 were clonogenic in soft agarose [85]. The average duration of exposure was 40 weeks. Most of the patients succumbed to complications of ascites fluid. At autopsy, tissues were collected for semiquantitation of macro- and micrometastases. Surprisingly, metastatic events were less than 50%, even the lung, which was the first capillary bed encountered by the tumor cells where only several single cells or micrometastases were seen without any macrometastasis [85]. Similarly in animal experiments, where highly metastatic cells were directly injected into the vascular system, metastasis occurs with a ratio of 1 in 10^4 cells [67].

Recently, however, the concept of cancer as a multistep progression, with metastatic potential arising late within a rare cell, has been challenged. According to Bernards and Weinberg (2002) [86], this model of tumor progression carries a striking conceptual inconsistency: the genes that specify the final step in tumor progression –metastasis- would not seem to confer increased proliferative benefit at the primary site. They argue that, there is no reason to think that a metastatic phenotype enables cells to proliferate more effectively within the primary tumor mass, thereby increasing their representation in the overall tumor-cell population [86].

Therefore, it is likely that the tendency to metastasize is largely determined by the identities of the mutant alleles that are acquired realtively early in the multistep tumorigenesis. According to Bernards and Weinberg (2002), the genes that are known to confer selective advantages early on may be the same genes that, further down the line, empower metastasis [86]. This means that even relatively small/early stage primary tumor cell populations may already have the ability to metastasize to distant sites in the body. In this context, an analogy can be drawn between metastatic spread of the cancer cells and migration of the birds. Although migratory birds have the capacity to fly all through out the summer, they would only migrate when their environment starts to get barren due changing climate. ❯ *Fig. 23-3.*

For example in pancreatic cancer, once sufficient desmoplastic tissue accumulates in the tumor stroma, the dynamics of the microenvironment may shift into a more hostile one for

⬛ Fig. 23-3

The impact of a hostile microenvironment on cancer cell behavior: Reduction of blood circulation not only results in hypoxia but also in a reduction of the nutrients. In response to their microenvironment, cancer cell show significant morphologic and behavioral changes. When pancreatic cancer cells are kept in high nutrient containing medium in a Boyden chamber to assess their invasiveness (a, 200x magnification), they preserve their rounded shape and invade moderately. In contrast, when the nutrient content of the medium is decreased, cancer cells undergo significant morphological changes (b, 200x magnification) similar to those of epithelial-mesenchymal transition and become highly invasive.

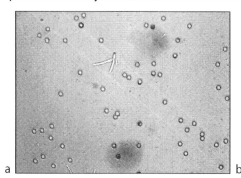
a

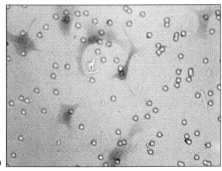
b

cancer. Since fibrosis leads to a hypoxic-barren milieu and increased TGF-ß1 activity can mitigate tumor growth, the initial r-selection (fastest one dominates the population) of cancer clones would be overtaken by K-selection (fittest one survives), choosing more aggressive phenotypes [4,87]. The selection pressure applied on the cancer cells is the combined effect of the other cancer and normal cells, defense systems of the host and gradual filling of the environmental vacuum that can provide nutritional support for only a certain number of cells. In this hostile micro-environment, aggressive clones may further evolve by acquiring new mutations due to hypoxia-driven genetic instability, resulting in enhanced invasiveness and metastasis, culminating in a poorer outcome. Or they may use their already existing abilities to move into another site where the microenvironment is less challenging. Therefore the changing microenvironment may initiate an escape mechanism within the cancer population.

In line with this argument, Gatenby and Gillies (2008) have proposed that carcinogenesis requires tumor populations to surmount distinct microenvironmental proliferation barriers that arise in the adaptive landscapes of normal and premalignant populations growing from epithelial surfaces [20]. Somatic evolution of invasive cancer can then be viewed as a sequence of phenotypical adaptations to these barriers. Thus, the genotypical and phenotypical heterogeneity of cancer populations is explained by an equivalence principle in which multiple strategies can successfully adapt to the same barrier. This model provides a theoretical framework in which the diverse cancer genotypes and phenotypes can be understood according to their roles as adaptive strategies to overcome specific microenvironmental growth constraints [20].

The role of the microenvironment goes probably even beyond what has been so far discussed to a point where stroma is actively involved in the carcinogenesis of epithelial cells. Perturbations of the normal mesenchymal–epithelial interactions can lead to unregulated growth, as evidenced by several studies in mammary fibroblast–epithelial cell interactions.

Normal, but not tumor associated, fibroblasts were able to inhibit the growth of a transformed mammary epithelial cell line in vitro [63]. Conversely, irradiated mammary fat pads containing only stromal elements induced a normally nontumorigenic transformed epithelial cell line to develop large tumors within the murine breast tissue, suggesting radiation-induced changes in the stroma disrupted its normal growth inhibitory effects on epithelial cells [88].

Interestingly, data from the 1980's preceding chemo-radiotherapy show that preoperative radiotherapy alone increases postoperative metastatic recurrence of PDAC [89]. On cultivated human PSC, radiation is a strong inducer of fibrosis, as seen by increased production and deposition of collagen type-I and fibronectin both in vivo and in vitro [4]. Although radiation inhibits cell proliferation and induces apoptosis in most of the tumor cells, it paradoxically promotes in vitro and in vivo invasiveness and metastasis of cancer cells by activating several mechanisms, including MMP-2, E-cadherin, α-catenin, integrins, HGF receptor/c-Met and MAPK pathways. The plausible link between these opposite effects can be the activated stroma. For example supernatants from irradiated PSC increased significantly pancreatic cancer cell lines invasiveness [4].

According to Schedin and Elias (2004) metastatic process has two rate limiting steps, both of which are in fact bottlenecks created by the tumor microenvironment: gaining access to the vasculature (or lymphatics) at the site of the primary tumor and tumor formation at the secondary site [67]. These observations suggest that a permissive tumor microenvironment is required for successful metastasis. Specifically, the microenvironment of the primary tumor needs to support tumor cell dissemination, motility, and local invasion into the vasculature (intravasation), whereas the microenvironment at the secondary site needs to support cell adhesion, proliferation, and neovascularization. The identification of these two rate-limiting steps to metastasis is consistent with the 'seed and soil' hypothesis originally put forth by Stephen Paget in 1889 [75]. Briefly, Paget proposed that the metastatic cell (the seed) requires an appropriate environment (the soil) for successful growth at the secondary site [67]. Recent evidence suggests that mesenchymal cells derived from the bone marrow and the native organ may create a suitable niche for the metastatic cells [90]. In other words, the seed is being transplanted into a secondary site with the appropriate soil. For both the primary and the secondary sites, one key role of the microenvironment that has gained prominent recognition is neovascularization. Tumors simply cannot progress without concomitant growth and organization of the stromal endothelial cells. It is likely that as tumor cells co-opt the PSC in their immediate vicinity, activated PSC may contribute to tumor neoangiogenesis with their potential to produce angiogenic substances like periostin and VEGF [10]. However, in comparison to normal pancreas where a fine capillary net is found in the periacinar spaces, peritumoral vessels are typically disorganized and leaky [12,17,80] ◉ Fig. 23-4.

The role played by the microenvironment in tumor development and dissemination extends far beyond the contribution of blood supply [15]. Additional mechanisms by which the microenvironment influences metastatic behavior of tumor cells are varied and include the following: changes in extracellular matrix (ECM) glycoprotein composition, which can alter cell adhesion, motility, proliferation, and apoptotic rates; altered ECM-degrading proteinase activities within the stroma, which presumably facilitate movement of tumorigenic cells by disrupting stromal barriers; and release of bioactive ECM fragments and/or growth factors that can promote or suppress neoplastic progression of both stromal and tumor cells [15,67]. Probably the stellate cell's over-activity and/or consequent desmoplasic changes of the microenvironment also contributes to the commonly encountered nerve alterations in pancreatic cancer [63]. Although these enlarged nerves are not tumor specific, and are also found in chronic pancreatitis

☑ Fig. 23-4

The impact of stromal activity in pancreatic cancer on the microvascular circulation and fine innervation of the pancreas: When the normal pancreatic tissue (a, b, c, 200x magnification) and pancreatic cancer (d, e, f, 200x magnification) are compared in terms of stellate cell activity (alpha smooth muscle actin expression, brown, a, d), capillary density (CD31 staining, brown, b, e) and nerve density (GAP-43 staining, brown, c, f), a significant difference is observed in all stainings. As the stellate cell activity increases (a, c), the fine endothelial staining of capillaries (b) is replaced by irregular staining of tumor vessels (e). In parallel, the fine periacinar nerve fibers (c) are disappearing as enlarged (d) nerves become visible in the fibrotic parts of the stroma, where cancer cells can be seen invading the perineural sheaths (arrows). Since all staining are specific, cancer cells, acini and the extracellular matrix remains unstained.

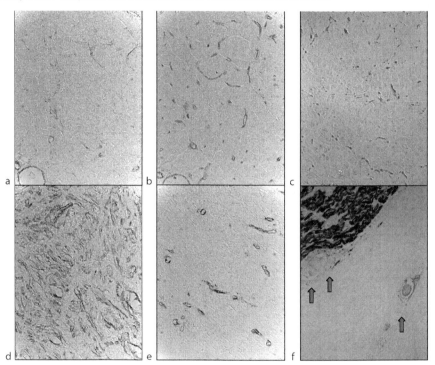

tissues as well as peritumoral normal tissues, they may provide another escape route for cancer cells out of the compact desmoplastic tissue of pancreatic cancer [21,91] ◉ Fig. 23-4.

In other words, an excessively tight extracellular matrix would provide a physical barrier for the cancer cell's motility; thereby hindering invasion and metastasis. Matrix metalloproteinases (MMP) have long been associated with metastases, poor prognosis, and the malignant phenotype of tumors [65]. Schneiderhan et al. (2007) have recently shown that PSC significantly contribute to MMP-2 secretion in the desmoplasia of pancreatic cancer in vivo and in vitro [71]. MMP-2 is found on PSC adjacent to cancer cells, and secretion of MMP-2 by PSC exceeds that of cancer cells by far [71]. As demonstrated in different carcinomas, EMMPRIN plays an important role in the interaction of carcinoma cells with mesenchymal cells and in pancreatic cancer progression [10,65,71]. EMMPRIN is thought to be released by tumor cells via microvesicle shedding which then binds to presently not identified receptors on PSC and induces the synthesis of matrix metalloproteinases, in particular of MMP-2 [71]. It has been recently demonstrated that MMP-2 is associated with the development of the desmoplasia of pancreatic cancer [65]. Interestingly however, although chronic pancreatitis tissues also exhibit a strong desmoplastic reaction which is comparable to that of PDAC tissues, EMMPRIN levels were not found to be significantly increased compared to normal pancreatic tissues [10]. In contrast, pancreatic neoplasms (serous cystic neoplasm, mucinous cystic neoplasm, intraductal papillary mucinous neoplasm and neuroendocrine tumors), regardless of whether they were desmoplastic or not, displayed significantly increased EMMPRIN expression [10]). According to Zhang et al., (2007) these findings suggest that increased EMMPRIN levels are more specific for cancer induced stromal activity rather than what is seen inflammation related activation seen in chronic pancreatitis [10].

Influences of tumor stroma may even extend beyond the primary tumor to facilitate spread of metastatic cells, as stromal cells derived from lymph nodes can increase the proliferation of tumor cells through the release of insulin-like growth factor and epidermal growth factor (EGF) [15,63,72]. Extracellular matrix proteins within the stroma also play a key role as hyaluronic acid facilitates the spread of breast cancer cells and the presence of the proteoglycan versican can predict lymph node recurrence of breast cancer [63]. Recently, Erkan et al. (2007) have shown that metastatic PDAC cells stimulate α-smooth muscle actin positive cells in secondary sites that produce periostin, collagen type-I and fibronectin [4]. In the liver and lymph node metastases, a similar pattern of α-SMA activity seen in the primary tumor was also detected around cancer cells. However, in contrast to the strong α-SMA positivity in these secondary sites, expression of all ECM proteins in the stroma around metastatic cells was found to be much less prominent than in the primary lesions [4]. The authors speculate that this difference, considering the temporal sequence of events, may merely reflect a shorter cancer–stromal cell interaction ❯ *Fig. 23-5.*

8 Perineural Invasion in Pancreatic Ductal Adenocaricnoma

Perineural invasion is frequently observed in pancreatic cancer and many nerves normally present in the retroperitoneum adjacent to the pancreas become engulfed by the desmoplastic reaction seen surrounding pancreatic cancer cells. Interestingly, the size of nerve fibers is increased within the areas of pancreatic fibrosis that characterizes chronic pancreatitis, which further supports the theory that stromal changes within the pancreas may precede the development of malignancy [63,91]. Nerve growth factor and its corresponding receptor TrkA are activated in chronic pancreatitis and nerve growth factor significantly increases pancreatic cancer cell growth and invasion in vitro and in vivo [63]. Similarly – artemin – another nerve growth factor with similar effects on pancreatic cancer cells, as well as its receptor GFRalpha3/RET are both over-expressed in chronic pancreatitis and PDAC associated chronic pancreatitis like changes [21].

Intrapancreatic nerve invasion should precede extrapancreatic perineural invasion. Nonetheless, considering the high frequency of intrapancreatic nerves ❯ *Fig. 23-4* if analyzed in detail, it should be impossible to find any case of PDAC without intrapancreatic perineural invasion, therefore the prognostic value of this finding is highly questionable. The clinically important aspect in pancreatic cancer is the invasion of the extrapancreatic nerve plexus which

■ Fig. 23-5

Immunohistochemistry analysis of stromal activation on the tumor-epithelial interface in primary and metastatic sites: To demonstrate the interplay between cancer cells, stellate cells and the extracellular matrix, consecutive sections were probed with the typical stellate cell activation marker (alpha-smooth muscle actin, brown staining, a, b, c, 50x magnification) and a stellate cell specific extracellular matrix protein (periostin, brown staining, d, e, f, 50x magnification). Red arrows mark the activated stellate cell's interface with normal tissue (a) in chronic pancreatitis-like changes of the peritumoral pancreas. Notice that periostin (d) positivity of the PSC precedes their alpha smooth muscle actin expression in the periacinar spaces (ellipse) marking the actual invasive front of the activated stroma. Strongest periostin expression in the peritumoral stroma is consistently found around the degenerating acini where tubular complexes are forming (square). In the fibrotic stroma of pancreatic cancer, stellate cells are highly active in the immediate vicinity of cancer cells (b), where they produce a periostin-rich ECM (e). In the liver metastasis of pancreatic cancer, there is an increased activity of hepatic stellate cells on the invasive front of the cancer (c). Nevertheless, in comparison to the primary tumor this stellate cell activity does not result in a strong periostin expression (f).

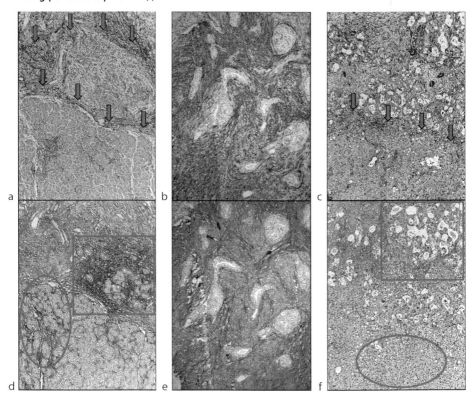

is found around the major arteries. Such an invasion causes abdominal pain and preclude curative resection thereby decreasing patient survival [92] ◉ *Fig. 23-6*. Noto et al. (2005) resected six patients with PDAC together with superior mesenteric artery and vein with a curative attempt, and performed cumbersome immunohistochemical analysis to trace the

◘ Fig. 23-6

Perineural invasion around the major abdominal arteries is a negative prognostic factor that leads to inoperability and local recurrence: The contrast enhanced computed tomography of a pancreatic tail-corpus tumor shows the typical hypodense tumor in the early arterial phase compared with the normal pancreas (white arrows). The inset on the left upper corner shows a thickened celiac plexus around the artery (red arrows). The inset on the right upper corner shows perineural invasion of cancer cells (black arrows, 50x magnification) at histological examination of the tissue obtained around the proper hepatic artery, precluding the possibility of a curative resection.

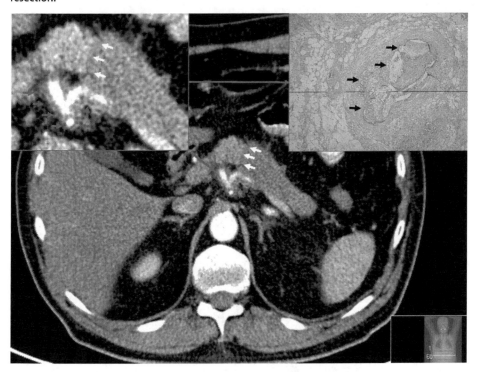

extension of the tumor around the artery [22]. They demonstrated that the neural invasion from the tumor expanded along the rear of the SMA along the inferior pancreaticoduodenal artery plexus in every case. Moreover, they also found lymphatic invasion in all patients, and concluded that lymph node involvement resulted from the metastases, but the neural involvement was due to the local invasion [22]. Despite the presence of several descriptive and in vitro studies, it is still not clear if there is a selective affinity of pancreatic cancer cells to the nerves, or if they are using the enlarged nerves, which are already there due to chronic pancreatitis like changes just because perineurium provides a lower physical resistance compared to the stiff extracellular matrix around it.

Therefore, although these results are interesting from a scientific point of view, it is likely that perineural invasion is an early event in PDAC where metastatic/invaive spread already exists in a subclinical way even in T1 tumors [92].

9 Assessment of the Stromal Contribution to Pancreatic Cancer Behavior: The Activated Stroma Index

In the late 80's, Pierce and Speers (1988) argued that a normal stroma can revert the early malignant changes in the epithelial component, or force a tumor to dormancy by providing an appropriate microenvironment [93]. Experimental data also demonstrate that even fully malignant cells can undergo phenotypic reversion, given the appropriate microenvironment [93]. This argument stems from the data showing that tissue interactions similar to cancer-stroma interaction determine the cell fate during embryogenesis. The fact that the connective tissue of an organ can dictate epithelial cell form and function is common knowledge in the field of developmental biology, where stromal–epithelial interactions have been studied for well over a century. On the contrary a permissive/activated stroma may further amplify the malignant potential of the epithelial cells. For example, Guerra et al. (2007) showed that mice harboring a conditional K-Ras mutation which was turned on after birth developed full-blown pancreatic cancers only after induction of pancreatitis [76].

The question of whether the desmoplasia is a reaction by the host to contain the tumor or whether it is the result of tumor–stromal interactions that promote tumorigenesis has been considered for decades. Although the majority of studies indicate a promotional role for stroma in tumor progression, Schedin and Elias (2004) argue that this may be due to an inclination for disease-based research to focus on causation i.e., the cancer cell but not the environment [67].

Unlike mostly well demarcated/capsulated neuroendocrine tumors of the pancreas, PDAC has typically an irregular shape with desmoplastic tissue extending beyond the cancerous core. Recently the PSC activity and various components of tumor stroma in PDAC have attracted attention of researchers. Watanabe et al. have reported that an extensive intratumoral fibro-blastic cell proliferation correlates with a poorer disease outcome in pancreatic cancer [94]. Hartel et al. (2004) have shown that patients with a better outcome have increased expression of connective tissue growth factor (CTGF) in fibroblasts surrounding the human pancreatic tumor cells [95]. CTGF has been implicated in the pathogenesis of fibrotic diseases, and its expression is predominant in PSC and is regulated by TGF-β.

Although the desmoplastic tissue in PDAC is a product of activated PSC, the highest ECM deposition is not always found where the highest stromal activity is detected. In peritumoral areas, PSC may outnumber the cancer cells without significant ECM deposition [66]. In contrast, vast amounts of desmoplastic tissue may contain only a few PSC. This variance may be due to the facts that pancreatic cancer cells can stimulate the PSC located very close to them more than others which are not in their immediate vicinity. With regard to the temporal sequence of events, α-SMA expression, which reflects PSC activity, should precede collagen deposition, as it is the product of the activated PSC. Through their production of matrix metalloproteinases, both PSC and cancer cells can degrade the previously deposited ECM. Thus, turnover of the ECM is a dynamic process, and immunohistochemical analysis of a specimen reveals areas with different disease duration and stromal activity.

Recently, Erkan et al. (2008) have quantified the amount of collagen deposition and PSC activity in 233 PDAC patients and showed that while increased PSC activity showed a tendency for a worsened prognosis, deposition of collagen was significantly correlated with a favorable outcome [66]. Although the activated PSC are the main producers of collagen, this paradoxical correlation with survival necessitates the use of an index comprising both parameters to evaluate the combined effect of the stroma on cancer behavior. Therefore "the activated stroma index (ASI)" was defined as the area of α-SMA staining (active component of the stroma) divided by the area of collagen staining (quiescent component of the stroma) measured in consecutive sections. When the whole cohort of 233 patients was divided into four quartiles according to the ASI, low stromal activity and high collagen deposition correlated with a better outcome (low ASI; median survival 25.7 months), whereas a high ASI indicating increased stromal activity but low collagen deposition correlated with poor survival (16.1 months). The median survival of patients in each quartile consistently decreased as the ASI increased, without a change in the distribution of gender, age, tumor size, nodal status (N), metastasis (M) and grade of the tumors. The median difference in survival between quartile 1 (low stromal activity) and quartile 4 (high stromal activity) was 9.6 months in favor of the former. Moreover in a multivariable Cox regression analysis ASI was found to be an independent prognostic marker in PDAC with an impact on patient survival as much as the lymph node status of the tumor [66].

Although it is known that cancer cells stimulate PSC in vitro to secrete more collagen, it is likely that the deposition and turnover of collagen in vivo depends on a multifactorial balance between PSC, cancer cells, and inflammatory cells, all of which produce significant amounts of matrix metalloproteinases. Therefore, it would be an oversimplification to reduce the stromal component of a tumor mass only to stellate cell activity and to collagen deposition and to disregard the impact of inflammatory and endothelial cells. Nevertheless, ASI as a surrogate marker for both the active and the quiescent components of the stroma proves to be a robust parameter reflecting the impact of the microenvironment on cancer behavior ❯ *Fig. 23-7.*

10 Targetting Pancreatic Cancer – Stroma Interactions as a Therapy Option

At the genetic level, pancreatic cancer is a well characterized neoplasm. By contrast, the molecular mechanisms linking the genetic changes to the aggressive nature of this disease remain poorly understood. One promising new development is the appreciation of the role of the cancer-associated stroma [4,79]. In the last decade isolation and in vitro cultivation of human and murine PSC have provided a useful tool for understanding which mechanisms regulate pancreatic cancer cell interactions with the adjacent stroma. For example, in order to metastasize successfully, tumor cells must invade local tissues. Thus, enzymes that are capable of disrupting stromal barriers, such as MMPs, were thought to be key mediators of invasion. Various MMPs are expressed by pancreatic cancer cells and transfection of tumor cells with MMP expression constructs increases their tumorigenicity and metastatic potential in both in vitro and in vivo models [15,63,65,67,71]. Based on these studies numerous inhibitors of MMPs have been designed that were effective in blocking tumorigenesis of MMP over-expressing tumor cells in mouse models. However, clinical trials evaluating the efficacy of MMP inhibitors in human cancers were disappointing, and in some cases MMP inhibition correlated with tumor progression. In fact, in human cancers most MMPs are synthesized by stromal cells rather than by the tumor cells [67,96]. Furthermore, some matrix proteolytic fragments have been identified that appear to act as tumor suppressors rather than tumor promoters. For example, angiostatin (a proteolytic fragment of plasminogen) and endostatin (a carboxyl-terminal fragment of collagen XVIII) are both endogenous inhibitors of angiogenesis, and suppress tumor growth in animal models [97]. Recently, the protease responsible

⬛ Fig. 23-7

The site-specific variation of stellate cell activity and collagen deposition: Since both staining are specific for the stroma, cancer cells (a, c) and the acini (b, d) remain unstained. The pancreatic stellate cell activity (alpha-smooth muscle actin expression, brown staining, a, b, 50x magnification) and consequent collagen deposition (aniline, c, d, blue staining, 50x magnification) shows a different pattern in the immediate vicinity of the cancer cells and in chronic pancreatitis like changes of the peritumoral stroma. Notice that the increased PSC activity results in a loose type of collagen deposition around the cancer structures (a, c), while the collagen deposited on the invasive front of the activated stroma in chronic pancreatitis like changes (b, d) results in a compact collagen deposition, suggesting the possibility of a defensive effort to encapsulate the cancer.

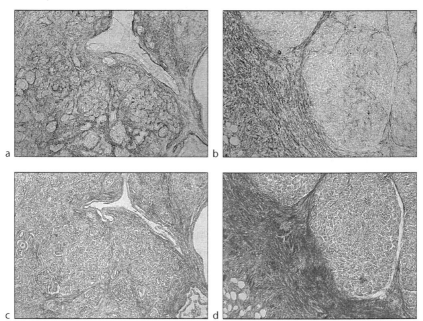

for the production of angiostatin in the Lewis lung carcinoma model was identified as MMP-2 [67,97]. These observations underline the indispensable role of the stromal component in regulating tumor behavior.

On the other hand, numerous in vitro studies using co-cultures of PSC with pancreatic cancer cells suggest that targeting the tumor stroma to uncouple cancer-PSC interactions is a reasonable strategy to treat pancreatic cancer. To accomplish this, selective inhibition of critical mediators of pancreatic cancer cell–stromal interactions, including TGF-ß, ECM proteins, and stellate cells provide valid options as it has been shown in other models [4,63].

Due to the diverse interaction between the PSC and the cancer cells, any agents that target pro-fibrotic growth factors, such as small molecule tyrosine kinase inhibitors that interfere with epidermal growth factor (EGF) receptor, FGF receptor, PDGF receptor, or IGF-1 receptor signaling, may be useful in suppressing the proliferation of pancreatic stellate cells [72]. A useful approach uncouple pancreatic cancer-stellate cell interactions could be the blockade/inhibition of pathways that are known to activate PSC [72]. For example, blockade of the intracellular signaling pathways downstream of the above mentioned receptors, is likely to provide a therapeutic benefit [57,63,72]. As summarized by Omary et al. (2007), there are also several reports from in vitro experiments with PSC that show key roles in the activation and/or proliferation process for several pathways, such as ERK1/2 MAPK, p38 MAPK, JNK, PI3K, PKC, and PPARγ [57]. In these studies, inhibition of most of these pathways results in attenuation of the activation and proliferation of PSC, but activation of PPARγ seems to block PSC activation [57,72]. It has also been reported that activated rat PSC express COX-2 when stimulated with TGF-β1 and other cytokines, as well as when stimulated with conditioned media from human pancreatic tumor cells [57,72]. Therefore, pharmacological inhibition of COX-2 and blockade of the TGF-β1 signaling decrease the expression of COX-2, α-SMA, and collagen type-I, suggesting that COX-2 might be a relevant therapeutic target for chronic pancreatitis and pancreatic cancer. Omary et al. (2007) further argues that efforts aimed at inducing PSC transdifferentiation from an activated to a quiescent state could also be attractive modalities [57]. For example, administration of vitamin A (retinol and its metabolites) induces culture-activated rat PSC to become quiescent [57].

Furthermore, targeting factors produced by stromal cells that are known to stimulate cancer cell growth and/or endothelial cell proliferation may also be a useful strategy. For example Fukasawa and Korc (2007) speculate that a so called VEGF trap may act to inhibit the VEGF-A–mediated proangiogenic signal that is produced by stromal cells [72]. Similarly, targeted blockade of hepatocyte growth factor, a pleiotrophic cytokine known to be produced primarily by stromal fibroblasts, inhibits the growth, invasion, and metastasis of various cancers including pancreatic cancer [98].

Recently there is a surge in the usage of animal experiments to better understand the importance of the stromal component of the tumor mass in cancer [55,70,84]. As an example, killing of tumor associated fibroblasts decreased cancer cell growth and greatly increased intratumoral intake of chemotherapeutic drugs in murine models of colon and breast cancers [99]. To accomplish this Loeffler et al. (2006) have constructed an oral DNA vaccine targeting fibroblast activation protein (FAP), which is specifically overexpressed by fibroblasts in the tumor stroma [99]. Through CD8+ T cell–mediated killing of tumor-associated fibroblasts, this vaccine successfully suppressed primary tumor cell growth and metastasis of multidrug-resistant murine colon and breast carcinoma. Furthermore, tumor tissue of FAP-vaccinated mice revealed markedly decreased collagen type I expression and up to 70% greater uptake of chemotherapeutic drugs. Most importantly, FAP-vaccinated mice treated with chemotherapy showed a 3-fold prolongation in lifespan and marked suppression of tumor growth, with 50% of the animals completely rejecting a tumor cell challenge. In the case of targeting fibrosis in pancreatic tumor models, a highly specific, fully human monoclonal antibody against CTGF (FG-3019), which activate PSC through their α5β1 integrin receptor, was shown to attenuate tumor growth, metastasis, and angiogenesis in an orthotopic mouse model of PDAC [72,100]. Therefore such strategies open a new venue for the combination of immuno- and chemotherapies in pancreatic cancer.

Taken together, these observations suggest that targeting the stroma in order to uncouple PCC–PSC interactions may interrupt multiple aberrant autocrine and paracrine pathways that promote pancreatic cancer cell growth, invasion, metastasis, and angiogenesis.

- The stroma, consisting of inflammatory, endothelial and stellate cells as well as the extracellular matrix, forms approximately 80% of the tumor mass in pancreatic cancer
- The activated stroma plays an important role in pancreatic cancer progression in vivo
- The isolation and routine in vitro cultivation of pancreatic stellate cells has provided a new avenue for understanding the interplay of tumor cells with their stroma
- There is a mutual interaction between tumor and stellate cells that contributes to growth, invasion and metastasis of tumor cells

Future Scientific Directions

- Development of more physiologic in vitro setups that overcome the limitations of the current two dimensional in vitro culture conditions which lack the extracellular component of the stroma
- Development of functional studies to clarify the molecular mechanisms of the recruitment of the immune cells into the tumor tissue and of their interactions with other stromal cells and the cancer cells
- Development of better animal models for investigating tumor-stromal interactions with the possibility to switch on and off the activity of different components of the stroma including inflammatory, endothelial and stellate cells

Clinical Implications

- The stroma of pancreatic cancer is an active player in tumor development and its response to conventional and targeted therapies
- The activated stroma index which shows the ratio of activated pancreatic stellate cells to the amount of collagen deposition is a strong and independent prognostic marker in pancreatic cancer
- Uncoupling pancreatic cancer and stellate cell interactions and/or targeting pancreatic stellate cells is a novel and promising therapeutic approach

References

1. Koong AC, Mehta VK, Le QT, Fisher GA, Terris DJ, Brown JM, Bastidas AJ, Vierra M: Pancreatic tumors show high levels of hypoxia. Int J Radiat Oncol Biol Phys 2000;48(4):919–922.
2. Reiser-Erkan C, Erkan M, Pan Z, Bekasi S, Giese NA, Streit S, Michalski CW, Friess H, Kleeff J: Hypoxia-inducible proto-oncogene Pim-1 is a prognostic marker in pancreatic ductal adenocarcinoma. Cancer Biol Ther 2008;7(9):1352–1359.
3. Masamune A, Kikuta K, Watanabe T, Satoh K, Hirota M, Shimosegawa T: Hypoxia stimulates pancreatic stellate cells to induce fibrosis and angiogenesis in pancreatic cancer. Am J Physiol Gastrointest Liver Physiol 2008;295(4):G709–G717.

4. Erkan M, Kleeff J, Gorbachevski A, Reiser C, Mitkus T, Esposito I, Giese T, Buchler MW, Giese NA, Friess H: Periostin creates a tumor-supportive microenvironment in the pancreas by sustaining fibrogenic stellate cell activity. Gastroenterology 2007;132(4): 1447–1464.

5. Armstrong T, Packham G, Murphy LB, Bateman AC, Conti JA, Fine DR, Johnson CD, Benyon RC, Iredale JP: Type I collagen promotes the malignant phenotype of pancreatic ductal adenocarcinoma. Clin Cancer Res 2004;10(21):7427–7437.

6. Coussens LM, Werb Z: Inflammation and cancer. Nature 2002;420(6917):860–867.

7. Michalski CW, Gorbachevski A, Erkan M, Reiser C, Deucker S, Bergmann F, Giese T, Weigand M, Giese NA, Friess H, Kleeff J: Mononuclear cells modulate the activity of pancreatic stellate cells which in turn promote fibrosis and inflammation in chronic pancreatitis. J Transl Med 2007;5:63.

8. Pollard JW: Tumour-educated macrophages promote tumour progression and metastasis. Nat Rev Cancer 2004;4(1):71–78.

9. Esposito I, Menicagli M, Funel N, Bergmann F, Boggi U, Mosca F, Bevilacqua G, Campani D: Inflammatory cells contribute to the generation of an angiogenic phenotype in pancreatic ductal adenocarcinoma. J Clin Pathol 2004;57(6):630–636.

10. Zhang W, Erkan M, Abiatari I, Giese NA, Felix K, Kayed H, Buchler MW, Friess H, Kleeff J: Expression of extracellular matrix metalloproteinase inducer (EMMPRIN/CD147) in pancreatic neoplasm and pancreatic stellate cells. Cancer Biol Ther 2007;6 (2):218–227.

11. Hanahan D, Weinberg RA: The hallmarks of cancer. Cell 2000;100(1):57–70.

12. Yancopoulos GD, Davis S, Gale NW, Rudge JS, Wiegand SJ, Holash J: Vascular-specific growth factors and blood vessel formation. Nature 2000;407 (6801):242–248.

13. Folkman J: angiogenesis. Annu Rev Med 2006; 57:1–18.

14. Hori A, Sasada R, Matsutani E, Naito K, Sakura Y, Fujita T, Kozai Y: Suppression of solid tumor growth by immunoneutralizing monoclonal antibody against human basic fibroblast growth factor. Cancer Res 1991;51(22):6180–6184.

15. Bissell MJ, Radisky D: Putting tumours in context. Nat Rev Cancer 2001;1(1):46–54.

16. Brown LF, Dvorak AM, Dvorak HF: Leaky vessels, fibrin deposition, and fibrosis: a sequence of events common to solid tumors and to many other types of disease. Am Rev Respir Dis 1989;140(4):1104–1107.

17. Kalluri R, Zeisberg M: Fibroblasts in cancer. Nat Rev Cancer 2006;6(5):392–401.

18. Carmeliet P: Angiogenesis in health and disease. Nat Med 2003;9(6):653–660.

19. Couvelard A, O'Toole D, Leek R, Turley H, Sauvanet A, Degott C, Ruszniewski P, Belghiti J, Harris AL, Gatter K, Pezzella F: Expression of hypoxia-inducible factors is correlated with the presence of a fibrotic focus and angiogenesis in pancreatic ductal adenocarcinomas. Histopathology 2005;46(6):668–676.

20. Gatenby RA, Gillies RJ: A microenvironmental model of carcinogenesis. Nat Rev Cancer 2008;8(1):56–61.

21. Ceyhan GO, Giese NA, Erkan M, Kerscher AG, Wente MN, Giese T, Buchler MW, Friess H: The neurotrophic factor artemin promotes pancreatic cancer invasion. Ann Surg 2006;244(2):274–281.

22. Noto M, Miwa K, Kitagawa H, Kayahara M, Takamura H, Shimizu K, Ohta T: Pancreas head carcinoma: frequency of invasion to soft tissue adherent to the superior mesenteric artery. Am J Surg Pathol 2005;29(8):1056–1061.

23. Balkwill F, Mantovani A: Inflammation and cancer: back to Virchow? Lancet 2001;357(9255):539–545.

24. Dvorak HF: Tumors: wounds that do not heal. Similarities between tumor stroma generation and wound healing. N Engl J Med 1986;315(26):1650–1659.

25. Whitcomb DC, Pogue-Geile K: Pancreatitis as a risk for pancreatic cancer. Gastroenterol Clin North Am 2002;31(2):663–678.

26. Dannenberg AJ, Subbaramaiah K: Targeting cyclooxygenase-2 in human neoplasia: rationale and promise. Cancer Cell 2003;4(6):431–436.

27. de Visser KE, Eichten A, Coussens LM: Paradoxical roles of the immune system during cancer development. Nat Rev Cancer 2006;6(1):24–37.

28. Mantovani A, Sozzani S, Locati M, Allavena P, Sica A: Macrophage polarization: tumor-associated macrophages as a paradigm for polarized M2 mononuclear phagocytes. Trends Immunol 2002;23(11): 549–555.

29. Domagala W, Striker G, Szadowska A, Dukowicz A, Weber K, Osborn M: Cathepsin D in invasive ductal NOS breast carcinoma as defined by immunohistochemistry. No correlation with survival at 5 years. Am J Pathol 1992;141(5):1003–1012.

30. Lin EY, Nguyen AV, Russell RG, Pollard JW: Colonystimulating factor 1 promotes progression of mammary tumors to malignancy. J Exp Med 2001;193(6):727–740.

31. Lewis CE, Pollard JW: Distinct role of macrophages in different tumor microenvironments. Cancer Res 2006;66(2):605–612.

32. Wilson TJ, Nannuru KC, Futakuchi M, Sadanandam A, Singh RK: Cathepsin G enhances mammary tumor-induced osteolysis by generating soluble receptor activator of nuclear factor-kappab ligand. Cancer Res 2008;68(14):5803–5811.

33. Sica A, Allavena P, Mantovani A: Cancer related inflammation: the macrophage connection. Cancer Lett 2008;267(2):204–215.

34. Galon J, Costes A, Sanchez-Cabo F, Kirilovsky A, Mlecnik B, Lagorce-Pages C, Tosolini M, Camus M, Berger A, Wind P, Zinzindohoue F, Bruneval P, Cugnenc PH, Trajanoski Z, Fridman WH, Pages F: Type, density, and location of immune cells within human colorectal tumors predict clinical outcome. Science 2006;313(5795):1960–1964.

35. Sica A, Schioppa T, Mantovani A, Allavena P: Tumour-associated macrophages are a distinct M2 polarised population promoting tumour progression: potential targets of anti-cancer therapy. Eur J Cancer 2006;42(6):717–727.

36. Curiel TJ, Coukos G, Zou L, Alvarez X, Cheng P, Mottram P, Evdemon-Hogan M, Conejo-Garcia JR, Zhang L, Burow M, Zhu Y, Wei S, Kryczek I, Daniel B, Gordon A, Myers L, Lackner A, Disis ML, Knutson KL, Chen L, Zou W: Specific recruitment of regulatory T cells in ovarian carcinoma fosters immune privilege and predicts reduced survival. Nat Med 2004;10(9):942–949.

37. Sica A, Bronte V: Altered macrophage differentiation and immune dysfunction in tumor development. J Clin Invest 2007;117(5):1155–1166.

38. Chu GC, Kimmelman AC, Hezel AF, DePinho RA: Stromal biology of pancreatic cancer. J Cell Biochem 2007;101(4):887–907.

39. Esposito I, Kleeff J, Bischoff SC, Fischer L, Collecchi P, Iorio M, Bevilacqua G, Buchler MW, Friess H: The stem cell factor-c-kit system and mast cells in human pancreatic cancer. Lab Invest 2002;82(11):1481–1492.

40. Esposito I, Friess H, Kappeler A, Shrikhande S, Kleeff J, Ramesh H, Zimmermann A, Buchler MW: Mast cell distribution and activation in chronic pancreatitis. Hum Pathol 2001;32(11):1174–1183.

41. Sattler M, Salgia R: Targeting c-Kit mutations: basic science to novel therapies. Leuk Res 2004;28 (Suppl 1): S11–S20.

42. Gulubova MV: Structural examination of tryptase- and chymase-positive mast cells in livers, containing metastases from gastrointestinal cancers. Clin Exp Metastasis 2003;20(7):611–620.

43. Gordon JR, Galli SJ: Promotion of mouse fibroblast collagen gene expression by mast cells stimulated via the Fc epsilon RI. Role for mast cell-derived transforming growth factor beta and tumor necrosis factor alpha. J Exp Med 1994;180(6):2027–2037.

44. Albrecht M, Frungieri MB, Kunz L, Ramsch R, Meineke V, Kohn FM, Mayerhofer A: Divergent effects of the major mast cell products histamine, tryptase and TNF-alpha on human fibroblast behaviour. Cell Mol Life Sci 2005;62(23):2867–2876.

45. Gaca MD, Pickering JA, Arthur MJ, Benyon RC: Human and rat hepatic stellate cells produce stem cell factor: a possible mechanism for mast cell recruitment in liver fibrosis. J Hepatol 1999;30(5):850–858.

46. Zimnoch L, Szynaka B, Puchalski Z: Mast cells and pancreatic stellate cells in chronic pancreatitis with differently intensified fibrosis. Hepatogastroenterology 2002;49(46):1135–1138.

47. Monti P, Leone BE, Marchesi F, Balzano G, Zerbi A, Scaltrini F, Pasquali C, Calori G, Pessi F, Sperti C, Di Carlo V, Allavena P, Piemonti L: The CC chemokine MCP-1/CCL2 in pancreatic cancer progression: regulation of expression and potential mechanisms of antimalignant activity. Cancer Res 2003;63(21):7451–7461.

48. Kleeff J, Kusama T, Rossi DL, Ishiwata T, Maruyama H, Friess H, Buchler MW, Zlotnik A, Korc M: Detection and localization of Mip-3alpha/LARC/Exodus, a macrophage proinflammatory chemokine, and its CCR6 receptor in human pancreatic cancer. Int J Cancer 1999;81(4): 650–7.

49. Balaz P, Friess H, Kondo Y, Zhu Z, Zimmermann A, Buchler MW: Human macrophage metalloelastase worsens the prognosis of pancreatic cancer. Ann Surg 2002;235(4):519–527.

50. Aoyagi Y, Oda T, Kinoshita T, Nakahashi C, Hasebe T, Ohkohchi N, Ochiai A: Overexpression of TGF-beta by infiltrated granulocytes correlates with the expression of collagen mrna in pancreatic cancer. Br J Cancer 2004;91(7):1316–1326.

51. Fukunaga A, Miyamoto M, Cho Y, Murakami S, Kawarada Y, Oshikiri T, Kato K, Kurokawa T, Suzuoki M, Nakakubo Y, Hiraoka K, Itoh T, Morikawa T, Okushiba S, Kondo S, Katoh H: CD8+ tumor-infiltrating lymphocytes together with CD4+ tumor-infiltrating lymphocytes and dendritic cells improve the prognosis of patients with pancreatic adenocarcinoma. Pancreas 2004;28(1):e26–e31.

52. Hiraoka N, Onozato K, Kosuge T, Hirohashi S: Prevalence of FOXP3+ regulatory T cells increases during the progression of pancreatic ductal adenocarcinoma and its premalignant lesions. Clin Cancer Res 2006;12(18):5423–5434.

53. Nummer D, Suri-Payer E, Schmitz-Winnenthal H, Bonertz A, Galindo L, Antolovich D, Koch M, Buchler M, Weitz J, Schirrmacher V, Beckhove P: Role of tumor endothelium in CD4+ CD25+ regulatory T cell infiltration of human pancreatic carcinoma. J Natl Cancer Inst 2007;99(15):1188–1199.

54. Clark CE, Hingorani SR, Mick R, Combs C, Tuveson DA, Vonderheide RH: Dynamics of the immune reaction to pancreatic cancer from inception to invasion. Cancer Res 2007;67(19):9518–9527.

55. Bachem MG, Schunemann M, Ramadani M, Siech M, Beger H, Buck A, Zhou S, Schmid-Kotsas A, Adler G: Pancreatic carcinoma cells induce fibrosis by stimulating proliferation and matrix synthesis of stellate cells. Gastroenterology 2005;128(4):907–921.

56. Mollenhauer J, Roether I, Kern HF: Distribution of extracellular matrix proteins in pancreatic ductal adenocarcinoma and its influence on tumor cell proliferation in vitro. Pancreas 1987;2(1):14–24.

57. Omary MB, Lugea A, Lowe AW, Pandol SJ: The pancreatic stellate cell: a star on the rise in pancreatic diseases. J Clin Invest 2007;117(1):50–59.

58. Watari N, Hotta Y, Mabuchi Y: Morphological studies on a vitamin A-storing cell and its complex with macrophage observed in mouse pancreatic tissues following excess vitamin A administration. Okajimas Folia Anat Jpn 1982;58(4–6):837–858.

59. Lohr M, Trautmann B, Gottler M, Peters S, Zauner I, Maillet B, Kloppel G: Human ductal adenocarcinomas of the pancreas express extracellular matrix proteins. Br J Cancer 1994;69(1):144–151.

60. Gress TM, Menke A, Bachem M, Muller-Pillasch F, Ellenrieder V, Weidenbach H, Wagner M, Adler G: Role of extracellular matrix in pancreatic diseases. Digestion 1998;59(6):625–637.

61. Apte MV, Haber PS, Applegate TL, Norton ID, McCaughan GW, Korsten MA, Pirola RC, Wilson JS: Periacinar stellate shaped cells in rat pancreas: identification, isolation, and culture. Gut 1998;43(1):128–133.

62. Bachem MG, Schneider E, Gross H, Weidenbach H, Schmid RM, Menke A, Siech M, Beger H, Grunert A, Adler G: Identification, culture, and characterization of pancreatic stellate cells in rats and humans. Gastroenterology 1998;115(2):421–432.

63. Farrow B, Albo D, Berger DH: The role of the tumor microenvironment in the progression of pancreatic cancer. J Surg Res 2008;149(2):319–328.

64. Friedman SL: Hepatic stellate cells: protean, multifunctional, and enigmatic cells of the liver. Physiol Rev 2008;88(1):125–172.

65. Bachem MG, Zhou S, Buck K, Schneiderhan W, Siech M: Pancreatic stellate cells-role in pancreas cancer. Langenbecks Arch Surg 2008;393(6):891–900.

66. Erkan M, Michalski CW, Rieder S, Reiser-Erkan C, Abiatari I, Kolb A, Giese NA, Esposito I, Friess H, Kleeff J: The Activated Stroma Index Is a Novel and Independent Prognostic Marker in Pancreatic Ductal Adenocarcinoma. Clin Gastroenterol Hepatol 2008;6(10):1155–1161.

67. Schedin P, Elias A: Multistep tumorigenesis and the microenvironment. Breast Cancer Res 2004;6(2):93–101.

68. Ingber DE, Madri JA, Jamieson JD: Role of basal lamina in neoplastic disorganization of tissue architecture. Proc Natl Acad Sci U S A 1981;78(6):3901–3905.

69. Sohara N, Znoyko I, Levy MT, Trojanowska M, Reuben A: Reversal of activation of human myofibroblast-like cells by culture on a basement membrane-like substrate. J Hepatol 2002;37(2):214–221.

70. Vonlaufen A, Joshi S, Qu C, Phillips PA, Xu Z, Parker NR, Toi CS, Pirola RC, Wilson JS, Goldstein D, Apte MV: Pancreatic stellate cells: partners in crime with pancreatic cancer cells. Cancer Res 2008;68(7):2085–2093.

71. Schneiderhan W, Diaz F, Fundel M, Zhou S, Siech M, Hasel C, Moller P, Gschwend JE, Seufferlein T, Gress T, Adler G, Bachem MG: Pancreatic stellate cells are an important source of MMP-2 in human pancreatic cancer and accelerate tumor progression in a murine xenograft model and CAM assay. J Cell Sci 2007;120(Pt 3):512–519.

72. Korc M: Pancreatic cancer-associated stroma production. Am J Surg 2007;194(4 Suppl):S84–S86.

73. Duxbury MS, Ito H, Zinner MJ, Ashley SW, Whang EE: CEACAM6 gene silencing impairs anoikis resistance and in vivo metastatic ability of pancreatic adenocarcinoma cells. Oncogene 2004;23(2):465–473.

74. Lohr M, Schmidt C, Ringel J, Kluth M, Muller P, Nizze H, Jesnowski R: Transforming growth factor-beta1 induces desmoplasia in an experimental model of human pancreatic carcinoma. Cancer Res 2001;61(2):550–555.

75. Paget S: The distribution of secondary growths in cancer of the breast. 1889. Cancer Metastasis Rev 1989;8(2):98–101.

76. Guerra C, Schuhmacher AJ, Canamero M, Grippo PJ, Verdaguer L, Perez-Gallego L, Dubus P, Sandgren EP, Barbacid M: Chronic pancreatitis is essential for induction of pancreatic ductal adenocarcinoma by K-Ras oncogenes in adult mice. Cancer Cell 2007;11(3):291–302.

77. Olumi AF, Grossfeld GD, Hayward SW, Carroll PR, Tlsty TD, Cunha GR: Carcinoma-associated fibroblasts direct tumor progression of initiated human prostatic epithelium. Cancer Res 1999;59(19):5002–5011.

78. Jaakkola P, Mole DR, Tian YM, Wilson MI, Gielbert J, Gaskell SJ, Kriegsheim A, Hebestreit HF, Mukherji M, Schofield CJ, Maxwell PH, Pugh CW, Ratcliffe PJ: Targeting of HIF-alpha to the von Hippel-Lindau ubiquitylation complex by O2-regulated prolyl hydroxylation. Science 2001;292(5516):468–472.

79. Kleeff J, Beckhove P, Esposito I, Herzig S, Huber PE, Lohr JM, Friess H: Pancreatic cancer microenvironment. Int J Cancer 2007;121(4):699–705.

80. Jain RK: Transport of molecules in the tumor interstitium: a review. Cancer Res 1987;47(12):3039–3051.

81. Schuch G, Kisker O, Atala A, Soker S: Pancreatic tumor growth is regulated by the balance between positive and negative modulators of angiogenesis. Angiogenesis 2002;5(3):181–190.

82. Kindler HL, Niedzwiecki D, Hollis D, Oraefo E, Schrag D, Hurwitz H, McLeod HL, Mulcahy MF, Schilsky RL, Goldberg RM: Cancer and Leukemia Group B, A double-blind, placebo-controlled, randomized phase III trial of gemcitabine (G) plus bevacizumab (B) versus gemcitabine plus placebo (P) in patients (pts) with advanced pancreatic cancer (PC): A preliminary analysis of Cancer and Leukemia Group B (CALGB), in 43rd ASCO Annual Meeting. 2007: Chicago, IL.

83. Fearon ER, Vogelstein B: A genetic model for colorectal tumorigenesis. Cell 1990;61(5):759–767.

84. Tuveson DA, Hingorani SR: Ductal pancreatic cancer in humans and mice. Cold Spring Harb Symp Quant Biol 2005;70:65–72.

85. Tarin D, Price JE, Kettlewell MG, Souter RG, Vass AC, Crossley B: Mechanisms of human tumor metastasis studied in patients with peritoneovenous shunts. Cancer Res 1984;44(8):3584–3592.

86. Bernards R, Weinberg RA: A progression puzzle. Nature 2002;418(6900):823.

87. Pianka ER: On r- AND K-SELECTION. American Naturalist 1970;104:592–597.

88. Barcellos-Hoff MH, Ravani SA: Irradiated mammary gland stroma promotes the expression of tumorigenic potential by unirradiated epithelial cells. Cancer Res 2000;60(5):1254–1260.

89. Ishikawa O, Ohigashi H, Imaoka S, Sasaki Y, Iwanaga T, Matayoshi Y, Inoue T: Is the long-term survival rate improved by preoperative irradiation prior to Whipple's procedure for adenocarcinoma of the pancreatic head? Arch Surg 1994;129(10): 1075–1080.

90. Valtieri M, Sorrentino A: The mesenchymal stromal cell contribution to homeostasis. J Cell Physiol 2008;217(2):296–300.

91. Ceyhan GO, Bergmann F, Kadihasanoglu M, Erkan M, Park W, Hinz U, Giese T, Muller MW, Buchler MW, Giese NA, Friess H: The neurotrophic factor artemin influences the extent of neural damage and growth in chronic pancreatitis. Gut 2007;56(4):534–544.

92. Reiser-Erkan C, Gaa J, Kleeff J: T1 Pancreatic Cancer With Lymph Node Metastasis and Perineural Invasion of the Celiac Trunk. Clin Gastroenterol Hepatol 2008;6(11):e41–e42.

93. Pierce GB, Speers WC: Tumors as caricatures of the process of tissue renewal: prospects for therapy by directing differentiation. Cancer Res 1988;48 (8):1996–2004.

94. Watanabe I, Hasebe T, Sasaki S, Konishi M, Inoue K, Nakagohri T, Oda T, Mukai K, Kinoshita T: Advanced pancreatic ductal cancer: fibrotic focus and beta-catenin expression correlate with outcome. Pancreas 2003;26(4):326–333.

95. Hartel M, Di Mola FF, Gardini A, Zimmermann A, Di Sebastiano P, Guweidhi A, Innocenti P, Giese T, Giese N, Buchler MW, Friess H: Desmoplastic reaction influences pancreatic cancer growth behavior. World J Surg 2004;28(8):818–825.

96. Bramhall SR, Schulz J, Nemunaitis J, Brown PD, Baillet M, Buckels JA: A double-blind placebo-controlled, randomised study comparing gemcitabine and marimastat with gemcitabine and placebo as first line therapy in patients with advanced pancreatic cancer. Br J Cancer 2002;87(2):161–167.

97. Sund M, Zeisberg M, Kalluri R: Endogenous stimulators and inhibitors of angiogenesis in gastrointestinal cancers: basic science to clinical application. Gastroenterology 2005;129(6):2076–2091.

98. Ohuchida K, Mizumoto K, Murakami M, Qian LW, Sato N, Nagai E, Matsumoto K, Nakamura T, Tanaka M: Radiation to stromal fibroblasts increases invasiveness of pancreatic cancer cells through tumor-stromal interactions. Cancer Res 2004;64(9):3215–3222.

99. Loeffler M, Kruger JA, Niethammer AG, Reisfeld RA: Targeting tumor-associated fibroblasts improves cancer chemotherapy by increasing intratumoral drug uptake. J Clin Invest 2006;116 (7):1955–1962.

100. Russo FP, Alison MR, Bigger BW, Amofah E, Florou A, Amin F, Bou-Gharios G, Jeffery R, Iredale JP, Forbes SJ: The bone marrow functionally contributes to liver fibrosis. Gastroenterology 2006;130(6):1807–1821.

24 Genetic Susceptibility and High Risk Groups for Pancreatic Cancer

William Greenhalf · John Neoptolemos

1	*Introduction*	*566*
2	*Inherited Genotypes and the Progression Model*	*567*
2.1	Oncogenes, Tumor Suppressors and Telomerase Activation: The Natural Order of Mutation?	567
2.2	Germ Line Mutations of Tumor Suppressors and DNA Repair Genes	568
2.3	A Choice of Progression Models: Which is the Best Fit?	569
2.3.1	Jumping the Queue in the PanIN Progression	569
2.3.2	Intraductal Papillary Mucinous Neoplasms (IPMNs): A Whole New Starting Point	570
2.3.3	Mutation: What, When and Where?	570
2.4	Pancreatitis and Progression Models	572
2.5	Diabetes and Progression Models	573
2.6	Classifying Predisposition: Artificial Genetic Boundaries, Real Differences in the Nature of Progression	577
2.6.1	Monogenic Direct Predisposition	577
2.6.2	Polygenic Direct Predisposition	582
2.6.3	Monogenic Indirect Predisposition	584
2.6.4	Polygenic Indirect Predisposition	585
2.7	Screening Results and Progression	586
3	*Specificity: Why the Pancreas?*	*587*
3.1	Gene-Environment Interactions	587
3.1.1	Tobacco	588
3.2	Familial Pancreatic Cancer (FPC)	589
4	*Susceptibility and Age*	*590*
4.1	Anticipation	590
5	*Outcome and Targeted Therapy*	*591*
6	*General Resources*	*591*

J. P. Neoptolemos, R. Urrutia, J. L. Abbruzzese, M. W. Büchler (eds.), *Pancreatic Cancer*,
DOI 10.1007/978-0-387-77498-5_24, © Springer Science+Business Media, LLC 2010

Abstract: Cancer develops because of a series of unfortunate events. The order of events defines a progression from normal cells through premalignant lesions to malignancy. A limited number of possible forms of progression are possible and initiation of this progression does not mean that a cancer will develop. The improbable events will have to happen in particular types of cells, quite probably at specific points in development. Cancer is a common disease only because the product of a large number of small probabilities is multiplied by the very large number of susceptible cells. The probability and consequences of mutation, epigenetic changes, infection, and other nonmalignant diseases are all determined by interaction between genotype and environment. On this basis many genes are involved in determining cancer risk; most of these have common allelic variants; subtle differences in the efficiency of these genes will impact on the probability of tumorigenic events. In combination, these will make large differences not just to the chance of developing cancer but also to the pathway that will lead to that cancer and the prognosis for the patient. This multigene effect is by far the most important element of genetic susceptibility, but it is unlikely to result in a significant family history of cancer. As pancreatic cancer is relatively uncommon, a family history spanning multiple generations is indicative of a rare (mutant) variant in a single gene. In reality, the consequence of inheriting such a high-risk allele will be dependent on a broader genetic context, and therefore, there is no such thing as a truly monogenic predisposition; but in certain families cancer does segregate with specific mutant alleles. In this chapter the way in which germline variation influences different stages of pancreatic cancer progression is discussed in order to explain why certain individuals should be considered as high risk. This has consequences for the management of a patient after cancer diagnosis but also for surveillance and screening, which will be covered in more detail in a separate chapter.

1   Introduction

All forms of cancer are always influenced by genes. Most, if not all, genes have polymorphic alleles, some alleles being more efficient and some less. The consequences of these subtle differences in activity are difficult to model, particularly as they may offer advantages in some respects and disadvantages in others. This provides a complex background for the process of natural selection, for example, inheritance of one particular allele of the *Tp53* tumor suppressor has been proposed to increase the chance of cancer but improve long-term longevity [1]. The effect of individual polymorphisms, even in such a major player as *Tp53*, will usually be imperceptible, but in combination inheritance of relatively common allelotypes may make the difference between whether or not a malignancy develops. This is supported by a meta analysis of candidate gene studies that showed that approximately one-third of polymorphisms investigated had a significant association with cancer [2]. The surprisingly large number of alleles that have been shown to have a significant impact on breast cancer risk in a whole genome study also provides empirical evidence for the importance of common alleles in defining cancer risk [3]. Quite literally this could be a matter of life and death, but the specific risk for each allele will be so small that knowledge of this impact is easy to dismiss as being of no practical use. Even on an academic basis, susceptibility based on multiple alleles is difficult to identify as it is customary to consider genetic susceptibility only in terms of a familial trait. Occurrence of the same combination of multiple alleles of unlinked genes in a single family is very unlikely unless the combination occurs in identical multiplets (e.g., twins). Even in identical twins, it is rare to see the same cancer [4] suggesting that environmental factors play a significant role in defining cancer risk in most cases [5,6]. Nevertheless, familial clusters do exist and in many cases the strength of the cluster does indicate something more than shared environment or pure coincidence. When the cluster occurs in a single generation, it can be explained by a relatively small number of risk alleles coming together from the two sides of the family, but when a rare tumor type (such as pancreatic cancer) occurs in multiple generations, this is strong evidence for a single high-risk allele or at least a collection of very closely linked risk alleles. In very rare cases family history suggests that inheritance of a single allele will make development of cancer almost inevitable [7]. These represent the autosomal dominant conditions that are discussed in this chapter.

In addition to the complex relationship between genetic susceptibility and environmental exposure there is also a complex relationship between cancer and other forms of disease. Viral infections may lead directly to transfer of genetic material associated with cancer [8]. Alternatively the pathology of viral and bacterial infection may predispose to cancer [9]. Diseases that cause inflammation generally increase cancer risk [10] and diabetes mellitus has been shown to be involved with various forms of cancer, in most cases, either as a risk factor or a symptom [11,12], although in prostate cancer type 2 diabetes appears to be protective [13–15]. The probability of developing viral infections [16], inflammatory diseases [17], or diabetes [18], and the way in which these diseases will impact on cancer [19–23] will, to some extent, depend on genotype.

In this chapter the way in which an inherited genotype will impact on the nature of tumorigenesis of the exocrine pancreas is discussed. For the purposes of simplicity the term pancreatic cancer can be taken as synonymous with pancreatic ductal adenocarcinoma unless otherwise specified; neuroendocrine tumors are not covered. This discussion is framed in the context of environmental exposure and benign disease all of which must be considered in risk stratification. In chapter 51 the way in which risk stratification can be used for primary screening of participants in screening trials will be discussed in greater detail.

2 Inherited Genotypes and the Progression Model

2.1 Oncogenes, Tumor Suppressors and Telomerase Activation: The Natural Order of Mutation?

Morphological states have been observed in most epithelial cancers that are assumed to lie between the normal cell and invasive carcinoma. The classic example is the polyp, adenoma, carcinoma series in colorectal cancer [24]. Evidence that these do represent a progression from normal to malignant was provided at the molecular level by the fact that the assumed sequence of morphological changes was matched by a logical progression of molecular changes, starting with just oncogene activation in the earliest lesions, then increasing numbers of tumor suppressors being inactivated along with oncogene activation in the later lesions [24]. In the case of pancreatic ductal adenocarcinoma, the progression model is best exemplified by the Pancreatic Intraepithelial Neoplasia (PanIN) lesions [25]. PanIN1 are the simplest form being just elongated mucin producing cells with little atypia. These lesions are associated with mutations in the proto-oncogene *K-Ras* [26]. PanIN-2 have increased nuclear size and loss of cellular polarity, and these are associated with *K-Ras* mutations in combination with loss of the tumor suppressor p16 [27]. PanIN3 lesions have budding off of cells into the ductal lumen and these have *K-Ras*, *CDKN2A (p16)* and *Tp53* mutations [26]. Telomere length is already reduced in PanIN1 [28]. Erosion of these protective ends will increase genetic instability accelerating the accumulation of mutations [29] but compromising clonal survival [30]. In order for the tumor to become established, telomere erosion needs to be limited. This is normally achieved by telomerase activation later in the progression [31].

PanIN progression fits nicely with a simple model of carcinogenesis whereby cells are induced to divide by an oncogene, giving more opportunity for mutation, and hence, checkpoint control is lost and apoptosis suppressed in some cells. This allows further expansion of a clonal populations from which immortal cells arise via the expression of telomerase [32,33]. This is also supported by a mouse model wherein a mutant form of K-Ras is expressed in all cells derived from the pancreatic bud cell (i.e., ductal, islet and acinar cells) [34]. Such mice develop PanIN-like lesions and eventually tumors with somatic tumor suppressor mutations [35,36].

2.2 Germ Line Mutations of Tumor Suppressors and DNA Repair Genes

Syndromes with inherited predisposition for cancer do not usually involve inheritance of germ line mutations of oncogenes. The reason for this is simple, activation of an oncogene will generally have a dominant effect. To pass on a mutation, the carrier must not only survive in utero but also must reach reproductive age. An active oncogene expressed in every cell of the body is not conducive to such long-term survival. Syndromes linked to inheritance of oncogenes do exist, but they are rare and the nature of the penetrance is complex. The best known example is the inheritance of the RET proto-oncogene in Multiple Endocrine Neoplasia type 2A (MEN2A) [37]. MEN2A carriers are able to tolerate inheritance of the activated oncogene, because the mutant isoform of the protein is not generally expressed in normal tissue [38,39]. A mutation in a potential oncogene (*palladin*) has been proposed to be involved in autosomal dominant predisposition to pancreatic cancer in a single large family [40]. Although this mutation has also been reported in a further family [41], it is not seen in the majority of pancreatic cancer families [42]. At the time of writing the role of palladin in pancreatic tumorigenesis remained controversial and no other inherited oncogenic mutation had been shown to explain predisposition for pancreatic cancer. Far more common is the inheritance of single mutated allele in a tumor suppressor gene. These are generally recessive alleles and the generally accepted model for tumor development following inheritance of such a mutant allele is the second hit model whereby a mutant allele becomes penetrant after somatic loss of the wild-type (normal) allele [43]. There are a number of cancer syndromes involving inheritance of a mutant allele of a tumor suppressor that may predispose to pancreatic cancer. Examples are given below:

1. Familial Multiple Mole Melanoma (FAMMM) often involves inheritance of mutations in the *CDKN2A* (p16) tumor suppressor [44].
2. Familial Adenomatous Polyposis (FAP) can involve mutation of the *APC* tumor suppressor [45].
3. Peutz-Jeghers Syndrome can involve mutation of the *STK11* tumor suppressor [46].
4. Li-Fraumeni Syndrome can involve mutations of the p53 or CHK2 tumor suppressors [47].

Even more frequently observed are associations between pancreatic cancer and inherited mutations of genes involved in DNA repair. The relatively frequent occurrence of germ-line mutations of DNA repair genes in familial cancers contrasts strongly with the somatic mutation profile of sporadic cancers; where DNA repair mutations are rare and mutations of oncogenes are common [48,49]. It is possible that DNA repair mutations, like germ line mutations in classical tumor suppressor genes, only become penetrant when a second, wild-type allele is lost by somatic mutation. However, a heterozygous mutation may also lead to a reduced efficiency of DNA repair, increasing the chance of somatic mutations [50,51]. The association of DNA repair genes with pancreatic cancer can be as part of a more general cancer syndrome such as Human Non-Polyposis Colon cancer (HNPCC) which is caused by muta-tions in a variety of mismatch repair genes [52] and Breast–Ovarian syndrome (BrOv), which can result from mutations in the recombination repair proteins BRCA1/2 [53]. However, there is also a well-documented association of sporadic cases of pancreatic cancer with polymorph-isms in DNA repair genes [54], including a reported association with variants in the Fanconi-Anemia genes FANCG and FANCC [55–57]. Although these reports indicate a low penetrance effect for Fanconi-Anemia variants, the association between pancreatic cancer and Fanconi Anemia genes appears to go beyond this. FANCD1 is BRCA2, which, as already described, is associated with pancreatic cancer in BrOv but is also associated in other families with what appears to be highly penetrant autosomal dominant predisposition specifically for pancreatic cancer [58].

2.3   A Choice of Progression Models: Which is the Best Fit?

The nature of predisposition may influence the nature of tumorigenesis, for example, in colorectal cancer tumors arising as a result of germline mutations in mismatch repair genes occur in the absence of multiple polyps (as seen in human non-polyposis colon cancer, HNPCC) [59], while germline mutations in the APC gene lead to multiple polyps and then colorectal cancer [45]. Furthermore, in the original Voglestein paper, which outlined a progres-sion model in colorectal cancer, loss of heterozygosity at the APC locus was not observed in any adenomas from 7 FAP patients, but was observed in 30% of adenomas from 33 sporadic cases. Suggesting that the role of the APC gene in the progression is different in at least some patients with a predisposition to cancer than it is in the majority of "sporadic cases."

2.3.1   Jumping the Queue in the PanIN Progression

A number of authors have questioned whether the simple model for a progression from PanIN1 to PanIN2 and then PanIN3 before the development of carcinoma is the only way that PanIN lesions develop into pancreatic cancer. PanIN lesions are relatively common in patho-logical samples from patients with cancer [60] and benign diseases [61], which clearly indicates that the majority of such lesions do not develop into cancers [62]. Even in mouse models individual PanIN like lesions produced by expression of mutant K-Ras only rarely progress to carcinoma [36]. This has led to the proposal that there are multiple pathways for PanIN lesions to progress to carcinoma. One is the pathway already described involving K-Ras mutations as the initiating event, but in most instances this results in growth arrest and cellular senescence. The alternative route involves initial mutation of tumor suppressors in morphologically normal cells with subsequent mutation of an oncogene leading directly to a PanIN3 type lesion [62]. Different forms of genetic predisposition will influence which type of mutation is the most likely initiator of tumorigenesis and hence which form of progression is most likely.

2.3.2 Intraductal Papillary Mucinous Neoplasms (IPMNs): A Whole New Starting Point

In the pancreas there are alternative precancerous lesions that may be able to progress to pancreatic cancer without the requirement for PanINs. Intraductal papillary mucinous neoplasms (IPMNs), as the name suggests, are intraductal tumors with mucinous columnar epithelial cells, which often, but not always, have papillary projections. Patients with IPMNs often go on to develop ductal adenocarcinomas. Ductal adenocarcinomas can arise subsequent to the surgical removal of an IPMN and in at least one case such an adenocarcinoma has been shown to have a different *K-Ras* genotype than the original lesion, suggesting a distinct origin for the carcinoma and the benign lesion [63]. This is consistent with the observation of PanIN lesions associated with IPMNs in some patients [64]. However, resection does greatly reduce the risk of carcinoma following detection of an IPMN [65], and hence, it is probable that progression can also be directly from a simple hyperplastic IPMN through an adenomatous form into genuine carcinoma, very similar to the progression seen in colorectal cancer [66]. Four forms of IPMN have been identified with progressively more severe atypia: In order from the lowest to the highest grade these are called Gastric, Intestinal, Pancreatobiliary and Oncocytic [67]. In addition, IPMNs can be subcategorized into main-duct and branch-duct forms depending on location. The main-duct forms seem to be more aggressive [68], although even branch-duct forms, if left untreated, will often develop into invasive carcinoma [69]. The molecular changes that occur during the IPMN progression appear similar to those seen in PanIN lesions: As with PanINs, *K-Ras* mutations seem to occur in even the simplest IPMN lesions with *CDKN2A (p16)* and *Tp53* mutations accumulating in more advanced forms [70]. Also, as with PanINs, telomeres shorten in the early forms of IPMN and telomerase is normally switched on as the premalignant lesions cross over into being genuine carcinomas [71]. Even promoter methylation seems to change in IPMNs in a similar way to the changes observed during PanIN progression [72,73]. Nevertheless, morphologically IPMNs, particularly the Oncocytic and Pancreatobiliary forms, are quite distinct from PanINs. Also IPMNs have a different pattern of expression [74]. This raises the question of how similar molecular changes lead to such divergent morphological forms.

2.3.3 Mutation: What, When and Where?

The simplest forms of IPMN and PanIN are both characterized by *K-Ras* mutation [26,70], and therefore it would be reasonable to hope that transgenic animals expressing mutant K-Ras would develop similar lesions. Pancreatic ductal adenocarcinoma is the most common form of pancreatic cancer and morphologically appears to be of ductal origin. Furthermore both IPMN [65] and PanINs [75] appear to have intraductal origins, and hence, it would be logical to express the oncogene in ductal cells. However, the expression of mutant K-Ras in mature ductal cells under the cytokeratin 19 promoter did not produce any PanIN lesions or adenocarcinoma [76]. When oncogenic K-Ras is expressed directly from the acinar specific elastase promoter [77] or from the Mist1 promoter, which is also expressed in mature acinar rather than mature ductal cells [78], mucinous papillary lesions very similar to human IPMNs result, but no PanIN. However, as already described, a murine model carrying oncogenic K-Ras under its own promoter gets PanIN like lesions if it is targeted to the common precursor cells of islet, acinar and ductal cells [34]. Another mouse model where PanIN lesions are seen has been described by Guerra et al. It is a mouse expressing mutant K-Ras under a tetracycline repressible promoter, expression requires an initial recombination event resulting from expression of Cre recombinase using the elastase promoter [79]. Superficially, this would seem to be functionally similar to the direct expression of mutant K-Ras from the elastase promoter, which was previously shown to result in IPMN-like lesions but no PanINs. However, it is possible that in some cells the elastase promoter is active in development but not continuously thereafter. If a cellular population expands from an elastase producing progenitor until it reaches some critical stage when mutant K-Ras expression will commit to development of a PanIN lesion, and if this stage is marked by absence of elastase expression, then it is easy to see why K-Ras under direct control of the elastase promoter would not cause PanINs and why constitutive expression after activation in the elastase producing progenitor would. In the Guerra model Cre recombinase is not expressed in ductal or islet cells but it is expressed not only in acinar cells but also in centroacinar cells [79]. Centroacinar cells are the Notch expressing putative progenitor cells that lie at the edge of the pancreatic duct and the acinus. When mutant Ras expression was inhibited using 4-OHT through development and up to 10 days after birth, these mice did not develop PanINs or adenocarcinomas unless pancreatitis was induced [79]. A possible explanation of this is that centroacinar cells differentiate to a ductal cell type during development of the mouse, but after the mouse reaches maturity this differentiation does not occur unless regeneration of tissue is required following pancreatitis. If mutant Ras is expressed during this transition PanIN and subsequently adenocarcinoma will develop.

Further evidence for the way in which the progression model depends on cellular context is provided by coexpression of TGF-α under an elastase promoter in a mouse expressing mutant K-Ras in all pancreatic lineages from its own promoter. In the absence of TGF-α only PanIN lesions are seen but coexpression of the growth factor in acinar cells gives rise to a combination of IPMN and PanIN-like lesions [80]. This suggests that mutant K-Ras in acinar cells when activated with TGF-α produces IPMN, but mutant K-Ras in some other cell lineage is enough (even in the absence of TGF- α) to produce PanIN. Evidence that the centroacinar cell is this PanIN-prone lineage is provided from yet another mouse model. In this model there is pancreas-specific knockout of the PTEN tumor suppressor. Loss of PTEN results principally in expansion of undifferentiated precursor cells to give Tubular Complex (TC) [81]. Occasionally PanIN-like lesions and even carcinomas develop in these PTEN knockout mice, seemingly originating with regions of TC [81]. The authors concluded from expression patterns and location of the TC that this metaplasia originated from centroacinar cells.

The morphological differences between IPMNs and PanINs could therefore result from where and when mutant proteins are expressed rather than just which mutant proteins are expressed. Hypothetically, a K-Ras mutation in an acinar cell would lead to expansion of a cell population which may develop into an IPMN. In contrast, oncogenic activation within the centroacinar cell, or the TC that develops from it, will give PanIN lesions.

Different forms of genetic predisposition could influence where and when somatic mutations are expressed and hence influence the morphology of the precancerous lesion.

2.4 Pancreatitis and Progression Models

Genetic predisposition may be indirect, for example, via an increased likelihood of pancreatitis and hence of cancer [82,83]. There is a general link between inflammatory diseases and cancer [84], for example, inflammatory bowel disease results in a tenfold increased risk of colorectal cancer [85] and *Helicobacter pylori* increases the risk of gastric cancer in a manner dependent on the nature of the resultant gastritis [86]. Notably, there is no evidence for an increased risk for cancer in the pancreas, which does not suffer an inflammatory response to *H. pylori* [87]. The increased risk of pancreatic cancer in patients with chronic pancreatitis depends on the etiology and the period of time with inflammation. With alcohol-related pancreatitis there is an approximately 2% cancer risk after 10 years and 4% after 20 years [88,89], while the risk conferred by autoimmune pancreatitis appears to be negligible [90]. All forms of pancreatitis may have a genetic component, but there is a syndrome with autosomal dominant predisposition (hereditary pancreatitis). This seems to be associated with an approximately 40% lifetime risk of pancreatic cancer [82,91,92].

There is an almost unlimited supply of mechanism by which inflammation could predispose to cancer. The cellular environment during inflammation will contain various cytokines and growth factors that could result in hyperplasia, providing dividing cells that could suffer the critical mutation that would commit them to tumorigenesis. Inflammation also involves the migration of inflammatory cells to regions with low partial pressures of oxygen and as a consequence activation of HIF-1 activity. This will provide a driver for angiogenesis supporting growth of cancer cells [93]. Similarly, infiltrating inflammatory cells express matrix metalloproteases (MMPs) which will facilitate cellular migration and potentially tumor cell growth [94]. MMP production and increased angiogenesis would be expected to increase the rate of tumor development and metastasis, but would not directly increase the chance of initiating tumorigenesis. In contrast the chance of a mutation will be increased by the generation of reactive oxygen and nitrogen species [95]. Similarly, increased activity of Activation Induced Cytidine Deaminase (AID) would be expected to increase the number of initiating events. AID has been proposed as a link between inflammation and cancer in the gastritis-gastric cancer and the ulcerative colitis-colorectal cancer associations. AID functions normally in the necessary hypermutation of immunoglobulin genes but in chronic inflammation may lead to mutations in tumor suppressors and oncogenes [10]. Inflammation involves a large number of different cell types. Tumor Associate Macrophages (TAMs) clearly have a particularly close link with cancer, but this connection is probably the result of feedback with an existing tumor, once again possibly increasing aggression but not initiation of cancer [93]. A key mediator that may lie upstream of the carcinoma in progression and that may link pancreatitis and carcinoma is the pancreatic stellate cell (PSC). PSC are activated by proinflammatory cytokines such as IL-1/6, TNF, and TGF-β1. The activated stellate cell will then release numerous factors that can induce the hyperplasia that could provide the mutant cells that develop into carcinoma [96]. For example, TGF-α is released from PSCs, and this is associated with upregulation of the Notch signaling pathway, which in turn is associated with acinar-ductal transdifferentiation [96,97].

Inflammation could therefore influence tumorigenesis in a number of different ways: promoting proliferation of nonmalignant "normal" cells as a field from which malignant cells can develop; causing differentiation of a population of cells so that development of malignancy is more likely; increasing the probability of mutation; or providing an environment in which an existing population of malignant cells can expand. As already described, the nature of the driving force towards tumor development will influence the form of progression and the genetic background will determine how likely this is to occur.

IPMNs seem to cause pancreatitis rather than pancreatitis causing IPMN [98], in contrast, PanIN lesions seem to arise more often in patients with pancreatitis [99] than in patients with no pancreatic disease [61]. Although narrowing of the pancreatic duct due to PanIN hyperplasia could contribute to obstructive pancreatitis [61], the most obvious explanation of the association between PanINs and pancreatitis is that the inflammation contributes to the development of the neoplasia. Another form of lesion associated with pancreatitis is TC. Expansion of undifferentiated precursor cells seems to result from upregulation of Notch signaling during tissue regeneration following an attack of acute pancreatitis [100] and possibly after occlusion of ducts in chronic pancreatitis [101]. TC may provide the background from which PanIN lesions arise, or possibly represents an independent precursor lesion [102,103]. Consensus guidelines on PanIN lesions found in mouse models differentiate PanIN originating in the pancreatic duct from those apparently originating from a region of acinar-duct cell transdifferentiation, i.e., formation of TC [104]. The former is assumed to represent the predominant form of progression in human pancreatic cancer, but it cannot be excluded that the latter form of progression occurs in at least some cases [103].

2.5   Diabetes and Progression Models

Genetic predisposition may also be linked to cancer indirectly via diabetes mellitus. Type 2 diabetes mellitus (insulin resistance [105]) is often diagnosed before a diagnosis of pancreatic cancer [106–109]. Much of this apparent elevated risk results from the fact that insulin resistance is a very early symptom of pancreatic cancer [106,110]. However, in a meta analysis of 36 published trials, diabetes mellitus was still shown to be a risk factor for cancer even if only patients with long-term diabetes (≥ 5 years) were considered (odds ratio of 1.5) [107]. Similarly, a systematic review identified a small, but significant, elevated risk in type 1 diabetes [111], which is immune mediated or idiopathic destruction of β-cell [112]. Both type 1 diabetes [112] and type 2 diabetes [18] have a significant genetic component. Furthermore, one of the best characterized families with an apparent autosomal dominant predisposition specifically for pancreatic cancer, Family X from the Seattle region of the USA, is characterized by endocrine failure as well as cancer risk [113]. Many members of Family X have been recruited into a screening program and have undergone resection before development of adenocarcinoma. An unusually high level of both PanIN and IPMN lesions were seen in the resected pancreata.

The association of pancreatic cancer and diabetes could be via an initial localized increase in insulin [114]. This would occur in the initial stages of type 2 diabetes and also pancreatitis-associated diabetes. This would not be part of the natural progression of disease in type 1 diabetes. The possibility that the link between type 1 diabetes and pancreatic cancer is via the use of exogenous insulin cannot be excluded [115], nor can the possibility of a common genetic predisposition for cancer and diabetes as discussed in the following section, however, insulin does increase the growth of cancer cells [116], so it is a likely mediator of tumorigenesis. Insulin acts through the insulin receptor increasing glucose uptake. Insulin can also bind to the IGF-1 receptor, albeit far less efficiently than Insulin Like Growth Factor, and this will also induce cell division. The IGF-1 receptor is expressed in pancreatic carcinoma cells [117] and can be induced (at least in rat models) on centroacinar cells [118]. IGF-1 receptor level

Table 24-1

Genes with germline variants associated with pancreatic cancer

Gene	Nature of mutation[a]	Role[b]	Syndrome[c]	Other cancers[d]	Associated condition[e]	Strength[f]	Environmental dependence[g]
BRCA2 [58]	Loss of function	DNA repair (Recombination)[b]	Breast Ovarian FPC	Breast, ovarian, prostate	Direct	Monogenic	Independent
Palladin [40]	Gain of function	Motility	FPC with endocrine failure	None	Direct?	Monogenic	Independent
MLH1, MSH2, MSH6 [122]	Loss of function	DNA repair (mismatch)	HNPCC	Colorectal	Direct	Monogenic	Independent
BRCA1 [123]	Loss of function	DNA repair (Recombination)	Breast Ovarian	Breast, ovarian	Direct	Monogenic	Independent
CDKN2A (p16) [124]	Loss of function	Tumor suppressor	FAMMM	Melanoma	Direct	Monogenic	Independent
STK11 [125]	Loss of function	Tumor suppressor	Peutz-Jeghers	Various gastrointestinal	Direct	Monogenic	Independent
APC [45]	Loss of function	Tumor suppressor	FAP	Colorectal	Direct	Monogenic	Independent
Tp53 [126]	Loss of function	Tumor suppressor	Li-Fraumeni	Various	Direct	Monogenic	Independent
ATM? [127] Disputed [128]	Loss of function	DNA repair (Recombination)	Ataxia Telangiectasia	Leukemia, Lymphoma [128]	Direct	Monogenic	Independent?
PRSS1 [82] (R122H/N29I)	Gain of function	Protease	Hereditary pancreatitis	None	Pancreatitis	Monogenic	Independent
FANCC [57]	Loss of function	DNA repair (Recombination)	Fanconi's Anemia (Recessive)	Leukemia, head and neck, esophageal [129]	Direct	Polygenic	Independent?
MGMT [54]	Polymorphism	DNA repair (Base modification)	None	Colorectal (minor allele protective) [130]	Direct	Polygenic	Independent?

Gene	Type	Function	Syndrome	Cancer association	Risk mechanism		
XRCC 1,2,3 [54, 131]	Polymorphism	DNA Repair (Recombination)	None	None	Direct	Polygenic	Smoking? [132]
APE1 [54]	Polymorphism	DNA Repair (BER)[b]	None	No independent link – possible multigene dependence [132]	Direct	Polygenic	Independent?
XPD [133]	Polymorphism	DNA Repair (NER)[b]	Xeroderma pigmentosum (Recessive)	Skin, lung [134]	Direct	Polygenic	Independent?
CYP1A1 [135]	Polymorphism	Xenobiotic	None	Lung, liver, esophageal [2]	Direct	Polygenic	Smoking
CYP1A2 [136]	Polymorphism	Xenobiotic	None	Lung, liver [137]	Direct	Polygenic	Smoking
NAT1 [136]	Polymorphism	Xenobiotic	None	Myeloma, lung, bladder [138]	Direct	Polygenic	Smoking
MTHFR [139]	Polymorphism	Folate metabolism	Homocystinuria (Recessive)	Colorectal, leukemia [140]	Direct	Polygenic	Independent?
MTRR [141]	Polymorphism	Folate metabolism	None related to cancer risk	Colorectal, leukemia? [142]	Direct	Polygenic	Independent?
FasL [143]	Polymorphism	Apoptosis (Intercellular signaling)	None	Esophageal [144]	Direct	Polygenic	Independent?
Caspase8 [143]	Polymorphism	Apoptosis (Intracellular signaling)	None	Glioma [145]	Direct	Polygenic	Independent?
PRSS1 [82] (A16V)	?	Protease	Hereditary pancreatitis?	None	Pancreatitis	Polygenic?	Independent?
PSTI(SPINK1) [146]	Polymorphism	Protease inhibitor	None	None	Pancreatitis	Polygenic	Independent?

□ Table 24-1 (continued)

Gene	Nature of mutation[a]	Role[b]	Syndrome[c]	Other cancers[d]	Associated condition[e]	Strength[f]	Environmental dependence[g]
CFTR [147]	Polymorphism	Chloride channel	Cystic fibrosis (Recessive)	Gastrointestinal [148]	Pancreatitis	Polygenic	Independent?
KCNQ1 [18]	Polymorphism	Potassium channel	None	None	Diabetes mellitus (Type 2)	Polygenic	Independent?
HLA-A/B [149]	Polymorphism	Immune response	None related to cancer risk	Various infection related cancers [150]	Diabetes mellitus (Type 1)	Polygenic	Independent?
UGT1A7 [151] Disputed [152]	Polymorphism	Xenobiotic	None	Disputed [152]	Pancreatitis?	Polygenic	Independent?
TNF-α [153]	Polymorphism	Cytokine	None	Gastric and other infection related cancers [154]	Pancreatitis?	Polygenic	Independent?
RANTES(CCL5) [153]	Polymorphism	Cytokine	None	Gastric and other infection related cancers [155]	Pancreatitis?	Polygenic	Independent?
CCR5 [153]	Polymorphism	Cytokine	None	Cervical (HPV related)?	Pancreatitis?	Polygenic	Smoking

[a]Loss of function means that the germline mutation stops an allele working, leading to dependence on the other allele for the gene function. Gain of function means that the mutation has a phenotype even when present in a heterozygote with a wild-type copy of the gene. Polymorphism means that the variant associated with cancer is present in a substantial proportion of the population with no overt phenotype, but may cause a subtle decrease (or increase) in the efficiency of the gene

[b]Proteins often have multiple functions. This list just describes a category that best fits each gene. DNA repair is described in basic terms, and recombination is meant to include any mechanism used to repair double strand breaks, NER is nucleotide excision repair and BER is base excision repair

[c]Syndromes are defined clinically. Some syndromes result from more than one mutation and some mutations are causative of more than one syndrome. Syndromes are autosomal dominant unless otherwise stated

[d]Principal cancers other than pancreatic ductal adenocarcinoma linked to germ line variants in the gene

[e]Where cancer risk is associated with another disease state and the other disease is associated with the variant in the gene

[f]Monogenic if at least one family has been shown to have cancer predisposition that segregates with the mutation. Polygenic if the variant is associated with apparently sporadic disease or with cancer in only a single generation

[g]Defined as independent unless the association with a genetic variant is only seen in combination with specific environmental exposures

also increases during pancreatitis [119]. The most likely effect of hyperinsuliaemia would therefore be hyperplasia. Hyperplasia in the form of tubular complex appears to progress to carcinoma via PanIN lesions, but no increased incidence of PanIN lesions has been recorded in diabetic patients. In contrast, IPMNs have been reported at an unusually high level in diabetic patients [120]. Also in patients with IPMN (either branch or main duct), diabetes is a predictor of malignancy [121], suggesting that the impact of diabetes is on progression to IPMN and from IPMN to carcinoma.

2.6   Classifying Predisposition: Artificial Genetic Boundaries, Real Differences in the Nature of Progression

⊗ *Table 24-1* shows a list of genes with allelic variants that have been associated with pancreatic cancer. In the table, these genes are divided into monogenic and polygenic and further divided according to whether the impact of allelic variation is directly on cancer risk or indirectly via a benign disease. As discussed in the following sections, these are very blurred distinctions.

2.6.1   Monogenic Direct Predisposition

Everyone is familiar with the concept that it is easier to break things than to make them work better; this is particularly true in genetic terms. Millions of years of evolution have resulted in optimized DNA repair and tumor suppressor genes. Random mutations are unlikely to result in any further improvement. In contrast, many missense and nearly all nonsense or frameshift mutations will result in a less efficient protein. Even some changes outside of coding regions will give reduction in efficiency. Under normal circumstances, it is likely that such mutations will be irrelevant as the other allele will produce a perfectly functional protein and regulatory pathways will ensure that levels of the functional protein are adequate to perform all required tasks. This means that the carriers of such mutations will be able to survive and prosper even if the mutation is in the germline. In order for the mutation to be passed on all that is necessary is that the mutation remains silent through development and does not cause too great a catastrophe before the carrier reaches reproductive age.

Knudson hypothesized in the 1970s that inherited mutations may predispose to cancer while maintaining silence long enough to be transferred to offspring, by the simple expedient of the mutation being recessive and cancer progression being facilitated in later life by random loss of the dominant wild-type allele [156]. Molecular analysis has confirmed this mechanism in numerous cancer syndromes [157–159]. If loss of the wild type allele occurs in a progenitor cell, this will give rise to a field of cells which are more likely to undergo somatic mutation (in the case of loss of a DNA repair gene) or where subsequent chance mutation of an oncogene will be tolerated. In either case cancer is now more likely. A phenotype that is inherited each and every time a particular allele is inherited is referred to as dominant. The phenotype discussed in this chapter is an increased chance of developing cancer. Although not all carriers of a defective allele in a tumor suppressor or DNA repair gene will develop cancer, every carrier has a greater chance of developing cancer and so the resultant syndrome will be dominant. In this sense, all monogenic predisposition to pancreatic cancer will be dominant, and as the method of penetrance requires loss of a wild-type allele, this will usually be autosomal dominant.

As discussed earlier, predisposition does not mean that there is a family history. Even if a single mutant allele does predispose to pancreatic cancer, this will not necessarily be manifest, as progression will still require a further series of random events. These random events may not happen before the carrier succumbs to another cause of death. A familial association is therefore unlikely unless the gene involved plays a pivotal role in tumorigenesis or the mutation in some way increases the chance of progression rather than just eliminating the need for one particular somatic mutation. The most obvious way that this could happen is haploid insufficiency of a DNA repair gene; this would mean that although DNA repair can be mediated by the heterozygote and this may be adequate to allow successful passage through development, mutations would be more likely. For example, heterozygous lymphocytes with one defective copy of either the *BRCA1* or *BRCA2* gene have been shown to be less efficient at recombination repair than their homozygous wild-type equivalent [50,51,160].

■ Fig. 24-1

Progression and different forms of genetic susceptibility. In the middle of the diagram, cells of the dorsal and ventral pancreatic bud are shown to develop into the three cellular lineages of the pancreas: Islet, acinar, and ductal. Centroacinar cells also develop from the bud cells and these maintain the ability to differentiate into ductal cells even in the mature pancreas. Mutation of the *K-Ras* oncogene in acinar cells is shown to lead to IPMN. The centroacinar cell is shown developing into Tubular Complex (TC) stimulated by pancreatitis. If *K-Ras* is mutated in these cells this leads to PanIN lesions. Environmental exposure leads to somatic mutations in TC, PanIN, or IPMN, allowing progression to carcinoma and eventual invasive malignancy. Germline mutations and polymorphisms influence each stage of progression. Single mutations which influence progression in isolation are shown at the top of the figure divided into: DNA repair; tumor suppressor; or oncogenes. In most cases, these are inherited as heterozygotes, becoming penetrant due to either reduced efficiency of the gene (haploid insufficiency) or loss of the wild-type allele. Haploid insufficiency will have an effect from the beginning of development, any mutation that results will be inherited by all progeny cells including those that form IPMN and PanIN lesions. Allelic loss is likely to occur during expansion of preneoplastic lesions, and by chance some IPMN and PanIN will have allelic loss and others will not. The putative oncogene *palladin* is shown at the top right of the figure. This may be maintained non-penetrant because the mutant form is not expressed outside of cells already in the process of tumorigenesis. Alternatively palladin may have some undefined tumor suppressor role. At the bottom left of the figure is monogenic predisposition to pancreatitis via the *PRSS1* mutations R122H or N29I. Above this is polygenic predisposition for cancer either through: Increased probability of somatic mutations; increasing proliferation of cellular populations to provide a field for cancer development; or by reducing the chance of tumor suppression during progression. On the right side of the figure is polygenic predisposition that can indirectly increase the probability of pancreatic cancer development, by increasing the chance of either pancreatitis or diabetes mellitus. Pancreatitis is shown as increasing the risk of pancreatic cancer by leading to the development of TC and by providing an environment for PanIN progression via Pancreatic Stellate Cells (PSC). Diabetes mellitus is shown in the figure to be linked to pancreatic cancer via localized hyperinsulinaemia. This could result during the early phases of type 2 diabetes or pancreatitis-induced diabetes. No explanation is given for the link between type 1 diabetes and pancreatic cancer. The arguments supporting each component of this figure are given in the main text along with supporting bibliography.

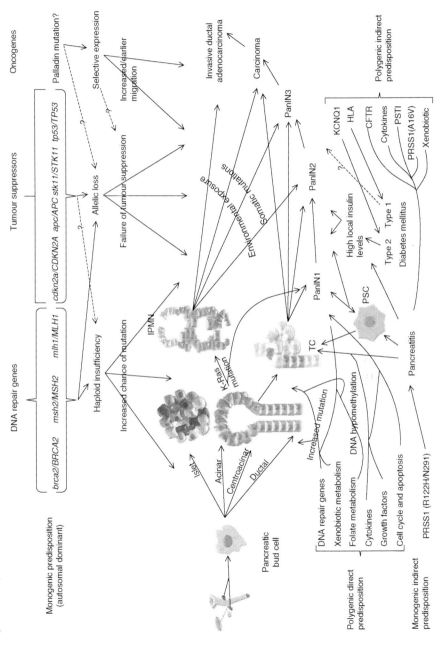

■ Fig. 24-1 (continued)

Slow accumulation of mutations in the heterozygous cell could make progression much more likely. This could even extend to accumulation of mutations during meiosis and thus allow passage of progressively more cancer risk to subsequent generations (as will be discussed later). It is also conceivable that haploid insufficiency could lead to hyperplasia, increasing the chance of somatic mutations and allelic loss.

Predisposition could result from increased chance that a preneoplastic lesion will develop and/or by increasing the chance that any preneoplastic lesion that does form will develop into a carcinoma. Due to haploid insufficiency loss of a single allele of a DNA repair gene could be expected, from the earlier argument, to increase the chance of mutations occurring before the development of PanIN or IPMN lesions. The precursor cell of any preneoplastic lesion (whether IPMN or PanIN) could therefore develop with multiple mutations already resident. These would expand with each preneoplastic lesion resulting in a far greater chance of the lesion developing into a carcinoma (see ❯ Fig. 24-1). In contrast, mutation of a tumor suppressor might increase the chance of a preneoplastic lesion developing (by increasing hyperplasia) or might remain completely silent until the second allele is lost. Allelic loss would be more probable during expansion of a pre-neoplastic lesion (IPMN or PanIN) and therefore would not expand with every benign lesion. Some lesions could develop into carcinoma (hence the predisposition) but the majority of preneoplastic lesions would not. Phenotypically, mutation of a tumor suppressor would be expected to result in a greater number of pre-neoplastic lesions than mutation of a DNA repair gene. This is supported in colorectal cancer by the observation that mutations of the tumor suppressor *APC* cause polyposis (FAP) but mutations of DNA mismatch repair genes cause nonpolyposis colorectal cancer (HNPCC) [45,59].

The discussion thus far has assumed inheritance of a recessive or partially recessive mutant allele. However, in 2006 a variant of the *palladin* gene was found to segregate with pancreatic cancer in a large US kindred (Family X). Palladin is a phosphoprotein that belongs to a family of cytoskeletal proteins and has been shown to support the normal organization of cytoskeletal actin [161]. The mutation (P239S) was reported to promote cell migration and alters cytoskeletal structure; this is a dominant phenotype and might be expected to be prometa-static. If this is the mechanism by which cancer predisposition is conferred, then it could be assumed to act at the far end of progression (see ❯ Fig. 24-1), perhaps even beyond the point at which a carcinoma has formed in situ. This would not alter the chance that a precancerous lesion forms and it is difficult to see how such a mechanism would lead to autosomal

⬛ Fig. 24-2

Tumor type specific predisposition due to BRCA2 mutations in different genetic contexts. Different populations will have different patterns of polymorphisms. In reality cancer risk will be influenced by hundreds of genes, but in this figure this is simplified to just 10. These are represented as high (Hi) and low (Lo) risk alleles. The first 5 are assumed to predispose to breast, ovarian, and prostate cancer; the second 5 specifically target the pancreas. None of the combinations of risk alleles will be likely to result in cancer on its own, but in this figure it is assumed that any 3 high-risk alleles combined with a BRCA2 mutation will give cancer. In the upper family tree, there are more breast/ovarian risk alleles, and hence, every carrier of a BRCA2 mutation (shown with a glow) develop cancer; breast cancer in the case of women and prostate cancer in men. In the second family tree, there are more pancreas-risk alleles and carriers develop pancreatic cancer. In the last tree, there are too few risk alleles to give cancer, but there is one carrier who has homozygotic BRCA2 mutations; this carrier develops Fanconi's anemia.

Fig. 24-2 (continued)

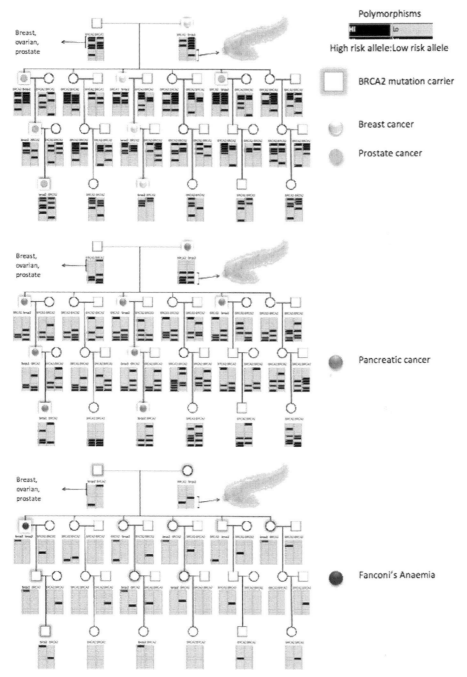

dominant cancer predisposition unless the formation of precancerous lesions was relatively common. PanIN1 lesions have been observed in 60% of postmortem samples from people without pancreatic disease over the age of 60 [61], but more advanced lesions were not identified. The *palladin* mutation is assumed to cause cancer in nearly all carriers within Family X; therefore, either Family X is particularly prone to preneoplastic lesions due to a polygenic background common to all members, or the *palladin* mutation must be increasing initiation of tumorigenesis by an undefined mechanism. As already described, there are an unusually high level of both PanIN and IPMN lesions in the resected samples obtained from Family X [113]. As all the resected samples came from mutation carriers, it is unclear whether this is the result of the *palladin* mutation or whether it is a general characteristic of the family that allows the mutation to become penetrant. It is also unclear how, if the *palladin* mutation is dominant and cancer promoting, it would not cause a more severe phenotype; for example, causing developmental problems. A possible answer to this last question is that maybe the mutant form of palladin is not expressed at high levels until after initiation of tumorigenesis. In general palladin appears to be expressed widely with no particular cancer specificity [162]. However, our own unpublished data (manuscript in preparation) suggest that splice variants of *palladin* that would include the putative mutation site do show some level of tumor specificity. It may be that this expression starts in PanIN or IPMN lesions.

2.6.2   Polygenic Direct Predisposition

It is dangerous to describe any form of cancer predisposition as monogenic, in reality no mutation will act independently of the rest of the genome. In this chapter the term monogenic is used merely to describe those mutations where at least some families exist in which cancer risk segregates with a mutation, but such families may well have multiple additional risk alleles. It is probable that no two family members have exactly the same combination of risk alleles but apparent segregation of predisposition with the high-risk mutation may result because all combinations of polymorphisms occurring in that family are adequate to give discernable cancer risk if present with the mutation, but no combination gives discernable risk without the high-risk mutation (see ❷ Fig. 24-2). Mutations of *BRCA2*, mismatch repair genes, *Tp53*, *STK11*, *APC*, and *CDKN2A (p16)* all result in an apparently autosomal dominant predisposition for cancer (including pancreatic cancer). However, the phenotypes of each of these mutations are extremely variable and the exact same mutation can lead to very different phenotypes in different families. For example, mutations in *BRCA2* can result in a Breast-Ovarian syndrome with an overwhelming predisposition for breast and ovarian cancer in women and a marked increase in prostate cancer risk in men, but in other families the predisposition for breast and ovarian cancer is not evident and in contrast there is a high risk of pancreatic cancer (a form of familial pancreatic cancer) [163]. In other families, still there is a recessive syndrome (Fanconi's anemia) where cancer risk is not normally overt in carriers but instead there is anemia combined with a risk of various forms of cancer including leukemias, esophageal, vulva, head and neck, and brain cancers [129]; but only in those individuals with two mutant alleles [164]. In all these cases the cancer predisposition is probably monogenic (carriers of the mutation have a greater risk of cancer than noncarriers) but a broader genetic background is probably required to define the penetrance of the mutations. In other genes the effect of mutations or polymorphisms may be so subtle that a definable risk is only identifiable by the most sophisticated of association studies that take into account multiple other environmental and genetic factors [165,166]. Because the effect is so moderate, such variations may be tolerated even if the variant allele is dominant. It is even possible that such variations only increase cancer risk if they are found in combination with variants in other genes. For example, mutation of a salvage pathway enzyme may only be significant in combination with a second mutation of an enzyme in the central metabolic pathway.

Modeling the effect of combinations of alleles in different genes is a challenge, but represents something of a Holy Grail for cancer risk assessment. As with the original Holy Grail, it is an item of faith that one day this goal will be achieved although it is unclear what route should be taken and it is uncertain what the prize will be. Conceptually, one day we will be able to combine all genomic and environmental data from an individual and accurately estimate their cancer risk. In order to do this the following forms of gene–gene and gene–environment interactions will need to be considered:

1. Additive – Combined risk is the sum of each risk taken separately
2. Multiplicative – Combined risk is the product of each risk taken separately
3. Synergistic – Combined risk is greater than the sum or product of each risk depending on the model used
4. Subadditive – Combined risk is greater than or equal to either risk taken separately, but not as great as predicted if the risks are independent
5. Dependent – Risk is only evident for factors if they are present in combination
6. Antagonistic – Risk in combination is less than at least one of the risks when taken separately

Pancreatic cancer risk due to *BRCA1* and *BRCA2* has been included within the risk for other cancer in the BOADICEA model of genetic susceptibility assuming multiplicative interactions [167]. In contrast, synergy between the risks of smoking, family history, and diabetes was established using an additive model [168]. There is clearly still a long way to go before cancer risks from all the polymorphisms in ◉ *Table 24-1* can be combined to accurately predict pancreatic cancer risk, but it is encouraging that the individual risks of prostate cancer for six polymorphism, as calculated in a single gene study, could be used relatively accurately to estimate risk in combination using an additive model [169].

FAS Ligand and Caspase 8 are both involved in the extrinsic pathway of apoptosis. Particular alleles of each have been shown to protect against pancreatic cancer [143]. The risks can be combined in a multiplicative model relatively accurately. There is also evidence that risks from other alleles of FASL and Caspase 8 can be combined with smoking or diabetes risks, again with a multiplicative model [143].

Given the relationship between inflammation and pancreatic cancer, it is reasonable to assume that polymorphisms of cytokines may influence cancer risk and that this should be related to inflammation. Therefore, when researchers failed to identify any association between pancreatic cancer and polymorphisms in the cytokines TNF-α, RANTES, or CCR5, it was entirely logical to continue further and to subdivide the test and control groups according to incidence of pancreatitis. A significant association was seen between all the polymorphisms and pancreatic cancer in patients with pancreatitis, but there was no association with cancer when comparing patients and controls without pancreatitis [153]. There was also an association between polymorphisms of the three cytokines and pancreatitis in patients with cancer, but not in the group without cancer. This interaction with pancreatitis is complex, it is still possible that the link to cancer is via risk of pancreatitis, but the fact that the association with pancreatitis was only seen in patients with cancer suggests that it is more likely that the polymorphisms actually influence the risk of cancer following inflammatory disease. To add yet another level of complexity, the association of the CCR5 polymorphism and cancer may be smoking dependent as well as pancreatitis dependent [153]. Similarly, a rare polymorphism of the nucleotide excision repair gene *XPD* is protective against pancreatic cancer, but only in ever smokers [133], suggesting (not surprisingly) that *XPD* acts downstream of smoking in determining cancer risk.

Ohnami et al. [141] looked at 227 single nucleotide polymorphisms (SNPs) in 46 enzymes selected, because they were involved in xenobiotic (carcinogen/drug) metabolism, DNA repair, or stress response. Only two SNPs were shown to be robustly associated with pancreatic cancer, both SNPs were in the same gene. The gene was Methionine Synthase Reductase (*MTRR*) and had been selected on the basis that it is involved in drug metabolism. However, the role of *MTRR* in folate metabolism may be more important as a mechanism for DNA methylation than in xenobiotic metabolism. DNA methylation mainly occurs at CpG islands. Many of these are in promoter regions and methylation is normally associated with reduction in expression. There is less methylation in cancer than in normal tissue, but certain tumor suppressor genes (including *CDKN2A*) have increased CpG island methylation in cancers [170]. Hypomethylation is a feature of pancreatic cancer [171] but hypermethylation of tumor suppressors is an early event in the PanIN progression [72]. In a cell line assay of CpG island methylation Ohnami et al. showed that the allele of *MTRR* associated with cancer risk gave lower levels of methylation than a low risk allele [141]. Another gene involved in folate metabolism has also been shown to have polymorphisms associated with pancreatic cancer risk (methylenetetrahydrofolate reductase, *MTHFR*) [139], and again the high-risk allele seems to be associated with lower rather than higher methylation.

It is impossible to make a generalization about how polygenic effects will impact on progression. The effects of each variant will be small and may start early in development. On the other hand low penetrant genotypes may only become significant after commitment to tumorigenesis. In this respect, it is interesting to observe that polymorphisms of the cell cycle proteins aurora and *CDKN2A*(p16) do not necessarily impact on the probability of developing cancer but are associated with earlier onset [172]. This suggests that there is a long period (years) between commitment and development of the carcinoma.

2.6.3 Monogenic Indirect Predisposition

As already described, both pancreatitis and diabetes mellitus are associated with a risk of pancreatic cancer, but only pancreatitis has an etiology with autosomal dominant predisposition. This is the syndrome known as hereditary pancreatitis (HP). Although HP is by definition autosomal dominant it has an extremely variable clinical course. Some patients suffer debilitating early onset acute attacks, followed by rapid progression to chronic disease, usually with both exocrine and endocrine failure; others (even within the same family) have late onset with mild attacks and little or no pancreatic failure. Some mutation carriers (approximately 20%) do not report any attacks at all [82]. A diagnosis of HP rather than sporadic pancreatitis has great significance in terms of screening or surveillance for cancer. Alcohol-induced chronic pancreatitis results in a relatively modest elevated risk of pancreatic cancer, but HP gives a greater than 40% lifetime risk. An explanation of this could be the duration of inflammation, but as reporting of symptoms varies and attacks may be subclinical, in practical terms knowledge that symptoms are due to HP should alter the management of a patient regardless of perceived duration of symptoms.

Mutations in the *PRSS1* gene cause HP, *PRSS1* encodes cationic trypsinogen, a zymogen of the protease trypsin. The most common mutations in HP are R122H, N29I, and A16V but many families have been described with clinically defined hereditary pancreatitis where there is no *PRSS1* mutation [82]. Also, as already described, many families harboring A16V do not fit the criteria for HP (autosomal dominant disease). It is widely assumed that the substitution of histidine for arginine in the R122H mutant protein results in a reduction in the destruction of autoactivated trypsinogen [173–175], thus giving a more prolonged activation of the protease and cellular damage (hence inflammation). The mechanism linking N29I with pancreatitis is similar in that increased trypsin activity is the end result, although in the case of N29I this is probably due to increased autoactivation [175]. The A16V mutation was originally found in three individuals with presumed idiopathic pancreatitis and in one said to have HP. The A16V mutation was also identified in seven first-degree relatives of these patients but only one had clinically apparent pancreatitis, suggesting that this mutation may be associated with pancreatitis in association with variants in other genes or particular environmental exposure [82].

If HP is linked to pancreatic cancer purely via the association of inflammation, then progression would be expected to be via PanIN lesions rather than IPMN. However, the link may be more complex, possibly including a direct link between cancer and the *PRSS1* mutations. Also, there appears to be a further increase in cancer risk in HP patients who develop diabetes mellitus [92] and diabetes mellitus appears to be more closely linked to the development of IPMN than PanINs.

2.6.4 Polygenic Indirect Predisposition

CFTR is associated with the monogenic recessive syndrome cystic fibrosis, but heterozygotes for mutations of *CFTR* have a well-documented increased risk of pancreatitis [147]. The association with pancreatic cancer is much more ambiguous, although it is logical that an association occurs via pancreatitis [166]. Similarly polymorphisms of the trypsin inhibitor PSTI [146] and the A16V variant of *PRSS1* both show a complex multigenic association with pancreatitis and therefore with cancer [82].

Another way in which genotype could influence the risk of pancreatitis and therefore cancer would be by increasing activation of chemical entities (xenobiotics) that act on the pancreas to induce pancreatitis or by reducing inactivation of such xenobiotics. UDP glucuronosyltransferases inactivate many drugs and metabolites by conjugating them to a glucuronidate moiety. A polymorphism of the UDP glucuronosyltransferase UGT1A7 was shown to be associated with pancreatitis and pancreatic cancer, but only in smokers [151]. It was not clear in the original study whether the link with cancer was via pancreatitis, but this is a possibility. However, this data and other reports on this UGT1A7 polymorphism have since been criticized due to possible unbalanced allelic amplification during PCR [152].

A polymorphism of KCNQ1, a pore-forming subunit of a voltage-gated potassium channel, is associated with type 2 diabetes mellitus and thus presumably with pancreatic cancer (although this is yet to be established) [18]. A possible link between type 2 diabetes and cancer would be via an increased localized level of insulin following development of insulin resistance [114]. In contrast type 1 diabetes involves destruction of β-cells without any development of insulin resistance, and therefore, the link with cancer is unlikely to be via hyperinsulinaemia.

An alternative possibility is that the genetic background that predisposes to type 1 diabetes also predisposes to pancreatic cancer. Type 1 diabetes is linked to polymorphisms in components of the Major Histocompatability Complex, specifically HLA-B and/or HLA-A [149]. Class I HLA have been linked to various forms of cancer, but usually these have involved infection, for example, *H. pylori* infection linked to gastric cancer [176], HPV infection in cervical cancer [150], and hepatitis B linked to hepatocellular cancer [177]. There is evidence for a link between hepatitis B infection and pancreatic cancer [178] but this link is not very strong.

Twin studies have shown only 20–60% concordance for type 1 disease, suggesting a strong gene–environment interaction. Type 2 diabetes is predominantly linked to obesity and environment plays a much more significant role than genotype. It is possible that the link between diabetes and cancer is via shared environment or a shared genetic susceptibility to a particular environmental exposure. Obesity has been linked to pancreatic cancer [179] and there are a number of genetic factors that influence obesity, and hence, variants of these genes could be shared risk factors for both cancer and type 2 diabetes.

Progression of cancer as a result of pancreatitis would be expected to be via PanIN lesions while progression as a result of diabetes mellitus would be expected to be via IPMN (as already described). However, the genetic contribution to the benign diseases might have an impact on the way in which progression occurs. For example, *CFTR*-related pancreatitis may have a very different clinical progression than alcohol-related pancreatitis, and as a consequence, the nature of cancer risk may be very different [147].

2.7   Screening Results and Progression

In the foregoing discussion, predictions have been made about how genetic susceptibility may impact on cancer progression. Traditionally such predictions have been difficult to test in a clinical setting. The problem being that pancreatic cancer is such a deadly disease because it is difficult to detect at an early stage and to study the early development of pancreatic cancer, detection of early stage cancers and preneoplastic lesions is necessary. However, there are now a number of groups carrying out screening of patients with a strong genetic predisposition to cancer. Initial results have been published by the Johns Hopkins and Washington groups. The German National Case Collection of Familial Pancreatic Cancer (FaPaCa) and the European Registry of Hereditary Pancreatitis (EUROPAC) work together in a European Union funded project, which at the time of writing had not published the results of the screening program. Similarly, the Moffitt cancer center had not published results but had outlined their protocols. These screening programs are discussed in chapter 51, but in this chapter it is relevant to discuss the types of lesion identified.

The results of the Washington group have already been mentioned as this program has focused on Family X, the large family with a palladin mutation. From a total cohort of 75 patients, 15 had abnormalities on imaging, all of whom had surgery. Histology results revealed PanIN-3 lesions in ten individuals and the remaining five specimens contained PanIN-2 [180]. From 11 Family X members described in detail, all had mucinous metaplasia in small interlobular ducts [113]. The Johns Hopkins group have screened 72 members of families with apparent familial pancreatic cancer (FPC) and six individuals with Peutz-Jegher's syndrome (PJS). Seven participants had a total pancreatectomy following imaging [181]. One PJS patient had an IPMN with no PanIN. One FPC patient with a *BRCA2* mutation also had

IPMN with no PanIN. Another FPC patient had IPMN and PanIN1 lesions. Three FPC patients had IPMN and PanIN3. One FPC patient had PanIN2 with no IPMN. A further *BRCA2* carrier in an FPC family was advised of IPMN-like lesions on the basis of imaging, but developed metastatic cancer before returning for surgery and hence no histological confirmation was possible. Interestingly all seven FPC patients who underwent pancreatectomy showed histological signs of chronic pancreatitis and the patient who developed metastatic disease also showed signs of chronic pancreatitis on imaging [181].

This is clearly a very small number of histological samples to draw any conclusions from. Also surgery was provoked by identification of abnormalities by imaging, perhaps biasing towards presence of IPMN. Nevertheless, the results do suggest that mutations in both *BRCA2* and *STK11* (the causative mutation in PJS) can result in IPMN, possibly as an intermediate step in the development of adenocarcinoma. It is worth noting that mutation of the *APC* gene can also lead to the development of IPMN [182]. *STK11*, which encodes for a serine-threonine protein kinase [183,184] that is involved in regulation of cell proliferation and polarity [185], also has a crucial role in the regulation of the AMP-activated protein kinase energy homeostasis cascade [186,187]. *STK11* mutants fail to activate GSK 3Beta, preventing it from inhibiting the Wnt signaling pathway [188,189] and many mutations also cause loss of interaction with PTEN [190]. In a drosophila model, *STK11* appears to be necessary for chromosome segregation [191]. *BRCA2*, as already described, is involved with other Fanconi Anemia genes in homologous recombination repair. It is unclear why either of these mutations might predispose more to progression through IPMN than through PanIN lesions. In the other FPC cases, the causative germline mutation is unknown. At least one of the FPC patients seems to have a predisposition linked more closely to PanIN lesions than IPMN, suggesting a different mechanism of cancer predisposition than is seen with *STK11*, *BRCA2*, or *APC* mutations.

3   Specificity: Why the Pancreas?

As described in ❯ *Table 24-1*, most genes that have been linked to pancreatic cancer have also been linked to other forms of malignancy. It is possible that in many cases the type of cancer an individual develops is a matter of chance, but at least in the case of *BRCA2* mutation carriers this is difficult to reconcile with the clustering of specific types of cancer within individual families [163]. It seems more likely that a shared genetic background or shared environment modulates the effect of *BRCA2* mutation to target the pancreas in particular individuals (see ❯ *Fig. 24-2*). If this is true for *BRCA2*, it could also be true for the effects of other mutations and polymorphisms. In some cases the link is obvious, as already described, pancreatitis and diabetes mellitus have a special relationship to the pancreas, it is therefore logical that genetic factors that interact with either benign disease will have a certain level of specificity for pancreatic cancer. In other cases the link with the pancreas is less obvious.

3.1   Gene-Environment Interactions

If it is true that genotype always influences cancer risk, it is equally true that environmental exposure will also always be a factor. Chemical mutagens are the most obvious carcinogens; these will contribute to a progression of somatic mutations and will therefore determine the penetrance of genetic susceptibility. As enzymes are involved both in activating and detoxifying these chemicals and enzymes are encoded by genes, the impact of carcinogens will, to an extent, be determined by genotype. In this chapter, chemicals that may be linked to cancer are described as xenobiotics and the enzymes that either activate or eliminate these compounds as xenobiotic processing enzymes or simply as xenobiotic enzymes. This will cover enzymes that elsewhere are described as carcinogen activating or drug metabolizing. Xenobiotic enzymes are divided into those involved in phase I or phase II metabolism and transport enzymes which are involved in import or export of xenobiotics into or out of cells. Phase I enzymes metabolize the xenobiotic, mainly by oxidation, often activating carcinogens but also they can directly detoxify xenobiotics or target them to phase II enzymes. Phase II enzymes conjugate the xenobiotic, or its metabolite, to small molecular weight organic compounds such as glutathione, generally detoxifying the metabolite [192].

Epidemiological studies indicate a range of compounds that are associated with pancreatic cancer. Some are directly mitogenic, potentially causing hyperplasia and hence making the initiation of tumorigenesis more likely as a result of mutation during DNA replication. Mitogenic compounds are rare, but include anabolic steroids and hormonal components of the contraceptive pill. Oral contraceptives and anabolic steroids are well-established risk factors for various forms of cancer [193]. Sex hormone receptors have been identified in pancreatic carcinomas, although, epidemiological evidence for a link between use of hormones and pancreatic cancer has not been convincingly presented. This may reflect the relatively minor role for sex hormones in the normal physiology of the pancreas. Most carcinogens are mutatgens, and the pattern of tumors caused by different mutagens varies greatly. This may be due to differences in exposure but may also reflect fundamental differences in the process of carcinogenesis or processing of chemical entities in different organs. By far the most significant source of carcinogens associated with pancreatic cancer is tobacco.

3.1.1 Tobacco

There is synergy between the pancreatic cancer risks from tobacco, the risks from diabetes, and the risk from a family history [168]. This suggests that genotype strongly influences the risk from smoking. The cancer risk associated with hereditary pancreatitis is increased further by smoking [194] suggesting that there is also a three way interaction between genotype, pancreatitis, and smoking.

Tobacco smoke contains at least 60 known mutagens, these can be divided into polycyclic aromatic hydrocarbons (PAH), nitrosamines, aromatic amines, and trace metals [195]. PAHs and N-nitrosamines are converted to DNA damaging agents by components of the P-450 system [196], which is comprised of phase I xenobiotic enzymes. This system is most active in the liver. It is therefore surprising that the link between pancreatic cancer and smoking is much more apparent than the link between smoking and hepatocellular carcinoma. It is possible that despite processing of PAHs and other tobacco carcinogens in the liver, exposure of the active metabolites is higher in the pancreas. Tobacco-related carcinogens do reach the pancreas in humans and do cause damage to DNA [197,198]. It is unclear what causes this exquisite sensitivity of pancreatic tissue, but it is possible that this is the result of the particular xenobiotic enzymes expressed in pancreatic tissue. Certainly, although the P450 system is primarily active in liver, it is also active in numerous other tissues and the profile of different

P450 isoforms varies greatly in different extrahepatic sites [199], but less is known about pancreas than other tissues. Various levels of the phase II xenobiotic enzyme GST are found in the pancreas [200,201]. It is perhaps significant that one of the five genes that codes for a form of GST-μ (GSTM1) seems to be completely silent in pancreas [200]. Interestingly, people who have two null alleles of GSTM1 have higher levels of PAH DNA adducts in their leukocytes and lung tissue [202,203] and have a higher incidence of lung [204] and possibly liver cancer [205]. If there is a natural lack of GSTM1 in pancreas and this is an explanation of the organs particular sensitivity to tobacco, this could explain why there is no real link with the GSTM1 null polymorphisms and pancreatic cancer [206], there is not likely to be an effect of reducing what is not there.

Many phase I xenobiotic metabolizing enzymes appear to be upregulated in pancreatitis [207]. This could help to explain the synergy between the cancer risks of pancreatitis and smoking that have been proposed (but not clearly demonstrated) by some authors [168]. In contrast, phase I enzymes are expressed less in diabetics than in individuals with normal endocrine function [208], despite the much more clearly defined synergy between cancer risk from diabetes and from smoking [168]. This could be explained by a more complex relationship between the cytochrome P450 (CYP) drug-metabolizing enzyme system and carcinogens than simply a matter of activation. Modification of xenobiotic compounds may activate or deactivate toxins depending on the specific toxin and the activity of phase II enzymes. All CYP enzymes and the NADPH cytochrome P-450 oxidoreductase appear to be preferentially expressed in islet cells [209]. Death of islet cells during the course of diabetes and changes in blood supply to the islets could result in a detrimental chain of events that actually increases the bio-availability of carcinogens dependent on the pattern of expression in the surrounding tissue [208], which in turn will depend on genotype. Polymorphisms that reduce activity of either *CYP1A1* [135] or *CYP1A2* [136] or polymorphisms that increase N-acetyltransferase *NAT1* [136] are all associated with pancreatic cancer and there is synergy between the polymorphisms of *CYP1A2* and *NAT1* [136], suggesting that it is the pattern of phase I enzyme expression rather than simply the level that counts.

3.2 Familial Pancreatic Cancer (FPC)

FPC is a syndrome with multiple cases of pancreatic cancer in a pattern consistent with autosomal dominant inheritance. FPC was initially described in 1987 with the first cohort of FPC families presented in 1989 [210]. The definition of FPC has gradually strengthened to exclude families that belong to other cancer syndromes (e.g., Breast-Ovarian syndrome), or hereditary illnesses such as HP [211]. It is quite possible to have more than one case of pancreatic cancer in a family without any monogenic predisposition. Thus selection of families retrospectively, on the basis of multiple cases of cancer, could give a false appearance of an autosomal dominant disease. Approximately one in ten American pancreatic cancer patients reported first-degree relatives with pancreatic cancer [212,213]. In a case-control study of individuals under the age of 75 admitted to Ospedale Magiore, [214] the relative risk of a pancreatic cancer patient reporting a first-degree relative with pancreatic cancer was 3.3 fold that of controls (95% CI: 1.42–2.44). A subsequent American case-control study indicated similar relative risks (3.2, 95% CI: 1.8–5.6) [215]. In 20% of FPC families a mutation in the BRCA2 gene has been shown to segregate with the disease [58], but for the majority of

FPC families, no disease gene has been identified. Apart from BRCA2 the only other FPC mutation is the *palladin* variant identified in Family X. The palladin gene was identified as a possible FPC gene following a linkage study that relied on a surrogate of pancreatic dysplasia for pancreatic cancer. Patients with dysplasia were identified by screening within Family X. Using this approach, a region at the end of chromosome 4, which gave two point LOD scores of greater than 3, was identified [216]. The minimum defined area was 4q32–34 and by sequencing candidate genes the P239S variant in palladin was identified [40]. However, recent work from the EUROPAC/FaPaCa study groups [217] and the National Familial Pancreas Tumor Registry [218] suggest that the 4q32–34 locus is unlikely to account for a significant proportion of families [42,162]. The search for other FPC genes is ongoing, exploiting novel mathematical models to account for the ambiguity in defining carrier status [219] and SNP arrays to increase the efficiency of linkage and association studies [220].

4 Susceptibility and Age

From the very earliest reports of familial cancer syndromes early onset has been taken as characteristic of genetic susceptibility [221]. There is no question that this is true for many forms of cancer and has often been assumed to be the case in inherited pancreatic cancer. However, analysis of precocious pancreatic cancer has not revealed germline mutations in any genes and has rarely identified familial associations [222]. Genetic variation certainly makes a difference to age of onset, with earlier onset associated with various polymorphisms of cell cycle genes [223,224], but notably these polymorphisms have not been shown to have an association with the development of cancer but just with the onset. In contrast, mutations such as BRCA2, which appear to give monogenic predisposition appear in patients with late as well as early onset [58]. However, although late onset is entirely consistent with familial pancreatic cancer, there is a trend for progressively earlier onset in kindred with successive generations (anticipation).

4.1 Anticipation

In simple terms, the onset of pancreatic cancer within FPC families occurs at an increasingly young age in consecutive generations [213,225]. The fact that average age of onset remains consistent with the sporadic disease is explained by earlier generations having a later age of onset than is normal, compensated for by the younger onset in later generations. This could be explained by various forms of bias, but meticulous statistical analysis suggests that the phenomenon is real [219]. The process of anticipation seems to extend over a limited number of generations. A possible explanation of this is a process of meiotic mutations occurring in the FPC families, high level mutation possibly resulting from haploid insufficiency of some DNA repair enzyme. Some of these mutations will be linked to the FPC mutation, and therefore, accumulation of extra mutations will segregate with pancreatic cancer predisposition, making the onset earlier, analogous to the consequence of polymorphisms of cell cycle genes as already described. The additional mutations will represent risk polymorphisms similar to those shown in ❯ *Fig. 24-2*. Limitation of the anticipation will occur because at some point either the pattern of risk alleles will give a form of cancer other than pancreatic or the carriers will not survive in utero [219].

5   Outcome and Targeted Therapy

Knowledge of genetic predisposition is of more than academic interest. In chapter 51 risk stratification will be described, high-risk groups are essential for a successful screening program, which will identify early tumors at a curable stage. In addition to risk stratification, knowledge of the particular form of genetic predisposition could allow targeting of chemotherapy. Germ line polymorphisms of base excision repair genes influence outcome in addition to possibly predisposing to cancer [226]. This is supported by the fact that ATM, ATR, and CHK1/2 polymorphisms have been proposed to be key determinants of response to gemcitabine and radiotherapy [227]. Particular forms of predisposition may also offer personalized forms of chemotherapy, for example, patients with BRCA2 mutations may be exquisitely sensitive to PARP inhibitors [228].

6   General Resources

In addition to the references cited in the text, readers can make use of the following online resources:

Registries of families with inherited pancreatic diseases
    http://www.europac-org.eu/
    http://pathology.jhu.edu/pancreas/PartNFPTR.php
Information on pancreatic cancer including free downloads
    http://www.moldiagpaca.eu/
List of mutation associated with chronic pancreatitis
    http://www.uni-leipzig.de/pancreasmutation/
Atlas of Genetics and Cytogenetics in Oncology and Haematology
    http://atlasgeneticsoncology.org/Kprones/HeredPancrCanID10068.html

---

Key Practice Points

Cancer syndromes associated with pancreatic cancer include: Breast-Ovarian cancer syndromes (BrOv) which can result from mutations in *BRCA1/2*; Familial Multiple Mole Melanoma (FAMMM), which often involves inheritance of mutations in *CDKN2A* (p16); Familial Adenomatous Polyposis (FAP), which often involves *APC* mutations; Peutz-Jeghers Syndrome which can involve mutation of *STK11* tumor suppressor; Human Non-Polyposis Colon cancer (HNPCC) which is caused by mutations in a variety of mismatch repair genes; Li-Fraumeni Syndrome, which can involve mutations of the p53 or CHK2 tumor suppressors; also Fanconi-Anemia associated with FANCG and FANCC genes

- If the nature of predisposition can be identified it should influence which clinical trials a patient is suitable for and whether a family member should be included on a screening program.

- Most genetic predisposition will not result in a family history of pancreatic cancer, research based testing for genetic polymorphisms is worthwhile to further classify the level of risk associated with variants.
- Specific cancer associated mutations may have different effects in different families because of other genetic factors. For example, *BRCA2* mutations may principally predispose to pancreatic cancer in one family and principally for breast cancer in another. An identified mutation must therefore be considered in the context of family history before recommending the most appropriate form of screening.

Published Guidelines

The International Agency for Research on Cancer (IARC) Unclassified Genetic Variants Working Group published guidelines in October 2008 on the way to classify genetic variants linked to cancer, who to test and recommendations on appropriate surveillance [229]. In summary:

- Genetic variants are classified between 1 (<0.1% chance of being pathogenic) and 5 (>99% chance of being pathogenic).
- Clinical testing of relatives should only be carried out in class 4 or above (>95% chance of being pathogenic)
- Surveillance is recommended for known carriers of class 3 or above (>50% chance of being pathogenic)
- Research testing is recommended for class 2 to 4 (1–99% chance of being pathogenic)

The working group proposed that panels of experts on each cancer predisposition syndrome should meet to designate appropriate surveillance and cancer management guidelines. Guidelines were published for screening and counseling HP patients in 2001 [230] and more generally for all high-risk groups in 2007 [231]. These will be discussed in more detail in the next chapter.

Future Research Directions

- Linkage studies using SNP arrays to identify further high-risk mutations in families with a strong cancer history
- Association studies using high density SNP arrays to identify low penetrant risk factors
- In silico modeling combined with sound epidemiological studies and molecular analysis of germline DNA from pancreatic cancer patients to quantify risk from combinations of markers.
- Prospective studies of family members in high-risk families to stratify risk.

References

1. Donehower LA: p53: guardian AND suppressor of longevity? Exp Gerontol 2005;40:7–9.
2. Dong LM, Potter JD, White E, et al.: Genetic susceptibility to cancer: the role of polymorphisms in candidate genes. JAMA 2008;299:2423–2436.
3. Easton DF, Pooley KA, Dunning AM, et al.: Genome-wide association study identifies novel breast cancer susceptibility loci. Nature 2007;447:1087–1093.
4. Rao BK, Noor O, Thosani MK: Identical twins with primary cutaneous melanoma presenting at

the same time and location. Am J Dermatopathol 2008;30:182–184.

5. Isaksson B, Jonsson F, Pedersen NL, et al.: Lifestyle factors and pancreatic cancer risk: a cohort study from the Swedish Twin Registry. Int J Cancer 2002; 98:480–482.

6. Lichtenstein P, Holm NV, Verkasalo PK, et al.: Environmental and heritable factors in the causation of cancer – analyses of cohorts of twins from Sweden, Denmark, and Finland. N Engl J Med 2000; 343:78–85.

7. Grocock CJ, Vitone LJ, Harcus MJ, et al.: Familial pancreatic cancer: a review and latest advances. Adv Med Sci 2007;52:37–49.

8. Dayaram T, Marriott SJ: Effect of transforming viruses on molecular mechanisms associated with cancer. J Cell Physiol 2008;216:309–314.

9. Amieva MR, El-Omar EM: Host-bacterial interactions in Helicobacter pylori infection. Gastroenterology 2008;134:306–323.

10. Hussain SP: Inflammation and cancer: is aid aiding? Gastroenterology 2008;135:736–737.

11. Inoue M, Iwasaki M, Otani T, et al.: Diabetes mellitus and the risk of cancer: results from a large-scale population-based cohort study in Japan. Arch Intern Med 2006;166:1871–1877.

12. Kuriki K, Hirose K, Tajima K: Diabetes and cancer risk for all and specific sites among Japanese men and women. Eur J Cancer Prev 2007;16:83–89.

13. Calton BA, Chang SC, Wright ME, et al.: History of diabetes mellitus and subsequent prostate cancer risk in the NIH-AARP Diet and Health Study. Cancer Causes Control 2007;18:493–503.

14. Gong Z, Neuhouser ML, Goodman PJ, et al.: Obesity, diabetes, and risk of prostate cancer: results from the prostate cancer prevention trial. Cancer Epidemiol Biomarkers Prev 2006;15:1977–1983.

15. Kasper JS, Giovannucci E: A meta-analysis of diabetes mellitus and the risk of prostate cancer. Cancer Epidemiol Biomarkers Prev 2006;15:2056–2062.

16. Zhou J, Smith DK, Lu L, et al.: A non-synonymous single nucleotide polymorphism in IFNAR1 affects susceptibility to chronic hepatitis B virus infection. J Viral Hepat 2008;16:45–52.

17. Reiner AP, Barber MJ, Guan Y, et al.: Polymorphisms of the HNF1A gene encoding hepatocyte nuclear factor-1 alpha are associated with C-reactive protein. Am J Hum Genet 2008;82:1193–1201.

18. Yasuda K, Miyake K, Horikawa Y, et al.: Variants in KCNQ1 are associated with susceptibility to type 2 diabetes mellitus. Nat Genet 2008;40: 1092–1097.

19. Chan PK, Cheung TH, Lin CK, et al.: Association between HLA-DRB1 polymorphism, high-risk HPV infection and cervical neoplasia in southern Chinese. J Med Virol 2007;79:970–976.

20. Kato I, van Doorn LJ, Canzian F, et al.: Host-bacterial interaction in the development of gastric precancerous lesions in a high risk population for gastric cancer in Venezuela. Int J Cancer 2006;119:1666–1671.

21. Garrity-Park MM, Loftus EV, Jr., Bryant SC, et al.: Tumor necrosis factor-alpha polymorphisms in ulcerative colitis-associated colorectal cancer. Am J Gastroenterol 2008;103:407–415.

22. Sandhu MS, Luben R, Khaw KT: Self reported non-insulin dependent diabetes, family history, and risk of prevalent colorectal cancer: population based, cross sectional study. J Epidemiol Community Health 2001;55:804–805.

23. Gudmundsson J, Sulem P, Steinthorsdottir V, et al.: Two variants on chromosome 17 confer prostate cancer risk, and the one in TCF2 protects against type 2 diabetes. Nat Genet 2007;39:977–983.

24. Vogelstein B, Fearon ER, Hamilton SR, et al.: Genetic alterations during colorectal-tumor development. N Engl J Med 1988;319:525–532.

25. Maitra A, Adsay NV, Argani P, et al.: Multicomponent analysis of the pancreatic adenocarcinoma progression model using a pancreatic intraepithelial neoplasia tissue microarray. Mod Pathol 2003;16:902–912.

26. Biankin AV, Kench JG, Dijkman FP, et al.: Molecular pathogenesis of precursor lesions of pancreatic ductal adenocarcinoma. Pathology 2003; 35:14–24.

27. Wilentz RE, Geradts J, Maynard R, et al.: Inactivation of the p16 (INK4A) tumor-suppressor gene in pancreatic duct lesions: loss of intranuclear expression. Cancer Res 1998;58:4740–4744.

28. van Heek NT, Meeker AK, Kern SE, et al.: Telomere Shortening Is Nearly Universal in Pancreatic Intraepithelial Neoplasia. Am J Pathol 2002;161: 1541–1547.

29. Chin L, Artandi SE, Shen Q, et al.: p53 deficiency rescues the adverse effects of telomere loss and cooperates with telomere dysfunction to accelerate carcinogenesis. Cell 1999;97:527–538.

30. Raynaud CM, Sabatier L, Philipot O, et al.: Telomere length, telomeric proteins and genomic instability during the multistep carcinogenic process. Crit Rev Oncol Hematol 2008;66:99–117.

31. Hiyama E, Kodama T, Shinbara K, et al.: Telomerase activity is detected in pancreatic cancer but not in benign tumors. Cancer Res 1997;57:326–331.

32. Hahn WC, Counter CM, Lundberg AS, et al.: Creation of human tumour cells with defined genetic elements. Nature 1999;400:464–468.

33. Hahn WC, Dessain SK, Brooks MW, et al.: Enumeration of the simian virus 40 early region elements necessary for human cell transformation. Mol Cell Biol 2002;22:2111–2123.

34. Hingorani SR, Petricoin EF, Maitra A, et al.: Preinvasive and invasive ductal pancreatic cancer and its early detection in the mouse. Cancer Cell 2003;4:437–450.

35. Hingorani SR, Wang L, Multani AS, et al.: Trp53R172H and KrasG12D cooperate to promote chromosomal instability and widely metastatic pancreatic ductal adenocarcinoma in mice. Cancer Cell 2005;7:469–483.

36. Tuveson DA, Shaw AT, Willis NA, et al.: Endogenous oncogenic K-ras(G12D) stimulates proliferation and widespread neoplastic and developmental defects. Cancer Cell 2004;5:375–387.

37. Mulligan LM, Eng C, Healey CS, et al.: Specific mutations of the RET proto-oncogene are related to disease phenotype in MEN 2A and FMTC. Nat Genet 1994;6:70–74.

38. Le Hir H, Charlet-Berguerand N, de Franciscis V, et al.: 5′-End RET splicing: absence of variants in normal tissues and intron retention in pheochromocytomas. Oncology 2002;63:84–91.

39. Le Hir H, Charlet-Berguerand N, Gimenez-Roqueplo A, et al.: Relative expression of the RET9 and RET51 isoforms in human pheochromocytomas. Oncology 2000;58:311–318.

40. Pogue-Geile KL, Chen R, Bronner MP, et al.: Palladin mutation causes familial pancreatic cancer and suggests a new cancer mechanism. PLoS Med 2006;3:e516.

41. Zogopoulos G, Rothenmund H, Eppel A, et al.: The P239S palladin variant does not account for a significant fraction of hereditary or early onset pancreas cancer. Hum Genet 2007;121:635–637.

42. Slater E, Amrillaeva V, Fendrich V, et al.: Palladin mutation causes familial pancreatic cancer: absence in European families. PLoS Med 2007;4:e164.

43. Testa JR, Hino O: Tumor suppressor genes and the two-hit model of recessive oncogenesis: celebrating Alfred Knudson's 80th birthday. Genes Chromosomes Cancer 2003;38:286–287.

44. Lynch HT, Brand RE, Hogg D, et al.: Phenotypic variation in eight extended CDKN2A germline mutation familial atypical multiple mole melanoma-pancreatic carcinoma-prone families: the familial atypical mole melanoma-pancreatic carcinoma syndrome. Cancer 2002;94:84–96.

45. Groen EJ, Roos A, Muntinghe FL, et al.: Extra-intestinal manifestations of familial adenomatous polyposis. Ann Surg Oncol 2008;15:2439–2450.

46. Latchford A, Greenhalf W, Vitone LJ, et al.: Peutz-Jeghers syndrome and screening for pancreatic cancer. Br J Surg 2006;93:1446–1455.

47. Vahteristo P, Tamminen A, Karvinen P, et al.: p53, CHK2, and CHK1 genes in Finnish families with Li-Fraumeni syndrome: further evidence of CHK2 in inherited cancer predisposition. Cancer Res 2001;61:5718–5722.

48. Wood LD, Parsons DW, Jones S, et al.: The genomic landscapes of human breast and colorectal cancers. Science 2007;318:1108–1113.

49. Jones S, Zhang X, Parsons DW, et al.: Core signaling pathways in human pancreatic cancers revealed by global genomic analyses. Science 2008;321:1801–1806.

50. Trenz K, Lugowski S, Jahrsdorfer U, et al.: Enhanced sensitivity of peripheral blood lymphocytes from women carrying a BRCA1 mutation towards the mutagenic effects of various cytostatics. Mutat Res 2003;544:279–288.

51. Trenz K, Rothfuss A, Schutz P, et al.: Mutagen sensitivity of peripheral blood from women carrying a BRCA1 or BRCA2 mutation. Mutat Res 2002;500:89–96.

52. Aarnio M, Sankila R, Pukkala E, et al.: Cancer risk in mutation carriers of DNA-mismatch-repair genes. Int J Cancer 1999;81:214–218.

53. Venkitaraman AR: Cancer susceptibility and the functions of BRCA1 and BRCA2. Cell 2002;108:171–182.

54. Jiao L, Bondy ML, Hassan MM, et al.: Selected polymorphisms of DNA repair genes and risk of pancreatic cancer. Cancer Detect Prev 2006;30:284–291.

55. Couch FJ, Johnson MR, Rabe K, et al.: Germ line Fanconi anemia complementation group C mutations and pancreatic cancer. Cancer Res 2005;65:383–386.

56. Rogers CD, van der Heijden MS, Brune K, et al.: The genetics of FANCC and FANCG in familial pancreatic cancer. Cancer Biol Ther 2004;3:167–169.

57. van der Heijden MS, Yeo CJ, Hruban RH, et al.: Fanconi anemia gene mutations in young-onset pancreatic cancer. Cancer Res 2003;63:2585–2588.

58. Hahn SA, Greenhalf B, Ellis I, et al.: BRCA2 germline mutations in familial pancreatic carcinoma. J Natl Cancer Inst 2003;95:214–221.

59. Lynch HT, Lynch JF: Hereditary nonpolyposis colorectal cancer. Semin Surg Oncol 2000;18:305–313.

60. Hisa T, Suda K, Nobukawa B, et al.: Distribution of intraductal lesions in small invasive ductal carcinoma of the pancreas. Pancreatology 2007;7:341–346.

61. Detlefsen S, Sipos B, Feyerabend B, et al.: Pancreatic fibrosis associated with age and ductal papillary hyperplasia. Virchows Arch 2005;447:800–805.

62. Real FX, Cibrian-Uhalte E, Martinelli P: Pancreatic cancer development and progression: remodeling the model. Gastroenterology 2008;135:724–728.

63. Komori T, Ishikawa O, Ohigashi H, et al.: Invasive ductal adenocarcinoma of the remnant pancreatic body 9 years after resection of an intraductal papillary-mucinous carcinoma of the pancreatic head:

a case report and comparison of DNA sequence in K-ras gene mutation. Jpn J Clin Oncol 2002;32: 146–151.

64. Biankin AV, Kench JG, Biankin SA, et al.: Pancreatic intraepithelial neoplasia in association with intraductal papillary mucinous neoplasms of the pancreas: implications for disease progression and recurrence. Am J Surg Pathol 2004;28: 1184–1192.

65. Bassi C, Sarr MG, Lillemoe KD, et al.: Natural history of intraductal papillary mucinous neoplasms (IPMN): current evidence and implications for management. J Gastrointest Surg 2008;12:645–650.

66. Hruban RH, Takaori K, Klimstra DS, et al.: An illustrated consensus on the classification of pancreatic intraepithelial neoplasia and intraductal papillary mucinous neoplasms. Am J Surg Pathol 2004;28:977–987.

67. Furukawa T, Kloppel G, Volkan Adsay N, et al.: Classification of types of intraductal papillary-mucinous neoplasm of the pancreas: a consensus study. Virchows Arch 2005;447:794–799.

68. Sugiyama M, Suzuki Y, Abe N, et al.: Management of intraductal papillary mucinous neoplasm of the pancreas. J Gastroenterol 2008;43:181–185.

69. Uehara H, Nakaizumi A, Ishikawa O, et al.: Development of ductal carcinoma of the pancreas during follow-up of branch duct intraductal papillary mucinous neoplasm of the pancreas. Gut 2008;57:1561–1565.

70. Wada K: p16 and p53 gene alterations and accumulations in the malignant evolution of intraductal papillary-mucinous tumors of the pancreas. J Hepatobiliary Pancreat Surg 2002;9:76–85.

71. Hashimoto Y, Murakami Y, Uemura K, et al.: Telomere shortening and telomerase expression during multistage carcinogenesis of intraductal papillary mucinous neoplasms of the pancreas. J Gastrointest Surg 2008;12:17–28; discussion 9.

72. Sato N, Fukushima N, Hruban RH, et al.: CpG island methylation profile of pancreatic intraepithelial neoplasia. Mod Pathol 2008;21:238–244.

73. Sato N, Ueki T, Fukushima N, et al.: Aberrant methylation of CpG islands in intraductal papillary mucinous neoplasms of the pancreas. Gastroenterology 2002;123:365–372.

74. Adsay NV, Merati K, Andea A, et al.: The dichotomy in the preinvasive neoplasia to invasive carcinoma sequence in the pancreas: differential expression of MUC1 and MUC2 supports the existence of two separate pathways of carcinogenesis. Mod Pathol 2002;15:1087–1095.

75. Kloppel G, Luttges J: The pathology of ductal-type pancreatic carcinomas and pancreatic intraepithelial neoplasia: insights for clinicians. Curr Gastroenterol Rep 2004;6:111–118.

76. Brembeck FH, Schreiber FS, Deramaudt TB, et al.: The mutant K-ras oncogene causes pancreatic periductal lymphocytic infiltration and gastric mucous neck cell hyperplasia in transgenic mice. Cancer Res 2003;63:2005–2009.

77. Grippo PJ, Nowlin PS, Demeure MJ, et al.: Preinvasive pancreatic neoplasia of ductal phenotype induced by acinar cell targeting of mutant Kras in transgenic mice. Cancer Res 2003;63:2016–2019.

78. Tuveson DA, Zhu L, Gopinathan A, et al.: Mist1-KrasG12D knock-in mice develop mixed differentiation metastatic exocrine pancreatic carcinoma and hepatocellular carcinoma. Cancer Res 2006; 66:242–247.

79. Guerra C, Schuhmacher AJ, Canamero M, et al.: Chronic pancreatitis is essential for induction of pancreatic ductal adenocarcinoma by K-Ras oncogenes in adult mice. Cancer Cell 2007;11:291–302.

80. Siveke JT, Einwachter H, Sipos B, et al.: Concomitant pancreatic activation of Kras(G12D) and Tgfa results in cystic papillary neoplasms reminiscent of human IPMN. Cancer Cell 2007;12:266–279.

81. Stanger BZ, Stiles B, Lauwers GY, et al.: Pten constrains centroacinar cell expansion and malignant transformation in the pancreas. Cancer Cell 2005; 8:185–195.

82. Howes N, Lerch MM, Greenhalf W, et al.: Clinical and genetic characteristics of hereditary pancreatitis in Europe. Clin Gastroenterol Hepatol 2004;2: 252–261.

83. Threadgold J, Greenhalf W, Ellis I, et al.: The N34S mutation of SPINK1 (PSTI) is associated with a familial pattern of idiopathic chronic pancreatitis but does not cause the disease. Gut 2002;50: 675–681.

84. Mantovani A, Allavena P, Sica A, et al.: Cancer-related inflammation. Nature 2008;454:436–444.

85. Itzkowitz SH, Yio X: Inflammation and cancer IV. Colorectal cancer in inflammatory bowel disease: the role of inflammation. Am J Physiol Gastrointest Liver Physiol 2004;287:G7–G17.

86. Imagawa S, Yoshihara M, Ito M, et al.: Evaluation of gastric cancer risk using topography of histological gastritis: a large-scaled cross-sectional study. Dig Dis Sci 2008;53:1818–1823.

87. de Martel C, Llosa AE, Friedmana GD, et al.: Helicobacter pylori infection and development of pancreatic cancer. Cancer Epidemiol Biomarkers Prev 2008;17:1188–1194.

88. Lowenfels AB, Maisonneuve P, Cavallini G, et al.: Pancreatitis and the risk of pancreatic cancer. International Pancreatitis Study Group. N Engl J Med 1993;328:1433–1437.

89. Malka D, Hammel P, Maire F, et al.: Risk of pancreatic adenocarcinoma in chronic pancreatitis. Gut 2002;51:849–852.

90. Ghazale A, Chari S: Is autoimmune pancreatitis a risk factor for pancreatic cancer? Pancreas 2007; 35:376.

91. Lowenfels AB, Maisonneuve P, DiMagno EP, et al.: Hereditary pancreatitis and the risk of pancreatic cancer. International hereditary pancreatitis study group. J Natl Cancer Inst 1997;89:442–446.

92. Rebours V, Boutron-Ruault MC, Schnee M, et al.: Risk of pancreatic adenocarcinoma in patients with hereditary pancreatitis: a national exhaustive series. Am J Gastroenterol 2008;103:111–119.

93. Sica A, Allavena P, Mantovani A: Cancer related inflammation: The macrophage connection. Cancer Lett 2008;267:204–215.

94. Manicone AM, McGuire JK: Matrix metalloproteinases as modulators of inflammation. Semin Cell Dev Biol 2008;19:34–41.

95. Leung PS, Chan YC: Role of oxidative stress in pancreatic inflammation. Antioxid Redox Signal 2008;11:135–165.

96. Algul H, Treiber M, Lesina M, et al.: Mechanisms of disease: chronic inflammation and cancer in the pancreas – a potential role for pancreatic stellate cells? Nat Clin Pract 2007;4:454–462.

97. Miyamoto Y, Maitra A, Ghosh B, et al.: Notch mediates TGF alpha-induced changes in epithelial differentiation during pancreatic tumorigenesis. Cancer Cell 2003;3:565–576.

98. Talamini G, Zamboni G, Salvia R, et al.: Intraductal papillary mucinous neoplasms and chronic pancreatitis. Pancreatology 2006;6:626–634.

99. Rosty C, Geradts J, Sato N, et al.: p16 Inactivation in pancreatic intraepithelial neoplasias (PanINs) arising in patients with chronic pancreatitis. Am J Surg Pathol 2003;27:1495–1501.

100. Siveke JT, Lubeseder-Martellato C, Lee M, et al.: Notch signaling is required for exocrine regeneration after acute pancreatitis. Gastroenterology 2008;134:544–555.

101. Bhanot U, Kohntop R, Hasel C, et al.: Evidence of Notch pathway activation in the ectatic ducts of chronic pancreatitis. J Pathol 2008;214:312–319.

102. Bockman DE: Transition to pancreatic cancer in response to carcinogen. Langenbecks Arch Surg 2008;393:557–560.

103. Esposito I, Seiler C, Bergmann F, et al.: Hypothetical progression model of pancreatic cancer with origin in the centroacinar-acinar compartment. Pancreas 2007;35:212–217.

104. Hruban RH, Adsay NV, Albores-Saavedra J, et al.: Pathology of genetically engineered mouse models of pancreatic exocrine cancer: consensus report and recommendations. Cancer Res 2006;66:95–106.

105. Lillioja S, Mott DM, Spraul M, et al.: Insulin resistance and insulin secretory dysfunction as precursors of non-insulin-dependent diabetes mellitus. Prospective studies of Pima Indians. N Engl J Med 1993;329:1988–1992.

106. Chari ST, Leibson CL, Rabe KG, et al.: Probability of pancreatic cancer following diabetes: a population-based study. Gastroenterology 2005; 129:504–511.

107. Huxley R, Ansary-Moghaddam A, Berrington de Gonzalez A, et al.: Type-II diabetes and pancreatic cancer: a meta-analysis of 36 studies. Br J Cancer 2005;92:2076–2083.

108. Wang F, Herrington M, Larsson J, et al.: The relationship between diabetes and pancreatic cancer. Mol Cancer 2003;2:4.

109. Silverman DT, Schiffman M, Everhart J, et al.: Diabetes mellitus, other medical conditions and familial history of cancer as risk factors for pancreatic cancer. Br J Cancer 1999;80:1830–1837.

110. Chari ST, Leibson CL, Rabe KG, et al.: Pancreatic cancer-associated diabetes mellitus: prevalence and temporal association with diagnosis of cancer. Gastroenterology 2008;134:95–101.

111. Stevens RJ, Roddam AW, Beral V: Pancreatic cancer in type 1 and young-onset diabetes: systematic review and meta-analysis. Br J Cancer 2007;96: 507–509.

112. Daneman D: Type 1 diabetes. Lancet 2006;367: 847–858.

113. Meckler KA, Brentnall TA, Haggitt RC, et al.: Familial fibrocystic pancreatic atrophy with endocrine cell hyperplasia and pancreatic carcinoma. Am J Surg Pathol 2001;25:1047–1053.

114. Kleeff J, Beckhove P, Esposito I, et al.: Pancreatic cancer microenvironment. Int J Cancer 2007;121: 699–705.

115. Bowker SL, Majumdar SR, Veugelers P, et al.: Increased cancer-related mortality for patients with type 2 diabetes who use sulfonylureas or insulin. Diabetes Care 2006;29:254–258.

116. Ding XZ, Fehsenfeld DM, Murphy LO, et al.: Physiological concentrations of insulin augment pancreatic cancer cell proliferation and glucose utilization by activating MAP kinase, PI3 kinase and enhancing GLUT-1 expression. Pancreas 2000;21:310–320.

117. Balaz P, Friess H, Buchler MW: Growth factors in pancreatic health and disease. Pancreatology 2001;1:343–355.

118. Nagasao J, Yoshioka K, Amasaki H, et al.: Expression of nestin and IGF-1 in rat pancreas after streptozotocin administration. Anat Histol Embryol 2004;33:1–4.

119. Karna E, Surazynski A, Orlowski K, et al.: Serum and tissue level of insulin-like growth factor-I (IGF-I) and IGF-I binding proteins as an index of pancreatitis and pancreatic cancer. Int J Exp Pathol 2002;83:239–245.

120. Tanaka M: Important clues to the diagnosis of pancreatic cancer. Rocz Akad Med Bialymst 2005;50:69–72.

121. Fujii T, Ishikawa T, Kanazumi N, et al.: Analysis of clinicopathological features and predictors of malignancy in intraductal papillary mucinous neoplasms of the pancreas. Hepatogastroenterology 2007;54:272–277.

122. Geary J, Sasieni P, Houlston R, et al.: Gene-related cancer spectrum in families with hereditary nonpolyposis colorectal cancer (HNPCC). Fam Cancer 2008;7:163–172.

123. Al-Sukhni W, Rothenmund H, Eppel Borgida A, et al.: Germline BRCA1 mutations predispose to pancreatic adenocarcinoma. Hum Genet 2008;124:271–278.

124. Lynch HT, Fusaro RM, Lynch JF, et al.: Pancreatic cancer and the FAMMM syndrome. Fam Cancer 2008;7:103–112.

125. Hearle N, Schumacher V, Menko FH, et al.: Frequency and spectrum of cancers in the Peutz-Jeghers syndrome. Clin Cancer Res 2006;12:3209–3215.

126. Birch JM, Alston RD, McNally RJ, et al.: Relative frequency and morphology of cancers in carriers of germline TP53 mutations. Oncogene 2001;20:4621–4628.

127. Su Y, Swift M: Mortality rates among carriers of ataxia-telangiectasia mutant alleles. Ann Intern Med 2000;133:770–778.

128. Olsen JH, Hahnemann JM, Borresen-Dale AL, et al.: Cancer in patients with ataxia-telangiectasia and in their relatives in the nordic countries. J Natl Cancer Inst 2001;93:121–127.

129. Rosenberg PS, Alter BP, Ebell W: Cancer risks in Fanconi anemia: findings from the German Fanconi Anemia Registry. Haematologica 2008;93:511–517.

130. Hazra A, Chanock S, Giovannucci E, et al.: Large-scale evaluation of genetic variants in candidate genes for colorectal cancer risk in the Nurses' Health Study and the Health Professionals' Follow-up Study. Cancer Epidemiol Biomarkers Prev 2008;17:311–319.

131. Jiao L, Chang P, Firozi PF, et al.: Polymorphisms of phase II xenobiotic-metabolizing and DNA repair genes and in vitro N-ethyl-N-nitrosourea-induced O6-ethylguanine levels in human lymphocytes. Mutation Res 2007;627:146–157.

132. Hung RJ, Hall J, Brennan P, et al.: Genetic polymorphisms in the base excision repair pathway and cancer risk: a HuGE review. Am J Epidemiol 2005;162:925–942.

133. Jiao L, Hassan MM, Bondy ML, et al.: The XPD Asp312Asn and Lys751Gln polymorphisms,

134. Manuguerra M, Saletta F, Karagas MR, et al.: XRCC3 and XPD/ERCC2 single nucleotide polymorphisms and the risk of cancer: a HuGE review. Am J Epidemiol 2006;164:297–302.

135. Duell EJ, Holly EA, Bracci PM, et al.: A population-based, case-control study of polymorphisms in carcinogen-metabolizing genes, smoking, and pancreatic adenocarcinoma risk. J Natl Cancer Inst 2002;94:297–306.

136. Li D, Jiao L, Li Y, et al.: Polymorphisms of cytochrome P4501A2 and N-acetyltransferase genes, smoking, and risk of pancreatic cancer. Carcinogenesis 2006;27:103–111.

137. Agundez JA: Cytochrome P450 gene polymorphism and cancer. Curr Drug Metab 2004;5:211–224.

138. Agundez JA: Polymorphisms of human N-acetyltransferases and cancer risk. Curr Drug Metab 2008;9:520–531.

139. Li D, Ahmed M, Li Y, et al.: 5,10-Methylenetetrahydrofolate reductase polymorphisms and the risk of pancreatic cancer. Cancer Epidemiol Biomarkers Prev 2005;14:1470–1476.

140. Mao R, Fan Y, Jin Y, et al.: Methylenetetrahydrofolate reductase gene polymorphisms and lung cancer: a meta-analysis. J Hum Genet 2008;53:340–348.

141. Ohnami S, Sato Y, Yoshimura K, et al.: His595Tyr polymorphism in the methionine synthase reductase (MTRR) gene is associated with pancreatic cancer risk. Gastroenterology 2008;135:477–488.

142. Sharp L, Little J: Polymorphisms in genes involved in folate metabolism and colorectal neoplasia: a HuGE review. Am J Epidemiol 2004;159:423–443.

143. Yang M, Sun T, Wang L, et al.: Functional variants in cell death pathway genes and risk of pancreatic cancer. Clin Cancer Res 2008;14:3230–3236.

144. Sun T, Miao X, Zhang X, et al.: Polymorphisms of death pathway genes FAS and FASL in esophageal squamous-cell carcinoma. J Natl Cancer Inst 2004;96:1030–1036.

145. Bethke L, Sullivan K, Webb E, et al.: The common D302H variant of CASP8 is associated with risk of glioma. Cancer Epidemiol Biomarkers Prev 2008;17:987–989.

146. Masamune A, Kume K, Shimosegawa T: Differential roles of the SPINK1 gene mutations in alcoholic and nonalcoholic chronic pancreatitis. J Gastroenterol 2007;42Suppl 17:135–140.

147. Cohn JA, Neoptolemos JP, Feng J, et al.: Increased risk of idiopathic chronic pancreatitis in cystic fibrosis carriers. Hum Mutat 2005;26:303–307.

148. Neglia JP, FitzSimmons SC, Maisonneuve P, et al.: The risk of cancer among patients with cystic

fibrosis. Cystic fibrosis and cancer study group. N Engl J Med 1995;332:494–499.

149. Nejentsev S, Howson JM, Walker NM, et al.: Localization of type 1 diabetes susceptibility to the MHC class I genes HLA-B and HLA-A. Nature 2007;450:887–892.

150. Madeleine MM, Johnson LG, Smith AG, et al.: Comprehensive analysis of HLA-A, HLA-B, HLA-C, HLA-DRB1, and HLA-DQB1 loci and squamous cell cervical cancer risk. Cancer Res 2008;68:3532–3539.

151. Ockenga J, Vogel A, Teich N, et al.: UDP glucuronosyltransferase (UGT1A7) gene polymorphisms increase the risk of chronic pancreatitis and pancreatic cancer. Gastroenterology 2003;124:1802–1808.

152. te Morsche RH, Drenth JP, Truninger K, et al.: UGT1A7 polymorphisms in chronic pancreatitis: an example of genotyping pitfalls. Pharmacogenomics J 2008;8:34–41.

153. Duell EJ, Casella DP, Burk RD, et al.: Inflammation, genetic polymorphisms in proinflammatory genes TNF-A, RANTES, and CCR5, and risk of pancreatic adenocarcinoma. Cancer Epidemiol Biomarkers Prev 2006;15:726–731.

154. Zhang J, Dou C, Song Y, et al.: Polymorphisms of tumor necrosis factor-alpha are associated with increased susceptibility to gastric cancer: a meta-analysis. J Hum Genet 2008;53:479–489.

155. Liou JM, Lin JT, Huang SP, et al.: RANTES-403 polymorphism is associated with reduced risk of gastric cancer in women. J Gastroenterol 2008; 43:115–123.

156. Knudson AG, Jr.: Retinoblastoma: a prototypic hereditary neoplasm. Semin Oncol 1978;5:57–60.

157. Ollikainen M, Hannelius U, Lindgren CM, et al.: Mechanisms of inactivation of MLH1 in hereditary nonpolyposis colorectal carcinoma: a novel approach. Oncogene 2007;26:4541–4549.

158. Seki M, Tanaka K, Kikuchi-Yanoshita R, et al.: Loss of normal allele of the APC gene in an adrenocortical carcinoma from a patient with familial adenomatous polyposis. Hum Genet 1992;89:298–300.

159. Willems AJ, Dawson SJ, Samaratunga H, et al.: Loss of heterozygosity at the BRCA2 locus detected by multiplex ligation-dependent probe amplification is common in prostate cancers from men with a germline BRCA2 mutation. Clin Cancer Res 2008;14:2953–2961.

160. Scott D, Barber JB, Levine EL, et al.: Radiation-induced micronucleus induction in lymphocytes identifies a high frequency of radiosensitive cases among breast cancer patients: a test for predisposition? Br J Cancer 1998;77:614–620.

161. Parast MM, Otey CA: Characterization of palladin, a novel protein localized to stress fibers and cell adhesions. J Cell Biol 2000;150:643–656.

162. Salaria SN, Illei P, Sharma R, et al.: Palladin is overexpressed in the non-neoplastic stroma of infiltrating ductal adenocarcinomas of the pancreas, but is only rarely overexpressed in neoplastic cells. Cancer Biol Ther 2007;6:324–328.

163. Greer JB, Whitcomb DC: Role of BRCA1 and BRCA2 mutations in pancreatic cancer. Gut 2007; 56:601–605.

164. Berwick M, Satagopan JM, Ben-Porat L, et al.: Genetic heterogeneity among Fanconi anemia heterozygotes and risk of cancer. Cancer Res 2007;67: 9591–9596.

165. Bugni JM, Han J, Tsai MS, et al.: Genetic association and functional studies of major polymorphic variants of MGMT. DNA repair 2007;6: 1116–1126.

166. Malats N, Casals T, Porta M, et al.: Cystic fibrosis transmembrane regulator (CFTR) DeltaF508 mutation and 5T allele in patients with chronic pancreatitis and exocrine pancreatic cancer. PANKRAS II Study Group. Gut 2001;48:70–74.

167. Antoniou AC, Cunningham AP, Peto J, et al.: The BOADICEA model of genetic susceptibility to breast and ovarian cancers: updates and extensions. Br J Cancer 2008;98:1457–1466.

168. Hassan MM, Bondy ML, Wolff RA, et al.: Risk factors for pancreatic cancer: case-control study. Am J Gastroenterol 2007;102:2696–2707.

169. Hsu FC, Lindstrom S, Sun J, et al.: A multigenic approach to evaluating prostate cancer risk in a systematic replication study. Cancer Genet Cytogenet 2008;183:94–98.

170. Vucic EA, Brown CJ, Lam WL: Epigenetics of cancer progression. Pharmacogenomics 2008;9:215–234.

171. Sato N, Maitra A, Fukushima N, et al.: Frequent hypomethylation of multiple genes overexpressed in pancreatic ductal adenocarcinoma. Cancer Res 2003;63:4158–4166.

172. Chen J, Li D, Wei C, et al.: Aurora-A and p16 polymorphisms contribute to an earlier age at diagnosis of pancreatic cancer in Caucasians. Clin Cancer Res 2007;13:3100–3104.

173. Sahin-Toth M: The pathobiochemistry of hereditary pancreatitis: studies on recombinant human cationic trypsinogen. Pancreatology 2001;1:461–465.

174. Sahin-Toth M, Toth M: Gain-of-function mutations associated with hereditary pancreatitis enhance autoactivation of human cationic trypsinogen. Biochem Biophys Res Commun 2000;278: 286–289.

175. Sahin-Toth M: Human cationic trypsinogen. Role of Asn-21 in zymogen activation and implications in hereditary pancreatitis. J Biol Chem 2000;275: 22750–22755.

176. Hirata I, Murano M, Ishiguro T, et al.: HLA genotype and development of gastric cancer in patients

with Helicobacter pylori infection. Hepatogastroenterology 2007;54:990–994.

177. Ramezani A, Hasanjani Roshan MR, Kalantar E, et al.: Association of human leukocyte antigen polymorphism with outcomes of hepatitis B virus infection. J Gastroenterol Hepatol 2008;23:1716–1721.

178. Hassan MM, Li D, El-Deeb AS, et al.: Association between hepatitis B virus and pancreatic cancer. J Clin Oncol 2008;26:4557–4562.

179. Larsson SC, Permert J, Hakansson N, et al.: Overall obesity, abdominal adiposity, diabetes and cigarette smoking in relation to the risk of pancreatic cancer in two Swedish population-based cohorts. Br J Cancer 2005;93:1310–1315.

180. Carlson C, Greenhalf W, Brentnall TA: Screening of hereditary pancreatic cancer families. In The Pancreas: An Integrated Textbook of Basic Science, Medicine and Surgery. H-G Beger, M Buchler, R Kozarek, et al. (eds.). Oxford: Blackwell 2008: 636–642.

181. Canto MI, Goggins M, Hruban RH, et al.: Screening for early pancreatic neoplasia in high-risk individuals: a prospective controlled study. Clin Gastroenterol Hepatol 2006;4:766–781; quiz 665.

182. Maire F, Hammel P, Terris B, et al.: Intraductal papillary and mucinous pancreatic tumour: a new extracolonic tumour in familial adenomatous polyposis. Gut 2002;51:446–449.

183. Hemminki A, Markie D, Tomlinson I, et al.: A serine/threonine kinase gene defective in Peutz-Jeghers syndrome. Nature 1998;391:184–187.

184. Jenne DE, Reimann H, Nezu J, et al.: Peutz-Jeghers syndrome is caused by mutations in a novel serine threonine kinase. Nat Genet 1998;18:38–43.

185. Boudeau J, Sapkota G, Alessi DR: LKB1, a protein kinase regulating cell proliferation and polarity. FEBS letters 2003;546:159–165.

186. Woods A, Johnstone SR, Dickerson K, et al.: LKB1 is the upstream kinase in the AMP-activated protein kinase cascade. Curr Biol 2003;13: 2004–2008.

187. Forcet C, Etienne-Manneville S, Gaude H, et al.: Functional analysis of Peutz-Jeghers mutations reveals that the LKB1 C-terminal region exerts a crucial role in regulating both the AMPK pathway and the cell polarity. Hum Mol Genet 2005;14:1283–1292.

188. Ossipova O, Bardeesy N, DePinho RA, et al.: LKB1 (XEEK1) regulates Wnt signalling in vertebrate development. Nat Cell Biol 2003;5:889–894.

189. Lin-Marq N, Borel C, Antonarakis SE: Peutz-Jeghers LKB1 mutants fail to activate GSK-3beta, preventing it from inhibiting Wnt signaling. Mol Genet Genomics 2005;273:184–196.

190. Mehenni H, Lin-Marq N, Buchet-Poyau K, et al.: LKB1 interacts with and phosphorylates PTEN: a functional link between two proteins involved in cancer predisposing syndromes. Hum Mol Genet 2005;14:2209–2219.

191. Bonaccorsi S, Mottier V, Giansanti MG, et al.: The Drosophila Lkb1 kinase is required for spindle formation and asymmetric neuroblast division. Development 2007;134:2183–2193.

192. Iyanagi T: Molecular mechanism of phase I and phase II drug-metabolizing enzymes: implications for detoxification. Int Rev Cytol 2007;260:35–112.

193. Giannitrapani L, Soresi M, La Spada E, et al.: Sex hormones and risk of liver tumor. Ann NY Acad Sci 2006;1089:228–236.

194. Lowenfels AB, Maisonneuve P, Whitcomb DC, et al.: Cigarette smoking as a risk factor for pancreatic cancer in patients with hereditary pancreatitis. Jama 2001;286:169–170.

195. Hoffmann D, Hoffmann I: The changing cigarette, 1950–1995. J Toxicol Environ Health 1997;50: 307–364.

196. Guengerich FP: Metabolism of chemical carcinogens. Carcinogenesis 2000;21:345–351.

197. Wang M, Abbruzzese JL, Friess H, et al.: DNA adducts in human pancreatic tissues and their potential role in carcinogenesis. Cancer Res 1998;58:38–41.

198. Hecht SS: DNA adduct formation from tobacco-specific N-nitrosamines. Mutation Res 1999;424: 127–142.

199. Bieche I, Narjoz C, Asselah T, et al.: Reverse transcriptase-PCR quantification of mRNA levels from cytochrome (CYP)1, CYP2 and CYP3 families in 22 different human tissues. Pharmacogenet Genomics 2007;17:731–742.

200. Nishimura M, Naito S: Tissue-specific mRNA expression profiles of human phase I metabolizing enzymes except for cytochrome P450 and phase II metabolizing enzymes. Drug Metab Pharmacokinet 2006;21:357–374.

201. Ulrich AB, Schmied BM, Standop J, et al.: Differences in the expression of glutathione S-transferases in normal pancreas, chronic pancreatitis, secondary chronic pancreatitis, and pancreatic cancer. Pancreas 2002;24:291–297.

202. Alexandrov K, Cascorbi I, Rojas M, et al.: CYP1A1 and GSTM1 genotypes affect benzo[a]pyrene DNA adducts in smokers' lung: comparison with aromatic/hydrophobic adduct formation. Carcinogenesis 2002;23:1969–1977.

203. Rojas M, Cascorbi I, Alexandrov K, et al.: Modulation of benzo[a]pyrene diolepoxide-DNA adduct levels in human white blood cells by CYP1A1, GSTM1 and GSTT1 polymorphism. Carcinogenesis 2000;21:35–41.

204. Carlsten C, Sagoo GS, Frodsham AJ, et al.: Gluta-thione S-transferase M1 (GSTM1) polymorphisms and lung cancer: a literature-based systematic HuGE review and meta-analysis. Am J Epidemiol 2008;167:759–774.

205. White DL, Li D, Nurgalieva Z, et al.: Genetic variants of glutathione S-transferase as possible risk factors for hepatocellular carcinoma: a HuGE systematic review and meta-analysis. Am J Epidemiol 2008;167:377–389.

206. Liu G, Ghadirian P, Vesprini D, et al.: Polymorphisms in GSTM1, GSTT1 and CYP1A1 and risk of pancreatic adenocarcinoma. Br J Cancer 2000; 82:1646–1649.

207. Standop J, Schneider M, Ulrich A, et al.: Differences in immunohistochemical expression of xenobiotic-metabolizing enzymes between normal pancreas, chronic pancreatitis and pancreatic cancer. Toxicol Pathol 2003;31:506–513.

208. Standop J, Ulrich AB, Schneider MB, et al.: Differences in the expression of xenobiotic-metabolizing enzymes between islets derived from the ventral and dorsal anlage of the pancreas. Pancreatology 2002;2:510–518.

209. Standop J, Schneider MB, Ulrich A, et al.: The pattern of xenobiotic-metabolizing enzymes in the human pancreas. J Toxicol Environ Health A 2002;65:1379–1400.

210. Lynch HT, Lanspa SJ, Fitzgibbons RJ, Jr., et al.: Familial pancreatic cancer (Part 1): Genetic pathology review. Nebr Med J 1989;74:109–112.

211. Greenhalf W, Malats N, Nilsson M, et al.: International Registries of Families at High Risk of Pancreatic Cancer. Pancreatology 2008;8:558–565.

212. Klein AP, Beaty TH, Bailey-Wilson JE, et al.: Evidence for a major gene influencing risk of pancreatic cancer. Genet Epidemiol 2002;23:133–149.

213. Rulyak SJ, Lowenfels AB, Maisonneuve P, et al.: Risk factors for the development of pancreatic cancer in familial pancreatic cancer kindreds. Gastroenterology 2003;124:1292–1299.

214. Fernandez E, La Vecchia C, D'Avanzo B, et al.: Family history and the risk of liver, gallbladder, and pancreatic cancer. Cancer Epidemiol Biomarkers Prev 1994;3:209–212.

215. Tersmette AC, Petersen GM, Offerhaus GJ, et al.: Increased risk of incident pancreatic cancer among first-degree relatives of patients with familial pancreatic cancer. Clin Cancer Res 2001;7:738–744.

216. Eberle MA, Pfutzer R, Pogue-Geile KL, et al.: A new susceptibility locus for autosomal dominant pancreatic cancer maps to chromosome 4q32–34. Am J Hum Genet 2002;70:1044–1048.

217. Earl J, Yan L, Vitone LJ, et al.: Evaluation of the 4q32–34 locus in European familial pancreatic cancer. Cancer Epidemiol Biomarkers Prev 2006; 15:1948–1955.

218. Klein AP, de Andrade M, Hruban RH, et al.: Linkage analysis of chromosome 4 in families with familial pancreatic cancer. Cancer Biol Ther 2007;6:320–323.

219. McFaul C, Greenhalf W, Earl J, et al.: Anticipation in familial pancreatic cancer. Gut 2006;55:252–258.

220. Zhang K, Qin Z, Chen T, et al.: HapBlock: haplotype block partitioning and tag SNP selection software using a set of dynamic programming algorithms. Bioinformatics 2005;21:131–134.

221. Lynch HT, Harris RE, Guirgis HA, et al.: Early age of onset and familial breast cancer. Lancet 1976;2:626–627.

222. Bergmann F, Aulmann S, Wente MN, et al.: Molecular characterisation of pancreatic ductal adenocarcinoma in patients under 40. J Clin Pathol 2006;59:580–584.

223. Chen J, Killary AM, Sen S, et al.: Polymorphisms of p21 and p27 jointly contribute to an earlier age at diagnosis of pancreatic cancer. Cancer Lett 2008.

224. Chen J, Anderson M, Misek DE, et al.: Characterization of apolipoprotein and apolipoprotein precursors in pancreatic cancer serum samples via two-dimensional liquid chromatography and mass spectrometry. J Chromatogr A 2007.

225. Rieder H, Sina-Frey M, Ziegler A, et al.: German national case collection of familial pancreatic cancer – clinical-genetic analysis of the first 21 families. Onkologie 2002;25:262–266.

226. Li D, Li Y, Jiao L, et al.: Effects of base excision repair gene polymorphisms on pancreatic cancer survival. Int J Cancer 2007;120:1748–1754.

227. Okazaki T, Jiao L, Chang P, et al.: Single-nucleotide polymorphisms of DNA damage response genes are associated with overall survival in patients with pancreatic cancer. Clin Cancer Res 2008; 14:2042–2048.

228. Bryant HE, Schultz N, Thomas HD, et al.: Specific killing of BRCA2-deficient tumours with inhibitors of poly(ADP-ribose) polymerase. Nature 2005;434: 913–917.

229. Plon SE, Eccles DM, Easton D, et al.: Sequence variant classification and reporting: recommendations for improving the interpretation of cancer susceptibility genetic test results. Hum Mutat 2008;29:1282–1291.

230. Ulrich CD: Pancreatic cancer in hereditary pancreatitis: consensus guidelines for prevention, screening and treatment. Pancreatology 2001;1:416–422.

231. Brand RE, Lerch MM, Rubinstein WS, et al.: Advances in counselling and surveillance of patients at risk for pancreatic cancer. Gut 2007;56: 1460–1469.

25 Inherited Pancreatic Endocrine Tumors

Jens Waldmann · Peter Langer · Detlef K. Bartsch

1	**Multiple Endocrine Neoplasia Type 1 (MEN1)** **603**
1.1	Introduction 603
1.2	Natural History of PETs in Patients with MEN1 604
1.3	Clinical Management 605
2	**Gastrinoma** **606**
2.1	Clinical Symptoms 606
2.2	Diagnostic Procedures 606
2.3	Treatment 607
2.4	Prognosis 608
3	**Insulinoma** **608**
3.1	Prognosis 608
3.2	Clinical Symptoms 608
3.3	Diagnostic Procedures 609
3.4	Treatment 610
4	**Vipomas and Glucagonomas** **611**
4.1	Clinical Symptoms 611
4.2	Diagnostic Procedures 611
4.3	Treatment 611
5	**Non-Functioning PETs** **611**
5.1	Clinical Symptoms 612
5.2	Diagnostic Procedures 612
5.3	Treatment 612
6	**Treatment of Liver Metastases in MEN1 Associated PETs** **612**
6.1	Screening and Surveillance in MEN1 Patients 613
7	**Von-Hippel-Lindau Syndrome (VHL)** **613**
7.1	Introduction 613
7.2	Prognosis 614
7.3	Clinical Symptoms 614

J. P. Neoptolemos, R. Urrutia, J. L. Abbruzzese, M. W. Büchler (eds.), *Pancreatic Cancer*,
DOI 10.1007/978-0-387-77498-5_25, © Springer Science+Business Media, LLC 2010

7.4   Diagnostic Procedures 615
7.5   Treatment 615
7.6   Screening and Surveillance 615

8   *Neurofibromatosis (NF) Type 1* 615
8.1   Introduction 615
8.2   Prognosis 616
8.3   Clinical Spectrum and Symptoms 616
8.4   Diagnostic Procedures 617
8.5   Treatment 617
8.6   Screening and Surveillance 618

Abstract: Pancreatic neuroendocrine tumors (PETs) may arise sporadically or in the setting of an inherited tumor syndrome. These syndromes encomprise the multiple endocrine neoplasia type 1 (MEN1), the Von-Hippel-Lindau (VHL)-syndrome and Neurofibromatosis type 1 (NF-1). The prevalence and the different entities of PETs differ significantly between these syndromes resulting in distinct treatment and screening recommendations.

Treatment of PETs in the setting of an inherited tumor syndrome should consider the natural history of the disease, clinical symptoms and the potential for malignant transformation which has to be taken into account individually for every patient.

1 Multiple Endocrine Neoplasia Type 1 (MEN1)

1.1 Introduction

MEN1 is an autosomal dominant inherited disease caused by germline mutations in the *Menin* gene on chromosome 11q13. It has a penetrance of over 90% by the age of 40 years and the incidence is estimated to be between 2 and 20 per 100,000 [1,2]. As first described by Wermer in 1954 affected patients display an "adenomatosis of endocrine glands" [3]. Before 1997, when the *Menin* gene was identified, an involvement of more than two characteristically affected organs was suspicious for MEN1. Patients can develop endocrine lesions in the parathyroid glands, the pancreas or duodenum, the anterior pituitary gland and the adrenals, respectively. The wide spectrum of tumors also includes neuroendocrine tumors of thymus and bronchial tree, foregut carcinoids, lipomas, cutaneus fibromas and thyroid neoplasms (❯ *Table 25-1*).

Clinical symptoms which are associated with hormone excess comprise in declining frequency hypercalcemia, nephrolithiasis, petic ulcer disease, hypoglycemia, visual field loss, galoctorrhea-amenorrhea and rarely Cushing's syndrome. The onset of the different manifestations varies considerably, although hypercalcemia is frequently the first manifestation by the age of 20, followed by Zollinger-Ellison syndrome between 30 and 40 years of age [4,5].

Primary hyperparathyroidism is observed in up to 97% of MEN1 patients and the parathyroids are therefore the most frequent affected glands. Pancreatico-duodenal endocrine tumors (PETs) the second frequent manifestation with a frequency of 60–80% [6,7]. After medical treatment of ulcer disease has improved by introducing protonpump inhibitors (PPI), malignant PETs became the most important determinant of survival in MEN1 patients [8,9]. PETs could be either functioning (Gastrinoma, Insulinoma VIPoma, Glucagonoma) or non-functioning. Gastrinomas, which are mostly located in the duodenal wall, account for 60% of functioning PETs followed by insulinoma with approximately 20%.

Patients with MEN1 have a decreased life-expectancy, with a 50% probability of death by the age 50. The major determinant of survival are neurondocrine carcinomas and malignant gastrinomas, since up to 50% develop liver or other distant metastases [8,10]. The surgical management of PETs in MEN1 patients remain controversial, because they have unique features compared to sporadic PETs. They are multiple and distributed through the entire pancreas, which has been proven in autopsy studies and studies with resected specimen of MEN1 patients [11,12]. However total pancreatectomy seem to be an "overtreatment" in theses patients and pancreoprivic diabetes might be a life-threatening condition. Nevertheless an aggressive surgical treatment is favored by most experts.

⬛ Table 25-1

Expression of MEN1

Affected organ	Tumor	Frequency (%)	Hormone	Clinical syndrome
Parathyroid gland	Hyperplastic parathyroid	88–97	Parathormon	Primary Hyperthyroidism
Pancreas and Duodenum	Gastrinoma	46	Gastrin	ZES
	Insulinoma	20	Insulinoma	Hypoglycemia
	NFPET	30–80	PP	None, local tumor growth
	VIPoma	1	VIP	WDH
	Glucagenoma	3	Glucagon	Glucagonoma-S.
Pituitary gland	Prolactinoma	20–60	Prolactin	Galactorrhea
	nf		None	Visual loss
Adrenal gland	nf	20–60	None	None
	f		Aldosteron, Cortisol	Cushing-, Conn-S.
Thymus	NET	2	CgA	
Lung	NET	3	Serotonin,CgA	Carcinoid-S.
Stomach	NET	3	CgA	
Skin	Lipoma	60	None	None
	Fibroma	20	None	None

ZES: Zollinger-Ellison-Syndrome, nfPET: non-functioning pancreaticoduodenal neuroendocrine tumor, PP: Pancreatic Polypeptide, VIP: vasoactive intestinal polypeptide, WDH: watery diarrhea and hypokalemia, nf: non-functioning, NET: neuroendocrine tumor, CgA: Chromogranin A, S: syndrome

Lifelong screening which should include regular imaging studies and careful hormonal assessments, is supposed to detect malignant transformation at the earliest stage and is therefore strongly emphasized by Brandi and colleagues on the NIH consensus conference in Bethesda [13]. In addition, if MEN1 is suspected based on the personal and family history a genetic testing of the index patient regarding a *MEN1* gene mutation should be performed after genetic counseling. The identification of a *MEN1* mutation in the index patient gives the possibility of a predictive genetic testing of family members after obligate genetic counseling. Mutation-positive family members should be enrolled in controlled screening programs, whereas mutation-negative family members can be omitted from such screening.

1.2   Natural History of PETs in Patients with MEN1

The natural history of PETs in MEN1 patients is still difficult to define due to the variability and the rarity of the disease. Approximately 50% of MEN1-associated pancreatic neoplasms are functional and cause symptoms by a hypersecretion of distinct hormones (e.g., gastrin, insulin). Non-functioning PETs (NFPETs) are responsible for the other 50% of PETs and are characterized by the absent of peptide hypersecretion (a part from Pancreatic Polypepide (PP)). They rarely become symptomatic in patients due to local tumor growth and advanced disease and are commonly detected during regular screening. PETs in MEN1 patients are multiple (up to 15) and NFPETs often coexists besides a clinically dominant functioning lesion. Since 60–80% of MEN1 patients develop PETs and these tumors represent the most common disease related cause of death, the identification and management of these lesions requires high awareness.

Gastrinoma is the most common functional PET in MEN1 patients and in contrast to its sporadic counterpart located in over 90% with in the duodenal wall underlying the mucosa [14]. Duodenal tumors are often small measuring from 1 to 10 mm and had developed lymph node metastases in 40–60% at the time of diagnosis [15,16]. However distant metastases to liver and bones are less frequent than in sporadic disease and MEN1 associated gastrinoma is suggested to follow a less aggressive course compared to its sporadic counterpart [17,18]. Nevertheless Gibril et al. report also an aggressive gastrinoma phenotype in approximately 25% of MEN1 patients which is associated with large (>30 mm) pancreatic tumors, high serum gastrin levels and liver and bone metastases [19].

Insulinoma is the second most frequent functioning PET in MEN1 patients with a prevalence of 10–20% [20]. Malignancy has been rarely reported and may develop in up to 9% of patients [21]. Coexistence with gastrinoma is observed in approximately 10% [22], although one tumor is dominating the hormone excess and consequently the clinical syndrome.

Non-functioning PETs with a prevalence of 30–80% are defined by the absence of hormone or peptide hypersecretion apart from PP [23]. These lesions are increasingly diagnosed, based on modern imaging modalities in controlled screening programs. The malignant potential of these tumors varies considerably, but the tumor size seems to be a predictor for malignant transformation. In small retrospective series an incidence of 20% lymph node metastases (LNM) in tumors larger than 1 cm and an incidence of LM of 30% in tumors larger than 2 cm have been reported, which means vice versa that LNM and LM have not been observed in tumors smaller than 1 cm [23,24]. The increasing number of resected NFPETs in prospective controlled screening programs revealed that malignancy is rarely observed in tumors smaller than 10 mm. Follow-up studies with endoscopic ultrasound suggested that most small NFPETs grow very slowly but they definitely own a malignant potential [25].

Vipomas occur rarely, are almost exclusively malignant and located in the pancreatic body or tail. Patients suffer from watery-diarrhea with severe electrolyte disbalances, especially if they present already with liver metastases.

Glucagonomas develop in less than 3% of MEN1 patients and glucagon excess is not necessarily associated with a clinical syndrome. Especially small tumors (<3 cm) are often asymptomatic, but tumors arc usually large and tend to be malignant in up to 80% [26,27]. In cases with diffuse metastases migratory, necrolytic skin rash, glossitis, stomatitis, angular cheilitis, diabetes, severe weight loss and diarrhea may occur (⊙ *Table 25-1*).

1.3   Clinical Management

Regarding the surgical management of MEN1 associated PETs the diagnostic work up and the surgical strategy have to be adopted to the tumor entity. However, some controversies exist regarding the extent, timing and benefit of pancreatic resections in MEN1 patients, especially

■ Table 25-2

Screening in MEN1

Screening in MEN1 patients	
Biochemical (annually)	
Parathyroid Glands	Calcium, parathormone
PET	Gastrin, Pancreatic Polypeptide, Chromogranin A
Pituitary Gland	Prolactin, IGF-1, ACTH
Midgut Carcinoids	5-HIAA (24-h Urine)
Tests and Imaging	
Insulinoma	Fasting test
Gastrinoma	Secretin provocation test
MRI Abdomen	If tumor is suspected or every 2–3 ys
SRS	If tumor is suspected or every 2–3 ys
MRI pituitary gland	Hormone excess, visual loss or every 5 ys
EUS	If tumor is suspected or every 2–3 ys
CT chest	If tumor is suspected or every 5 ys

PET: pancreaticoduodenal neuroendocrine tumor, IGF-1: Insulin-like Growth factor 1, ACTH: adrenocorticotropic hormone, 5-HIAA: 5-hydroxyindolacetic acid, ys: years, MRI: magnetic resonance imaging, SRS: somatstatin-receptor scintigraphy, CT: computed tomography

since profound evidence based data are still lacking. However, a consensus conference has proposed guidelines for the treatment of MEN1-PETs [28].

2 Gastrinoma

2.1 Clinical Symptoms

The clinical appearance of MEN1 associated Zollinger-Ellison syndrome is similar to its sporadic counterpart (see previous chapter). It is characterized by abdominal pain due to peptic ulcers, heartburn with or without diarrhea. Hypercalcemia increases symptoms in MEN1 patients with concomitant primary hyperparathyroidism. Quite the contrary is observed in patients after parathyroid surgery with hypocalcemia resulting in milder symptoms and even false negative secretin provocation tests. This has led to the recommendation to first cure the pHPT before the resection of gastrinoma [31].

2.2 Diagnostic Procedures

The diagnosis is established by clinical symptoms, an elevated serum gastrin level in the presence of acid in the stomach (pH < 4) and a positive secretin-provocation test (see sporadic gastrinoma). After the biochemical diagnosis is established the further work up should include endoscopic ultrasound (EUS), somatostatin-receptor-scintigraphy (SRS), magnetic resonance imaging (MRI) or computed tomography (CT) scan. In contrast to sporadic gastrinoma MEN1 associated gastrinomas are predominantly localized in the first and second portion of the duodenum (50% vs. >90%) and in the majority less than 10 mm in size. Therefore, they often cannot be localized preoperatively by EUS, SRS or CT scan. However, EUS is warranted to detect additional PETs which are frequently present as well as to detect peripancreatic lymph node metastases. MRI and CT scan provide useful information on the anatomy and serve for an exact preoperative staging, especially lymph node and liver metastases. SRS can verify the endocrine nature of the pancreatic lesion and is the best imaging tool to detect metastatic spread (e.g. liver, lymph node, bone or lung). Although an exact preoperative localization of MEN1-gastrinoma is often impossible, the gastrin source can be regionalized by a selective arterial secretin injection test (Imamura technique) [32]. This regionalization facilitates the decision for the adequate surgical procedure which might include a pylorus-preserving partial pancreatico-duodenectomy.

2.3   Treatment

The management of ZES in MEN1 patients is controversial reaching from medical treatment with proton pump inhibitors alone to extensive pancreatic resections. This controversy has several reasons. It has been demonstrated, that the occurrence of liver metastases as the major prognostic determinant depends on the tumor size in pancreatic gastrinomas. The prevalence of liver metastases was 4% in tumors <1 cm in size and 62% in tumors in tumor ≥3 cm diameter [33]. The presence of liver metastases is associated with a decrease of the 10-year survival from 96 to 30% [30]. Thus, some authors advocate surgery only in tumors larger than 3 cm. However, 90% of MEN1 gastrinomas are small (<1 cm) and located in the duodenum. The association between size and the risk of liver metastases has to be established for duodenal gastrinomas. It has also been shown, that medically treated ZES patients developed liver metastases more frequently than surgical managed patients (29% vs. 5%) [17]. On the other hand MEN1-ZES can rarely be cured by surgery [16]. Most experts, including our group, recommend an aggressive surgical approach as soon as the biochemical diagnosis of ZES is established. The goal of this philosophy is to prevent the development of liver metastases and to improve long-term survival, although biochemical cure might not be achieved.

Surgery is indicated in patients with MEN-ZES when diffuse metastatic spread has been excluded by preoperative imaging and a coexisting pHPT has been cured before. At surgery a duodenotomy and excision of palpable tumors, enucleation of pancreatic head tumors and spleen-preserving distal pancreatectomy to the level of the portal vein with peripancreatic lymphadenectomy as recommended by Thompson et al. [34] is considered the standard procedure. The biochemical cure rate of this procedure is low and varies between 0 and 33%, but the development of liver metastases in the follow-up does not exceed 16% (◉ *Table 25-3*). Therefore, we and other groups proposed a pylorus-preserving partial pancreatico-duodenectomy (PPPD) for MEN1-ZES. The rationale is that MEN1 is a genetically determined disease and that the ZES will recur as long as the target organ duodenum exists. In addition, it has been shown, that MEN1 associated gastrinomas are associated with hyperplastic gastrin cell lesions and very small gastrin-producing microtumors less than 500 μm in diameter [35] which cannot be removed by local excision since they are not palpable. Finally, 95% of MEN1 gastrinomas are located within the gastrinoma triangle and occur multiple (see Figure X Chapter Fendrich) [61]. PPPD has been evaluated in smaller case series and achieved biochemical cure rates up to 90% [23]. However, before PPPD can be suggested as standard procedure in MEN1 patients with ZES much more data need to be

⬛ Table 25-3

Results after surgical excision of MEN1 associated gastrinoma (ST: secretin provocation test; LM: liver metastases)

Authors	Patients (n)	ST normal (%)	LM (%)
Thompson [43]	40	9 (33)	1 (2.5)
Norton [63]	48	0 (0)	3 (6)
Grama [21]	6	0 (0)	1 (16)
McFarlane [33]	10	0 (0)	0 (0)
Mignon [22]	29	1 (3.5)	5 (13)
Bartsch [64]	8	2 (25)	0 (0)
Total	141	12 (8.5)	9 (6.3)

analyzed, especially the longterm-side effects have to be carefully evaluated. Pancreatic-preserving duodenectomy might be another favorable alternative [31], but it is an technically even more demanding procedure than PPPD and the morbidity is high.

In recurrent or persistent MEN1 associated ZES surgery has to be carefully indicated in every patient.

The decision depends on the severity of ZES, the type of the initial procedure and the presence of lymph node or liver metastases. Given the relatively slow progression of the disease the reoperation should avoid the situation of a total pancreatico-duodenectomy, since the side effects of this procedure might be more life-threatening than the ZES.

2.4   Prognosis

Compared to sporadic gastrinomas, MEN1 associated gastrinomas have a more favorable prognosis [29]. The overall survival of operated MEN1 associated gastrinomas is excellent with 10- and 20-years survival rates of 96 and 85%, although 40–60% of patients have lymph node metastases at initial laparotomy [16,17].

3   Insulinoma

3.1   Prognosis

Biochemical cure is achieved in 57–100% of cases in the absence of diffuse metastatic spread to the liver (❱ Table 25-4). MEN1 patients with insulinoma are usually younger (20–30 years) than patients with sporadic insulinoma (40–60 years). Malignancy is rarely reported and occurs in up to 9%.

3.2   Clinical Symptoms

Symptoms are mainly caused by hypoglycemia and are described in detail in the chapter of sporadic pancreatic endocrine tumors.

◘ Fig. 25-1

Specimen after Pylorus-preserving pancreaticoduodenectomy (PPPD) in a MEN1 patient with ZES. (arrows indicate two small gastrinoma, P: Papilla vateri).

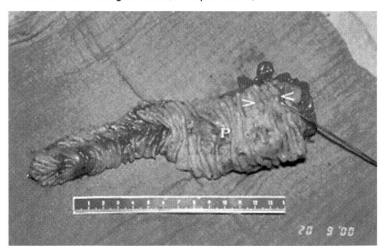

◘ Table 25-4

Results after pancreatic surgery in MEN1 associated insulinoma

Authors	Surgery	PD/TP	DP	E	Cure	LM
Demeure [37]	6	0	5	1	84%	0
Grama [21]	7	0	NA	NA	57%	1
O'Riordain [62]	18	1	12	5	89%	0
Thompson [6]	7	0	7	0	100%	0
Lowney [7]	10	NA	NA	NA	NA	1
Bartsch [64]	6	1	2	3	100%	0
Laimore [24]	3	1	NA	NA	NA	NA
Total	57	3	26	9	57–100%	2

PD: Pancreaticoduodenectomy, TP: Total Pancreatectomy, DP: Distal Pancreatic resection, E:Enucleation, NA: Not available, LM: livermetastases

3.3   Diagnostic Procedures

The biochemical diagnosis is established by a positive fasting test, defined by a pathological insulin-glucose-index and symptomatic hypoglycemia. CT, MRI, SRS and US demonstrated a decreased sensitivity (0–60%) in the preoperative localization compared to EUS (60–95%) (see sporadic insulinomas). Most MEN1 patients have multiple, frequently non-functioning tumors in the pancreas making the identification of the insulinoma difficult. Therefore, the surgical procedure in MEN1 associated insulinomas differs substantially from that of sporadic insulinomas, which often require only enucleation.

3.4   Treatment

Like in sporadic insulinoma surgery is always indicated, if the biochemical diagnosis of organic hyperinsulism is established and diffuse metastatic disease is excluded by imaging, since there is no adequate medical treatment to control the insulin excess. The standard procedure in MEN1 insulinoma comprise complete exploration of the pancreas, bidigital palpation, IOUS followed by a distal spleen-preserving pancreatectomy to the level of the vena portae and enucleation of pancreatic head tumors (❯ Fig. 25-2). Enucleation of single tumors

⬛ Fig. 25-2

Situs and specimen after distal pancreatic resection in a MEN1 patient with multiple NFPETs and insulinoma in pancreatic head (PH: pancreatic head, VMS: superior mesenteric vein, PV: portal vein).

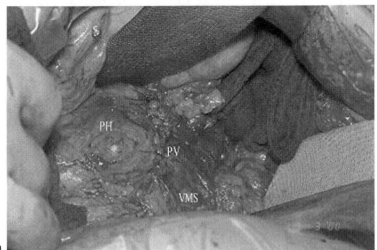

a

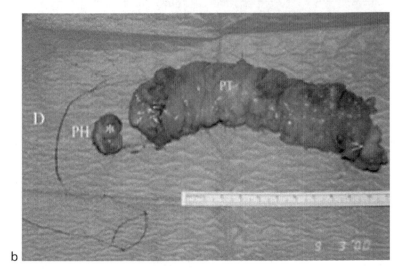

b

should be avoided as multiple tumors are observed in 80–100% [36]. If malignancy is suspected by gross invasion or lymph node metastases a peripanceatic lymphadenectomy should be performed.

4   Vipomas and Glucagonomas

Vipomas and glucagonomas are rare functional PETs in MEN1 patients occuring in 1–3% of patients. Malignancy is frequently observed with 66% and 50–80%, respectively.

4.1   Clinical Symptoms

VIPoma is associated with profuse watery-diarrhea and hypotension, also referred to as WDHA-syndrome. Tumors are often large (>5 cm) and liver metastases are frequently present at the time of diagnosis. Glucagon-excess infrequently causes specific symptoms, but gluca-genoma, usually large at diagnosis may cause abdominal pain due to local tumor growth. In case of diffuse metastases a migratory, necrolytic skin rash might be the leading symptom. In addition, glossitis, stomatitis, angular cheilitis, diabetes and severe weight loss may occur.

4.2   Diagnostic Procedures

The biochemical diagnosis is based on the measurement of elevated serum-levels for VIP or glucagon. Preoperatively CT or MRI and SRS should be performed to obtain an adequate staging.

4.3   Treatment

Recommendations for surgical procedures are rather based on general proposals, than on following oncologic principles a widespread experience. The only chance of cure is the complete surgical resection, as these tumors are frequently malignant. Glukagonomas and Vipomas are mainly located in the pancreatic body or tail making a distal splenopancreatectomy with peripancreatic lymph node dissection the procedure of choice. In case of pancreatic head VIPoma or glucagonoma a PPPD should be performed. Debulking procedures are indicated if more than 90% of the fluid mass was can be resected, since they lead to an improvement of the clinical syndrome caused by the hormone excess.

5   Non-Functioning PETs

The incidence of NFPETs in MEN1 patients varies from 30 to 80% [23,37,38]. NFPETs in MEN1 patients have been reported to be malignant in 30–50% and are less frequently malignant than their sporadic counterparts with 70% [10,21,39]. Retrospective data on sporadic NFPETs have revealed that 20% of patients with tumors larger >1 cm had lymph node metastases and 30% of patients with tumors >2 cm had liver metastases, respectively. However, there is no conclusive association between tumor size and the risk of malignancy in

MEN1 associated NFPETs. Even small (10–20 mm) NFPETs with lung and liver metastases have been reported in MEN1 [27]. This has lead to an aggressive surgical strategy to prevent the development of distant metastases. In sporadic NFPETS a lack of specific symptoms results in a delayed diagnosis associated with a poorer overall survival compared to functioning PETs [40]. This is different in MEN1 associated NFPETs, since these will be nowadays diagnosed early by regular screening.

5.1   Clinical Symptoms

Symptoms are commonly unspecific, as hormone excess related symptoms are lacking. In large tumors local tumor growth associated symptoms such as jaundice, abdominal pain or discomfort and weight loss may frequently occur.

5.2   Diagnostic Procedures

After a careful biochemical evaluation in order to detect hormone oversecretion, especially in regard to subclinical ZES, imaging should include CT or MRI of the abdomen, SRS and EUS. EUS is the superior preoperative imaging modality in MEN1 patients, especially if the tumor size is below 10 mm. It has to be highlighted that NFPETs in MEN1 are often multiple and may be associated with functioning tumors.

5.3   Treatment

The timing and extent of surgery is an ongoing discussion. Skogseid advocate the most aggressive approach with surgical exploration in case of biochemical evidence, even if imaging fail to visualize pancreatic lesions [37,41]. Thompson and Bartsch proposed surgery in NFPETs and MEN1 if the visualized tumor measures more than 10 mm. The threshold of 10 mm is based on a 20% incidence of lymph node metastases in NFPETs larger than 10 mm [24]. Both groups emphasize distal pancreatectomy at the level of the portal vein, enucleation of tumors located in the pancreatic head and a regional lymphadenectomy (◉ Fig. 25-2). The rational of these recommendations is to remove PETs in an early stage of disease to prevent the development of distant metastases. Fraker and Norton suggested surgery in NFPETs exceeding 2–3 cm, since this size might be correlated with an increased risk for the development of liver metastases [42].

6   Treatment of Liver Metastases in MEN1 Associated PETs

Liver and other distant metastases are the most important predictor of survival in patients with MEN1-PETs. The treatment in MEN1 patients with advanced disease attempts to reduce symptoms related to the hormone excess and to repress the tumor progression. Treatment options for metastastic MEN1 associated PETs are the same as for sporadic PETs, which are summarized in detail in the chapter of sporadic pancreatic endocrine tumors. If possible, cytoreductive surgery should be performed, even if a multivisceral resection is necessary. Other treatment options comprise biotherapy with somatostatin analogs and interferon, chemotherapy (streptozosin, doxorubicin), embolization and chemoembolization, radiofrequency ablation, laser induced tumor ablation, liver transplantation, peptide receptor radiotherapy with *177* Lu and *90* Y octreotid and selective intraarterial radiotherapy [44–50].

In patients with ZES and metastasic, non-resectable distant metastases, symptoms can be controlled by high dose administration of proton-pump-inhibitors.

6.1   Screening and Surveillance in MEN1 Patients

Genetic testing for a *MEN1* mutation is suggested in patients suspicious for MEN1. The identification of a *MEN1* mutation in the index patient gives the possibility of a predictive genetic testing of family members. A predictive genetic testing requires obligate a genetic counseling prior testing. Mutation-positive family members should be enrolled in controlled screening programs according to a consensus conference [28], whereas mutation-negative family members can be spared from further investigations. However, in approximately 10% of patients with MEN1 a MEN1 mutation cannot be identified.

Regular screening should include biochemical parameters and imaging procedures every 3–5 years according to the NIH consensus conference. Hormonal assessment should include PP, gastrin and CgA, Calcium, intact parathormone and secretin stimulation test (ZES). CT scan is useful as initial diagnostic tool to identify lesions in pancreas, adrenal glands, thymus and lung. However, its accuracy in detecting PETs is very limited, as duodenal tumors will always and PETs smaller than 10 mm will often missed. SRS and EUS are superior in the detection of PETs in MEN1 patients (● *Table 25-2*). Regular screening intends to detect glands involved in the disease at their earliest stage, especially to prevent the development of advanced metastatic disease by timely interventions. However, this potential benefit has yet to be prooved in prospective controlled studies.

Guidelines for screening are provided by the NIH Consensus conference in 2001 [28] and by the National Comprehensive Cancer Center in 2003 (www.nccn.org).

7   Von-Hippel-Lindau Syndrome (VHL)

7.1   Introduction

The VHL-syndrome is an autosomal dominant inherited syndrome that most commonly causes retinal, spinal, adrenal, renal and pancreatic lesions. The annual incidence is estimated to be 1 of 36,000 with a more than 90% penetrance by age 65 years. The VHL-gene, located at chromosome 3p25–26, is coding a tumor suppressor gene which plays a pivotal role in the transduction of hypoxia driven signals. Over 250 mutations have been reported to be associated with the VHL-syndrome and the mutated VHL-protein leads to an increased transcription of hypoxia-induced genes. This results in an increased growth and survival of endothelial and stromal cells and lastly promotes their malignant transformation.

Regarding morbidity, the most serious lesions are hemangioblastomas and retinal angiomata as they impair the vision and other neurological functions. Mortality is most often determined by renal cell carcinoma and malignant PETs. VHL has been classified in four distinct phenotypes by the National Cancer Institute (● *Table 25-5*) which represent the four clinical phenotypes 1, 2A, 2B and 2C based on the different lesions [51]. Pancreatic neoplasms only occur in phenotypes 1 and 2B.

◻ Table 25-5

Phenotypes of VHL (CNS: central nervous system)

Phenotype-Classification in families with VHL	
Type	**Phenotype**
Type 1	Retinal hemangioblastoma
	CNS hemangioblastoma
	Renal cell carcinoma
	Pancreatic neoplasms and cysts
Type 2A	Pheochromocytomas
	Retinal hemangioblastomas
	CNS hemangioblastomas
Type 2B	Pheochromocytomas
	Retinal hemangioblastomas
	CNS hemangioblastomas
	Renal cell carcinoma
	Pancreatic neoplasm and cysts
Type 2C	Pheochromocytomas

7.2 Prognosis

The lifetime expectancy in VHL-patients was less than 50 years before surveillance protocols were developed. The major cause of death is renal cell carcinoma. Pancreatic lesions occur in 50–77% of VHL patients, most commonly pancreatic cysts and cystadenomas. The development of distant metastases of these both type of lesions have not been reported. Pancreatic endocrine tumors (PETs) are less common (5–17%), but own a malignant potential. Pancreatic cysts or serous cystadenoma may coexist, but PETs are usually smaller and solid. The median age of diagnosis is approximately 36 years and PETs are mostly non-functioning. The most frequent sites of metastases are the liver and bones. Libutti reported that 17% of VHL-patients with PETs had distant metastases or developed them during follow up [52]. The probability for malignancy increases with a tumor size of more than 30 mm from 0 to 20% [53].

7.3 Clinical Symptoms

The most common pancreatic lesions are pancreatic cysts, which are present in 17–56% of VHL-patients [54]. These lesions exhibit no malignant potential. Pancreatic cysts are detected commonly by CT scan of the abdomen during routinely imaging in asymptomatic patients. They rarely produce duodenal compression and abdominal discomfort, if the entire pancreas is multicystic.

Serous cystadenoma is uncommon, but has been reported to be associated with VHL. Lesions typically grow slowly and malignant transformation in the setting of VHL has not been reported. Serous cystadenomas may lead to endocrine or exocrine insufficiency as well as to stenosis of the bile duct if they grow to substantial size by compressing the pancreatic parenchyma.

Since almost all PETs in VHL are non-functioning, they are clinically inapparent and will be generally detected during screening. Fifty percent of PETs in VHL-patients are located in the pancreatic head, whereas 25% each are located in the pancreatic corpus and tail, respectively.

7.4   Diagnostic Procedures

A hormonal assessment is not necessary since PETs in VHL patients are non-functional. Imaging can be managed by CT scan or MRI, and EUS which is superior in the detection of PETs smaller than 10 mm. A pheochromocytoma has to be excluded before scheduling VHL-patients for pancreatic surgery.

7.5   Treatment

As stated by Melmon and Rosen 1964 "the cystic lesions of the pancreas and the kidney should be left alone" [55]. If cystadenoma or pancreatic cysts are symptomatic due to a compression of the bile duct or the duodenum pancreatic resection may be necessary.

There are no evidence-based guidelines in respect to the time point and the extent of surgery for PETs in VHL patients. It has been suggested that the probability for malignancy increases significantly if the tumor size exceeds 30 mm compared to tumors which are less than 3 cm [53]. Lesions between 10 and 30 mm require a personally adopted approach with respect to patients age, comorbidity and growth kinetics. Functioning PETs and lesions exceeding 30 mm require surgical resection. Based on small series most experts recommend follow-up by MRI, CT or EUS every 12 months for lesions smaller than 10 mm. The surgical strategy should aim to preserve as much pancreatic parenchyma as possible. Therefore, most experts recommend enucleation whenever feasible. Intraoperative ultrasound is obligatory to visualize the relationship of the tumor to the main pancreatic duct and major vessels. A laparoscopic approach is justified in preoperatively imaged lesions, if they are located in the pancreatic body/tail or in the ventral surface of the pancreatic head.

7.6   Screening and Surveillance

Although recent studies contributed to the understanding of phenotype-genotype correlation, mutation based screening has yet not been recommended. Most experts warrant routine screening aiming all VHL-associated lesions. In respect to the endocrine manifestations screening for pheochromocytoma in VHL-type 2 patients encompire an assessment of catecholamine excretion in 24-h urine, MRI and MIBG-scan annually starting by the age of 10. Non-functioning PETs are screened by MRI or EUS every 1–2 years starting by age 10–20. Screening recommendations of the National Cancer Institute are enlisted in ⊙ *Table 25-6*.

8   Neurofibromatosis (NF) Type 1

8.1   Introduction

Neurofibromatosis encomprises a group of hereditary conditions predisposing to neurocutaneus manifestations. The genetically most amenable conditions are neurofibromatosis type 1 and 2.

◻ Table 25-6

Recommendation for screening in VHL patients (US: ultrasound)

Recommended Screening in VHL-patients	
Diagnostic test	Start age/intervals
Ophthalmoscopy	6/annually
24-h urinary Metanephrins	10/annually
MRI of craniospinal axis	12/annually
MRI of auditory canals	in symptomatic patients
US of abdomen	15–18/annually
MRI of abdomen	11–20/annually
Audiologic funtional tests	in symptomatic patients

Neurofibromatosis type 1 is associated with pheochromocytoma, pancreaticoduodenal neuro-endocrine tumors (PET) and other tumor manifestations affecting the central and peripheral nervous system. Neurofibromatosis type 2 is characterized by bilateral acoustic neurinomas, whereas pheochromocytomas and PETs are not part of this syndrome.

Neurofibromatosis type 1 affects 1 in 3,000 live births and 50% are caused by spontaneous mutations. The penetrance is almost 100%, but the clinical phenotype varies considerably. A phenotype-genotype correlation has not been defined so far. The *NF-1* gene is located on chromosome 17q11.2 and is coding for *neurofibromin* gene which acts as a tumor suppressor gene. *Neurofibromin* appears to be involved in the activation of the protoncogene *p21-Ras* and belongs to the family of Ras-GTPases. Mutations of *neurofibromin* can result in a loss of inactivation of *p21-Ras*, in other words the oncogene becomes activated.

The NIH criterias for neurofibromatosis lead to a safe diagnosis if two or more of the criterias listed in ◉ *Table 25-7* are present [56].

8.2   Prognosis

Compared to the healthy population NF-1 patients exhibit a 4-times increased risk for malignant tumors, especially carcinomas and sarcomas. An analysis of death certificates in the US revealed a decreased lifetime expectancy of 20 years compared to the general population with a mean age of death of 50 years for males and 54 years for females, respectively. The relative risk for connective and soft tissue carcinomas was increased by 34-fold [57].

8.3   Clinical Spectrum and Symptoms

Besides benign and malignant tumors of the peripheral and central nervous system typical cutaneus manifestation as cafe-au-lait spots and freckling of non-sun exposed areas occur. Twenty-five percent develop an involvement of the gastro-intestinal tract, most common intestinal fibromas. Furthermore pheochromocytoma (3–13%) and rarely PETs have been

■ Table 25-7
◘ Table 25-7

NIH criteria for neurofibromatosis (NF)

NIH diagnostic criterias for NF type 1
Cardinal Clinical Features (Any Two or More Are Required for Diagnosis)
6 or more café-au-lait macules over 5 mm in greatest diameter in prepubertal individuals and over 15 mm in greatest diameter in postpubertal individuals
2 or more neurofibromas of any type or 1 plexiform neurofibroma
Freckling in the axillary or inguinal regions
Optic glioma
2 or more Lisch nodules (iris hamartomas)
A distinctive osseous lesion such as sphenoid dysplasia or thinning of the long bone cortex with or without pseudarthrosis
A first degree relative (parent, sibling, or offspring) with NF1 by the above criteria

reported to be associated to the disease [58]. Only four cases of PETs have been reported in the literature. The gastrointestinal involvement which is observed in 25% of NF-1 patients includes hyperplasia of the plexus myentericus, neurofibromas, gastrointestinal stromal tumors (GIST), adenocarcinomas, pheochromocytomas, tumors of the papilla vateri and PETs. Klein analyzed 37 cases of periampullary neoplasms and found that the majority originates from the papilla (54%), followed by the duodenum (38%) and the pancreas (8%). Neuroendocrine tumors were observed more frequently (41%) than neurofibromas (30%) [59].

Somatostatinoma is a distinct entity of periampullary neoplasms and most often causes symptoms of duodenal obstruction such as jaundice, weight loss, abdominal pain and gastrointestinal bleeding. A somatostatinoma syndrome related to a somatostatin excess with hyperglycemia, cholecystolithiasis and imperfect digestion has yet not been reported in NF1 patients. Pancreatic neoplasms are rare, but they are usually visualized by ultrasonography, EUS, CT scan or MRI.

8.4   Diagnostic Procedures

With regard to periampullary neuroendocrine tumors endoscopy, endocopic retrograde cholangiopancreaticography and EUS should be the first line diagnostic tools followed by CT or MRI. Pancreatic neoplasms require EUS, CT or MRI and SRS as an adequate preoperative staging.

8.5   Treatment

Since PETs in NF-1 patients are rare, recommendations for their treatment are only based on small case series and reach at most evidence level 4. Duodenal somatostatinomas smaller than 2 cm can be treated by local excision, since distant metastases have yet not been reported. If the tumor exceed 2 cm PPPD might be the procedure of first choice. PETs larger than 2 cm in the NF-1 patient require the same treatment as the ductal adenocarcinoma, which implies a distal pancreatic resection for PETs located in the pancreatic tail and body or a PPPD for PETs located in the pancreatic head or the duodenum [63–65].

8.6　Screening and Surveillance

Screening in NF-1 patients has not been defined and general recommendations are lacking. Due to the low incidence of pheochromocytoma (0,1–5,7%) and PETs (1%) regular screening is not generally recommended [56,60].

Key Practice Points

MEN1
- Genetic screening and counseling is mandatory
- Patients should be referred to specialized centers
- Patients should be enrolled in regular screening programs
- Gastrinoma is the most frequent functional PET
- Malignant neuroendocrine tumors are the most common cause of death

Gastrinoma in MEN1
- Assess gastrin in every MEN1 patient
- Predominant duodenal localization
- Surgery in case of the biochemical diagnosis after diffuse metastatic spread is excluded
- Duodenotomy and lymphadenectomy are essential (PPPD is an option)
- Resect liver metastases

Insulinoma in MEN1
- Preoperative localization is not necessary
- Distal pancreatectomy and enucleation of pancreatic head tumors are mandatory
- Only enucleation is not adequate

NFPETs in MEN1
- EUS is superior to CT and MRI
- NFPETs are multiple
- Surgical treatment if the size exceed 10 mm
- Distal pancreatic resection and enucleation of pancreatic head tumors is the standard procedure

Published Guidelines

MEN1
- NIH consensus conference, Bethesda 2001 [28]
- National Comprehensive Cancer Center 2003 (www.nccn.org)

VHL
- NCI (www.cancer.org)

Nf
- NIH consensus conference 1988 an update 1990 [56,60]

Future Research Directions

- Prospective randomized multi-center trials are required to assess the use of regular screening on a EBM-level
- Evaluation of pancreaticoduodenectomy as standard procedure for MEN1 associated ZES

References

1. Ki Wong F, Burgess J, Nordenskjold M, Larsson C, Tean Teh B: Multiple endocrine neoplasia type 1. Semin Cancer Biol 2000;10(4):299–312.

2. Burgess JR, Greenaway TM, Shepherd JJ: Expression of the MEN-1 gene in a large kindred with multiple endocrine neoplasia type 1. J Intern Med 1998; 243(6):465–470.

3. Wermer P: Genetic aspects of adenomatosis of endocrine glands. Am J Med 1954;16:363–371.

4. Trump D, Farren B, Wooding C, Pang JT, Besser GM, Buchanan KD, Edwards CR, Heath DA, Jackson CE, Jansen S, Lips K, Monson JP, O'Halloran D, Sampson J, Shalet SM, Wheeler MH, Zink A, Thakker RV: Clinical studies of multiple endocrine neoplasia type 1 (MEN1). Qjm 1996;89(9):653–669.

5. Roy PK, Venzon DJ, Shojamanesh H, Abou-Saif A, Peghini P, Doppman JL, Gibril F, Jensen RT: Zollinger-Ellison syndrome. Clinical presentation in 261 patients. Medicine (Baltimore) 2000;79(6):379–411.

6. Thompson NW: Management of pancreatic endocrine tumors in patients with multiple endocrine neoplasia type 1. Surg Oncol Clin N Am 1998; 7(4):881–891.

7. Lowney JK, Frisella MM, Lairmore TC, Doherty GM: Pancreatic islet cell tumor metastasis in multiple endocrine neoplasia type 1: correlation with primary tumor size. Surgery 1998;124(6):1043–8; discussion 1048–1049.

8. Doherty GM, Olson JA, Frisella MM, Lairmore TC, Wells SA, Jr., Norton JA: Lethality of multiple endocrine neoplasia type I. World J Surg 1998; 22(6):581–6; discussion 586–587.

9. Dean PG, van Heerden JA, Farley DR, Thompson GB, Grant CS, Harmsen WS, Ilstrup DM: Are patients with multiple endocrine neoplasia type I prone to premature death? World J Surg 2000; 24(11):1437–1441.

10. Carty SE, Helm AK, Amico JA, Clarke MR, Foley TP, Watson CG, Mulvihill JJ: The variable penetrance and spectrum of manifestations of multiple endocrine neoplasia type 1. Surgery 1998;124(6): 1106–13; discussion 1113–1114.

11. Pipeleers-Marichal M, Donow C, Heitz PU, Kloppel G: Pathologic aspects of gastrinomas in patients with Zollinger-Ellison syndrome with and without multiple endocrine neoplasia type I. World J Surg 1993;17(4):481–488.

12. Thompson NW, Lloyd RV, Nishiyama RH, Vinik AI, Strodel WE, Allo MD, Eckhauser FE, Talpos G, Mervak T: MEN I pancreas: a histological and immunohistochemical study. World J Surg 1984; 8(4):561–574.

13. Brandi ML: Multiple endocrine neoplasia type 1. Rev Endocr Metab Disord 2000;1(4):275–282.

14. Donow C, Pipeleers-Marichal M, Schroder S, Stamm B, Heitz PU, Kloppel G: Surgical pathology of gastrinoma. Site, size, multicentricity, association with multiple endocrine neoplasia type 1, and malignancy. Cancer 1991;68(6):1329–1334.

15. Gibril F, Schumann M, Pace A, Jensen RT: Multiple endocrine neoplasia type 1 and Zollinger-Ellison syndrome: a prospective study of 107 cases and comparison with 1009 cases from the literature. Medicine (Baltimore) 2004;83(1):43–83.

16. Norton JA, Fraker DL, Alexander HR, Venzon DJ, Doppman JL, Serrano J, Goebel SU, Peghini PL, Roy PK, Gibril F, Jensen RT: Surgery to cure the Zollinger-Ellison syndrome. N Engl J Med 1999;341(9):635–644.

17. Norton JA, Fraker DL, Alexander HR, Gibril F, Liewehr DJ, Venzon DJ, Jensen RT: Surgery increases

survival in patients with gastrinoma. Ann Surg 2006;244(3):410–419.

18. Yu F, Venzon DJ, Serrano J, Goebel SU, Doppman JL, Gibril F, Jensen RT: Prospective study of the clinical course, prognostic factors, causes of death, and survival in patients with long-standing Zollinger-Ellison syndrome. J Clin Oncol 1999;17(2):615–630.

19. Gibril F, Venzon DJ, Ojeaburu JV, Bashir S, Jensen RT: Prospective study of the natural history of gastrinoma in patients with MEN1: definition of an aggressive and a nonaggressive form. J Clin Endocrinol Metab 2001;86(11):5282–5293.

20. Rasbach DA, van Heerden JA, Telander RL, Grant CS, Carney JA: Surgical management of hyperinsulinism in the multiple endocrine neoplasia, type 1 syndrome. Arch Surg 1985;120(5):584–589.

21. Grama D, Skogseid B, Wilander E, Eriksson B, Martensson H, Cedermark B, Ahren B, Kristofferson A, Oberg K, Rastad J, et al.: Pancreatic tumors in multiple endocrine neoplasia type 1: clinical presentation and surgical treatment. World J Surg 1992; 16(4):611–8; discussion 618–619.

22. Mignon M, Cadiot G: Diagnostic and therapeutic criteria in patients with Zollinger-Ellison syndrome and multiple endocrine neoplasia type 1. J Intern Med 1998;243(6):489–494.

23. Bartsch DK, Fendrich V, Langer P, Celik I, Kann PH, Rothmund M: Outcome of duodenopancreatic resections in patients with multiple endocrine neoplasia type 1. Ann Surg 2005;242(6):757–64; discussion 764–766.

24. Lairmore TC, Chen VY, DeBenedetti MK, Gillanders WE, Norton JA, Doherty GM: Duodenopancreatic resections in patients with multiple endocrine neoplasia type 1. Ann Surg 2000;231(6):909–918.

25. Kann PH, Balakina E, Ivan D, Bartsch DK, Meyer S, Klose KJ, Behr T, Langer P: Natural course of small, asymptomatic neuroendocrine pancreatic tumours in multiple endocrine neoplasia type 1: an endoscopic ultrasound imaging study. Endocr Relat Cancer 2006;13(4):1195–1202.

26. Mignon M, Ruszniewski P, Podevin P, Sabbagh L, Cadiot G, Rigaud D, Bonfils S: Current approach to the management of gastrinoma and insulinoma in adults with multiple endocrine neoplasia type I. World J Surg 1993;17(4):489–497.

27. Thakker RV: Multiple endocrine neoplasia type 1. Endocrinol Metab Clin North Am 2000;29(3): 541–567.

28. Brandi ML, Gagel RF, Angeli A, Bilezikian JP, Beck-Peccoz P, Bordi C, Conte-Devolx B, Falchetti A, Gheri RG, Libroia A, Lips CJ, Lombardi G, Mannelli M, Pacini F, Ponder BA, Raue F, Skogseid B, Tamburrano G, Thakker RV, Thompson NW, Tomassetti P, Tonelli F, Wells SA, Jr., Marx SJ: Guidelines for diagnosis and therapy of MEN type 1 and type 2. J Clin Endocrinol Metab 2001; 86(12):5658–5671.

29. Cadiot G, Vuagnat A, Doukhan I, Murat A, Bonnaud G, Delemer B, Thiefin G, Beckers A, Veyrac M, Proye C, Ruszniewski P, Mignon M: Prognostic factors in patients with Zollinger-Ellison syndrome and multiple endocrine neoplasia type 1. Groupe d'Etude des Neoplasies Endocriniennes Multiples (GENEM and groupe de Recherche et d'Etude du Syndrome de Zollinger-Ellison (GRESZE). Gastroenterology 1999;116(2):286–293.

30. Weber HC, Venzon DJ, Lin JT, Fishbein VA, Orbuch M, Strader DB, Gibril F, Metz DC, Fraker DL, Norton JA, et al.: Determinants of metastatic rate and survival in patients with Zollinger-Ellison syndrome: a prospective long-term study. Gastroenterology 1995;108(6):1637–1649.

31. Thompson NW: The surgical management of hyperparathyroidism and endocrine disease of the pancreas in the multiple endocrine neoplasia type 1 patient. J Intern Med 1995;238(3):269–280.

32. Imamura M, Minematsu S, Tobe T, Adachi H, Takahashi K: Selective arterial secretin injection test for localization of gastrinoma. Nippon Geka Gakkai Zasshi 1986;87(6):671–679.

33. MacFarlane MP, Fraker DL, Alexander HR, Norton JA, Lubensky I, Jensen RT: Prospective study of surgical resection of duodenal and pancreatic gastrinomas in multiple endocrine neoplasia type 1. Surgery 1995;118(6):973–979; discussion 979–980.

34. Thompson NW: Surgical treatment of the endocrine pancreas and Zollinger-Ellison syndrome in the MEN 1 syndrome. Henry Ford Hosp Med J 1992; 40(3–4):195–198.

35. Anlauf M, Perren A, Kloppel G: Endocrine precursor lesions and microadenomas of the duodenum and pancreas with and without MEN1: criteria, molecular concepts and clinical significance. Pathobiology 2007;74(5):279–284.

36. Demeure MJ, Klonoff DC, Karam JH, Duh QY, Clark OH: Insulinomas associated with multiple endocrine neoplasia type I: the need for a different surgical approach. Surgery 1991;110(6):998–1004; discussion 1004–1005.

37. Skogseid B, Eriksson B, Lundqvist G, Lorelius LE, Rastad J, Wide L, Akerstrom G, Oberg K: Multiple endocrine neoplasia type 1: a 10-year prospective screening study in four kindreds. J Clin Endocrinol Metab 1991;73(2):281–287.

38. Sheppard BC, Norton JA, Doppman JL, Maton PN, Gardner JD, Jensen RT: Management of islet cell tumors in patients with multiple endocrine

neoplasia: a prospective study. Surgery 1989;106(6): 1108–1117; discussion 1117–1118.

39. Fendrich V, Langer P, Celik I, Bartsch DK, Zielke A, Ramaswamy A, Rothmund M: An aggressive surgical approach leads to long-term survival in patients with pancreatic endocrine tumors. Ann Surg 2006;244(6):845–851; discussion 852–853.

40. Kouvaraki MA, Shapiro SE, Cote GJ, Lee JE, Yao JC, Waguespack SG, Gagel RF, Evans DB, Perrier ND: Management of pancreatic endocrine tumors in multiple endocrine neoplasia type 1. World J Surg 2006;30(5):643–653.

41. Skogseid B, Oberg K, Eriksson B, Juhlin C, Granberg D, Akerstrom G, Rastad J: Surgery for asymptomatic pancreatic lesion in multiple endocrine neoplasia type I. World J Surg 1996;20(7): 872–6; discussion 877.

42. Thompson NW: Current concepts in the surgical management of multiple endocrine neoplasia type 1 pancreatic-duodenal disease. Results in the treatment of 40 patients with Zollinger-Ellison syndrome, hypoglycaemia or both. J Intern Med 1998;243(6):495–500.

43. Norton JA: Surgery and prognosis of duodenal gastrinoma as a duodenal neuroendocrine tumor. Best Pract Res Clin Gastroenterol 2005;19(5):699–704.

44. Sarmiento JM, Heywood G, Rubin J, Ilstrup DM, Nagorney DM, Que FG: Surgical treatment of neuroendocrine metastases to the liver: a plea for resection to increase survival. J Am Coll Surg 2003;197(1):29–37.

45. Chamberlain RS, Canes D, Brown KT, Saltz L, Jarnagin W, Fong Y, Blumgart LH: Hepatic neuroendocrine metastases: does intervention alter outcomes? J Am Coll Surg 2000;190(4):432–445.

46. Touzios JG, Kiely JM, Pitt SC, Rilling WS, Quebbeman EJ, Wilson SD, Pitt HA: Neuroendocrine hepatic metastases: does aggressive management improve survival? Ann Surg 2005; 241(5):776–783; discussion 783–785.

47. Kouvaraki MA, Ajani JA, Hoff P, Wolff R, Evans DB, Lozano R, Yao JC: Fluorouracil, doxorubicin, and streptozocin in the treatment of patients with locally advanced and metastatic pancreatic endocrine carcinomas. J Clin Oncol 2004;22(23):4762–4771.

48. Eriksson B, Oberg K: An update of the medical treatment of malignant endocrine pancreatic tumors. Acta Oncol 1993;32(2):203–208.

49. Arnold R, Trautmann ME, Creutzfeldt W, Benning R, Benning M, Neuhaus C, Jurgensen R, Stein K, Schafer H, Bruns C, Dennler HJ: Somatostatin analogue octreotide and inhibition of tumour growth in metastatic endocrine gastroenteropancreatic tumours. Gut 1996;38(3):430–438.

50. Frilling A, Weber F, Saner F, Bockisch A, Hofmann M, Mueller-Brand J, Broelsch CE: Treatment with (90) Y- and (177)Lu-DOTATOC in patients with metastatic neuroendocrine tumors. Surgery 2006;140 (6):968–76; discussion 976–977.

51. Lonser RR, Glenn GM, Walther M, Chew EY, Libutti SK, Linehan WM, Oldfield EH: von Hippel-Lindau disease. Lancet 2003;361(9374):2059–2067.

52. Libutti SK, Choyke PL, Bartlett DL, Vargas H, Walther M, Lubensky I, Glenn G, Linehan WM, Alexander HR: Pancreatic neuroendocrine tumors associated with von Hippel Lindau disease: diagnostic and management recommendations. Surgery 1998;124(6):1153–1159.

53. Marcos HB, Libutti SK, Alexander HR, Lubensky IA, Bartlett DL, Walther MM, Linehan WM, Glenn GM, Choyke PL: Neuroendocrine tumors of the pancreas in von Hippel-Lindau disease: spectrum of appearances at CT and MR imaging with histopathologic comparison. Radiology 2002;225(3):751–758.

54. Hough DM, Stephens DH, Johnson CD, Binkovitz LA: Pancreatic lesions in von Hippel-Lindau disease: prevalence, clinical significance, and CT findings. AJR Am J Roentgenol 1994;162(5):1091–1094.

55. Melmon KL, Rosen SW: Lindau's Disease. Review of the Literature and Study of a Large Kindred. Am J Med 1964;36:595–617.

56. Neurofibromatosis. Conference statement. National Institutes of Health Consensus Development Conference. Arch Neurol 1988;45(5):575–578.

57. Rasmussen SA, Yang Q, Friedman JM: Mortality in neurofibromatosis 1: an analysis using U.S. death certificates. Am J Hum Genet 2001;68(5):1110–1118.

58. Okada E, Shozawa T: Von Recklinghausen's disease (neurofibromatosis) associated with malignant pheochromocytoma. Acta Pathol Jpn 1984;34(2): 425–434.

59. Klein A, Clemens J, Cameron J: Periampullary neoplasms in von Recklinghausen's disease. Surgery 1989;106(5):815–819.

60. Mulvihill JJ, Parry DM, Sherman JL, Pikus A, Kaiser-Kupfer MI, Eldridge R: NIH conference. Neurofibromatosis 1 (Recklinghausen disease) and neurofibromatosis 2 (bilateral acoustic neurofibromatosis). An update. Ann Intern Med 1990;113 (1):39–52.

61. Stabile BE, Morrow DJ, Passaro E, Jr.: The gastrinoma triangle: operative implications. Am J Surg 1984;147(1):25–31.

62. O'Riordain DS, O'Brien T, van Heerden JA, Service FJ, Grant CS: Surgical management of insulinoma associated with multiple endocrine neoplasia type I. World J Surg 1994;18(4):488–493; discussion 493–494.

63. Harris GJ, Tio F, Cruz A Jr.: Somatostatinoma: a case report and review of the literature. J Surg Oncol 1987;36:8.
64. O'Brien TD, Chejfec G, Prinz RA: Clinical features of duodenal somatostatinomas. Surgery 1993;114:1144.
65. Eckhauser FE, Colletti LM, Somatostatinoma In Berger HB, Warshaw AL, Carr-Locke D, Russel C, Büchler MW, Neoptolemus JP, Stan MG: The pancreas, Blackwell science, London P, 1276.